Trends in
Autonomic
Pharmacology

Trends in Autonomic Pharmacology
Volume 1

Edited by

Stanley Kalsner, Ph.D.
Department of Pharmacology
School of Medicine
University of Ottawa
Ottawa, Ontario
Canada

Urban & Schwarzenberg • Baltimore-Munich 1979

Urban & Schwarzenberg, Inc.
7 E. Redwood Street
Baltimore, Maryland 21202
U.S.A.

Urban & Schwarzenberg
Pettenkoferstrasse 18
D-8000 München 2
GERMANY

Library of Congress Cataloging in Publication Data
Main entry under title:

, Trends in autonomic pharmacology.

Includes index.
1. Autonomic drugs. 2. Neuropharmacology.
I. Kalsner, Stanley, 1936–   II. Title:
Autonomic pharmacology. [DNLM: 1. Autonomic
drugs—Pharmacodynamics—Period. 2. Autonomic
nervous system—Drug effects—Period. 3. Pharmacology—Trends—Period. W1 TR403]
RM323.T73   615'.78   79-17275

ISBN 0-8067-1001-2 (Baltimore)
ISBN 3-541-71001-2 (Munich)

Printed in the United States of America

To my wife, Jenny, and our children, Lydia, Pamela and Louisa

Contents

Contributors

Bruno G. Benfey
Department of Pharmacology and
  Therapeutics
McGill University
Montreal, Quebec, Canada

Graeme Campbell
Department of Zoology
University of Melbourne
Melbourne, Australia

Denis Crankshaw
Department of Neurosciences
McMaster University
Hamilton, Ontario, Canada

Luigi Cubeddu X.
Department of Pharmacology
Central University of Venezuela
School of Pharmacy
Caracas, Venezuela

Michael J. Daly
Department of Pharmacology
Glaxo-Allenburys Research (Ware) Ltd.
Ware, Hertfordshire, England

Edwin E. Daniel
Department of Neurosciences
McMaster University
Hamilton, Ontario, Canada

Cheryl F. Dreyfus
Department of Anatomy
Columbia University
College of Physicians and Surgeons
New York, NY, USA

John Fozard
Centre de Recherche Merrell
  International
Strasbourg, France

Michael D. Gershon
Department of Anatomy
Columbia University
College of Physicians and Surgeons
New York, NY, USA

Ian L. Gibbins
Department of Zoology
University of Melbourne
Melbourne, Australia

Dennis G. Haylett
Department of Pharmacology
University College
London, England

Leon Hurwitz
Department of Pharmacology
University of New Mexico
School of Medicine
Albuquerque, NM, USA

Stanley Kalsner
Department of Pharmacology
University of Ottawa
School of Medicine
Ottawa, Ontario, Canada

Chiu-Yin Kwan
Department of Neurosciences
McMaster University
Hamilton, Ontario, Canada

Geoffrey P. Levy
Department of Pharmacology
Glaxo-Allenburys Research (Ware) Ltd.
Ware, Hertfordshire, England

Linda J. McGuffee
Department of Pharmacology
University of New Mexico
School of Medicine
Albuquerque, NM, USA

John H. McNeill
Division of Pharmacology and
  Toxicology
Faculty of Pharmaceutical Sciences
University of British Columbia
Vancouver, British Columbia, Canada

John F. Moran
Department of Biochemical
  Pharmacology
State University of New York at
  Buffalo
School of Pharmacy
Buffalo, NY, USA

Taube P. Rothman
Department of Anatomy
Columbia University
College of Physicians and Surgeons
New York, NY, USA

Heinz O. Schild
Department of Pharmacology
University College
London, England

José M. Trifaró
Department of Pharmacology and
  Therapeutics
McGill University
Montreal, Quebec, Canada

David J. Triggle
Department of Biochemistry
State University of New York at
  Buffalo
School of Medicine
Buffalo, NY, USA

David I. Wallis
Department of Physiology
University College
Cardiff, Wales

Preface

The aim of this series is to provide a means through which the diverse themes currently occupying researchers in autonomic pharmacology can be beneficially brought together for students and investigators alike. At present there is no compendium available that surveys on an ongoing basis the breadth and depth of current activity in a field noted for the variety of its interests, its innovations, and sometimes for its controversies. Autonomic pharmacology has never exhausted itself for long with stale problems nor allowed itself to wither; and its adherents continue to uncover new and fundamental concepts and techniques that have a broad range of applicability, sometimes to seemingly separate and remote disciplines.

The origins of scientific pharmacology are historically intertwined with those of autonomic pharmacology. They are exemplified by the early interest of investigators in the internal milieu, homeostasis, and the extrinsic control of organs by nerves, culminating in the concepts of neurochemical transmission, specific receptors for endogenous agonists, and the mechanisms of neurosecretion, cardiovascular function, and smooth muscle contraction.

Autonomic pharmacology has moved from its initial anatomical orientation through a long active phase of physiological exploration to its recent primarily biochemical mode of operation. It is an ambition of this series to emphasize for readers the necessity of an integrative approach to many of the current unresolved issues; that neither anatomy, biochemistry, nor physiology alone can resolve pharmacological problems is made abundantly clear in several of the articles included in this initial volume.

The title chosen for this series, incorporating as it does the word "Trends," may appear at first glance to suggest a concern with an insubstantial aspect of science. As one investigator commented, "It seems to imply a flitting passage and not necessarily something solid—which is what we want in a book"; or, as another said, it suggests an interest in material that is "fashionable." The choice of the title is deliberate. The Oxford English Dictionary defines *trend* as "the general course, tendency, or drift of action, thought," etc. The purpose of this series, then, is to evaluate issues and problems currently consuming a good deal of research, time, thought, and effort and also to illuminate areas that deserve more attention than they currently receive.

New ideas, approaches, or techniques have an intrinsic excitement, particularly when they appear to shed interpretive light on old problems or open up novel avenues for exploration. Sometimes a trend of thought develops on a particular problem shared by several investigators and takes hold seemingly independently of the vigor of the evidence available to support it. The premature expansion of a hypothesis and its implications, the so-called snowball effect, may be one consequence of this. Similarly, and for varied reasons, other developments fall on infertile ground or receive a mixed reception, and their essential worth remains uncommunicated. The evidence for or against a particular set of interpretations may be difficult to decipher and cumbersome to evaluate except for a very few workers immersed in the area.

The articles presented here range from concerns with patterns of nerve innervation to investigations of functional relationships between nerves, transmitter substances, and their effector organs. Also considered are the modes of secretion and combination of transmitters with receptors, the kinds and categories of receptors, response termination and tissue desensitization, and the identity of the sequence of steps culminating in effector response. In the selection of authors for each of the topics under review a significant criterion was that they be investigators active in the mainstream of the particular research they describe and that they possess the skill and foresight to analyze cogently not only recent developments but also the historical thrust of their respective areas. It is unavoidable that, to some extent, the choices reflect my own points of view. Undoubtedly some readers may argue with the emphasis made and the conclusions reached on individual topics. It is hoped that future volumes will provide a forum for alternative opinions.

An autobiographical sketch by a distinguished autonomic pharmacologist also is to be included in each volume so that we can have some insight into the personalities and scientific experiences of the people who have contributed so much to the development of the field. I am grateful to Dr. Schild for his contribution to this inaugural volume. I would also like to express my appreciation to Braxton Mitchell of Urban & Schwarzenberg, who accepted the need for this project and provided all necessary help toward its completion. I wish to thank Mr. Robert Dobson of my laboratory for his editorial assistance in putting together this volume and also Mr. Mohamad Suleiman for his continued technical support. To my wife Jenny, I offer my special thanks for the encouragement and support she gave me throughout the conception and preparation of this work.

Stanley Kalsner
Ottawa, Ontario
January 1979

Recollections and Reflections of an Autopharmacologist

Heinz O. Schild

I. AUTOPHARMACOLOGY

When the editor suggested that I write a personal introduction for this series entitled 'Reflections of an Autonomic Pharmacologist', I felt unqualified for the task; but it occurred to me that by training and experience I might be better qualified to discuss the related subject of autopharmacology, to which proposal the editor generously agreed.

Dale employed this term in the title of his autobiographical work "Adventures in Physiology with Excursions into Autopharmacology" (Dale,

1953). He made an important distinction with respect to autopharmaco-logical agents. One group he defined as "hormones in the true sense," pointing out that when Bayliss and Starling introduced the word *hormone* they intended it to apply to an active principle formed in one organ and carried by the blood to others in which it produced its specific pharmacodynamic effect. Dale considered it desirable, in the interest of clear thinking, to restrict the use of the word *hormone* to the meaning originally applied to it. In that sense he considered adrenaline the "perfect" type of vasomotor hormone; and he would allow vasopressin a presumptive claim, at least, to be included in the list. In a second group he placed agents that were also produced in the body with intense physiological activity; this activity, however, was normally restricted to the immediate neighborhood of their liberation. In that second sense he considered that histamine might function as a physiological capillary vasodilator—though, interestingly, he was too cautious ever to commit himself explicitly to a physiological role for histamine (or, for that matter, for adenylic acid, which he also discusses in terms of a potential physiological vasodilator).

Dale was always extremely careful in arguing from analogy. In discussing the likelihood that the concept of chemical transmission might be extended to central synapses he urged great caution and reliance only on "direct and critically scrutinized evidence."

Retrospectively I see the concept of autopharmacology—i.e., regulation of body functions by pharmacodynamic agents produced in the body—as the central plank of my own pharmacological thinking, although this has developed in unexpected directions. Certain developments—e.g., receptor theory—may have gone rather beyond what Dale would have considered "direct evidence," but on the whole I feel that Dale's auto-pharmacology has been the dominating influence on me as well as on a whole generation of pharmacologists.

I shall now touch upon some aspects of my own experimental work and pharmacological thinking, largely disregarding chronology.

II. EARLY LONDON EXPERIENCES

Arriving in Dale's laboratory in October 1932, I was struck by its marvelous organization and, more important, its powerful flow of ideas. Its exterior atmosphere was that of a typical old-fashioned physiological laboratory, with the smoked drum as mainstay. The laboratory consisted of a single oblong room with two or three operating tables. It formed part of the building of the National Institute for Medical Research, of which Dale was the overall director. The technical organization of the legendary F4 lab centred on Collison, the chief technician. Collison had to be informed the evening before of any experiment planned, which was then set out to perfec-

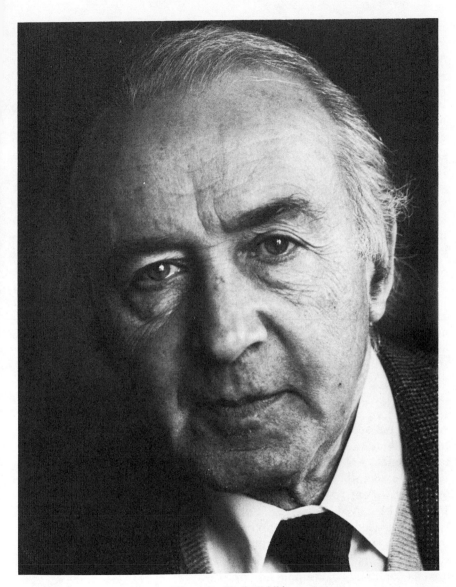

Figure 1. H. O. Schild.

tion next morning; but it was not advisable to change one's mind. It would be difficult to disentangle how many of the basic ideas emanated from the master himself—who was kept rather occupied, though by no means exclusively, by his administrative duties—and how much from such outstanding coworkers as Feldberg and Gaddum. I can remember these two first discussing and then performing the fundamental experiment of perfusion of the cat's superior cervical ganglion, which proved the nicotinic action of acetylcholine. I can remember Dale and Feldberg carrying out the experiment that proved that sweat secretion was cholinergic, although anatomically sweat glands are innervated by the sympathetic.

My own investigations during that year were on a more modest scale, but some proved to be forerunners to developments several years later. Dale had suggested to me an examination of Szent-Gyorgi's claim that the adrenal medulla contained a precursor of adrenaline with the same colorimetric activity but 10 times its biological activity. Having modified the colorimetric assay procedure, I came to the conclusion that the large discrepancy between colorimetric and biological (spinal cat) assay did not exist. Nevertheless, a much smaller discrepancy than that postulated by the Hungarian workers, of about 40%, stubbornly persisted. I could not explain this finding at the time, although it turned out to be the forerunner of a fundamental observation made several years later by Holtz: that the adrenal gland contained noradrenaline as well as adrenaline.

In the course of investigating the colorimetric assay of adrenaline a fluorescence assay for adrenaline was developed (Gaddum and Schild, 1933). The fluorescence assay was highly sensitive: adrenaline, oxygen, and alkali were the only ingredients required for the effect. The fluorescence assay was later perfected by Danish workers, since when it has become the standard method of adrenaline assay.

III. DRUG RECEPTORS

As I feel old age creeping up, I realize its many handicaps. When it comes to quick thinking, my grandson of eleven beats me. When it comes to working in the lab, I realize that I can't or won't do as many things by myself as I used to and that I must either give up or be dependent on outside assistance. In one respect, however, I feel more free than when I was young. I seem to have lived long enough to be able to change my mind.

The subject of drug receptors is one on which I have gradually changed by mind. I started by being rather skeptical, in the Dale tradition, of the receptor idea; but I have become a supporter, recognizing the great merit of even an admittedly oversimplified approach.

My incursion into quantitative pharmacology started with the pA_2 index of drug antagonism (Schild, 1947a). To measure the activity of drugs opposing bronchoconstriction I needed a measure of drug antagonism not dependent on comparison with another antagonist; and I selected a null measure, following on some old work by Clark and Raventos. The pA_2 index was a fairly stable measurement, independent of agonist strength and providing a quantitative measure of specificity. None of the likely antagonists proved completely specific; but many were relatively specific, mepyramine being 10,000 times more active when assessed by pA_2 against histamine than when tested against acetylcholine, and atropine 1,000 times more active against acetylcholine than against histamine. The original aim of pA_2 measurement was practical rather than theoretical. I was aware at the time of the Langmuir-Gaddum approach (Gaddum, 1937) to competitive antagonism but somewhat doubtful of its validity, and I was not unduly perturbed when my early pA_2 results did not conform with quantitative theoretical prediction (as it turned out later, this was due to nonattainment of full equilibrium).

In Chang and Gaddum's method of parallel quantitative assays (Chang and Gaddum, 1933), even minor differences in the structure of drugs were revealed by comparing their relative activities in different preparations. The question arose whether differences between drugs would also be revealed by differences in pA_2 values when they are tested with a common antagonist. Experiment showed that while some drugs could be readily differentiated by their pA_2 values, others could not be thus differentiated, equiactive doses producing the same pA_2 with the same antagonist (Schild, 1947b). This was the first indication to me of the existence of natural drug classes indistinguishable by antagonists.

Almost imperceptibly I drifted towards an approach based on the twin concepts of drug receptors and competitive antagonism in the Langmuir Gaddum guise. On the occasion of a controversy concerning various mathematical formulations of drug antagonism it struck me that competitive drug antagonism could be expressed succinctly in terms of a single antagonist affinity constant $K_2 = (x-1)/B$ (Schild, 1949), where x is the *dose ratio*. Later I adopted a logarithmic transformation that gave a straight line intersecting the abscissa at a point corresponding to pA_2 (Arunlakshana and Schild, 1959). This became a convenient general test for characterizing the simplest type of competitive drug antagonism. An example of its use in a class experiment is shown in Figure 2.

This general approach provided a means for the classification of both drugs and receptors if the following rules, derived from receptor theory, were applied (Schild, 1973): 1) When different agonists acting on the same receptors are tested with the same competitive antagonist, the affinity constant of the latter (or pA_2 value if the antagonism is truly competitive) should be the same; and 2) Identical receptors in different preparations should produce the same affinity constant (pA_2 value) with the same competitive antagonist.

The sort of difficulty that might arise in the rigid application of these rules was illustrated by some recent experiments carried out in conjunction with workers at Sandoz, Basle (Bertholet). The question was whether β-adrenoceptors in three different guinea pig tissues—auricle, trachea, and isolated fat cells—were identical. It was found experimentally that all three

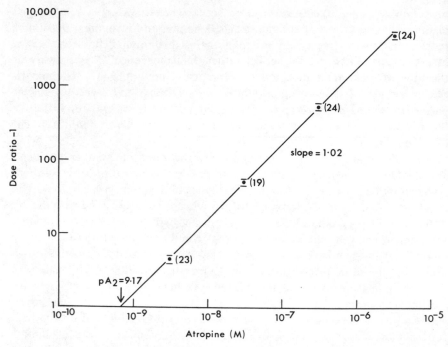

Figure 2. Antagonism of acetylcholine (ach) and atropine (atr). Competitive antagonism demonstrated by linear regression, slope = 1, when plotting log (dr-1) v. log conc atr. dr = dose ratio = (conc ach after atr) / (conc ach before atr). Contractions of guinea pig ileum. pA_2 = 9.2. Averaged student class results. (Data kindly provided by Dr. D. H. Jenkinson.)

isolated preparations gave perfect relations of competitive antagonism ('slope' = 1) when propranolol was tested with isoprenaline. However, whereas the pA_2 values for auricle and trachea were statistically indistinguishable, the pA_2 values for fat cell receptors were significantly lower—by about 0.5 log units. Could they be reasonably assumed to relate to the same receptor, or might the differences in pA_2 reflect subtle differences in the structure of lipolytic and other β-adrenoceptors?

A. Noncompetitive Antagonism

This term is nearly always a misnomer when applied to drug antagonism. Equations for noncompetitive antagonism in which agonist and antagonist both react competitively but with different receptors, or different parts of the same receptor (Schild, 1954), can readily be worked out, the resultant theoretical curves starting from a common origin with progressive decrease of slopes and maxima; but the interpretation of experimental curves of this kind is difficult. Difficulties are of two kinds: 1) *Unsurmountable* antagonist curves, as Gaddum called them, are not necessarily indicative of true noncompetitive antagonism. Indeed, this last probably occurs very rarely;

and 2) Assumptions regarding the receptor-response relationship are particularly hazardous when the log dose-response curves are not parallel. Some assumption regarding the relationship between receptor activation and response inevitably has to be made. In competitive antagonism with parallel log dose-response curves the usual assumption is that equal responses involve the activation of equal numbers of receptors. This assumption is applicable also to the Stephensen-Ariens-Furchgott extension of receptor theory. A corresponding assumption, that equal responses involve equal receptor numbers, may also be made when curves are non-parallel; but it is then rather more hazardous. An extreme assumption would be based on the old Clark theory that response is directly proportional to receptor occupation and that a maximal response corresponds to 100% receptor occupation, but this assumption is improbable and is seldom made nowadays. Nevertheless, when theory fails, empirical constants can usefully fill the gap; and it has become a common practice, especially in the drug industry, to characterize "noncompetitive" antagonists (i.e., those reducing dose-response maxima) in terms of the concentration needed to reduce the maximum of the log dose-response curve to one-half.

B. Histamine Receptors

I have long been interested in histamine receptors. Indeed, this interest can be said to have begun with studies of histamine antagonism long before I dreamt of receptors. I recall that, working with A. J. Clark in Edinburgh, I suggested to him that I should try to find a substance that would antagonize histamine in much the same way in which atropine antagonized acetylcholine. Clark said that it was a good idea. Instead of starting straight away to test various possible antagonists, I went to study a book by Feldberg and Schilf (1930), which we used to call the "Old Testament," because it contained everything that was then known about histamine. I noticed there that the Swiss biochemist Guggenheim had found that the isolated guinea pig gut became unresponsive to histamine after a dose of indolethylamine (tryptamine). Following this up, I found that tryptamine was an antagonist of histamine over a wide range of concentrations, that it was moderately specific in the sense that histamine was antagonized more than acetylcholine, and that it also inhibited the Dale-Schultz reaction. Nevertheless, tryptamine seemed a rather poor histamine antagonist; but when I tried to induce my friends in the field of chemistry to synthesize more specific histamine antagonists, I failed to persuade them to do so. Soon afterwards a group of French workers, under the able guidance of Fourneau, began evolving really effective antihistamines by gradual modification of chemical structure.

My interest in this field persisted, and many years later I tried to tackle the antihistamine problem with a theoretically sounder receptor outlook in order to discover whether antihistamines obeyed receptor "laws." In joint work with colleagues (Arunlakshana and Ash) it became obvious that one type of histamine action seemed to be exerted on a well-defined common receptor affected by typical antihistamines such as mepyramine. Histamine analogues varying in activity a thousandfold produced the same pA_2 values with mepyramine when tested on guinea pig gut; and several quite different pharmacological preparations gave the same pA_2 values when tested with histamine and mepyramine, evidence of a distinct histamine (H_1) receptor (Ash and Schild, 1966).

It became clear at the same time that other histamine effects, including stimulation of gastric acid secretion and relaxation of isolated rat uterus, were not exerted by way of H_1 receptors. The question arose whether these actions might be mediated by a well-defined second histamine receptor. Again I was faced with the tricky problem of receptor definition. How should receptors be defined? Should they be defined in terms of their affinity for competitive antagonists or by common activity ratios of agonists? How can the existence of a receptor be validated? We felt that it was necessary to validate a postulated new receptor by demonstrating identical antagonist affinity constants in several different preparations. In our case there was some evidence for a second histamine receptor based on similar agonist activity ratios when different histamine analogues were quantitatively tested for their relative activities in causing stimulation of gastric acid secretion and inhibition of rat uterus. However, the crucial evidence of a common competitive antagonist was missing. This evidence was eventually produced by Black and his team (Black et al., 1972), who synthesized new competitive H_2 receptor antagonists in a systematic investigation starting from the structure of histamine itself. In this work they used three test systems—guinea pig heart rate stimulation, rat uterus inhibition and rat gastric acid secretion—to ascertain that a new histamine receptor with common pA_2 values could indeed be identified.

C. Metal Receptors

The term *metal receptor* is unusual but perhaps justified as being analogous to metal enzymes. Certain enzymes require metals as cofactors for their full action; in the same way certain receptors require metals as cofactors to exert their full activity. An example of a metal receptor is the receptor for the S-S polypeptide vasopressin. The effect of vasopressin is potentiated by magnesium and greatly potentiated (over tenfold) by transition metals, cobalt, nickel, and manganese. The role of metal is not understood; but one possibility is that the polypeptide binds to the receptor in the normal way, while the metal coordinates with the receptor, forming an additional link between receptor and polypeptide that aids their apposition and interaction (Schild, 1969). This is a neglected field of receptor pharmacology, of potential interest for the future.

IV. HISTAMINE RELEASE

This "autopharmacological" subject has followed me throughout my career and provided the opportunity for a long and fruitful collaboration with my friend and colleague Jack Mongar. I recall some of the problems in this field.

A. Can Histamine Release Alone Account For the Anaphylactic Reaction of Smooth Muscle?

Figure 3 illustrates an attempt to answer this question. An isolated guinea pig uterus sensitized to ovalbumin was treated with large doses of histamine until it became refractory to it, failing to respond to histamine by contraction. The addition of the antigen, ovalbumin, to the bath at this stage nevertheless caused a maximal contraction (Schild, 1949). This experiment seems to suggest that although the guinea pig uterus responds to histamine and histamine is known to be released in the anaphylactic reaction of the uterus, the anaphylactic response of the uterus cannot be fully explained in terms of histamine. This experiment gave an early indication that factors other than histamine may be involved in the anaphylactic reaction of smooth muscle.

B. Is Histamine Involved in Human Bronchial Asthma?

An opportunity to deal with this question arose accidentally through observations made by Dr. Herxheimer on a patient who in spirometer tests reacted to pollen inhalation with an asthmatic attack. Subsequently this patient required surgical removal of a lobe of his lung because of bronchiectasis. Dr. Hawkins prepared isolated bronchial chains from the excised lobe. The bronchial chain preparations of this patient reacted like the classical preparation of the isolated sensitized guinea pig uterus, producing a powerful bronchoconstriction with the specific antigen, pollen extract, followed by desensitization to pollen but not to histamine (Schild et al., 1951). Histamine release from the patient's excised lungs by pollen extract was demonstrated by biological assay. Of particular interest was the finding that while the isolated bronchial chain responded to histamine added to the bath by a contraction that was readily antagonizable by antihistamines, bronchial-chain contractions elicited by pollen were not antagonizable by antihistamines unless extremely high concentrations were applied, supporting the clinical finding that antihistamines are ineffective in bronchial asthma.

C. Inhibition by Sympathomimetic Amines of Anaphylactic Histamine Release

An accidental finding made in another context showed that adrenaline inhibited antigen-induced histamine release in isolated sensitized Ringer-

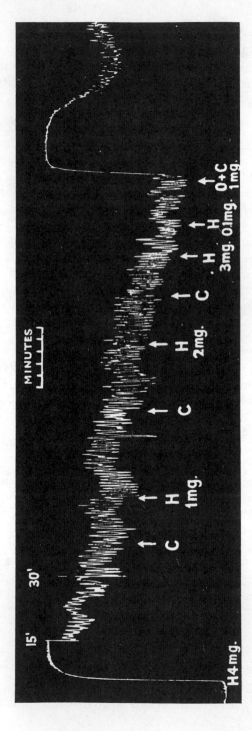

Figure 3. Anaphylactic contraction of isolated guinea-pig uterus sensitized to ovalbumin. Maximal contraction after addition of ovalbumin (O) in spite of desensitization to histamine (H). (C) = Control. (Data by H. O. S.)

perfused guinea pig lungs. Adrenaline was added to the perfusate immediately preceding addition of the antigen and was then oxidized to enable bioassay of any released histamine to be carried out. It was found that adrenaline produced a statistically highly significant reduction of anaphylactic histamine release (Schild, 1936).

These early observations have since been independently confirmed and are believed to be due to an "antianaphylactic" effect of beta adrenoceptor stimulation. In recent work with Dr. Assem, isoprenaline, in very low concentrations, inhibited anaphylactic histamine release, particularly strongly in passively sensitized chopped human lungs obtained at operation (Assen and Schild, 1971). We suggested that low concentrations of circulating adrenaline in human beings could provide an autoregulatory mechanism by which bronchial allergy might be controlled. These experiments suggest that when β-adrenoceptor stimulants are employed in bronchial asthma, they may exert a dual effect, part bronchodilator and part antianaphylactic.

D. Soluble Antigen-Antibody Complexes and Anaphylaxis

This investigation started when Dr. Broder from Canada brought to our laboratory soluble antigen-antibody complexes of bovine plasma proteins that he had himself prepared. When soluble complexes prepared in antigen excess were injected into isolated Ringer-perfused guinea pig lungs, they produced a powerful but transient bronchoconstriction and a simultaneous release of histamine and "slow-reacting substance of anaphylaxis" (SRSA) (Broder and Schild, 1965). After the first effect subsided, a second dose of antigen-antibody complex would produce a second effect. In one such experiment 10 successive doses of complex produced 10 successive episodes of bronchoconstriction and transmitter release. Normal gamma globulins are known to inhibit passive anaphylactic sensitization by blocking uptake sites; they also inhibited the bronchoconstrictor and transmitter releasing effects of Ag-Ab complexes.

Our interpretation of these effects was that these soluble Ag-Ab complexes might represent a foreshortened model of the anaphylactic reaction. In passive anaphylactic sensitization the normal sequence of events is likely to be as follows: 1) attachment of antibody to cell receptors; 2) attachment of antigen to antibody, and 3) intracellular reactions leading to transmitter release. With soluble complexes, stage 2 occurs *in vitro*. Stage 1 is foreshortened and is immediately followed by stage 3.

E. Mechanism of Anaphylaxis

A comprehensive hypothesis of the mechanism of transmitter release during the anaphylactic reactions has been the outcome of a series of experimental findings (Mongar and Schild, 1962). The basic assumption is of a two-stage reaction, the first a calcium-requiring activation stage, the second an energy-requiring stage of transmitter release. Some of the main experimental findings were as follows:

Calcium proved to be an important, indeed essential, requirement for anaphylactic histamine release which was completely blocked by calcium chelating agents. More recent work (Foreman and Mongar) suggests that anaphylactic histamine release may be initiated by the entry of calcium into mast cells. There is evidence that the antiasthma drug cromoglycate may produce its action by inhibiting this calcium entry.

Temperature was shown to be a critical factor, anaphylactic histamine release depending on the presence of a heat-labile intracellular component. A slight elevation above normal body temperature caused inactivation of the anaphylactic mechanism. The heat-labile component appears to be an intracellular protein denatured progressively at temperatures between 42.5 and 45 degrees.

Biochemical inhibitors. Although a complete biochemical analysis of the anaphylactic mechanism is still outstanding, Parrot's early conclusion that the anaphylactic reaction is an energy-requiring process has stood the test of tme. Our own studies showed that a large number of agents, including antipyretics, anesthetics, and metabolic inhibitors, inhibit anaphylactic histamine release in a dose-dependent manner. However, the effects of all these agents were unselective, causing a generalized depression of cell function, as evidenced by inhibition of smooth-muscle contractility and of oxygen consumption. We failed to discover a selective inhibitor of anaphylactic histamine release.

The discovery, by serendipity, of the clinical effectiveness of cromoglycate in bronchial asthma and of its capacity to inhibit histamine release in isolated preparations has initiated a new era in this field and a search for compounds with similar activities. Unfortunately, cromoglycate acts essentially locally; and the search for a systemically acting substitute is still continuing.

V. SOME ISOLATED VENTURES

The title of this section refers to some experiments originated in our laboratory that have, so far, failed to arouse much general interest.

A. Actions of Drugs in Depolarized Smooth Muscle

It has been known through the work of Bulbring and colleagues that the application of drugs to isolated smooth muscle gives rise to conducted electrical impulses that are abolished when the muscle is depolarized by immersion in potassium solution. Our experiments have shown that depolarized smooth-muscle preparations, although electrically silent, nevertheless remain capable of responding to drugs. Acetylcholine, histamine, and oxytocin caused contractions in potassium-depolarized smooth muscle; and adrenaline caused relaxation (Evans, Schild, and Thesleff, 1958). The essential requirement for both contraction and relaxation in depolarized smooth muscle was calcium. Interestingly, the same receptors appear to be involved in the action of drugs in depolarized smooth muscle as in drug action in normal nondepolarized preparations.

B. Vascular Permeability Factors

In conjunction with Drs. Willoughby, Boughton, and Spector, we have studied large-molecule capillary permeability factors extracted from lymphocytes and other tissues. In more recent studies with Drs. Davies and Hartley, large molecular proteins were prepared from spleen. Their subcutaneous injection into the rat produced dose-dependent increases in capillary permeability, evidenced by dye extravasation. When the permeability-increasing proteins were treated with chemical reagents capable of modifying protein endgroups, interesting changes in their permeability activities resulted. Reagents that destroyed the epsilon amino group of lysine abolished the permeability-increasing activity of the proteins, while reagents that inactivated the free carboxyl groups of dicarboxylic acids had the opposite effect, increasing permeability activity (Davies et al., 1974).

Other studies showed evidence that the permeability effects of these large-molecular proteins were produced indirectly, through the release of serotonin and histamine from mast cells. It seemed likely that the permeability effects of these proteins were due to an unusual type of pharmacological action associated with certain protein endgroups rather than with a specific molecule.

VI. BIOASSAY

Bioassay is an English disease; I shouldn't think it is taken seriously anywhere else. In Britain, it has acquired the connotation of "pharmacological measurement," which may explain why it is considered to form an essential part of a pharmacologist's training in England.

A. Biological Standardization

Bioassay grew out of the need to standardize pharmacologically active agents such as insulin, posterior pituitary extract, and digitalis, which could not otherwise be adequately measured. At an early stage Trevan introduced the idea of all-or-none responses, and it was realized that they formed symmetric normal (Gaussian) distributions, particularly if set out on a logarithmic dose axis. Two important developments were 1) the recognition that biological measurements must be comparative, by reference to a stable standard preparation; and 2) the recognition that statistics played an essential part in assessing the error limits of bioassays. The introduction of statistics into bioassay has been immensely important and has influenced all of pharmacology.

B. Pharmacological Analysis of Tissue Extracts

My introduction to the field of bioassay came through the analysis of the pharmacological properties of tissue extracts. It had been known since the 1920s that extracts of many mammalian tissues exerted a powerful depressor action, shown to be due to their content of acetylcholine and histamine. Subsequently other pharmacologically active principles such as prostaglandin and "substance P" were detected in mammalian tissue extracts.

During an investigation with Gaddum of the pharmacological actions of substance P contained in extracts of intestine, it became necessary to separate the depressor effects of substance P and of histamine, both present in intestinal extracts. They were separated by the device of boiling the tissue extract in strongly acid solution, which destroyed substance P, leaving histamine intact. This type of mixed chemical and biological approach has been employed, for example, in Code's method of measuring the histamine content of blood.

C. Bioassay of Histamine

One of my earliest lessons in pharmacology has been the salutary recognition of an abysmal ignorance of statistics. The incentive to remedy this arose in the following way. Various authors had suggested that reactive hyperemia, or hyperemia following muscular exercise, was due to an increased free-histamine content in blood. To test this suggestion in perfused hindlimbs of the dog, blood was extracted during vasodilatation and assayed for its histamine content by the conventional 'matching' assay. I felt dissatisfied with this type of assay, finding it difficult to convince myself that any variations in histamine content had not been due to chance. In the end I found a way out of this dilemma through a particular application of Fisher's analysis of variance, adapting it to a single-subject assay of histamine. I adapted the randomized block approach, the novelty being that randomization was effected in time instead of conventionally in space (Schild, 1942). Statistically controlled single-subject assays have since been widely used in pharmacology.

D. Analytical and Comparative Bioassays

It has become clear that bioassays can have two distinct and entirely different objectives. The aim of *analytical dilution assays* is to find the concentration of an unknown solution in terms of a standard, identical in composition or closely similar to it. Mathematical bioassay theory has been exclusively concerned with this type of bioassay, which is the only one purists would feel worth considering. Yet the importance of analytical bioassay, though remaining considerable, is, if anything, declining, because of the growing importance of affinity assays such as radioimmunoassays, by which extremely small quantities of biological materials can now be accurately measured.

A second type of bioassay exists that has been named, not very happily, *comparative assay*. It deals with the problem of comparing the biological effects of two chemically dissimilar substances, expressing the activity of one in terms of the other. This is bound to be a rather messy affair, since dose-response relations usually differ; but its practical importance is great, since comparative bioassays form the indispensable basis of all new drug development. A particular subtype is the comparative bioassay of different drugs in human beings. I shall discuss this in somewhat greater detail because of its relevance to quantitative pharmacology, quoting examples from the literature as well as from our own experience.

E. Assay of Antihistamines in Human Beings

The assay of antihistamines by Bain and colleagues (Bain, 1949), carried out on medical students, is a classic example of quantitative human bioassay and illustrates some of the difficulties and pitfalls encountered. These workers used as a quantitative index the diameter of intracutaneous histamine wheals after the parenteral administration of antihistamines. It was found inadequate to express the relative activities of antihistamines in terms of a single parameter. Three separate quotients were required, defined as 1) "mean potency quotient," based on the ratio of equiactive does; 2) "mean duration quotient", based on the time required for a drug action to be reduced by half; and 3) "mean therapeutic quotient," based on the total amount of drug required in 24 hours.

F. Comparison of Drugs in Human Uterus

The actions of oxytocic drugs in animals are unrepresentative; these drugs can be tested meaningfully only in women. In experiments with Dr. Myerscough we compared by external tocography the oxytocic effects of two ergot derivatives. The experimental design had severe inbuilt restrictions, only two postpartum days being available for each patient. A design of incomplete randomized blocks was employed in which variability between patients and within patients could be separately assessed. The outcome was that a precise activity ratio for the two drugs with exact fiducial limits could be calculated (Myerscough and Schild, 1958).

G. Comparison of Sedative Drugs in Human Beings

These experiments were carried out in two stages by Drs. Lader and Wing. In the first stage students in the pharmacology department were the sub-

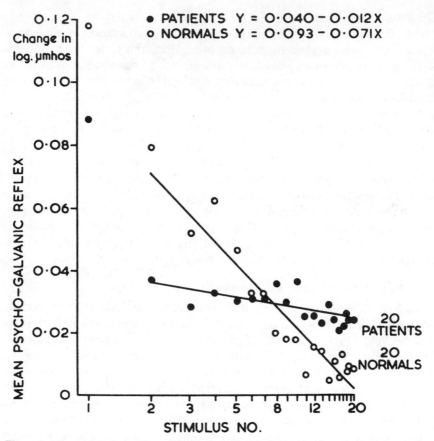

Figure 4. Rate of decline of "psychogalvanic reflex" in patients with pathological anxiety and in normal controls. (After Lader and Wing [1964]. J. Neurosurg. Psychiatr. London.)

jects, in the second stage psychiatric patients at the Maudsley Hospital. A more complex plan was required than in the previously quoted human bioassays. The experimental plan was based largely on the rate of habituation of the psychogalvanic reflex (PGR) to a repeated sound stimulus. The rate of habituation of the PGR and other measurable parameters were shown to be influenced by sedative drugs such as Librium and barbiturates, whose activities could thus be quantitatively assessed (Lader and Wing, 1964). An interesting finding (fig. 4) was that patients with pathological anxiety found it much more difficult to habituate than did normal controls, although their rate of habituation could be improved by sedative drugs.

H. Testing Analgesics in Human Beings

It is widely agreed that radiant heat and other methods of artificially induced pain cannot provide an adequate model for clinical pain. It is now considered preferable to test analgesics for their activities in situations of clinical pain, employing trained observers as intermediaries to question patients and obtain from them appraisals of pain relief. Such methods have been developed by Houde and colleagues in New York, who used a linear scale of pain relief on a logarithmic dose axis to measure the relative activities of analgesics in human beings (Houde, Wallenstein, and Beaver, 1966).

I. Value of Comparative Drug Assays in Human Beings: Therapeutic Ratio

Quantitative human drug assays have not been used a great deal by clinical pharmacologists, who have tended to regard them, with some justification, as somewhat crude and irrelevant to the clinical situation. Yet I suspect that they will be increasingly attempted, if only for the reason that, unless some parameter can be established by which two drugs are shown to be of equivalent potency, it is futile to try comparing them by a second parameter.

An interesting attempt to approach the vexed problem of the therapeutic ratio by means of quantitative human bioassays is that of Seed et al. (1958). These workers tested the relative analgesic activities of two morphine analogues by methods similar to those described above and compared them to their relative respiratory depressant activities. They found no statistically significant differences between the two relative activities; therefore by this criterion the two morphine analogues had the same therapeutic ratio in human beings.

VII. AUTOBIOGRAPHICAL SKETCH

I was born in a lovely spot, called Fiume, now Rijeka, right at the tip of the Adriatic where the frontier between the Western and Eastern Roman Empires is believed to have run. My education was correspondingly mixed up. I went to Italian and German schools and spoke English and French by the age of fourteen. I didn't learn much else to remember, but can still quote long passages from Dante by heart. I studied medicine in Munich, and in 1932, by a great piece of good luck, went to work with Dale in London. I was fortunate in not getting caught up in totalitarian regimes and was able to avoid fascism in Italy and nazism in Germany. My basic interest, curiously, was physics; but I became a pharmacologist by a sort of often-encountered compromise.

I had the good fortune of making many good friends among pharmacologists and physiologists, all of whom, I am happy to say, are still tremendously active. They include Georg Kahlson, Mauricio Rocha e Silva, Jack Mongar, Jim Black, Bob Furchgott, and Wilhelm Feldberg, with whom I have collaborated closely.

To end with, I would like to recall briefly, by some thumbnail recollections, a few pharmacologists who have greatly influenced me and who are no longer alive.

Dale. I have mentioned him before; he was a personality of tremendous force. I have elsewhere described the incident when I heard him say at the end of a successful experiment, "and if they don't believe me let *them* repeat the experiment." It was an expression of his conviction that if he did a single clear-cut experiment it was worth believing in.

Gaddum. Gaddum was an excellent mathematician; he would not rest unless he had personally solved a problem. He believed in doing the minimum number of experiments that was statistically required.

Clark. His chief characteristic was vigor. He used to sit in his office, with doors and windows wide open, talking to himself. I once tried to squeeze out a drop of my blood for a cholinesterase determination at a student lecture. Clark got impatient, grabbed a needle, and pierced his own finger so violently that he nearly pierced it through.

Straub. A nice chap, a kindly German boss, and certainly no Nazi. I once saw him with an unruly class of students who became immediately quiet when he said, "Not so much noise, it produces too much heat."

VIII. REFERENCES

Arunlakshana, O.: Schild, H.O.: Some Quantitative Uses of Drug Antagonists. Br J Pharmac 14(1959)48–58

Ash, A.S.F.; Schild, H.O.: Receptors Mediating Some Actions of Histamine. Br J Pharmac 27(1966)427–439

Assem, E.S.K.; Schild, H.O.: Inhibition of the Anaphylactic Mechanism by Sympathomimetic Amines. Int Arch Allergy 42(1971)576–589

Bain, W.A.: The Quantitative Comparison of Histamine Antagonists in Man. Proc Roy Soc Med 42(1949)615–623

Bertholet et al: A Study of β-adrenoceptors in the Guinea Pig, in preparation

Black, J.W.; Duncan, W.A.M.; Durant, C.J.; Ganellin, C.R.; Parsons, E.M.: Definition and Antagonism of Histamine H_2-Receptors. Nature 236(1972)385–390

Broder, I.; Schild, H.O.: The Action of Soluble Antigen-Antibody Complexes in Perfused Guinea Pig Lung. Immunology 8(1965)300–318

Chang, H.C.; Gaddum, J.H.: Choline Esters in Tissue Extracts. J Physiol 79(1933)255

Dale, H.H.: Adventures in Physiology with Excursions into Autopharmacology. Pergamon, London, 1953

Davies, H.; ff., S.; Hartley, R.E.; Schild, H.O.: Chemical Properties of High Molecular Weight Spleen Extract with Permeability Activity. Agents and Actions 4(1974)74–83

Evans, D.H.L.; Schild, H.O.; Thesleff, S.: Effects of Drugs on Depolarized Plain Muscle. J Physiol 143(1958)474–485

Feldberg, W.; Schilf, E.: Histamine. Springer, Berlin, 1930

Gaddum, J.H.: The Quantitative Effects of Antagonistic Drugs. J Physiol 89(1937)7P

Gaddum, J.H.; Schild, H.O.: A Sensitive Physical Test for Adrenaline. J Physiol 80(1933)9P

Houde, R.W.; Wallenstein, S.L.; Beaver, W.T.: Evaluation of Analgesics in Patients with Cancer Pain. In: Lasagna. Clinical Pharmacology 1, pp. 51–97, 1966

Lader, M.H.; Wing, L.: Habituation of the Psychogalvanic Reflex in Patients with Anxiety States and in Normal Subjects. J Neurol Neurosurg Psych 27(1964)210–218

Mongar, J.L.; Schild, H.O.: Cellular Mechanisms in Anaphylaxis. Physiol Rev 42(1962)226–270

Myerscough, P.R.; Schild, H.O.: Quantitative Assays of Oxytocic Drugs on the Human Post-partum Uterus. Brit J Pharmac 13(1958)207–212

Schild, H.O.: Histamine Release and Anaphylactic Shock in Isolated Lungs of Guinea-pigs. J Exp Physiol 26(1936)165–179

Schild, H.O.: A Method of Conducting a Biological Assay on a Preparation Giving Repeated Graded Responses Illustrated by the Estimation of Histamine. J Physiol 101(1942)115–130

Schild, H.O.: pA, A New Scale for the Measurement of Drug Antagonism. Br J Pharmac 2(1947a)189–206

Schild, H.O.: The Use of Drug Antagonists for the Identification and Classification of Drugs. Br J Pharmac 2(1947b)251–258

Schild, H.O.: The Experimental Evidence for the Use of Antihistamine Drugs in Allergic Conditions. Proc Roy Soc Med 42(1949a)623–625

Schild, H.O.: pA$_x$ and Competitive Drug Antagonism. Br J Pharmac 4(1949b)277–280

Schild, H.O.; Hawkins, D.F.; Mongar, J.L.; Herxheimer, H.: Reactions of Isolated Human Asthmatic Lung and Bronchial Tissue to a Specific Antigen. Lancet (1951)376

Schild, H.O.: Noncompetitive Drug Antagonism. J Physiol 124(1954)33P

Schild, H.O.: The Effect of Metals on the S-S Polypeptide Receptor in Depolarized Rat Uterus. Brit J Pharmac 36(1969)329–349

Schild, H.O.: Receptor Classification with Special Reference to β-adrenergic Receptors. In: Drug Receptors, pp. 29–36. Macmillan, London, 1973

Seed, J.C.; Wallenstein, S.L.; Houde, R.W.; Bellville, J.W.: A Comparison of the Analgesic and Respiratory Effects of Dihydrocodeine and Morphine in Man. Arch Int Pharmacodyn 96(1958)293–339

The Apparent Multiplicity
of Ganglionic Receptors

David I. Wallis

I. INTRODUCTION

There have been many reports in the last three decades of the presence of a considerable variety of "pharmacological receptors" at the synapses of autonomic ganglia. This trend towards an apparent multiplicity of receptors has led to considerable confusion about their nature and about their possible functional significance. It is pertinent to ask whether any of these receptors, other than those of the classical nicotinic kind, have any functional role in the transmission process. Is it perhaps the case that the identification of receptor after receptor at this synapse is the result of unwarranted conclusions? In this chapter I attempt to clarify this issue by considering the ways in which ganglion receptors have been identified, and I try to assess the degree to which they may be regarded as totally specific and the extent to which they may be considered functional.

Receptor shall mean a molecule or molecular complex that is capable of recognizing and selectively interacting with a neurotransmitter or other endogenous ligand and that, after binding it, is capable of generating some step that initiates the chain of events leading to the biological response (Kahn, 1976). Considerations of space have not allowed me to cover the literature exhaustively; I have tried to select what seem the most significant contributions in the field, ranging over a variety of sympathetic and parasympathetic ganglia. The majority of the work quoted may seem to derive from studies of mammalian sympathetic ganglia, especially of the superior cervical ganglion (scg). This is an inevitable consequence of the attention this particular ganglion has received. It must be borne in mind that species differences and differences between neurons in various ganglia may be sufficiently great to make generalizations invalid or at least unwise.

II. THE RANGE OF GANGLIONIC RECEPTORS: THE HISTORY OF THE TREND

That transmission is achieved through acetylcholine (ACh) acting upon nicotinic receptors is well established. Much more recent is evidence for the occurrence in sympathetic ganglia of other potential transmitter substances. Thus, catecholamines may be released from the small, intensely fluorescent (SIF) cells and, perhaps, from the dendrites or collaterals of the principal neurons; various polypeptides, such as substance P and somatostatin, may be present in, and perhaps be released from, networks of nerve terminals within ganglia (Table 3). Whether there are receptors for all of these substances on the ganglion cells has not been established. Further, it is now clear that at various synapses, including ganglionic and neuroeffector synapses, receptors may be located presynaptically. The physiological role of these presynaptic receptors may be to alter the amount of transmitter released by a nerve impulse. I refer to an action of this kind as a modulator action, even though this term is undeniably vague. Substances that modulate transmission may act either by altering transmitter release or by changing postsynaptic excitability; for this definition to be sufficiently restrictive, the modulator substance must arise within the body and under physiological, not pathological, conditions. A transmitter producing postsynaptic hyperpolarization or one inducing presynaptic inhibition might both be thought of as modulators in this sense.

A brief survey of the range and distribution of nonnicotinic ganglion receptors will provide the necessary historical perspective and will illustrate how the number of putative receptors has grown over the years. Information about their occurrence, the responses they mediate, their possible physiological role, and any information there may be about their location at the synapse is summarized in Tables 1-3. It will be significant for the subsequent discussion that a clear physiological function has not been established for many of these receptors. In some cases, the distribution of the receptors may be so wide that the notion of a physiological role for the receptors at all sites may be regarded with skepticism.

Dale and Laidlaw had realized as early as 1912 that responses to muscarinic agonists could be observed in sympathetic ganglia (Dale and Laidlaw, 1912) (Table 1). There is now very considerable evidence that muscarinic receptors can mediate slow depolarizations—the so-called slow epsp—and facilitate the transmission process; they may also be involved in specific transmission pathways through ganglia, which are readily revealed only during nicotinic receptor blockade (see also Fozard in this volume). Various reports have described a component in certain reflex responses that is resistant to nicotinic-receptor-blocking drugs and apparently mediated by muscarinic receptors. Freyburger et al. (1950) found this true of the pressor response of dogs and rabbits to asphyxia, but not true of the same response in cats and monkeys; it was also the case in dogs where the pressor response was evoked by an increase in intracranial pressure (Hilton and Steinberg, 1960). Physiological roles for these muscarinic receptors are well defined; but, as subsequent discussion shows, there are still questions to be answered about their exact status. The observations cover a range of ganglia and of species (Table 1). Rather less well confirmed is evidence that, in certain ganglia, muscarinic receptors located on ganglion cells may be part of a mechanism generating membrane hyperpolarization; these receptors may be the direct cause of the slow ipsp of amphibian ganglion cells (Weight & Padjen, 1973a,b).

There can be no doubt of the presence within ganglia of catecholamine receptors, for they have been demonstrated in so many ganglia and such a variety of species. The release of a catecholamine, perhaps dopamine or noradrenaline, from the ganglionic SIF cells and the involvement of these cells in inhibitory processes, either presynaptic in nature or dependent upon ganglion cell hyperpolarization (the slow ipsp), are topics that have received much attention recently and are dicussed in this volume by Fozard. They are touched upon in later sections of this chapter. Ganglionic α receptors are located both on ganglion cells and on the presynaptic terminals. It is likely that there are separate and distinct dopamine receptors in some ganglia, although the effects they mediate seem to be identical with those mediated by α receptors. There may also be ganglionic β receptors, but no claims have been made that these serve any physiological role; they induce excitatory rather than inhibitory effects. An additional role has been proposed for ganglionic dopamine receptors by Libet and his colleagues. They suggest their activation is able to enhance the depolarization mediated by muscarinic receptors.

Table 2 shows that there is substantial documentation for two other amine receptors at ganglionic synapses. Specific 5-HT receptors have been reported to be present in many ganglia and in many species. Since these receptors have been the subject of much of my recent work, a subsequent section in this chapter is especially concerned with the status of these receptors. There is good evidence to suggest that 5-HT receptors are not confined to the somadendritic regions of ganglion cells. As Table 2 indicates, under some circumstances they can facilitate transmission and under others depress transmission. In the intramural ganglia of the intestine, recent evi-

Table 1. Muscarinic and catecholamine ganglionic receptors

Receptor	Principal Ganglia Studied	Principal Species Studied	Response	Proposed Physiological Role	Location at Synapse
Muscarinic	scg	{ Cat, rabbit, rat, turtle	Excitation or facilitation of transmission[1] depolarization[2] slow epsp[3] inhibition[4] hyperpolarization[5] slow ipsp (?)[6]	a) Facilitation of transmission[7] b) Specific transmission pathway[8] c) Depression of transmission[4]	Somadendrites (?)
	Stellate	Dog, cat			
	Lumbar	Frog			
α	scg	{ Rabbit, cat, rat, Guinea pig	Inhibition[1] hyperpolarization[2] reduction of ACh release[3]	Depression of transmission[4]	Somadendrites, presynaptic terminals
	img	Guinea pig			
	lumbar	Frog			
	vesical parasympathetic	Cat			

References

[1] Dale and Laidlaw (1912); Koppanyi (1932); see also Trendelenburg (1967); Volle (1969); Haefely (1972); Nishi (1977).
[2] Brown (1966a); Koketsu, Nishi, and Soeda (1968); Dun, Nishi, and Karczmar (1976).
[3] Libet (1967); see also Haefely (1972); Nishi (1977).
[4] Pappano and Volle (1962).
[5] Takeshige et al. (1963); Brown (1966b); Weight and Padjen (1973a).
[6] Weight and Padjen (1973a,b).
[7] Eccles and Libet (1961); Libet (1964); Brimble and Wallis (1974); see also Volle (1969); Haefely (1972); Nishi (1977).
[8] Hilton and Steinberg (1966); Brown (1967); Flacke and Gillis (1968); Brown (1969); Chinn and Hilton (1976); Henderson and Ungar (1978).

			Excitation or facilitation of transmission[5] depolarization[6]		Somadendrites (?)
β	scg	Cat			
Dopamine	Prevertebral scg Lumbar	Dog {Rabbit, rat, cat, cow, monkey dog}	Inhibition[7] hyperpolarization[8] slow ipsp[9] reduction of ACh release[10]	Depression of transmission[11] Enhancement of muscarinic depolarization[12]	Somadendrites, presynaptic terminals

References

[1] Marrazzi (1939); Lundberg (1952); Matthews (1956); de Groat and Volle (1966a,b); Trendelenburg (1967); Aiken and Reit (1969); Kosterlitz and Lees (1972); de Groat and Saum (1972).

[2] Eccles and Libet (1961); Libet and Tosaka (1966); de Groat and Volle (1966a,b); Libet and Kobayashi (1969); Kobayashi and Libet (1970); Haefely (1969).

[3] Paton and Thompson (1953); Haefely (1969); Christ and Nishi (1969, 1971b); see also Kosterlitz and Lees (1972); Nishi (1977).

[4] Eccles and Libet (1961); Williams (1967); Siegrist et al. (1968); Williams and Palay (1969); Matthews and Raisman (1969); see also Haefely (1969); Kosterlitz and Lees (1972).

[5] Bulbring and Burn (1942); Bulbring (1944); Konzett (1956); Matthews (1956); Malméjac (1955); de Groat and Volle (1966a,b).

[6] de Groat and Volle (1966a,b); Haefely (1969).

[7] Dun and Nishi (1974); Williams (1973).

[8] Libet (1970); Dun, Kaibara, and Karczmar (1977).

[9] Libet (1970); Libet and Owman (1974).

[10] Dun and Nishi (1974).

[11] Libet and Tosaka (1969, 1970); Libet and Owman (1974); see also Libet (1976).

[12] Libet and Tosaka (1970); Libet, Kobayashi and Tanaka 1975.

NOTES:

scg, superior cervical ganglion; img, inferior mesenteric ganglion; c-smg, coeliac-superior mesenteric ganglion; ip, intramural parasympathetic ganglion; ACh, acetylcholine; α, α-adrenoceptor; β, β-adrenoceptor.

Table 2. 5-HT, histamine and GABA ganglionic receptors

Receptor	Principal Ganglia Studied	Principal Species Studied	Response	Proposed Physiological Role	Location at Synapse
5-HT	scg[1] Stellate[2] img[3] Lumbar[4] Ciliary[5] ip[6] Pelvic[7]	rabbit, cat, rat rat, cat cat dog, frog dog guinea pig cat, dog, rat	Excitation or facilitation of transmission[8] depolarization[9] depression of transmission[10]	Transmission modulator (?)[11] Excitatory transmitter in intestine[12]	Somadendrites[9] presynaptic terminals[13] axons[14]

References

[1] Robertson (1954); Trendelenburg (1956a, 1957); Jéquier (1965); de Groat and Volle (1966b).
[2] Hertzler (1961); Aiken and Reit (1969).
[3] Gyermek and Bindler (1962a,b).
[4] Watanabe and Koketsu (1973); Wallis and Willems, unpublished.
[5] Page and McCubbin (1953).
[6] Robertson (1953); Gaddum and Picarelli (1957); Hirst and Silinsky (1975).
[7] Gyermek (1962); Vanov (1965); Saum and de Groat (1973).
[8] Robertson (1954); Trendelenburg (1956a, 1957); Hertzler (1961); Gyermek and Bindler (1962a,b); Saum and de Groat (1973); Hirst and Silinsky (1975).
[9] de Groat and Volle (1966b); Haefely (1974); Wallis and Woodward (1973, 1975); Hirst and Silinsky (1975); North and Wallis (1977); Wallis and North (1978a,c).
[10] Jéquier (1965); Machova and Boska (1969); Saum and de Groat (1973); de Groat and Lalley (1973); Wallis and Woodward (1974).
[12] Bulbring and Gershon (1967); Gershon et al. (1977); Dreyfus, Sherman, and Gershon (1977).
[13] Wallis and Woodward (1975).
[14] Wallis and Nash, unpublished.

			Transmission modulator (?)	Somadendrites (?)
Histamine	scg[1] Stellate[2]	Cat, rabbit, rat Cat	Excitation or facilitation of transmission[3] depolarization[4] depression of transmission[5]	Transmission modulator (?)	Somadendrites (?)
GABA	scg[6] img[7] Lumbar[8]	Cat, rat Cat Frog	Depolarization[9] depression of transmission[10]	None (?)	Somadendrites (?) Presynaptic terminals and C fiber axons[11]

References

[1] Konzett (1952); Trendelenburg (1954, 1955); Trendelenburg (1967); Haefely (1972).
[2] Aiken and Reit (1969).
[3] Trendelenburg (1954, 1955, 1957); Iorio and McIsaac (1966); Brimble and Wallis (1973).
[4] Watson (1970); Haefely (1972); Wallis and North, unpublished.
[5] Gertner and Kohn (1959); Brimble and Wallis (1973).
[6] de Groat (1970); Adams and Brown (1973).
[7] Matthews and Roberts (1961).
[8] Koketsu, Shoji, and Yamamoto (1974).
[9] de Groat (1970); Bowery and Brown (1974); Adams and Brown (1975).
[10] de Groat (1970); Adams and Brown (1973, 1975); Koketsu et al. (1974).
[11] Koketsu et al. (1974); Brown and Marsh (1978).

NOTES:
5-HT, 5-hydroxytryptamine; GABA, γ-aminobutyric acid; other abbreviations as in table 1.

Table 3. Polypeptide ganglionic receptors

Receptor	Principal Ganglia Studied	Principal Species Studied	Response	Proposed Physiological Role	Location at Synapse
Angiotensin	scg[1] Stellate[2] ip[3]	Cat, rabbit, rat Cat Guinea pig	Excitation or facilitation of transmission[4] depolarization[5] altered ACh release[6] depression of tranmission[7]	None (?)	Somadendrites Presynaptic terminals[6]
Bradykinin	scg[8] Stellate[9]	Cat, rabbit, dog, rat Cat	Excitation or facilitation of transmission[10] depolarization[11] depression of transmission[12]	None (?)	Somadendrites (?)
Substance P	scg[13] img, c-smg[14] ip[15]	Cat Guinea pig, cat, rat Mouse	Excitation or facilitation of transmission[13] (?)	Present in nerve terminals (sensory collaterals ?) within ganglia	Somadendrites (?)
Vasoactive intestinal peptide	img, c-smg[16] ip[17]	Guinea pig (?)		Present in networks of nerve terminals within ganglia	
Enkephalin	img, c-smg[18] ip	Guinea pig rat		Present in networks of nerve terminals within ganglia	
Somatostatin	img, c-smg[19] ip[20]	Guinea pig Rat		Present in networks of nerve terminals within ganglia	

References

[1] Lewis and Reit (1965); Haefely, Hürlimann, and Thoenen (1966). Trendelenburg (1966); Watson (1970).
[2] Aiken and Reit (1968, 1969).

[3] Khairallah and Page (1961).

[4] Lewis and Reit (1965, 1966); Haefely et al. (1966); Trendelenburg (1966); Machova and Boska (1967); Aiken and Reit (1969); Wallis, Williams, and Wali (1978).

[5] Haefely (1970); Dun and Nishi (1975); Wallis and Woodward (unpublished).

[6] Panisset (1967).

[7] Haefely et al. (1965).

[8] Lewis and Reit (1965, 1966); Trendelenburg (1966); Haefely et al. (1966).

[9] Aiken and Reit (1969).

[10] Lewis and Reit (1965, 1966); Trendelenburg (1966); Haefely et al. (1966); Wallis and Woodward (1974).

[11] Haefely (1970).

[12] Haefely et al. (1965).

[13] Beleslin, Radmanov, and Varagic (1960).

[14] Hökfelt et al. (1977).

[15] Nilsson et al. (1975); Pearse and Polak (1975); Hökfelt et al. (1977).

[16] Hökfelt et al. (1977).

[17] Bryant et al. (1976).

[18] Elde et al. (1976); quoted by Hokfelt et al. (1977).

[19] Hökfelt et al. (1977).

[20] Hökfelt et al. (1975).

NOTES:

Abbreviations as in table 1.

dence implicates 5-HT as a transmitter substance of a population of intrinsic neurons.

Specific histamine receptors have been reported in some sympathetic ganglia, but apparently in a rather limited range of species. Brimble and Wallis (1973) described the presence of both H_1- and H_2-histamine receptors at the synapses of the rabbit scg. H_1 receptors mediated facilitation of transmission and H_2 receptors depression of transmission. However, the precise nature of the H_2 receptors is dubious, since identification depended on blockade by the relatively nonspecific H_2 antagonist burimamide. Attempts to confirm the presence of H_2 receptors with the more specific antagonists, metiamide and cimetidine, have not been successful (Strupinski and Wallis, unpublished). Further work is needed to clarify the situation.

GABA receptors on ganglion cells have been closely investigated, particularly by Brown and his colleagues. GABA is not normally released within the ganglion, and no physiological role is suggested for these receptors. Like several other receptors, they are not confined to the soma dendritic regions of the ganglion cells, since their presence on the presynaptic terminals has been reported in Amphibia and on the surface of the unmyelinated axons in the cervical sympathetic nerve of the rat.

Receptors for polypeptides (Table 3) have received less attention, possibly because of the tachyphylaxis these substances often seem to induce. The peptides for which most information exists are angiotensin and bradykinin; it is possible that their action may be both on ganglion cells and on presynaptic terminals. Thus, Panisset (1967) has reported a presynaptic action of angiotensin in cat ganglia, and the facilitatory action of bradykinin on rabbit ganglia has been interpreted as being presynaptic (Wallis and Woodward, 1974). The potent effects on transmission of these two peptides contrast with the erratic and limited depolarizations of the ganglion cell membrane they seem capable of evoking. Both peptides are capable of depressing and facilitating transmission under different circumstances.

The presence of specific receptors for the other polypeptides listed in Table 3 is much less well attested. They are included principally because very recent immunohistochemical studies have indicated that these polypeptides are present in fine networks of nerve terminals that are more prominent in certain autonomic ganglia than in others. There is no clear evidence that the polypeptides are released within ganglia. With the exception of receptors for enkephalin in the intramural ganglia of the intestine, there is virtually no evidence for the presence within autonomic ganglia of specific receptors for substance P; vasoactive intestinal peptide; somatostatin; or, in other ganglia, enkephalin. Current research will probably alter this state of affairs within the near future.

III. STATUS OF GANGLIONIC NONNICOTINIC RECEPTORS

The survey above shows clearly the trend toward a great multiplicity of receptors at the ganglionic synapse. Although some of these receptors can be characterized pharmacologically by using specific antagonists and by examining the activity of a range of compounds related to the natural agonist, this has not been done for many of the receptors. Further, characterization does not by itself satisfy the definition of *receptor* given in the introduction. For instance, even though the criterion for specificity may be met, it still remains unclear whether each receptor is linked to a specific mechanism leading to a biological response or whether it may merely interact with some subsidiary or modulatory site near the nicotinic receptor for ACh or with some macromolecule involved in the events producing the biological response to activation of nicotinic receptors. Before we can begin to resolve this problem, it is necessary to formulate as clearly as possible what we understand by *receptor* and the relationship this entity has with other membrane structures.

A. Relevance of Experimental Technique

One limitation to our knowledge of these receptors arises from the kinds of experimental technique that have been used. Much of the earlier work involved recording from effectors governed by postganglionic neurons whose cell bodies lie in the ganglion. For example, the nictitating membrane of the cat innervated from the scg has been extensively studied. The information this kind of technique yields is not only indirect, but also relates to only a very specific population of ganglion cells—those that innervate the membrane. Gross electrical recording from the ganglion, although it may yield important insights, cannot distinguish between populations of ganglion cells whose complement of receptors may differ. The receptors on particular cells can only be examined readily by intracellular recording, although technical ingenuity can allow comparisons to be made in other ways. For instance, Aiken and Reit (1969) were able to show by comparing cardioacceleration and sweating of the foot pad in cats, that adrenergic and cholinergic neurons in the cat stellate ganglion displayed a differential sensitivity to a range of substances. The indolealkylamine, 5-HT was a much more effective stimulant of cholinergic neurons, whereas acetylcholine and histamine were more effective on adrenergic neurons. The muscarinic agonist (4-(m-chlorophenylcarbamoyloxy)-2-butynyltrimethyl ammonium chloride, McN-A343), angiotensin, and bradykinin each stimulated the adrenergic neurons but not the cholinergic ones. Conceivably, the sensitivity of different noradrenergic neurons may also differ; alternatively, if the same population of cells may be activated by different preganglionic routes

(Wallis and North, 1978b), then one route may involve a muscarinic receptor component in the transmission process and the other may not. Henderson and Ungar (1978) have recently shown that, in the dog, sympathetic ganglionic transmission during the baroreceptor reflex is mediated by nicotinic receptors, whereas the transmission evoked by stimulation of carotid body chemoreceptors involves muscarinic receptors with a subsidiary nicotinic pathway.

What is required is intracellular recording coupled with a technique that will allow the identification of neurons in terms of the effector they innervate. Differences between the receptor complements of functionally different ganglionic synapses may then become more apparent. Even intracellular recording by itself cannot tell us about the minute distribution of these receptors over the cell surface. It can distinguish between a presynaptic and a postsynaptic location, but it cannot easily reveal whether the receptors are localized, say, to certain regions of the dendrites or to parts of the soma. Microscopic techniques are necessary for this; perhaps autoradiography combined with electron microscopy may eventually reveal the specific binding sites. Alternatively, the techniques of Harris, Kuffler, and Dennis (1971) might be more widely used. They observed single parasympathetic ganglion cells of the frog heart by using Nomarski optics; and, by employing extremely fine micropipettes, they demonstrated a much higher sensitivity of the postsynaptic membrane to ACh at the synaptic boutons than elsewhere over the cell surface.

B. Lability of Receptors

A factor that should also be considered is that the experimental technique may be unduly artificial; especially might this be true of *in vitro* techniques or where ganglia are perfused with physiological solutions rather than with blood. Trendelenburg (1956b) found that the cat scg, perfused *in situ*, had only 1/10 to 1/100 of the sensitivity of a ganglion with a normal blood supply to such substances as histamine, pilocarpine, and 5-HT, even though its sensitivity to nicotinic agents was not markedly changed. Hancock and Volle (1970) suggested that the acetylcholine receptors of the rat scg might be labile and altered by perfusion with physiological solutions. They observed that spike discharges evoked by muscarinic agents in ganglia with an intact blood supply were abolished by atropine but not by hexamethonium, whereas discharges in ganglia perfused with Locke solution were sensitive to both atropine and hexamethonium. It is important to bear in mind that changes in receptor specificity might be induced by particular experimental conditions. In general, however, most reports do not suggest that *in vitro* conditions themselves substantially alter the receptor population of ganglion cells.

Longer-term changes in the specificity or the distribution of receptors may be envisaged. Various authors have reported an increase in the sensitivity to muscarinic agonists of the denervated ganglion (Bokri, Fehér, and Mozsik, 1963; Takeshige and Volle, 1963). Dun, Nishi, and Karczmar (1976), using intracellular recording and microiontophoresis, explored the changes that occur in rabbit scg cells following preganglionic denervation. Nicotinic responses were reduced and muscarinic responses increased 2–3 weeks after denervation. These changes could not be explained by any alteration in the electrical properties of the cells, for there were none; a change in the affinity of the receptors was also discounted, because the K_a values for the complexing of ACh with the nicotinic or the muscarinic receptors had not altered. It was suggested that denervation may induce a change in the relative numbers of receptors, nicotinic receptors decreasing and muscarinic receptors increasing in number. In the case of these cells, the precise localization of the receptors is unknown, but nicotinic receptors at least might be expected to be concentrated on the subsynaptic regions of the cell membrane. In frog cardiac parasympathetic ganglion cells (Kuffler, Dennis, and Harris, 1971), extrasynaptic portions of the membrane become sensitive to focally applied ACh after denervation, suggesting a spread or an unmasking of receptors. Such a process might be occurring on the rabbit scg cells; but if so, the unmasked receptors would appear to be of the muscarinic type.

Changes in the receptor population with this kind of time course might involve replacement of receptors. Receptor macromolecules, like other membrane constituents, are believed to be in a state of continual turnover, although little seems to be known about the rates of turnover. Membrane proteins have a half-life of 30–60 h, with a range of 2 h–16 days (Schimke, 1975). Studying rat diaphragm in culture, Berg and Hall (1974) found that only 20% of ACh receptors were lost per 24 h from innervated muscle, but this loss increased to 80% when the muscle was denervated. Changes on denervation of ganglion cells might reflect not an alteration in a static receptor macromolecule but replacement with receptors with somewhat different distributions or characteristics.

C. Nature of Receptors

Recent ideas about receptor structure emphasize that they should be regarded as part of a complex entity. Some part of the complex must embody a ligand recognition site. Because the same recognition pattern may be associated with different responses, it is usual to imagine the complex as comprising at least two components—a recognition site and a catalytic or amplification site. These two functions could be embodied in the same macromolecule or in separate macromolecules (Triggle and Triggle, 1976). The amplification site may be some kind of ion channel or ionophore. The simplest assumptions about the binding site—i.e., that there exists a single, unique transmitter recognition site and that all the analogues and antagonists also bind to this same unique site, occupying greater or lesser areas of it according to the nature of the ligand—may not necessarily be applicable to all kinds of receptors (Triggle and Triggle, 1976). An alternative concept is that there are multiple, but overlapping, binding sites for various related ligands which produce their effects through interaction at topographically distinct sites from those involved in binding the transmitter molecule itself.

The next section explores certain of these points by reference to some of our recent findings on ganglionic 5-HT receptors. The observations on this particular receptor and their interpretation exemplify some of the problems that arise in deciding upon the nature, status, and function of ganglionic nonnicotinic receptors.

IV. GANGLIONIC 5-HT RECEPTORS

Crucial to the status of any receptor as a separate entity must be pharmacological distinctness. Ganglionic 5-HT receptors have usually been described as distinct from nicotinic receptors and as falling into that category of peripheral 5-HT receptors designated M because of the sensitivity of the 5-HT effects to morphine (Trendelenburg, 1967). Many authors have noted that excitatory actions of 5-HT at the ganglion are resistant to nicotinic blocking agents, such as hexamethonium (e.g., Trendelenburg, 1956; de Groat & Lalley, 1973; Wallis & Woodward, 1975; North & Wallis, 1977; Wallis & North, 1978a, 1978c). Selective blockade of the action of nicotinic agonists such as 1,1-dimethyl-4-phenylpiperazinium (DMPP) compared to that of 5-HT has also been demonstrated (Gyermek and Bindler, 1962b; Watson, 1970). It is, in fact, a characteristic of ganglionic responses to 5-HT, as well as to other nonnicotinic agents, that their effectiveness is apparently enhanced during the period of nondepolarizing blockade induced by nicotine (Trendelenburg, 1967). The 5-HT receptors of the cat scg are said to be insensitive to blockade by lysergic acid diethylamide (LSD), brom-LSD or phenoxybenzamine. Like the M receptors on intramural plexus neurons of the intestine, they are sensitive to blockade by morphine, methadone, and cocaine. However, the precise nature of this blockade may be questioned, since the responses of an effector organ were used to assess ganglionic actions. For instance, morphine may well have interfered with the release of noradrenaline at the nictitating membrane neuroeffector junction. This junction in the cat is peculiarly sensitive to morphine (Kosterlitz and Lees, 1972). Another reason why the specificity of the blockade may be doubted is that these agents interfere equally with the ganglionic actions of histamine, pilocarpine, angiotensin, and bradykinin (Trendelenburg, 1967). Further, the intra-arterial injection of small doses of calcium chloride into the scg, which does not affect the nicotinic response, abolishes the postganglionic discharge evoked by both methacholine, a muscarinic agonist, and 5-HT (Takeshige and Volle, 1964; Smith, 1966). As Trendelenburg (1967) has suggested, it is likely that these agents block a pathway common to the chain of events initiated by activation of the specific nonnicotinic receptors. They should not be regarded, therefore, as interacting with the ligand binding site proper, assuming that such entities exist for 5-HT and other nonnicotinic substances that excite or inhibit ganglion cells.

Although, on the above evidence, it would seem that ganglionic 5-HT receptors may be somewhat poorly characterized in terms of antagonists, other findings suggest a considerable degree of specificity. The 5-HT receptors of the cat inferior mesenteric ganglion (img) are antagonized selectively by 5-hydroxy-3-indoleacetamidine (Gyermek, 1964). Our own experiments on the rabbit scg show that a specific antagonist of 5-HT receptors is quipazine maleate (2-(1-piperazinyl)quinoline maleate). It has only a weak agonist action at the ganglion, although at other sites it has been described as an agonist at 5-HT receptors (Green, Youdin, and Grahame-Smith, 1976). Further, atropine prevents the ganglionic action of methacholine and other muscarinic agonists without affecting responses to 5-HT or histamine, while pyrilamine antagonizes the ganglionic action of histamine without affecting those of 5-HT or muscarinic agonists (Trendelenburg, 1967). The next section will suggest that ganglionic 5-HT receptors can be relatively well defined by comparison of the agonist activity of various analogues of 5-HT.

A. Potency of Chemically Related Substances

The nature of ganglionic 5-HT receptors has been investigated in the cat img *in situ* by Gyermek and his colleagues, who studied action potential discharge in a small number of postganglionic axons and, recently, in the isolated scg of the rabbit in my laboratory, using the sucrose gap technique to record change in resting membrane potential. The effects of 5-HT on single ganglion cells of the rabbit have also been described (North and Wallis, 1977; Wallis and North, 1978a, 1978c). The sucrose gap experiments, not yet complete, have shown that small modifications to the 5-HT molecule severely deplete its ability to depolarize the ganglion. The tissue is constantly superfused, and the best way of obtaining reproducible depolarizations is to inject 5-HT in a small volume of Krebs solution into the superfusion stream to the ganglion (Wallis and Woodward, 1975). 0.2 μmol 5-HT produces a depolarization around $\frac{2}{3}$ maximum; a rapid depolarization and repolarization are followed by an after-hyperpolarization (Fig. 1Ai).

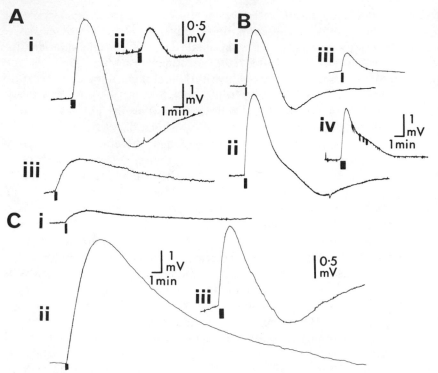

Figure 1. Records of change in membrane potential induced by 5-HT or related compounds. Rabbit scg's were mounted in a sucrose gap apparatus. Chart records, depolarization upwards. Black bars show duration of injection.
A. Responses to (i) 0.2 μmol 5-HT, (ii) 0.2 μmol 6-hydroxytryptamine (6-HT) and (iii) 2 μmol α methyl 5-HT (αM 5-HT), calibration as for (i).
B. Responses of ganglion cells and axons in the same preparation. (i) Ganglion, 0.05 μmol 5-HT; (ii) ganglion, 0.2 μmol 5-HT; (iii) axons, 0.1 μmol 5-HT; and (iv) axons, 0.4 μmol 5-HT.
C. Responses of ganglion to (i) 0.2 μmol 5-methoxydimethyltryptamine (5-MODMT), calibration as for (ii); (ii) 0.1 μmol bufotenine (5-HDMT); and (iii) 0.2 μmol 5-HT.

The relative activities of analogues of 5-HT can be expressed in terms of molar amounts equiactive with 5-HT, giving the equipotent molar ratio (epmr). The response of the analogue was matched as closely as possible by an appropriate amount of 5-HT. When the analogue failed to produce any response or produced one so small that it was difficult to measure against the baseline noise, the compound was described as inactive; an epmr greater than a certain value could be assigned to it by comparison with an amount of 5-HT generating a threshold response. The method allows comparison of activity; but it cannot distinguish, for instance, between reduced affinity for the receptors and reduced efficacy of the agonist.

Hydroxyl substitution of the indole nucleus seems crucial to activity at the ganglionic receptor. Thus, tryptamine (T) has less than 1/100 of the activity of 5-HT, with a mean epmr of 138. The position of the hydroxyl moiety is also important, because 6-hydroxytryptamine (6-HT) has about 1/25 of the activity of 5-HT; responses to the two amines are shown in Figure 1Ai, ii. The substitution of a second hydroxyl at carbon atom 6, as in 5-6 dihydroxytryptamine, results in an epmr of about 5. Unlike receptors of brain stem neurons in cats and rats (Bradley and Briggs, 1974), ganglionic 5-HT receptors are not excited by the 5-methoxy-derivative of tryptamine (5-MOT); like dopamine, 5-MOT induces a weak hyperpolarization of the ganglion.

The nature of the ethylamine side chain attached to carbon 3 of the indole nucleus is also crucial. The amino acid precursor of 5-HT, 5-hydroxytryptophan, was without activity in about a third of the ganglia tested (mean epmr ⏌145). Tryptophan is inactive. Melatonin, in which the side chain is acetylated and the indole nucleus carries a 5-methoxy group, is almost without activity (epmr ⏌360).

Hallucinogens such as LSD and mescaline may act at 5-HT receptors in the CNS. The indole moiety of LSD is fused within a heterocyclic ring system; it has about 1/40 the activity of 5-HT at the ganglion and often produces a biphasic response. Activity is very dependent upon the diethyl-amide part of the molecule, since lysergic acid itself is inactive. Mescaline has only about 1/400 the activity of 5-HT and sometimes evokes a weak hyperpolarization like 5MOT.

Of greater interest is the effect of side chain methylation. Methylation at the α-carbon atom considerably reduces activity, for α-methyl 5-HT has only about 1/25 that of 5-HT (Fig. 1Aiii). N-methylation produces dramatic changes in activity when more than one methyl group is introduced. N-methyl 5-HT gives responses similar to those evoked by 5-HT (Fig. 2Ai, ii) (epmr 1.4); 5-hydroxydimethyltryptamine or bufotenine (5-HDMT) gives responses of very much greater magnitude and duration than 5-HT (Fig. 1Cii, iii; Fig. 2Ai, iii) and is on average 5–6 times more active (epmr 0.19). The depolarization induced by 0.2 μmol can persist for 30 minutes. A change at carbon atom 5 very much affected this activity. 5-methoxy-dimethyltryptamine (5-MODMT) is only about 1/40 as active as 5-HT (Fig. 1Ci), whereas dimethyltryptamine, although it produces prolonged depolarizations, has 1/3 the activity of 5-HT (epmr 3) and 4-hydroxy-dimethyltryptamine (psilocin) is 1/100 as active as 5-HT. N-methylation of tryptamine increases its activity twofold, but it is still much less active than N-methyl 5-HT. Introduction of a methyl substituent in the indole nucleus at carbon atom 2 to give 2-methyl-N'N'-dimethyltryptamine greatly reduces activity (epmr ⏌120). However, the introduction of a third methyl group on the terminal nitrogen produces a quaternary ammonium compound and the most potent depolarizing agent we have tested on the ganglion, 5-hydroxy-N'N'N'-trimethyltryptamine or bufotenidine (5-HTMT). Depolari-

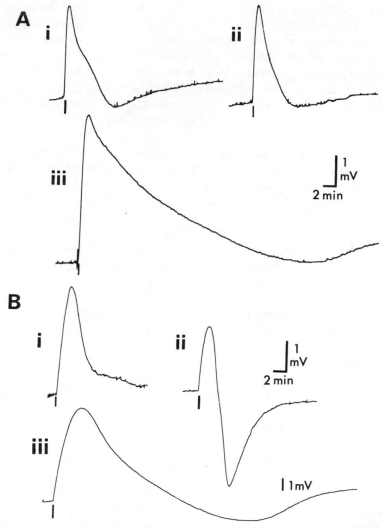

Figure 2. Sucrose gap records of change in membrane potential (as in Fig. 1).
A. Responses to (i) 0.1 µmol 5-HT, (ii) 0.1 µmol N-methyl 5-HT (NM 5-HT), and (iii) 0.05 µmol bufotenine (5-HDMT).
B. Responses to (i) 0.2 µmol 5-HT, (ii) 0.2 µmol dimethylphenylpiperazinium (DMPP), and (iii) 0.01 µmol N,N,N-trimethyl 5-HT (5-HTMT).

zations are of great magnitude and duration (Fig. 2Biii); its activity is 50 times that of 5-HT and about 10 times that of bufotenine. The di- and trimethyl derivatives are apparently much more active than standard nicotinic agonists as well, for acetylcholine in the presence of an anticholinesterase is roughly comparable in activity to 5-HT (Wallis and Woodward, 1975), and the epmr for trimethylammonium (against 5-HT) is about 2. We have generally used DMPP to induce depolarizations mediated via nicotinic receptors (epmr = 0.93 ± 0.16, mean ± SEM, n = 19). DMPP evokes responses characterized by a large after-hyperpolarization (Fig. 2Bii). Gyermek and Bindler (1962a), in contrast, reported that 5-HDMT, 5-HTMT, and NM5-HT were approximately equipotent with 5-HT in cat ganglia.

These preliminary data are only suggestive of the characteristics of the ganglionic 5-HT receptor site, but certain features distinguish it from hypothetical receptors in the CNS at which psychotomimetic drugs act (Carlstrom, Bergin, and Falkenberg, 1973). In the CNS, (a) the amino nitrogen atom may be alkylated and dimethylation gives higher hallucinogenic potency than monomethylation; (b) indolealkylamines with a completely unmethylated side chain have extremely low activity; and (c) the indole nucleus may be substituted with hydroxyl or methoxy groups in position 4 or 5. Thus, 5-MODMT is one of the most potent hallucinogens but is relatively inactive at the ganglion. Further, although methylation appears to increase activity of a molecule at the ganglionic receptor, it will be seen below that the dimethylated indoleamines have special properties that make it doubtful whether they are acting simply via 5-HT receptors.

There appears to be no straightforward way of establishing the conformation of the receptor-bound species of a ligand; the process of binding may result in a conformation unlike that found in solution or in the crystalline state. But if a group of indole compounds adopt similar conformations in crystal, they may display similar properties at the receptor. Carlstrom et al. (1973) have attempted to demonstrate that certain indolealkylamines active in the CNS adopt a conformation that has several particular features. Most of their steric information is based on X-ray crystallography. They emphasize that the rings are planar and the only conformational changes that can take place are rotations about single bonds in the side chain. They suggest that indolealkylamines fall into two groups, depending on whether the ethylamine side chain is fully extended or whether the amino nitrogen atom is rotated inward (i.e., is in the gauche position to the pyrrole ring). Many of the analogues inactive at the ganglion, and inactive also as hallucinogens, possess folded side chains, e.g., tryptamine and all tryptophans. DMT, 5-MODMT, psilocin, LSD, and bufotenine—as well as 5-HT itself, which exists in both conformations in the crystalline state—have extended side chains. Although an extended side chain may be a requirement for activity at ganglionic receptors, these would appear to be less permissive in other respects, e.g., the requirement for a hydroxyl at carbon #5. Not all these substances are highly active.

B. Distribution of 5-HT Receptors

The distribution of receptors over sympathetic neurons may be widespread. The terminals of preganglionic nerve fibres in the ganglion may possess 5-

HT receptors (Wallis and Woodward, 1975), as may cell bodies of preganglionic neurons in the cord (de Groat and Ryall, 1967). It can be shown that the nonmyelinated axons leaving the ganglion in the internal carotid nerve are also capable of being depolarized by 5-HT (Fig. 1Bi–iv), although the magnitude of this depolarization varies considerably from preparation to preparation. It appears that these axonal membranes possess 5-HT receptors in addition to their sparse population of nicotinic receptors (Kosterlitz, Lees, and Wallis, 1968). There are 5-HT receptors on the terminals of postganglionic sympathetic neurons, excitation of which results in release of noradrenaline (Fozard and Mobarok Ali, 1976). Although present on the same cells as the ganglionic 5-HT receptors, their sensitivity to 5-HT analogues appears to be different. Thus, for NM 5-HT the epmr is about 2 and for 5,6-dihydroxytryptamine around 5—values similar to those quoted above. However, rather than being 5 times more active than 5-HT, 5-HDMT showed a lower activity, epmr 2.3 (Fozard and Mobarok Ali, 1976).

C. Relation between 5-HT Receptors and Nicotinic Receptors

So far I have emphasized the distinctiveness of ganglionic 5-HT receptors by reference to our own work and to that of many others. However, there are reasons for supposing that the 5-HT receptor is quite intimately associated with the nicotinic receptor and might represent an adjacent binding site. Two arguments may favour this view. First, 5-HT depolarizations have several features in common with depolarizations evoked by nicotinic agents, including a rapid change in potential, a dependence on Na^+ ions and the development of an after-hyperpolarization—probably as a consequence of the electrogenic extrusion of Na^+ ions from the cell (Wallis and Woodward, 1975). Wallis and North (1978a,c) demonstrated that 5-HT increases membrane conductance and noted the similarities in the conductance changes initiated by 5-HT and ACh acting on nicotinic receptors. They probably involve Na^+, K^+, and, perhaps, Ca^{++} ions. There is a difference in the estimated reversal potentials, that for acetylcholine being about -12 mV (Dun et al., 1976), whereas that for 5-HT is about -24 mV (Wallis and North, 1978c) It is possible that nicotinic and 5-HT receptors activate, if not the same ion channels or ionophores, then perhaps a partially shared population of channels; ion channels not shared may account for the difference in reversal potentials.

The second line of argument depends on the mode of action of the di- and trimethylated derivatives of 5-HT (5-HDMT, 5-HTMT) and on antagonists at 5-HT and nicotinic receptors. Our observations show that the depolarizations evoked by these N-methylated substances are incompletely blocked by certain antagonists of 5-HT, such as quipazine, but are considerably reduced by nicotinic receptor blockers. Similar observations have been made in respect of 5-HDMT on the cat img (Gyermek and Bindler, 1962a), on the cat scg (Haefely, 1974), and on the terminals of the cardiac sympathetic nerves of the rabbit (Fozard and Mobarok Ali, 1978). It would appear that these two methylated derivatives have a dual action at the ganglion cell membrane, reacting with both nicotinic and 5-HT binding sites. The N-methylated end of a molecule already bound at a 5-HT receptor through its indole nucleus might conceivably react with a neighboring nicotinic receptor. The dual action presumably explains the extraordinarily high activity at very low concentrations of these amines, although an additional factor, not substantiated, might be the period of time for which the ion channels remain open.

Insofar as antagonists of ganglion 5-HT receptors have been identified, they are a diverse group of substances that do not necessarily have a close chemical affinity to the indolealkylamine. Whereas hexamethonium in high concentrations (250–550 μM) potentiates 5-HT depolarizations in some preparations (Wallis and Woodward, 1975), it depresses them in others. Perhaps high selectivity should not be expected with these concentrations. However, d-tubocurarine is known to antagonize certain responses to both ACh and 5-HT in invertebrate neurons (Gerschenfeld and Paupardin-Tritsch, 1974). Similarly, we find it blocks depolarizations to both 5-HT and DMPP. In the absence of complete quantitative information, it is impossible to be sure that these actions do not represent an interference with the ion channels or some other feature of the mechanism rather than binding at the ligand recognition site. It may be significant, as pointed out by Stone (1974), that there is a considerable similarity in structure between tubocurarine and several other antagonists effective at different receptors. In addition, there is now detailed evidence (Ascher, Marty, and Nield, 1978) to suggest that at some nicotinic receptors (perhaps including those of sympathetic ganglia [Blackman, 1970]), hexamethonium and curare do not act by competing for the ligand recognition site. These authors propose that the receptor channel complex in the presence of the ligand exists in two states, conducting and nonconducting; the antagonists act by combining with the conducting complex and converting it to a second kind of nonconducting complex. The site of reaction may be in the structure crossed by the permeating ions, so that the antagonists act as pore blockers. Channel blockade per se, although compatible with antagonism by curare of several transmitter ligands, needs further qualification before it can explain the complex results obtained for invertebrate nicotinic receptors (Ascher et al., 1978).

Gyermek and Bindler (1962b) considered a spectrum of antagonists, ranging from morphine, cocaine, brom-LSD, LSD, phenoxybenzamine, benzyloxygramine, and atropine to hexamethonium; one end of the spectrum is relatively selective for 5-HT receptors, the other for the nicotinic agonist, DMPP. Certain agents (brom-LSD, benzyloxygramine), although indolealkylamines, show little or no selectivity. Picrotoxin is another agent that blocks the excitatory actions of 5-HT at sympathetic ganglia (de Groat and Lalley, 1973), yet fails to act selectively at vesical autonomic ganglia (Saum and de Groat, 1973).

At present, ideas about the nature of ganglionic 5-HT receptors and their relation to both nicotinic receptors and ion channels can be only speculative. It does seem possible that the ion channels may be associated with multiple, but overlapping, binding sites. A portion of ion channels may have both nicotinic and 5-HT recognition sites associated with them; different antagonists may obscure a greater or lesser part of the multiple site-ion-channel complex. It will be important to discover whether any of the antagonists of 5-HT at these receptors are acting in a competitive fashion.

If the fluid mosaic membrane model (Singer and Nicolson, 1972) can be applied to the ganglion cell membrane, the ideas of Kahn (1976) about hormone receptors might be relevant. He supposes that receptors may be normally in an oligomeric state. The binding of a neurotransmitter ligand depolymerizes the receptor ligand subunit, which can then migrate in the fluid mosaic membrane until it interacts with an effector unit, in this case an ion channel. It might be the case that both ACh and 5-HT receptors can interact with the same, or some of the same, ion channels. Even if mobility of receptors within the membrane occurs, it is likely to be severely restricted to a membrane "domain," probably the subsynaptic region.

V. RECEPTOR FUNCTION AND ELECTROGENESIS

The classical mode of transmitter action, the mechanism perhaps involving several steps, is one in which a potential change is brought about by ions flowing down their electrochemical gradients. A transitory opening of ion channels follows the binding of ligand with receptor. It is, of course, not the only way in which the membrane potential or the excitability of the target cell may be altered. Possible mechanisms involve the stimulation of membrane ion pumps, which are believed to generate a potential without a detectable change in membrane resistance, and a decrease in the resting conductance of the cell membrane by the closure of ion channels. Both have been postulated for ganglion cells, and both may be linked to the activation of certain enzymes and thus will be highly dependent upon cell metabolism (Nishi, 1977). The mechanisms through which ganglionic presynaptic receptors achieve an alteration in transmitter release are largely mysterious, but they need not involve any change in resting membrane potential.

The nicotinic receptor-ion channel complex in the open conformation is permeable to Na^+ and K^+ ions. Calculations on somadendritic membrane of rabbit scg cells suggest that the Na conductance increase is about 1.8 times the K conductance increase; the reversal potential of the receptor-ion channel is about -12 mV (Dun et al., 1976). In cat scg, a lower reversal potential (-30 mV) has been reported (Skok, quoted by Nishi, 1977). There seems no compelling evidence (Triggle and Triggle, 1976) for postulating separate Na^+ and K^+ ion channels. As discussed in the previous section, 5-HT receptors appear to be associated with a very similar ion channel. Activation of ganglionic receptors appear to be associated with a very similar ion channel. Activation of ganglionic GABA receptors is also associated with an increase in conductance, the channel being specific for Cl^- ions (Adams and Brown, 1975). The ionic basis of the membrane potential changes induced by some of the other substances listed in Tables 1–3—e.g., histamine, polypeptides—is much less well established, although there is evidence that angiotensin increases Na^+ conductance in cat scg cells (Dun and Nishi, 1975).

Not only is the evidence for muscarinic receptors at the ganglion considerable; it also points unequivocally to some different mode of potential generation. First, the response displays a long latency, whether it is produced by the iontophoretic application of ACh or by intrinsic ACh as manifested in the slow epsp (Nishi, 1977). Second, there is no change in membrane resistance during the slow epsp or during the muscarinic response of rabbit cells; in frog cells membrane resistance may increase (Kobayashi and Libet, 1970). Third, the effects on the muscarinic response of displacing the membrane potential are incompatible with a conductance increase. However, the underlying mechanism is still poorly understood. Species differences and differences between cells in the same ganglion complicate the issue. Nishi, Soeda, and Koketsu (1969) found that the effect of changes in membrane potential on the slow epsp of the frog varies considerably between cells; in most cells, the membrane current associated with the slow epsp increases during depolarization and decreases during hyperpolarization, and the increase in membrane resistance during the slow epsp is found only when the cell is depolarized. Metabolic inhibitors, such as dinitrophenol, depress the slow epsp preferentially compared to the nicotinically mediated fast epsp or the slow ipsp (Kobayashi and Libet, 1968). Various hypotheses have been advanced to explain these findings; one involves a metabolically dependent electrogenic mechanism other than a Na^+ or Cl^- pump (Kobayashi and Libet, 1968) and another inactivation of the resting K^+ conductance (Weight and Votava, 1970). The observations of various authors are not in complete accord (Nishi, 1977); therefore it is not possible to decide between hypotheses at present. Either mechanism may be associated with an increase in intracellular cyclic guanosine 3',5'-monophosphate (cGMP), in which case interaction of the ligand with the muscarinic receptor will activate a membrane guanylate cyclase (Greengard and Kebabian, 1974; Weight, Petzold, and Greengard, 1974). A causal link between the increased levels of cGMP and the potential change has yet to be established.

The location of these acetylcholine effects cannot be regarded as certain. An action via muscarinic receptors is postulated, because atropine and other muscarinic blockers prevent the effects. However, these substances may not combine directly with the ACh binding site (Triggle and Triggle, 1976); further, Krnjevic (1978) has suggested that an intracellular action of ACh may reduce outward K^+ current in spinal motoneurons rather like tetraethylammonium, which blocks K^+ channels at the inner side of the membrane. The ganglionic slow epsp may be generated in this manner.

Preliminary observations (Wallis and North, unpublished) suggest that histamine may depolarize rabbit scg cells by inactivating K^+ conductance, since histamine reduces the positive after-potential, which follows the action potential and is dependent upon increased K^+ permeability, and usually increases membrane resistance.

Ganglionic α-adrenoceptors seem also associated with a potential generating mechanism that does not involve the opening of ion channels. They are generally regarded as responsible for the slow ipsp of mammalian cells (Nishi, 1977). The slow ipsp is diminished in amplitude by depolarization of the cells, enhanced by moderate hyperpolarization and not accompanied by any measurable change in membrane resistance (Kobayashi and Libet, 1968, 1970; Nishi and Koketsu, 1968). There is some disagreement about its sensitivity to ouabain and extracellular K^+ ions. Although it may be due to synaptic activation of an electrogenic Na^+ pump (Nishi, 1977), the evidence of Kobayashi and Libet (1968) and Lees and Wallis (1974) does not support this idea. Alternatively, some kind of ion pump other than the ouabain-sensitive Na-K one is involved (Kobayashi and Libet, 1968). The slow ipsp of frog cells may be induced by a fall in resting Na^+ conductance (Weight and Padjen, 1973b); but it may not be mediated by α receptors, as noted earlier. The slow ipsp of mammals may be evoked by dopamine released from interneurons and acting on α receptors (Libet, 1970; Libet & Owman, 1974; Fozard, this volume). The presence of specific dopamine receptors has not been established in most ganglia. Much, too, is unresolved concerning the underlying mechanisms. Although the activation of ganglionic dopamine receptors results in an increase in cyclic adenosine $3',5'$-monophosphate (cAMP) (Greengard and Kebabian, 1974), there is doubt whether this has anything to do with the generation of the slow ipsp. Indeed, cAMP injected directly into the cell (Gallagher and Shinnick-Gallagher, 1978) produces a depolarization rather than a hyperpolarization and a fall in membrane resistance, which seems incompatible with a role for cAMP as a second messenger in the mediation of the slow ipsp.

An action of one kind by a ligand on the ganglion cell membrane does not preclude other actions. Thus, ACh has an action via nicotinic and muscarinic receptors; 5-HT can generate hyperpolarizations in bullfrog cells when depolarizations are blocked by nicotine (Watanabe and Koketsu, 1973); and adrenaline and 5-HT enhance the activity of the electrogenic Na pump in amphibian cells in some unknown way (Shirasawa, Akasu, and Koketsu, 1976). Whether these actions are mediated by specific receptors has not been investigated.

The mechanisms associated with presynaptic receptors should now be considered. The evidence for nicotinic receptors on preganglionic terminals was reviewed by Nishi (1977). Activation of these receptors depolarizes the terminals, slightly lowers electrical threshold, attenuates action potentials invading the terminals (Ginsborg, 1971), and can occur during and after tetanic stimulation of the preganglionic fibers so that posttetanic hyperpolarization is to some extent counteracted (Nishi, 1977). There is release of stored ACh only when the terminals are exposed to relatively high concentrations of exogenous ACh; therefore it is unlikely that transmitter release occurs as a result of activation of these receptors (Collier and Katz, 1970). Presynaptic α-adrenoceptors reduce the number of quanta of ACh released by an action potential without changing the proportion of quanta released from the readily available pool (Christ and Nishi, 1971a,b). Because the electrical threshold of the terminal remains unchanged, the mechanism may not involve a change in membrane potential (Christ and Nishi, 1971b). Further, the effect is dissimilar to that produced by a reduction in extracellular Ca^{++} ions and may be dependent instead on an altered intracellular Na^+ ion concentration.

Receptors for both 5-HT (Wallis and Woodward, 1975) and GABA (Koketsu, Shoji, and Yamamoto, 1974) may be located on terminals at mammalian and amphibian ganglia, respectively. Both substances induce a depolarization of the terminals, GABA probably by a conductance increase to Cl^- ions. GABA reduces ACh release (Koketsu et al., 1974), but it is not known whether this is true of 5-HT. The significance of these and other presynaptic receptors is at the moment obscure, but it is possible that there are multiple presynaptic receptor sites parallelling the sites on the ganglion cell membrane.

VI. RECEPTORS AND GANGLIONIC FUNCTION

The evidence reviewed above indicates that receptors considered recognition sites are of many diverse kinds at ganglionic synapses. If this is accepted, what significance is to be attached to the existence of so wide a spectrum of receptors? Perhaps receptors for which there is a physiological role can be differentiated from the remainder, which are pharmacological curiosities.

This seems a distinction of doubtful value unless careful thought is given to the definition of *physiological*. Does a receptor that might be brought into use in an emergency state, but otherwise is not activated under physiological conditions, possess a physiological role or not? How easily can a physiological modulator role be established or disproved? Although nicotinic receptors are in general responsible for transmission, there is substantial evidence that some transmission is resistant to nicotinic receptor blockade (see above and Trendelenburg, 1967) and mediated through muscarinic receptors. The latter may play a physiological role in circumscribed routes through the ganglion (Henderson and Ungar, 1978). In addition, they may be more significant after some change in the nicotinic receptors or after other changes in the ganglion. Thus, muscarinic effects are most pronounced after nicotinic receptor blockade, after tetanic stimulation of preganglionic nerves, after treatment with anticholinesterases (Trendelenburg, 1967) or after activation of β-adrenoceptors (de Groat and Volle, 1966). Further, muscarinic receptors are likely to mediate changes in excitability through the slow epsp, thus serving a physiological modulator function. Most evidence suggests that they are classical muscarinic receptors situated on the outer cell membrane surface, possibly associated with guanylate cyclase. However, until binding studies can demonstrate this unequivocally, it seems wise to bear in mind Krnjevic's suggestion (1978) that such muscarinic effects may be mimicked in motoneurons by intracellular application of ACh. It remains to be seen whether ACh can pass through the ganglion cell membrane and whether atropine can significantly reduce this entry.

The variety of receptors to other substances suggests that a physiological role for each is unlikely. Some, it might be argued, could be part of a complex modulating system, perhaps only brought into play in emergency states or other special circumstances. It is reasonable to suppose that the α-adrenoceptors, either presynaptically or postsynaptically, might act as a negative feedback system diminishing sympathetic "drive" when ganglionic synapses are highly active. Catecholamines are released within the ganglion (Kosterlitz and Lees, 1972), and circulating catecholamines could reinforce their action. What has not been demonstrated is that this is of physiological significance, even during maximal sympathetic activity. Perhaps it should be regarded as a potential "brake" on sympathetic overactivity. Similarly, we argue (Wallis and Woodward, 1973) that circulating or locally released 5-HT might achieve a concentration capable of activating ganglionic receptors, especially in conditions such as carcinoid syndrome. This has yet to be demonstrated *in vivo*. In general, there seems far too great a variety of receptors for them all to be involved in a series of modulating systems. Other possibilities remain, for it is conceivable that many of the receptors are vestigial, i.e., that they are the vestiges of transmitter systems from an earlier stage of evolution. This idea receives no support, as far as I can tell, from comparative physiology. There is tentative evidence (Michelson, 1973) that, in nonvertebrate phyla such as the echinoderms, ACh receptors may be of an undifferentiated kind sensitive to both nicotinic and muscarinic blocking agents, but none to suggest that the autonomic nervous system utilised different kinds of chemical transmission during the course of evolution. Alternatively, it may be more plausible to consider that the membranes of autonomic neurons and perhaps other nerve cells possess small populations of receptors of quite different kinds, conferring on them the potentiality of responding to a wide range of biological transmitter molecules. Many of these receptors might be sites overlapping or related to the more significant nicotinic or muscarinic receptors. They would thus share some of the later steps in the process inducing the biological response, such as an ion channel or a membrane-bound enzyme. A substance interfering with one of these later steps would antagonise all ligands binding at the overlapping sites in a noncompetitive fashion. Such receptors would not be vestigial, for their presence would not need to signify that the ligand with which they reacted was, at some earlier stage of evolution, the transmitter at the synapse. Somewhat in the same vein, Brimble and Wallis (1973) suggest that the multiplicity of receptors "represented an inevitable but physiologically insignificant sensitivity of the mechanisms operating at the synapse to biologically active substances"; and Brown and Marsh (1978) suggest that GABA receptors may be "a ubiquitous component of mammalian unmyelinated nerve cell membranes."

VII. CONCLUSIONS AND THEORETICAL IMPLICATIONS

Certain tentative conclusions seem permissible, the first being that receptors should not be regarded as fixed entities in the membrane; they are likely to be labile. Thus, physical and chemical changes may be able to alter receptor conformation, surrounding binding sites or, by changing the physical state of membrane phospholipids, the surrounding membrane. Any of these events may be reflected in an apparent alteration in the receptor's characteristics. Benfey, elsewhere in this book, discusses the implications of the effects of temperature on the apparent interconversion of α- and β-adrenoceptors (Kunos and Szentivanyi, 1968). Perfusion of the cat scg with a solution low in K^+ ions produces an apparent change in the characteristics of nicotinic receptors (Perry and Reinert, 1954, 1955). The actions of ACh are no longer antagonized by pentamethonium, hexamethonium, or decamethonium. This effect is very similar to that seen in ganglia denervated 20–40 days previously, but with a normal blood supply; in denervated ganglia normality can be restored by perfusing with solutions rich in K^+ ions. Alteration of the binding sites close to the nicotinic receptor may be induced by changes in the concentration of ions in the extracellular fluid and, in the case of denervation, perhaps by other changes. Perfusion of rat ganglia with a physiological solution instead of blood results in the blocking of the effects of muscarinic agents by both hexamethonium and atropine, whereas with an intact blood supply only atropine is efficacious (Hancock and Volle, 1970). Thus, characteristics of a receptor and of adjacent binding sites may be strongly dependent upon the extracellular environment.

The changes seen on denervation may be explicable, not because the characteristics of some existing receptor have altered, but because the receptor population is gradually changed with the turnover of receptor glycoprotein. This might be the explanation for the apparent increase in the muscarinic and decrease in the nicotinic receptors that is reported by Dun et al. (1977). At the neuromuscular junction, it has been suggested that some factor related to "disuse" might be responsible for the appearance of a receptor population with different characteristics.

Second, the importance of the exact site at which antagonists act to interfere with a particular response must be stressed. Antagonists are precise tools for identification of a specific receptor only insofar as they bind to the recognition site itself. The concept of a receptor glycoprotein—which alters the conformation of an ion channel, perhaps through an intermediary—implies that antagonists can affect one of a number of sequential steps. The general scheme

$$R + L \rightleftharpoons R.L \rightarrow X \rightarrow \text{ion channel or ion pump}$$

where R is the receptor, R.L is the receptor-ligand complex, X is an intermediary molecule or ion, and arrows indicate "has an effect on," may be capable of describing the mechanisms believed to operate at the ganglionic synapse. It would include those where the intermediary induced a conformation change in an ion channel and those where X was a membrane-bound enzyme, generating cGMP, for instance, which might then activate a membrane ion pump. Sequential events and interaction of antagonists with sites (or events) other than R may account for a number of similarities noted for nonnicotinic ganglionic receptors by Trendelenburg (1967). For example, nonnicotinic stimulants typically evoke responses of long latency blocked by cocaine and by an increase in extracellular Ca^{++} ions; mutual cross-tachyphylaxis is observed with histamine, muscarinic agents, and 5-HT; and nonnicotinic stimulants are much more effective after repetitive stimulation of the preganglionic nerves. The role of Ca^{++} ions may be of particular interest. Trendelenburg (1967) concluded that Ca^{++} ions have an action very similar to cocaine and that cocaine blocks, not the receptor itself, but a pathway common to the chain of events elicited by activation of the specific receptors. Membrane Ca^{++} may also be crucial to the operation of nicotinic receptor-ion channels. Lièvremont, Tazieffe-Depierre, and their

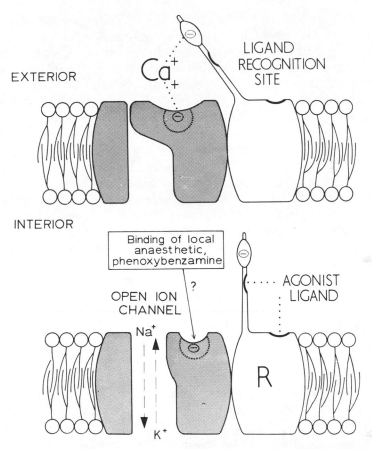

Figure 3. Diagrammatic representation of conformation change and displacement of calcium ion induced by ligand binding with consequent conformation change in an ion channel (after Lièvremont and Pascaud, 1972). R, receptor or binding site.

colleagues (for references see Triggle and Triggle, 1976) propose that depolarizing agents cause liberation of Ca^{++} ions from the endplate and that nondepolarizing antagonists prevent this mobilization. The bridging role of Ca^{++} ions is represented diagrammatically in Figure 3 in a much simplified version of their scheme (Lièvremont and Pascaud, 1972). One component of the receptor complex is an ACh-sensitive, Ca^{++}-binding lipoprotein; the critical step in the mediation of the response is displacement by the agonist, perhaps by an allosteric action, of Ca^{++} ions bound to the lipoprotein, which serve to maintain the ion channels in the closed state. Rebinding of Ca^{++} in the absence of the agonist causes the ion channels to close. Taylor (1973) also posits a central role for agonist-divalent cation exchange at endplate receptors. Local anesthetics such as cocaine can compete with Ca^{++}

for binding sites at various nicotinic receptors (Triggle and Triggle, 1976), antagonising the agonist ligand in a noncompetitive manner. This model might be applicable to both nicotinic and nonnicotinic receptors at the ganglion. Antagonism by local anaesthetics and Ca^{++}ions would be explicable in terms of their tendency to react with ion channel binding sites, so maintaining the closed conformation. It is of interest that phenoxybenzamine, which antagonises 5-HT responses at the ganglion and interferes with responses to histamine, ACh, and vasoactive peptides at various tissues (Triggle and Triggle, 1976), may bind at two distinct sites, one of which is a Ca^{++} uptake or binding site. At the ganglion, phenoxybenzamine may be effective because of an interaction with Ca^{++} binding sites. It may be that ganglionic receptors and the associated mechanisms generating the response fall into two main categories: 1) conductance-increase mechanisms; and 2) ion pump or channel closure mechanisms, possibly mediated by an enzyme. Some ligands such as ACh and 5-HT may be capable of operating through both mechanisms. Thus, the nicotinic and 5-HT receptors belong to category 1. If, as seems likely, the muscarinic, histamine, angiotensin, and perhaps a second 5-HT receptor belong to category 2, this would explain the cross-tachyphylaxis described by Trendelenburg (1967) between muscarinic agonists, histamine, angiotensin, and 5-HT.

These conclusions are purely qualitative and must at the moment remain highly tentative. It is hoped that they will lead to a more precise and quantitative approach. They serve to emphasize, I believe, that the very multiplicity of ganglionic receptors has been a spur towards a more flexible approach to our understanding of synaptic function and a stimulus to the investigation of processes that modulate transmission at the synapse. In 1967, Trendelenburg stated that "the role of acetylcholine in ganglionic transmission will have to be re-interpreted in accordance with the concept of 'multiple' receptors" (p. 52); and observations since that date have, on the whole, reinforced his conclusion. There seems little doubt that a great range of receptors, in the sense of recognition sites that can initiate some change in cell excitability, have been identified. Although they represent a potentially large range of modulatory mechanisms, it has yet to be demonstrated that activation of many of these receptors has physiological significance. At present, their importance may be as pointers to kinds of modulation that may operate at other synapses.

VIII. REFERENCES

Adams, P.R.; Brown, D.A.: Action of γ-Aminobutyric Acid (GABA) on Rat Sympathetic Ganglion Cells. Br J Pharmac 47(1973)639–640
Adams, P.R.; Brown, D.A.: Actions of γ-Aminobutyric Acid on Sympathetic Ganglion Cells. J Physiol (Lond) 250(1975)85–120

Aiken, J.W.; Reit, E.: Stimulation of the Cat Stellate Ganglion by Angiotensin. J Pharmac exp Ther 159(1968)107–114

Aiken, J.W.; Reit, E.: A Comparison of the Sensitivity to Chemical Stimuli of Adrenergic and Cholinergic Neurons in the Cat Stellate Ganglion. J Pharmac exp Ther 169(1969)211–223

Ascher, P.; Marty, A.; Nield, T.O.: The Mode of Action of Antagonists of the Excitatory Response to Acetylcholine in *Aplysia* Neurones. J Physiol (Lond) 278(1978)207–235

Beleslin, D.; Radmanov, B.; Varagic, V.: The Effect of Substance P on the Superior Cervical Ganglion of the Cat. Br J Pharmac 15(1960)10–13

Berg, D.K.; Hall, Z.W.: Fate of α-Bungarotoxin Bound to Acetylcholine Receptors of Normal and Denervated Muscle. Science, NY, 184(1974)473–474

Blackman, J.G.: Dependence on Membrane potential of the Blocking Action of Hexamethonium at a Sympathetic Ganglionic Synapse. Proc Univ Otag med Sch 48(1970)4–5

Bokri, E.; Fehér, O.; Mozsik, G.: Investigation of Denervation Supersensitivity in a Sympathetic Ganglion. Pflugers Arch ges Physiol 277(1963)347–356

Bowery, N.G.; Brown, D.A.: Depolarizing Actions of γ-Aminobutyric Acid and Related Compounds on Rat Superior Cervical Ganglion in Vitro. Br J Pharmac 50(1974)205–218

Bradley, P.B.; Briggs, I.: Further Studies on the Mode of Action of Psychotomimetic Drugs: Antagonism of the Excitatory Actions of 5-Hydroxytryptamine by Methylated Derivatives of Tryptamine. Br J Pharmac 50(1974)345–354

Brimble, M.J.; Wallis, D.I.: Histamine H_1 and H_2-Receptors at a Ganglionic Synapse. Nature 246(1973)156–158

Brimble, M.J.; Wallis, D.I.: The Role of Muscarinic Receptors in Synaptic Transmission and its Modulation in the Rabbit Superior Cervical Ganglion. Eur J Pharmac 29(1974)117–132

Brown, A.M.: Cardiac Sympathetic Adrenergic Pathways in which Transmission Is Blocked by Atropine Sulphate. J Physiol (Lond) 191(1967)271–288

Brown, A.M.: Sympathetic Ganglionic Transmission and the Cardiovascular Changes in the Defense Reaction in the Cat. Circulation Res 24(1969)843–849

Brown, D.A.: Effects of Hexamethonium and Hyoscine on the Drug-Induced Depolarization of Isolated Superior Cervical Ganglia. Br J Pharmac 26(1966a)521–537

Brown, D.A.: Electrical Responses of Cat Superior Cervical Ganglia in Vivo to Some Stimulant Drugs and Their Modification by Hexamethonium and Hyoscine. Br J Pharmac 26(1966b)538–551

Brown, D.A.; Marsh, S.: Action of GABA on Mammalian Peripheral Nerves. J Physiol (Lond) 280(1978)10

Bryant, M.D.; Polak, J.M.; Modlin, I.; Bloom, S.R.; Albuquerque, R.H.; Pearse, A.G.E.: Possible Dual Role for Vasoactive Intestinal Peptide as Gastrointestinal Hormone and Neurotransmitter Substance. Lancet i (1976)991–993

Bulbring, E.: The Action of Adrenaline on Transmission in the Superior Cervical Ganglion. J Physiol (Lond) 103(1944)55–67

Bulbring, E.; Burn, J.H.: An Action of Adrenaline on Transmission in Sympathetic Ganglia, Which May Play a Part in Shock. J Physiol (Lond) 101(1942)289–303

Bulbring, E.; Gershon, M.D.: 5-Hydroxytryptamine Participation in the Vagal Inhibitory Innervation of the Stomach. J Physiol (Lond) 192(1967)823–846

Carlstrom, D.; Bergin R.; Falkenberg, G.: Molecular Characteristics of Biogenic Monoamines and their Analogs. Quart Rev Biophys 6(1973)257–310

Chinn, C.; Hilton, J.G.: Selective Activation of Nicotinic and Muscarinic Transmission in Dog Cardiac Sympathetic Ganglia. Eur J Pharmac 40(1976)77–82

Christ, D.D.; Nishi, S.: Presynaptic Action of Epinephrine on Sympathetic Ganglia. Life Sci 8(1969)1235–1238

Christ, D.D.; Nishi, S: Site of Adrenaline Blockade in the Superior Cervical Ganglion of the Rabbit. J Physiol (Lond) 213(1971a)107–117

Christ, D.D.; Nishi, S.: Effects of Adrenaline on Nerve Terminals in the Superior Cervical Ganglion of the Rabbit. Br J Pharmac 41(1971b)331–338

Collier, B.; Katz, H.S.: The Release of Acetylcholine by Acetylcholine in the Cat's Superior Cervical Ganglion. Br J Pharmac 39(1970)428–438

Dale, H.H.; Laidlaw, P.P.: The Significance of the Suprarenal Capsules in the Action of Certain Alkaloids. J Physiol (Lond) 45(1912)1–26 de Groat, W.C.: The Actions of γ-Aminobutyric Acid and Related Amino Acids on Mammalian Autonomic Ganglia. J Pharmac exp Ther 172(1970)384-396

de Groat, W.C.; Lalley, P.M.: Interaction between Picrotoxin and 5-Hydroxytryptamine in the Superior Cervical Ganglion of the Cat. Br J Pharmac 48(1973)233-244

de Groat, W.C.; Ryall, R.W.: An Excitatory Action of 5-Hydroxytryptamine on Sympathetic Preganglionic Neurones. Exp Brain Res 3(1967)299-305

de Groat, W.C.; Saum, W.R.: Sympathetic Inhibition of the Urinary Bladder and of Pelvic Ganglionic Transmission in the Cat. J Physiol (Lond) 220(1972)297-314

de Groat, W.C.; Volle, R.L.: The Actions of the Catecholamines on Transmission in the Superior Cervical Ganglion of the Cat. J Pharmac exp Ther 154(1966a)1-13

de Groat, W.C.; Volle, R.L.: Interactions between the Catecholamines and Ganglionic Stimulating Agents in Sympathetic Ganglia. J Pharmac exp Ther 154(1966b)200-215

Dreyfus, C.F.; Sherman, D.L.; Gershon, M.D.: Uptake of Serotonin by Intrinsic Neurons of the Myenteric Plexus Grown in Organotypic Tissue Culture. Brain Res 128(1977)109-123

Dun, N.J.; Kaibara, K.; Karczmar, A.G.: Dopamine and Adenosine 3',5'-Monophosphate Responses of Single Mammalian Sympathetic Neurons. Science, NY, 197(1977)778-780

Dun, N.; Nishi, S.: Effects of Dopamine on the Superior Cervical Ganglion of the Rabbit. J Physiol (Lond) 239(1974)155-164

Dun, N.; Nishi, S.: Action of Angiotensin II on Mammalian Ganglion Cells. Pharmacologist 17(1975)223

Dun, N.; Nishi, S.; Karczmar, A.G.: Alteration in Nicotinic and Muscarinic Responses of Rabbit Superior Cervical Ganglion Cells after Chronic Preganglionic Denervation. Neuropharmacology 15(1976)211-218

Eccles, R.M.; Libet, B.: Origin and Blockade of the synaptic Responses of Curarized Sympathetic Ganglia. J Physiol (Lond) 199(1961)189-203

Elde, R.; Hökfelt, T.; Johansson, O.; Terenius, L.: Immunohistochemical Studies Using Antibodies to Leucine—Enkephalin: Initial Observations on the Nervous System of the Rat. Neuroscience 1 (1976)349-351

Flacke, W.; Gillis, R.A.: Impulse transmission via Nicotinic and Muscarinic Pathways in the Stellate Ganglia of the Dog. J Pharmac exp Ther 163(1968)266-276

Fozard, J.R.; Mobarok Ali, A.T.M.: Evidence for Tryptamine Receptors on Cardiac Sympathetic Nerves. Br J Pharmac 58(1976)276-277P

Fozard, J.R.; Mobarok Ali, A.T.M.: Dual Mechanism of the Stimulant Action of N,N-Dimethyl-5-Hydroxytryptamine(Bufotenine) on Cardiac Sympathetic Nerves. Eur J Pharmac 49(1978)25-30

Freyburger, W.A.; Gruhzit, C.C.; Rennick, B.R.; Moe, G.K.: Action of Tetraethylammonium on Pressure Response to Asphyxia. Amer J Physiol 163(1950)554-560

Gaddum, J.H.; Picarelli, Z.P.: Two Kinds of Tryptamine Receptor. Br J Pharmac 12(1957)323-328

Gallagher, J.P.; Shinnick-Gallagher, P.: Electrophysiological Effects of Nucleotides Injected Intracellularly into Rat Sympathetic Ganglion Cells. In.: Iontophoresis and Transmitter Mechanisms in the Mammalian Central Nervous System, pp. 152-154, ed. by R.W. Ryall and J.S. Kelly. Elsevier/North-Holland, Amsterdam-New York, 1978

Gershenfeld, H.M.; Paupardin-Tritsch, D.: On the Transmitter Function of 5-Hydroxytryptamine at Excitatory and Inhibitory Monosynaptic Junctions. J Physiol (Lond) 243(1974)457-481

Gershon, M.D.; Dreyfus, C.F.; Pickel, V.M.; Joh, T.H.; Reis, D.J.: Serotonergic Neurons in the Peripheral Nervous System: Identification in Gut by Immunohistochemical Localization of Tryptophan Hydroxylase. Proc Nat Acad Sci U.S.A. 74(1977)3086-3089

Gertner, S.B.; Kohn, R.: Effect of Histamine on Ganglionic Transmission. Br J Pharmac 14(1959)179-182

Ginsborg, B.L.: On the Presynaptic Acetylcholine Receptors in Sympathetic Ganglia of the Frog. J Physiol (Lond) 216(1971)237-246

Green, A.R.; Youdim, M.B.H.; Grahame-Smith, D.G.: Quipazine: Its Effects on Rat Brain, 5-Hydroxytryptamine Metabolism, Monoamine Oxidase Activity and Behaviour. Neuropharmacology 15(1976)173-179

Greengard, P.; Kebabian, J.W.: Role of Cyclic AMP in Synaptic Transmission in the Mammalian Peripheral Nervous System. Fed Proc 33(1974)1059-1067

Gyermek, L.: Action of 5-Hydroxytryptamine on the Urinary Bladder of the Dog. Arch int Pharmacodyn 87(1962)137–144

Gyermek, L.: Action of Guanidine Derivatives on Autonomic Ganglia. Arch int Pharmacodyn 150(1964)570–581

Gyermek, L.; Bindler, E.: Blockade of the Ganglionic Stimulant Action of 5-Hydroxytryptamine. J Pharmac exp Ther 135(1962a)344–348

Gyermek, L.; Bindler, E.: Action of Indole Alkylamines and Amidines on the Inferior Mesenteric Ganglion of the Cat. J Pharmac exp Ther 138(1962b)159–164

Haefely, W.: Effects of Catecholamines in the Cat Superior Cervical Ganglion and Their Postulated Role as Physiological Modulators of Ganglionic Transmission. Progr in Brain Res 31(1969)61–72

Haefely, W.: Some Actions of Bradykinin and Related Peptides on Autonomic Ganglion Cells. In: Bradykinin and Related Kinins, pp. 591–599. Plenum, New York, 1970

Haefely, W.: Electrophysiology of the Adrenergic Neuron. In: Catecholamines. Handbook of Experimental Pharmacology, Vol. 23, p. 661–725, ed. by H. Blaschko & E. Muscholl. Springer, Berlin-Heidelberg-New York, 1972

Haefely, W.: The Effects of 5-Hydroxytryptamine and Some Related Compounds on the Cat Superior Cervical Ganglion in Situ. Naunyn-Schmiedebergs Arch Pharmak 281 (1974)145–165

Haefely, W.; Hürlimann, A.; Thoenen, H.: Effects of Bradykinin and Angiotensin on Ganglionic Transmission. Biochem Pharmac 14(1965)1393

Haefely, W.; Hürliman, A.; Thoenen, H.: The Effect of Bradykinin and angiotensin on Ganglionic Transmission. In: Hypotensive Polypeptides, pp. 314–327, ed. by E.G. Erdös, N. Back, F. Sicuteri & A.F. Wilde. Springer, Berlin-Heidelberg-New York, 1966

Hancock, J.C.; Volle, R.L.: Cholinoceptive Sites in Rat Sympathetic Ganglia. Arch int Pharmacodyn 184(1970)111–120

Harris, A.J.; Kuffler, S.W.; Dennis, M.J.: Differential Chemosensitivity of Synaptic and Extrasynaptic Areas on the Neuronal Surface Membrane in Parasympathetic Neurons of the Frog, Tested by Microapplication of Acetylcholine. Proc Roy Soc Lond B 177(1971)541–553

Henderson, C.G.; Ungar, A.: Effect of Cholinergic Antagonists on Sympathetic Ganglionic Transmission of Vasomotor Reflexes from the Carotid Baroreceptors and Chemoreceptors of the Dog. J Physiol (Lond) 277(1978)379–385

Hertzler, E.C.: 5-Hydroxytryptamine and Transmission in Sympathetic Ganglia. Br J Pharmac 17(1961)406–413

Hilton, J.G.; Steinberg, M.: Effects of Ganglion and Parasympathetic Blocking Drugs upon the Pressor Response Elicited by Elevation of the Intracranial Fluid Pressure. J Pharmac exp. Ther 153(1966)285–291

Hirst, G.D.; Silinsky, E.M.: Some Effects of 5-Hydroxytryptamine, Dopamine and Noradrenaline on Neurones in the Submucous Plesus of Guinea-Pig Small Intestine. J Physiol (Lond) 251(1975)817–832

Hökfelt, T.; Efendic, S.; Hellerstrom, C.; Johansson, O.; Luft, R.; Arimura, A.: Cellular Localization of Somatostatin in endocrine-Like Cells and Neurons of the Rat with Special Reference to A_1 Cells of the Pancreatic Islets and to the Hypothalamus. Acta endocr Copnh Suppl 200(1975)5–41

Hökfelt, T.; Elfvin, L.-G.; Schultzberg, M.; Elde, R.; Goldstein, M.; Luft, R.: Occurrence of Somatostatin-Like Immuno-Reactivity in Some Peripheral Sympathetic Noradrenergic Neurones. Proc Matn Acad Sci USA 74(1977)3587–3591

Hökfelt, T.; Elfvin, L.-G.; Schultzberg, M.; Fuxe, K.; Said, S.I.; Mutt, V.; Goldstein, M.: Immunohistochemical Evidence of Vasoactive Intestinal Polypeptide-Containing Neurons and Nerve Fibres in Sympathetic Ganglia. Neuroscience 2(1977)885–896

Hökfelt, T.; Elfvin, L.-G.; Schultzberg, M.; Goldstein, M.; Nilsson, G.: On the Occurrence of Substance P-Containing Fibres in Sympathetic Ganglia. Immunohistochemical Evidence. Brain Res 132(1977)29–41

Hökfelt, T.; Johansson, O.; Kellerth, J-O.; Ljungdahl, A.; Nilsson, G.; Nygårds, A.; Pernow, B.: Immunohistochemical Distribution of Substance P. In: Substance P. Nobel Symposium, Vol. 37, ed. by U.S. Von Euler & B. Pernow. Raven, New York, 1977

Iorio, L.C.; McIsaac, R.J.: Comparison of the Stimulating Effects of Nicotine, Pilocarpine and Histamine on the Superior Cervical Ganglion of the Cat. J Pharmac exp Ther 151(1966)430–437

Jaramillo, J.; Volle, R.L.: Ganglionic Blockade by Muscarine, Oxotremorine and AHR-602. J Pharmac exp Ther 158(1967)80–88

Jéquier, E.: Effet de la Sérotonine sur la Transmission Synaptique dans le Ganglion Sympathique Cervical Isolé du Rat. Helv physiol pharmac Acta 23(1965)163–179

Kahn, C.R.: Membrane Receptors for Hormones and Neurotransmitters. J Cell Biol 70(1976)261–286

Khairallah, P.A.; Page, I.H.: Mechanisms of Action of Angiotensin and Bradykinin on Smooth Muscle in Situ. Am J Physiol 200(1961)51–54

Kobayashi, H.; Libet, B.: Generation of Slow Postsynaptic Potentials without Increases in Ionic Conductance. Proc Nat Acad Sci USA 60(1968)1304–1311

Kobayashi, H.; Libet, B.: Actions of Noradrenaline and Acetylcholine in Sympathetic Ganglion Cells. J Physiol (Lond) 208(1970)353–372

Koketsu, K.; Nishi, S.; Soeda, H.: Acetylcholine Potential of Sympathetic Ganglion Cell Membrane. Life Sci 7(1968)741–749

Koketsu, K.; Shoji, T.; Yamamoto, K.: Effects of GABA on Presynaptic Nerve Terminals in Bullfrog (Rana catesbiana) Sympathetic Ganglia. Experientia 30(1974)382–383

Konzett, H.: Sympathomimetica und Sympathicolytica am Isoliert Durchströmten Ganglion Cervicale Superius der Katze. Helv Physiol Pharmac Acta 8(1950)245–258

Konzett, H.: The Effect of Histamine on an Isolated Sympathetic Ganglion. J Mt Sinai Hosp 19(1952)149–153

Koppanyi, T.: Studies on the Synergism Antagonism of Drugs. I. The Non-Parasympathetic Antagonism between Atropine and the Miotic Alkaloids. J Pharmac exp Ther 46(1932)395–405

Kosterlitz, H.W.; Lees, G.M.: Interrelationship between Adrenergic and Cholinergic Mechanisms. In: Catecholamines. Handbook of Experimental Pharmacology, Vol. 23, pp. 762–812, ed. by H. Blaschko & E. Muscholl. Springer, Berlin-Heidelberg-New York, 1972

Kosterlitz, H.W.; Lees, G.M.; Wallis, D.I.: Resting and Action Potentials recorded by the Sucrose-Gap Method in the Superior Cervical Ganglion of the Rabbit. J Physiol (Lond) 195(1968)39–53

Krnjevic, K.: Intracellular Actions of a Transmitter. In: Iontophoresis and Transmitter Mechanisms in the Mammalian Central Nervous System, pp. 155–157, ed. by R.W. Ryall and J.S. Kelly. Elsevier/North-Holland, Amsterdam-New York, 1978

Kuffler, S.W.; Dennis, M.J.; Harris, A.J.: The Development of Chemosensitivity in Extrasynaptic Areas of the Neuronal Surface after Denervation of Parasympathetic Ganglion Cells in the Heart of the Frog. Proc Roy Soc B 177(1971)555–563

Kunos, G.; Szentivanyi, M.: Evidence Favouring the Existence of a Single Adrenergic Receptor. Nature 217(1968)1077–78

Lundberg, A.: Adrenaline and transmission in the Sympathetic Ganglion of the Cat. Acta Physiol Scand 26(1952)252–263

Lees, G.M.; Wallis, D.I.: Hyperpolarization of Rabbit Superior Cervical Ganglion Cells Due to Activity of an Electrogenic Sodium Pump. Br J Pharmac 50(1974)79–93

Lewis, G.P.; Reit, E.: The Action of Angiotensin and Bradykinin on the Superior Cervical Ganglion of the Cat. J Physiol (Lond) 179(1965)538–553

Lewis, G.P.; Reit, E.: Further Studies on the Actions of Peptides on the Superior Cervical Ganglion and Suprarenal Medulla. Br J Pharmac 26(1966)444–460

Libet, B.: SLow Synaptic Responses and Excitatory Changes in Sympathetic Ganglia. J Physiol (Lond) 174(1964)1–25

Libet, B.: Long Latent Periods and Further Analysis of Slow Synaptic Responses in Sympathetic Ganglia. J Neurophysiol 30(1967)494–514

Libet, B.: Generation of Slow Inhibitory and Excitatory Postsynaptic Potentials. Fed Proc 29(1970)1945–1956

Libet, B.: The SIF Cell as a Functional Dopamine-Releasing Interneuron in the Rabbit Superior cervical Ganglion. In: SIF Cells: Structure and Function of the Small Intensely Fluorescent Sympathetic Cells, pp. 163–177, ed. by O. Eranko, Fogarty Int. Centre Proc. No. 30, US Govt Printing Office, Washington, D.C., 1976

Libet, B.; Kobayashi, H.: Generation of Adrenergic and Cholinergic Potentials in Sympathetic Ganglion Cells. Science, NY, 164(1969)1530–1532

Libet, B.; Kobayashi, H.; Tanaka, T.: Synaptic Coupling into the Production and Storage of a Neuronal Memory Trace. Nature 258(1975)155–157

Libet, B.; Owman, Ch.: Concomitant Changes in Formaldehyde-Induced Fluorescence of Dopamine Interneurones and in Slow Inhibitory Postsynaptic Potentials of the Rabbit Superior Cervical Ganglion, Induced by Stimulation of the Preganglionic Nerve or by a Muscarinic Agent. J Physiol (Lond) 237(1974)635–662

Libet, B.; Tosaka, T.: Slow Postsynaptic Potentials Recorded Intracellularly in Sympathetic Ganglia. Fed Proc 25(1966)270

Libet, B.; Tosaka, T.: Slow Inhibitory and Excitatory Postsynaptic Responses in Single Cells of Mammalian Sympathetic Ganglia. J Neurophysiol 32(1969)43–50

Libet, B.; Tosaka, T.: Dopamine as a Synaptic Transmitter and Modulator in Sympathetic Ganglia: a Different Mode of Synaptic Action. Proc Nat Acad Sci USA 67(1970)667–673

Lièvremont, M.; Pascaud, M.: Étude de la Sensibilité Cholinergique à la jonction Neuromusculaire, Définition et Rôle Opérant Calcique. CR Acad Sci Ser D 274(1972)1345–1348

Machova, J.; Boska, D.: A Study of the Action of Angiotension on the Superior Cervical Ganglion in Comparison with Other Ganglion Stimulating Agents. Eur J Pharmac 1(1967)233–239

Machova, J.; Boska, D.: The Effect of 5-Hydroxytryptamine, Dimethylphenylpiperazinium and Acetylcholine on Transmission and Surface Potential in the Cat Sympathetic Ganglion. Eur J Pharmac 7(1969)152–158

Malméjac, J.: Action of Adrenaline on Synaptic Transmission and on Adrenal Medullary Secretion. J Physiol (Lond) 130(1955)497–512

Marrazzi, A.S.: Arenergic Inhibition of a Sympathetic Synapse. Am J Physiol 127 (1939)738–744

Matthews, M.R.; Raisman, G.: Two Cell Types in the Superior Cervical Ganglion of the Rat. J Anat (Lond) 103(1968)397–398

Matthews, R.J.: The Effect of Epineprine Levarterenol and dl-Isoproterenol on transmission in the Superior Cervical ganglion of the Cat. J Pharmac exp Ther 116(1956)433–443

Matthews, R.J.; Roberts, B.J.: The Effect of Gamma-Aminobutyric Acid on Synaptic Transmission in Autonomic Ganglia. J Pharmac exp Ther 132(1961)19–22

Michelson, M.J.: In: Comparative Pharmacology, Vol. I, ed. by M. J. Michelson, Pergamon, Oxford, 1973

Nilsson, G.; Larsson, L.I.; Håkansson, R.; Brodin, E.; Sundler, F.; Pernow, B.: Localization of Substance P-like Immunoreactivity on Mouse Gut. Histochemistry 43(1975)97–99

Nishi, S.: Cellular Pharmacology of Ganglionic transmission. In: Advances in general and Cellular Pharmacology, Vol. 1, p. 179–245, ed. by T. Narahashi and C.P. Bianchi. Plenum, New York-London, 1977

Nishi, S.; Koketsu, K.: Underlying Mechanisms of Ganglionic Slow IPSP and Post-Tetanic Hyperpolarization of Pre- and Postganglionic Elements. Proc Int Union Physiol Sci VII(1968)321

Nishi, S.; Soeda, H.; Koketsu, K.: Unusual Nature of Ganglionic Slow EPSP Studied by a Voltage Clamp Method. Life Sci 8(1969)33–42

North, R.A.; Wallis, D.I.: Intracellular Recording of the Effects of 5-hydroxytryptamine on Rabbit Superior Cervical Ganglion Cells. Br J Pharmac 59(1977)505–506P.

Page, I.H.; McCubbin, J.W.: The Variable Arterial Pressure Response to Serotonin in Laboratory Animals and Man. Circulat Res 1(1953)354–362

Panisset, J-C.: Effect of Angiotensin on the release of Acetylcholine from Preganglionic and Postganglionic Nerve Endings. Can J Physiol Pharm 45(1967)313–317

Pappano, A.J.; Volle, R.L.: The Reversal by Atropine of Ganglionic Blockade Produced by Acetylcholine. Life Sci 12(1962)677–682

Paton, W.D.M.; Thompson, J.W.: The Mechanism of Action of Adrenaline on the superior Cervical Ganglion of the Cat. Proc XIX Int Physiol Congr Montreal (1953)664–665

Pearse, A.G.E.; Polak, J.: Immunocytochemical localization of Substance P in Mammalian Intestine. Histochemistry 41(1975)373–375

Perry, W.L.M.; Reinert, H.: The effects of Preganglionic Denervation on the Reactions of Ganglion Cells. J Physiol (Lond) 126(1954)101–115

Perry, W.L.M.; Reinert, H.: On the Metabolism of Normal and Denervated Sympathetic Ganglion Cells. J Physiol (Lond) 130(1955)156–166

Robertson, P.A.: An Antagonism of 5-Hydroxytryptamine by Atropine. J Physiol (Lond) 121(1953)54–55P

Robertson, P.A.: Potentiation of HT by the True Cholinesterase Inhibitor 284 C51. J Physiol (Lond) 125(1954)37–38P

Saum, W.R.; de Groat, W.C.: The Action of 5-Hydroxytryptamine on the Urinary Bladder and on vesical Autonomic Ganglia in the Cat. J Pharmac exp Ther 185(1973)70–83

Schimke, R.T.: Turnover of Membrane Proteins in Animal Cells. In: Methods in Membrane Biology, Vol. III, pp. 201–236, ed. by E.D. Korn. Plenum, New York, 1975

Shirasawa, Y.; Akasu, T.; Koketsu, K.: effects of Adrenaline and Serotonin on the Pump Potential of Sympathetic Ganglion Cell Membrane in Bullfrogs. J Physiol Soc Japan 38(1976)270–272

Siegrist, G.; Dolivo, M.; Dunant, Y.; Foroglou-Kerameus, C.; Ribaupierre, Fr. de Rouiller, Ch.: Ultrastructure and Function of the Chromaffin Cells in the Superior Cervical Ganglion of the Rat. J Ultrastruct Res 25(1968)381–407

Singer, S.J.; Nicolson, G.L.: The Fluid Mosaic Model of the Structure of Cell Membranes. Science, NY 175(1972)720–731

Smith, J.C.: Pharmacologic Interactions with 4-(m-Chlorophenyl Carbamoyloxy)-2-butynyltrimethylammonium Chloride, a Sympathetic Ganglion Stimulant. J Pharmac exp Ther 153(1966)276–284

Stone, T.W.: Pharmacological Receptors and the Control of Cell Function. Arch. int. Pharmacodyn. 210(1974)365–373

Takeshige, C.; Pappano, A.J.; de Groat, W.C.; Volle, R.L.: Ganglionic Blockade Produced in Sympathetic Ganglia by Cholinomimetic Drugs. J Pharmac exp Ther 141(1963)333–342

Takeshige, C.; Volle, R.L.: Cholinoceptive Sites in Denervated Sympathetic Ganglia. J Pharmac exp Ther 141(1963)206–213

Takeshige, C.; Volle, R.L.: Similarities in the Ganglionic Actions of Calcium Ions and Atropine. J Pharmac exp Ther 145(1964)173–180

Taylor, D.B.: The Role of Inorganic Ions in Ion Exchange Processes at the Cholinergic Receptor of Voluntary Muscle. J Pharmac exp Ther 186(1973)537–551

Trendelenburg, U.: The Action of Histamine and Pilocarpine on the Superior Cervical Ganglia and the Adrenal Glands of the Cat. Br J Pharmac 9(1954)481–487

Trendelenburg, U.: The Potentiation of Ganglionic Transmission by Histamine and Pilocarpine. J Physiol (Lond) 129(1955)337–351

Trendelenburg, U.: The Action of 5-Hydroxytryptamine on the Nictitating Membrane and on the Superior Cervical Ganglion of the Cat. Br J Pharmac 11(1956a)74–80

Trendelenburg, U.: Modification of Ganglionic transmission through the Superior Cervical Ganglion of the Cat. J Physiol (Lond) 132(1956b)529–541

Trendelenburg, U.: The Action of Histamine, Pilocarpine and 5-Hydroxytryptamine on Transmission through the Superior Cervical Ganglion. J Physiol (Lond) 135(1957)66–72

Trendelenburg, U.: Observations on the Ganglion-Stimulating Action of Angiotensin and Bradykinin. J Pharmac exp Ther 154(1966)418–425

Trendelenburg, U.: Some Aspects of the Pharmacology of Autonomic Ganglion Cells. Ergebn Physiol 59(1967)1–85

Triggle, D.J.; Triggle, C.R.: Chemical Pharmacology of the Synapse. Academic, London-New York-San Francisco, 1976

Vanov, S.: Responses of the Rat Urinary Bladder in Situ to Drugs and to Nerve Stimulation. Br J Pharmac 24(1965)591–600

Volle, R.L.: Ganglionic transmission. Ann. Rev. Pharmacol. 9(1969)135–146

Wallis, D.I.; North, R.A.: Responses of Sympathetic Ganglion Cells of the Rabbit to 5-Hydroxytryptamine Recorded with Intracellular Electrodes. In: Iontophoresis and Transmitter Mechanisms in the Mammalian Central Nervous System, pp. 438–440, ed. by R.W. Ryall and J.S. Kelly. Elsevier/North-Holland, Amsterdam-New York, 1978a

Wallis, D.I.; North, R.A.: Synaptic Input to Cells of the Rabbit Superior Cervical Ganglion. Pflugers Archiv. 374(1978b)145–152

Wallis, D.I.; North, R.A.: The Action of 5-Hydroxytryptamine on Single Neurones of the Rabbit Superior Cervical Ganglion. Neuropharmacology 17(1978c)1023–1028

Wallis, D.I.; Williams, C.; Wali, F.A.: The Effect of 5-Hydroxytryptamine and Hexamethonium on Post-Train Facilitation in the Superior Cervical Ganglion. Eur J Pharmac 52(1978)17–25

Wallis, D.I.; Woodward, B.: The Depolarizing Action of 5-Hydroxytryptamine on Sympathetic Ganglion Cells. Br J Pharmac 49(1973)168P

Wallis, D.I.; Woodward, B.: The Facilitatory Actions of 5-Hydroxytryptamine and Bradykinin in the Superior Cervical Ganglion of the Rabbit. Br J Pharmac 51(1974)521–531

Wallis, D.I.; Woodward, B.: Membrane Potential changes Induced by 5-Hydroxytryptamine in the Rabbit Superior Cervical Ganglion. Br J Pharmac 55(1975)199–212

Watanabe, S.; Koketsu, K.: 5-HT Hyperpolarization of Bullfrog Sympathetic Ganglion Cell Membrane. Experientia 29(1973)1370–1372

Watson, P.J.; Drug Receptor Sites in the Isolated Superior Cervical Ganglion of the Rat. Eur J Pharmac 12(1970)183–193

Weight, F.F.; Padjen, A.: Acetylcholine and Slow Synaptic Inhibition in Frog Sympathetic Ganglion Cells. Brain Res 55(1973a)225–228

Weight, F.F.; Padjen, A.: Slow Synaptic Inhibition: Evidence for Synaptic Inactivation of Sodium Conductance in Sympathetic Ganglion Cells. Brain Res 55 (1973b)219–224

Weight, F.F.; Petzold, G.; Greengard, P.: Guanosine 3′,5′-Monophosphate in Sympathetic Ganglia: Increase Associated with Synaptic Transmission. Science, NY 186(1974)942–944

Weight, F.F.; Votava, J.: Slow Synaptic Excitation of sympathetic Ganglion Cells: Evidence for Synaptic Inactivation of Potassium Conductance. Science, NY 170(1970)755–758

Willems, J.L.: Dopamine-Induced Inhibition of Synaptic Transmission in Lumbar Paravertebral Ganglia of the Dog. Nauyn-Schmeideberg's Arch Pharmacol 279(1973)115–126

Williams, T.H.: Electronmicroscopic Evidence for an Autonomic Interneurone. Nature 214(1967)309–310

Williams, T.H.; Palay, S.L.: Ultrastructure of the Small Neurons in the Superior Cervical Ganglion. Brain Res 15(1969)17–34

The Mammalian Enteric Nervous System: A Third Autonomic Division

Michael D. Gershon, Cheryl F. Dreyfus, and Taube P. Rothman

In most textbooks of anatomy or physiology, the enteric nervous system is treated more or less as a component of the parasympathetic division of the autonomic nervous system (ANS). The enteric ganglia are presented as relay stations in the vagal or sacral pathways that mediate central nervous system (CNS) control of the gut. Nevertheless, as will be discussed more extensively below, this view has not always prevailed. Langley (1921), to whom we are indebted for much of our concept of the ANS, actually argued that the ANS ought to be divided not simply into the two divisions—sympathetic and parasympathetic—routinely recognized today, but into three divisions, with the enteric nervous system as the third division. He felt that it was very likely that many of the enteric ganglion cells did not even receive an input from the CNS and therefore could not serve as simple CNS-to-gut relays.

It is very difficult and probably also unprofitable to trace backward in the literature to try to determine why Langley's position passed from the commonly held view. During a period when interest in the enteric nervous system was fairly quiescent (except among pharmacologists, who have long recognized the value and convenience of studying the effect of neurally active drugs on the gut), exactly how the system was classified probably made rather little difference. However, recently there has been a renaissance of scientific interest in the enteric nervous system, and it is becoming apparent that the view of this system that appears in most texts is not only inadequate but probably detrimental to developing an understanding of neural control of the gut. It now appears that the enteric nervous system contains a previously unsuspected diversity of intrinsic neuronal types and has many structural and chemical features in common with the CNS. In fact, the more the enteric nervous system has been found to resemble the CNS, the less it seems to have in common with other regions of the peripheral nervous system.

In this review we will advance the thesis that Langley's classification of the enteric nervous system, as a third division of the ANS, should be retained or reinstated. In doing so, we will not try to summarize all the work done on the system since Langley. Instead, we will concentrate on the evidence for enteric neuronal diversity, the means of recognizing the various neurons, and particularly on the implications and potential of this neuronal diversity for future research in developmental neurobiology.

I. THE INNERVATION OF THE MAMMALIAN GASTROINTESTINAL TRACT

The general outline of the innervation of the gastrointestinal tract has been extensively reviewed (Schofield, 1968) and therefore will be described only briefly here. A section of the gut reveals two intrinsic neural plexuses; the submucosal (Meissner's), and the myenteric (Auerbach's). The submucosal plexus consists of small ganglia and their connectives and appears to be organized segmentally (Hirst and McKirdy, 1975). Conduction over long distances proximodistally apparently does not occur. The myenteric plexus is situated between the outer longitudinal and the inner circular smooth-muscle layers of the muscularis externa. This plexus consists of relatively large groups of intrinsic ganglion cells connected by bundles of axons, and it is organized to permit conduction over relatively long distances along the length of the gut (Yokoyama, Ozaki, and Kajitsuka, 1977). The two enteric plexuses are interconnected (Baumgarten, Holstein, and Owman, 1970; Gabella, 1972).

Most descriptions of the ANS include two separate preganglionic outflows from the central nervous system (CNS) to the gut, discussed in the following paragraphs.

A. Parasympathetic and Sympathetic Innervations

1. Parasympathetic innervation Preganglionic parasympathetic fibers from the tenth cranial or the sacral nerves travel in the vagus or pelvic nerves, respectively, and synapse on postganglionic neurons within the enteric nervous system. Although traditionally this innervation has been considered excitatory, recent observations indicate that some of the preganglionic fibers synapse with intrinsic neurons that inhibit the motility of the gut (Martinson and Muren, 1963; Campbell, 1970; Gabella, 1972). The excitatory postganglionic neurons are at least predominantly cholinergic (Campbell, 1970).

2. **Sympathetic innervation** The sympathetic preganglionic outflow originates from the intermediolateral cell column of all the thoracic and the first three lumbar segments of the spinal cord. Cell bodies of the postganglionic sympathetic neurons are situated extrinsic to the gut, in the prevertebral ganglia. These neurons are adrenergic. With only one known exception in mammals, the proximal colon of the guinea pig (Costa and Gabella, 1971), all the axons of adrenergic axons reach the gut from prevertebral ganglia in perivascular nerves, and there are no intrinsic adrenergic perikarya. The overwhelming majority of perivascular axons to the gut are adrenergic, although cholinergic fibers in this sympathetic supply have been described (Drakontides and Gershon, 1972). Since cholinergic axons develop earlier in ontogeny than do adrenergic axons (Gershon and Thompson, 1973), their effects dominate when perivascular nerves are stimulated in newborn animals; cholinergic nerves excite and adrenergic relax gastrointestinal smooth muscle (Campbell, 1970).

B. The Intrinsic Enteric Nervous System

As noted above, this traditional description of the ANS probably does not completely describe the enteric innervation. In his early reviews of the ANS, Langley (1921) divided the system into three divisions, giving separate status to the vast discrepancy between the very large number of ganglion cells in the enteric plexuses and the very much smaller number of fibers in the vagus nerve as that nerve passed through the diaphragm. There are fewer than 20,000 vagal fibers and over 6,000,000 ganglion cells (Irwin, 1931). Langley thus doubted that many of those ganglion cells in the gut could receive a vagal input or were connected to the CNS at all. Thus, although sympathetic and parasympathetic fibers clearly reached the gut, it was not reasonable to describe the bulk of the enteric innervation in terms of the craniosacral or thoracolumbar outflows that define the parasympathetic and sympathetic divisions of the ANS.

Since Langley's work, considerable additional evidence has accumulated that indicates the separateness of the enteric innervation. Trendelenburg showed, as early as 1917, that neurally mediated reflex activity could be elicited by increasing mucosal pressure *in vitro* (Trendelenburg, 1917). This reflex, consisting of a descending wave of oral excitation and anal relaxation analogous to the activity described for the gut *in vivo* by Bayliss and Starling (1899, 1900, 1901), implies the existence of a complete reflex pathway within the intrinsic components of the enteric nervous system. That is, the gut must have within it sensory receptors, primary afferent neurons (distinct from dorsal-root or cranial-nerve ganglia that are not present in *in vitro* preparations), and integrative neurons as well as motor neurons. Trendelenburg's work has been confirmed many times since 1917, and considerable work has been done on the analysis of the neural pathways involved (Bulbring, Lin, and Schofield, 1958; Kosterlitz and Lees, 1964).

1. **Distinguishing features of the enteric nervous system** Certain morphological features of the intrinsic enteric innervation also distinguish the gut from other peripheral organs. Unlike other peripheral organs, but like the CNS, the gut exhibits the following characteristics:

a. There are pseudounipolar and bipolar sensory neurons located in the submucosal plexus (Schofield, 1968). These neurons respond to pressure or distention on the mucosal surface (Bulbring et al., 1958). Elsewhere in the nervous system, sensory neurons of this type are found only in dorsal-root or cranial-nerve ganglia.

b. Unlike other peripheral nerves or ganglia, neurons in the myenteric plexus are not supported by endoneurial, perineurial, or epineurial connective tissue sheaths, but receive internal support from glial elements resembling the astroglia of the CNS. There is no collagen within the myenteric plexus (Gabella, 1971, 1972; Cook and Burnstock, 1976a, b).

c. There is little extracellular space in the myenteric plexus. In this respect, its appearance is similar to that of the CNS (Gabella, 1972).

d. A blood–myenteric plexus barrier to small protein molecules, similar to the blood-brain barrier of the CNS, has been demonstrated. Tight junctions between the endothelial cells of capillaries that supply neuronal elements in the plexus, which itself is devoid of capillaries, compose this barrier (Gershon and Bursztajn, 1978). Perivascular macrophages back up the endothelial barrier.

e. Within the enteric nervous system there exists a multiplicity of transmitter substances. In addition to acetylcholine (ACh) and norepinephrine (NE), there is evidence that 5-HT (see below) and possibly adenosine triphosphate (ATP) are transmitters there (Burnstock, 1972). Prostaglandins (Dajani, Roge, and Bertermann, 1975), somatostatin (Hokfelt et al., 1975), substance P (Hokfelt et al., 1974; Hokfelt et al., 1977b), vasoactive intestinal peptide (VIP) (Bryant et al., 1976; Fuxe et al., 1977; Larsson, 1977; Schultzberg et al., 1978) and enkephalin (Elde et al., 1976; Schultzberg et al., 1978) may also be enteric neurotransmitters or modulators of neurotransmission; and 5-HT and these peptides have all been found in intrinsic enteric neurons (Schultzberg et al., 1978).

Therefore, the enteric nervous system represents a self-contained unit that should be thought of today as Langley did originally—as a separate division of the ANS. In several ways, particularly with its multiplicity of neuronal types, the enteric nervous system resembles the CNS. However, the enteric nervous system is far less complicated than the CNS; and, unlike the CNS, for purposes of investigation the gut can be removed and isolated *in vitro*. The advantages of such a system are obvious. In addition to biochemical, electrophysiological, pharmacological, and morphological studies, small segments of intestinal muscle with adherent myenteric and/or submucosal plexus, or segments of fetal intestine, can be grown in orga-notypic tissue culture (Rikimaru, 1971; Cook and Peterson, 1974; Dreyfus, Bornstein, and Gershon, 1977a; Dreyfus, Sherman, and Gershon, 1977b; Schultzberg et al., 1978). Under these conditions, the extrinsic innervation degenerates, and intrinsic neurons can be examined separately.

2. **Neurotransmitters in the enteric nervous system**

  a. *Acetylcholine* (**ACh**) ACh is the neurotransmitter of preganglionic parasympathetic vagal and sacral fibers and also of the postganglionic neurons located in the myenteric plexus (Dale, 1937a, b). Therefore, cholinergic axons within the myenteric plexus may be of either intrinsic or extrinsic origin. Specific drugs can be used either to block (e.g., hexametho-nium) or excite (e.g., DMPP or nicotine) the nicotinic ganglionic receptors for acetylcholine. Different drugs antagonize (e.g., atropine) or excite (e.g., muscarine) the muscarinic receptors for ACh. One such drug is 3-quinuclidinyl benzylate (QNB), which is a potent central and peripheral muscarinic antagonist (Albanus, 1970). The compound ^{3}H-QNB is com-mercially available and has been used to demonstrate muscarinic receptors in the CNS (Yamamura, Kuhar, and Snyder, 1974; Yamamura and Snyder, 1974a) and in the gut (Yamamura and Snyder, 1974b). Unfortunately, the alpha neurotoxins, such as alpha-bungarotoxin, found in snake venoms, which bind to the nicotinic receptor at the neuromuscular junction, do not bind to the nicotinic receptors of enteric ganglia and cannot be used to demonstrate these receptors (Bursztajn and Gershon, 1977). The precursor, ^{3}H-choline is taken up by cholinergic axons and is enzymatically converted within them to ACh. Since, in the gut, only neural elements have a high affinity uptake mechanism for choline and this uptake is closely linked to the synthesis of ACh (Pert and Snyder, 1974; Kuhar and Murrin, 1978), ACh production is an excellent marker for the identification of enteric cholinergic neurons (Richter and Marchbanks, 1971). It is far more specific than is the cytochemical detection of the enzyme responsible for the inacti-vation of ACh, acetylcholinesterase (ACh-esterase) (Gunn, 1971; Kyosola, Veijola, and Rechardt, 1975). Another excellent marker for cholinergic innervation is the activity of the enzyme choline acetyltransferase (Fonnum, 1969).

  b. *Nonadrenergic Intrinsic Inhibitory Transmitter* When cholinergic excitatory innervation is blocked, stimulation of vagal or sacral nerves provokes an inhibitory (relaxant) response of the gut that is not due to stimulation of adrenergic fibers (Martinson, 1965; Burnstock, Campbell, and Rand, 1966; Campbell, 1966). Nonadrenergic relaxation of the gut can also be induced by electrical field stimulation of isolated innervated preparations or by raising mucosal pressure. Several lines of evidence, discussed in the paragraphs following, indicate that the vagal, sacral, and intrinsically induced inhibitory responses are very different from adrenergic relaxation (Martinson, 1965; Burnstock et al., 1966; Campbell, 1966; Burnstock, 1972).

(*1*) The nonadrenergic inhibitory response is elicited at lower frequencies of stimulation than are required to relax the gut by stimulation of adrenergic nerves.

(*2*) Adrenergic neuron blocking agents (such as guanethidine) or a combination of alpha-and beta-adrenoceptor antagonists do not inhibit nonadrenergic relaxation.

(*3*) Stimulation of intestine grown in organotypic tissue culture elicits a relaxant response after the extrinsic adrenergic fibers have degenerated, indicating that nonadrenergic inhibitory neurons are intrinsic to the gut (Rikimaru, 1971).

(*4*) During ontogeny, inhibitory responses develop long before adrenergic nerves reach the gut (Gershon and Thompson, 1973). These inhibitory responses must therefore be nonadrenergic. It should be noted that the sympathetic perivascular nerves do not become inhibitory to the gut until after birth, although some adrenergic fibers can be detected in the fetal gut (Burn, 1968; Gershon and Thompson, 1973).

Although ATP has been proposed, on good evidence, as the neurotransmitter of nonadrenergic inhibitory neurons, which have therefore been called "purinergic" (Burnstock, 1972), it should not yet be definitely stated that this substance is the nonadrenergic inhibitory transmitter, since contrary reports have appeared (Spedding, Sweetman and Weetman, 1975). Recently, a plexus of enteric nerves has been found that becomes brightly fluorescent after incubation with quinacrine. Quinacrine-fluorescent nerves are not adrenergic or cholinergic, and they are found only in those locations that have nonadrenergic inhibitory nerves. Quinacrine fluorescence (Olson, Alund, and Norberg, 1976) has therefore been proposed as a marker for the histofluorescent detection of these putatively "purinergic" neurons.

c. *Norepinephrine* (*NE*) As stated above, the cell bodies of origin of all the adrenergic axons in the gut of most species lie outside the gut itself. Adrenergic fibers reach the intestinal wall via the perivascular nerves, where they may either directly relax smooth muscle (Gershon, 1967b) or interfere with release of ACh (Jacobowitz, 1965; Norberg and Sjoqvist, 1966; Paton and Vizi, 1969). NE reduces the release of ACh from the gut through an action on alpha-adrenoceptors (Kosterlitz, Lydon, and Watt, 1970). A mutually inhibitory, reciprocal, adrenergic-cholinergic axoaxonic synapse has recently been identified in the myenteric plexus (Manber and Gershon, 1978, 1979).

Several methods are available for the identification of adrenergic axonal varicosities. Catecholamines (CA) can be visualized by fluorescence microscopy after exposure of dried tissue to formaldehyde gas of appropriate water content (formaldehyde-induced fluorescence, or FIF) (Falck et al., 1962; Hamberger, 1967) or exposure to glyoxylic acid (Bloom and Battenberg, 1976; Dreyfus, Gershon, and Crain, 1978). The catecholamine-containing axon terminals also have a high affinity for ^{3}H-NE that is due to the presence of a reuptake mechanism for the transmitter's inactivation. This permits the axons to be shown by radioautography. In addition, after fixation with sodium or potassium permanganate, small vesicles with electron-dense cores (40–60 mn) can be seen with the electron microscope in adrenergic terminal varicosities (Figure 1) (Hokfelt, 1971; Bloom, 1973). Moreover, analogues of CA (e.g., 5-hydroxydopamine [5-HD] [Thoenen and Tranzer, 1968]; 6-hydroxydopamine [6-HD] [Richards and Tranzer, 1969]) are taken up as false neurotransmitters by adrenergic axons. The 5-HD forms a recognizable electron opaque substance that marks the terminal, and 6-HD can be used acutely to label (Cobb and Bennett, 1971) or chronically to destroy adrenergic axon terminals (Tranzer and Richards, 1971). The chemical sympathectomy induced by 6-HD is useful either for the identification or for the elimination of the adrenergic innervation. In addition, pharmacological agents that block adrenergic receptors and drugs that prevent the reuptake of NE are also available, and both alpha- and beta-adrenoceptors have been assayed by using labeled ligands. The mixed alpha-agonist-antagonist ^{3}H-dihydroergocryptine has been used to evaluate alpha-adrenoceptor activity in nervous tissue and smooth muscle (U'Prichard and Snyder, 1977; Williams, Mullikin, and Lefkowitz, 1976). Beta-adrenoceptors have been probed with fluorescent antagonists, such as 9-amino-acridino propranalol, which permit histological receptor identification (Atlas and Levitzki, 1977; Atlas and Segal, 1977), or with labeled ligands, such as ^{125}I-hydroxybenzylpindolol (Brown et al., 1976; Bylund, Charness and Snyder, 1977) or ^{3}H-dihydroalprenalol, which permit radioligand assay of beta-adrenoceptors (Alexander, Davis, and Lefkowitz, 1975).

    d. Prostaglandins and Peptides Prostaglandins (Dajani et al., 1975) and peptides have been proposed as neurotransmitters or neuromodulatory agents in the enteric nervous system. Peptides, which have been found by using immunocytochemical methods within neurons of the CNS, have similarly been found in enteric neurons. These peptides include enkephalin (Elde et al., 1976; Schultzberg et al., 1978) somatostatin (Hokfelt et al., 1975), substance P (Hokfelt et al., 1974; Hokfelt et al., 1977b; Nilsson et al., 1975), and vasoactive intestinal polypeptide (VIP) (Bryant et al., 1976; Fuxe et al., 1977; Larsson, 1977; Schultzberg et al., 1978). Each of the four peptides can still be demonstrated in the enteric nervous system grown for 3

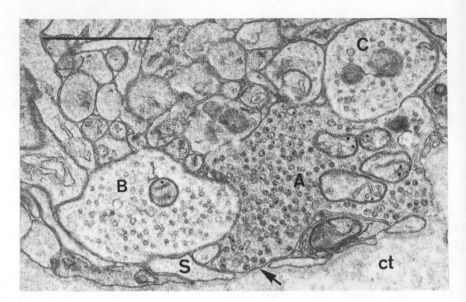

Figure 1. An electron micrograph of the guinea pig myenteric plexus at the interface with connective tissue space that separates the plexus from the longitudinal layer of smooth muscle. The tissue has been fixed with $KMnO_4$. An adrenergic terminal varicosity can be recognized at (A) from its content of small dense core vesicles (average diameter 48 ± 2 [SE] nm). Terminal varicosities at B and C contain small lucent vesicles (average diameter 45 ± 2 [SE] nm) and therefore have the morphological appearance of cholinergic varicosities. At the arrow, varicosity A is bare to the connective tissue space (ct) and is not enclosed by surrounding Schwann elements (S). Such a terminal's opening to the connective tissue space is probably a point of transmitter release for diffusion to and action on the smooth muscle. Note the direct apposition of varicosities B and C on A. Such appositions may be the morphological representation of axoaxonic contacts where reciprocal adrenergic-cholinergic neuromodulation takes place. The marker (upper left) = 1.0 µm. (From Manber and Gershon, 1979).

weeks in organotypic tissue culture (Schultzberg et al., 1978). Therefore, at least some of the cell bodies of each of these peptide-containing neurons must lie within the wall of the gut itself. Research on the role of the peptides or prostaglandins has just recently been started, and relatively little is known of their actions on enteric neurons. However, these studies have been begun; and rapid advances can be expected, although the physiological role of these substances cannot yet be outlined. The guinea pig ileum contains opiate receptors that can be assayed with appropriate radioligands. Presumably these receptors relate to the enkephalin-containing enteric neurons. These receptors have made the gut a valuable model system for opiate research, and the gut model has greatly facilitated the discovery of enkephalin (Hughes, 1975).

 e. 5-Hydroxytryptamine (5-HT-serotonin)   There are two known stores of serotonin in the vertebrate gut: the mucosa (Erspamer, 1966) and the enteric nervous system (Gershon, 1968; Robinson and Gershon, 1971). The 5-HT found in enterochromaffin cells in the mucosa is nonneuronal. It may play a modulating role in the initiation of the neurally mediated peristaltic reflex (Bulbring and Crema, 1958; Bulbring and Lin, 1958). Pressure on the mucosa, caused by material passing downward through the lumen, may stimulate mucosal sensory receptors to release 5-HT from enterochromaffin cells.

Until the mid-1960s, it was not believed that a peripheral serotonergic innervation existed in mammals. However, in the 1950s (Gaddum, 1953; Gaddum and Picarelli, 1957) and the 1960s, receptors for 5-HT were discovered in the guinea pig ileum; and several investigators reported that 5-HT stimulated ganglia in the myenteric plexus (Brownlee and Johnson, 1963; Gershon, 1967a; Bianchi et al., 1968; Paton and Zar, 1968). Further evidence then led to the hypothesis that 5-HT is an enteric neurotransmitter. A listing of this evidence follows:

(1) *Evidence supporting the existence of serotonergic neurons in the mammalian enteric nervous system*

(a)   5-HT stimulates both excitatory and intrinsic inhibitory enteric neurons (Bulbring and Gershon, 1967; Kottegoda, 1969; Bianchi, Beani, and Crema, 1970; Furness and Costa, 1973). Pharmacological and physiological evidence indicates that 5-HT receptors are located on myenteric and submucosal ganglion cells (Brownlee and Johnson, 1963; Gershon, 1967a; Hirst and Silinsky, 1975). In fact, there is direct evidence that 5-HT releases ACh from the myenteric plexus (Adam-Vizi and Vizi, 1978). Since this release is antagonized by tetrodotoxin, it is apparent that 5-HT releases ACh by activating enteric ganglion cells. Electrophysiological evidence indicates that 5-HT mimics the effects of transmitter released by stimulation of myenteric axons (Dingledine, Goldstein, and Kendig, 1974; Mayer and Wood, 1978; Wood and Mayer, 1978a; Wood and Mayer, 1979a, b). For example, intracellular recordings show a characteristic long, slow depolarization in response to 5-HT that is identical to the effects of stimulation of the inputs (connectives) of the myenteric ganglia (Wood and Mayer, 1978a; Mayer and Wood, 1978; Wood and Mayer, 1979a, b). Wood and Mayer (1978b) have postulated that the serotonergic nerves function to "gate" the passage of information between myenteric ganglia. They found that the somata of myenteric ganglion cells are relatively inexcitable. Thus, activity remains isolated in the dendrites of these cells except when the axosomatic serotonergic innervation increases the somal excitability by increasing membrane resistance. Under these conditions dendritic excitation is seen as able to excite the soma and therefore the axon of the ganglion cell, thereby leading to the conduction of ganglionic activity out of the ganglion to other regions of the myenteric plexus.

(b)   The effect of nerve stimulation (the slow depolarization) is abolished by antagonism of the action of 5-HT (Mayer and Wood, 1978; Wood and Mayer, 1978a).

(c)   The gut releases 5-HT when stimulated electrically (Bulbring and Gershon, 1967; Furness and Costa, 1973; Schulz and Cartwright, 1974). The release of 5-HT is Ca^{+2}-dependent and blocked by high Mg^{+2} and tetrodotoxin (Jonakait et al., 1978).

(d)   A population of enteric neurons has serotonergic marker properties. A list of such properties is shown below:

(2)   *Properties of enteric serotonergic neurons*

(a)   A population of enteric neurons contains and stores 5-HT. This was shown by administering L-tryptophan and inhibiting MAO *in vivo* and then microspectrophotofluorometrically analyzing the pattern of formaldehyde-induced histofluorescence of the myenteric plexus (Robinson and Gershon, 1971; Dreyfus et al., 1977a). Neurons grown in culture do not require such enhancement of serotonin content to be demonstrable by histofluorescence (Dreyfus et al., 1977a).

(b)   A population of enteric neurons *in situ* or in culture can synthesize ^{3}H-5-HT from the dietary precursor amino acid, ^{3}H-L-tryptophan (Dreyfus et al., 1977a).

(c)   Neurons of the myenteric and submucosal plexuses contain immunochemically demonstrable tryptophan hydroxylase (Gershon et al., 1977).

(d)   Enteric neurons have a mechanism adequate for inactivating 5-HT serving as a neurotransmitter. This mechanism is a highly specific uptake of the amine (Gershon and Altman, 1971; Gershon, Robinson, and Ross, 1976). The uptake mechanism has the following properties:

(i)   It is sodium-dependent.

(ii)   It is saturable.

(iii) It is temperature-dependent.

(iv)   It is energy-dependent and is effectively blocked by inhibitors of anaerobic metabolism.

(v)   The uptake is highly specific to 5-HT. Thus, affinity for the uptake site is eliminated by removal of the aliphatic side chain of 5-HT and is reduced 100-fold by methylation of the aliphatic amine, removal of the ring 5-hydroxyl, or substitution of 6-HT for 5-HT. The uptake of 5-HT is not inhibited by analogues lacking these features, such as LSD (Gershon et al., 1976).

(vi)   The uptake of 5-HT by enteric neurons is powerfully and competitively antagonized by fluoxetine (Lilly 110140) (Gershon and Jonakait, 1979), a drug that also specifically inhibits the uptake of 5-HT by CNS serotonergic axons (Wong et al., 1974).

(vii)   The uptake mechanism appears to be limited to serotonergic neurons. Consequently, 5-HT uptake is unaffected by prior chemical sympathectomy (Gershon and Altman, 1971), and the 5-HT uptake mechanism precedes that of NE in mammalian ontogeny (Rothman, Ross, and Gershon, 1976).

(viii)   The uptake of 5-HT, and the facility with which ^{3}H-5-HT can be fixed in tissue (whereas metabolites wash out) permits the radioautographic localization of the enteric axons that take up and bind 5-HT (Gershon and Ross, 1966a, b; Gershon and Altman, 1971; Rothman et al., 1976; Dreyfus et al., 1977b). Radioautography is also a valuable marker for CNS serotonergic neurons (Descarries, Beaudet, and Watkins, 1975; Chan-Palay, 1975).

(e)   The enteric serotonergic neurons are intrinsic to the gut itself. That is, the enteric serotonergic axons are not derived from vagal or sympathetic neurons that project to the gut, but from neurons whose cell bodies lie within the enteric nerve plexuses. Therefore, the enteric serotonergic neurons survive for extended periods of time in organotypic tissue culture while the extrinsic innervation, cut off in culture from its cell bodies, degenerates (Dreyfus et al., 1977a, b; Gershon et al., 1977). Moreover, there are no serotonergic axons in the vagus nerves (Dreyfus et al., 1977b).

(f)   The enteric serotonergic neurons contain a specific serotonin-binding protein (SBP) (Jonakait et al., 1977). This protein is similar to the SBP also found in CNS serotonergic neurons (Tamir and Huang, 1974; Tamir and Kuhar, 1975).

(g)   A population of enteric neurons release ^{3}H-5-HT and SBP simultaneously on electrical stimulation of the gut (Jonakait et al., 1978). This release is Ca^{+2}-dependent and is antagonized by high Mg^{+2} and tetrodotoxin. Endogenous 5-HT is also released under similar conditions (Gershon and Tamir, unpublished observation). Since the specific activity of released ^{3}H-5-HT is higher than that in the tissue, newly taken up ^{3}H-5-HT must be preferentially released by enteric serotonergic neurons.

(h)   The varicosities of enteric neurons can be isolated by a combination of differential and density-gradient centrifugation techniques from homogenates of the myenteric plexus (Jonakait and Gershon, 1976; Jonakait et al., 1979). These autonomic synaptosomes differ from the synaptosomes of the CNS in that they, like the autonomic varicosities from which they are derived, contain no presynaptic membrane specializations. They are also obtained without adhering postsynaptic membrane specializations. However, in common with CNS synaptosomes, they do contain clusters of synaptic vesicles and mitochondria, but no microtubules. These isolated varicosities of enteric neurons both contain 5-HT and take up 5-HT from an ambient medium.

The gut also has a high-affinity, saturable uptake mechanism for the amino acid L-tryptophan (Dreyfus et al., 1977a). Studies with cell fractionation techniques indicate that axon terminals are responsible for this uptake (Jonakait et al., 1979). It is likely that this uptake is associated in gut, as in brain (Aghajanian, Kuhar, and Roth, 1973), with biosynthesis of 5-HT. Tryptophan hydroxylase, the rate-limiting step in the biosynthesis of 5-HT, *in vitro*, has a K_m of about 50 μM (Dreyfus et al., 1977a). This is the approximate concentration of L-tryptophan in tissues. Thus the rate of 5-HT biosynthesis will depend heavily on changes in the L-tryptophan concentration. This explains why administration of L-tryptophan to animals increases the 5-HT content of the myenteric plexus and makes the amine demonstrable by histofluorescence (Dreyfus et al., 1977a). There is a difference between the tryptophan hydroxylase of axons and that of cell bodies. The axonal enzyme is sensitive to inhibition by parachlorophenylalanine (PCPA), whereas the perikaryal enzyme is not (Aghajanian and Asher, 1971). Therefore, if PCPA and L-tryptophan are given simultaneously, the 5-HT concentration is increased in cell bodies, but not in axons; and the cell bodies of serotonergic neurons can be individually visualized (without interference by overlying axons). Serotonergic axons and cell bodies have been differentially localized in both brain and gut by using L-tryptophan and PCPA in combination with histofluorescence (Aghajanian and Asher, 1971; Dreyfus et al., 1977a).

Thus it seems reasonable to conclude that there are serotonergic neurons in the enteric nervous system. Many methods are available for their study.

C. Sectional Summary

Although Langley's view of the enteric nervous system as a separate but equal division of the ANS is not widely prevalent today, there is good reason to reinstate it. It seems likely that many enteric neurons do not receive inputs from the CNS and function as components of an intrinsic nervous system that can display reflex activity and that enjoys considerable autonomy. Moreover, the enteric nervous system has many features that are different from other regions of the PNS and that resemble the CNS. These features include anatomical characteristics such as the internal architecture of the myenteric plexus and a blood–myenteric-plexus barrier. They also include a diversity of intrinsic neuronal types reflected in the relative abundance of enteric neurotransmitters. Identified or putative enteric neurotransmitters include small molecules, ACH, NE, and 5-HT, a purine, and the neuropeptides, VIP, enkephalin, somatostatin, and substance P. The forces that control the development of these diverse neuronal types have not yet been worked out; but considerable insight not only into development, but also into the critical role played by the enteric nervous system in bowel function, may be derived from an examination of the condition congenital megacolon or Hirschsprung's disease.

II. CONGENITAL MEGACOLON (HIRSCHSPRUNG'S DISEASE)

A. In Human Beings

Hirschsprung's disease is a birth defect occurring in infants and children, with an incidence between 1:2,000 and 1:10,000 (0.02%) in the general population (Bodian and Carter, 1963). Symptoms of the disease include extreme constipation, the inability to defecate, distention and enlargement of the colon, bleeding, vomiting, and malnutrition (LaMont and Isselbacher, 1977). It occurs in siblings in 3.6% of cases and also may occur in conjunction with a number of familial hereditary diseases thought to be derived from defects in neural crest development (Bolande, 1975). Megacolon (enlargement of the colon) occurs secondarily, proximal to the segment of distal colon, rectum, and/or anal canal that is narrow because of the congenital absence within this segment of intrinsic enteric ganglion cells (Tittel, 1901; Whitehouse and Kernohan, 1948; Zuelzer and Wilson, 1948; Bodian, Stephens, and Ward, 1949; Okamato and Ueda, 1967; Boley, 1975; Kadair, Sims, and Critchfield, 1977). Myenteric and submucosal ganglion cells (derived from neural crest during embryogenesis) are both lacking (Okamoto and Ueda, 1967; Gannon, Noblett, and Burnstock, 1969). Apparently normal intrinsic excitatory and inhibitory ganglion cells are present in the dilated portion of colon proximal to the constricted area. However, the inability of the constricted segment to manifest normal propulsive motility produces proximal distention and dilatation that, in severe cases, can extend through the entire colon. A hypoganglionic transitional zone, conical in shape, is usually interposed between the constricted and the dilated segments of gut (Smith, 1967; Baumgarten, Holstein, and Stelzner, 1973b). Although devoid of ganglion cells, the aganglionic segment is innervated, in humans, by many unmyelinated intramuscular adrenergic fibers (Ehrenpreis, 1966; Gannon et al., 1969; Garret, Howard, and Nixon, 1969; Webster, 1974). This pattern is abnormal, since adrenergic axons normally are largely confined to the myenteric plexus and do not, except in the taenia coli (where they are found in connective tissue septae), grow into and among the fibers of the smooth muscle layer. Cholinergic nerve fibers that either are extrinsic (preganglionic) in origin or are ingrowths of neurites from intrinsic postganglionic cholinergic neurons in the normally ganglionated neighboring segment are also abundant in the aganglionic bowel (Kamijo, Hiatt, and Koelle, 1953; Adamo, Marples, and Trounce, 1960; Niemi,

Kouvalainen, and Hjeht, 1961; Garrett et al., 1969; Meier-Ruge et al., 1972; Webster, 1974). Therefore, although aganglionic, the affected segments are *not* denervated.

B. In Mice

Congenital megacolon has been reported to arise as a an autosomal recessive genetic trait in several strains of laboratory mice. Like humans, mutant mice exhibit all the symptoms resulting from the segmental absence of intrinsic ganglion cells in the colon (Lane, 1966; Webster, 1974; Richardson, 1975; Wood, 1979). The genetic trait is often, although not always, associated with other recognizable phenotypic expressions, particularly coat color.

Megacolon in mice was first reported by Derrick and St. George-Grambauer (1957). Histological studies revealed the absence of enteric ganglia from the lower colon. It should be noted that in mice the term *colon* refers to the entire large intestine distal to the cecum, because in these animals there is no clear-cut separation between distal colon and rectum. Ganglia normally extend to about 1 mm from the sphincter of striated muscle surrounding the anal canal (Webster, 1973). The next reports of megacolon in mice were that of Bielschowsky and Schofield (1960, 1962) who found that 10% of mice with piebald (white and tan) coat color (strain s/s NZY) were also deficient in enteric ganglia and had constricted segments of colon measuring 2–7 mm in length. Much experimentation has now been done on two mutant strains of mice reported by Lane in 1966 (Lane, 1966). Each is characterized by changes in coat pigmentation and megacolon in the homozygous state. Homozygotes of the piebald-lethal (S^1) strain have black eyes and a white coat with patches of black pigment. Because they develop fatal megacolon within the first few days of life, the establishment of breeding colonies of these mice is difficult. The second mutant with megacolon, the lethal spotted (L^s), resembles the S^1/S^1 homozygote except that the ears and tail are less pigmented. However, the colored L^s/L^s homozygotes often survive for longer periods than do S^1/S^1 mice (Lane, 1966). These animals can live to breeding age and are fertile. Cross-breeding homozygote L^s/L^s mice produces litters in which all members develop megacolon (Lane, 1966; Bolande and Towler, 1972; Webster, 1974; Bolande, 1975). The lethal spotted mice exhibit the same symptoms and pathology as do human patients with Hirschsprung's disease. The colon is filled with fecal matter except for the short aganglionic segment, approximately 7–10 mm in length, proximal to the anus (Lane, 1966; Bolande, 1975). Above this segment, the colon is maximally distended with fecal pellets. The transitional hypoganglionic zone, interposed between the aganglionic and dilated colon, is approximately 1–2 cm in length.

In general, the murine and human megacolons are similar, except that the hyperinnervation by adrenergic fibers within the aganglionic segment, associated with Hirschsprung's disease, has not been reported in mice. Nevertheless, adrenergic axons do, as in the human, invade the aganglionic tissue of the mice (Baumgarten, 1967; Bolande and Towler, 1972; Webster, 1974; Bolande, 1975; Wood, 1979). Moreover, the availability of L^s/L^s mutant mice and their ability to survive with megacolon long enough to be bred and colonized makes them particularly suitable for studies of the differentiation of the intrinsic innervation of the mammalian gut.

Other experimental models are also available. Congenital megacolon has been produced experimentally in dogs (McElhannon, 1960; Hukuhara, Kotani, and Sato, 1961), in rats (Imamura et al., 1975), and in rabbits.

C. Etiology

Several alternative proposals have been put forward concerning the etiology of megacolon. These include an inhibitory action of NE released by the large numbers of adrenergic fibers in the constricted colonic segment (Baumgarten et al., 1973b). However, since cholinergic excitatory fibers are also present in the aganglionic bowel, this explanation seems unlikely. Likewise, the proposal that spasm is caused by denervation hypersensitivity (Cannon's law [Cannon, 1939]) is probably also incorrect, because aganglionic segments are neither denervated nor supersensitive to either ACh or NE (Penninckx and Kerremans, 1975). Thus the absence of intrinsic ganglion cells, resulting in a lack of coordinated neural activity, leads to a functional obstruction of the bowel. The intrinsic enteric ganglia must therefore be critical to normal propulsive activity. Methods of diagnosis (Swenson, Fisher, and MacMahon, 1955; Dobbins and Bill, 1965; Aldrich and Campbell, 1968; Campbell and Noblett, 1969) and treatment of the disease by surgical excision of the constricted segment (Swenson and Bill, 1948) have been successfully developed.

Bodian (1952) proposed that the lack of ganglion cells is due to a genetically determined disturbance occurring during embryonic development, and Huther (1954) and Swenson (1950, 1955) both believed that a pelvic source of neuroblasts exists and is defective in patients with megacolon. Since both lethal spotted mice and piebald-lethal mice have pigmentary abnormalities as well as defects in the formation of enteric ganglia, Mayer (1965) and Mayer and Maltby (1964) have proposed that both mutants have abnormal neural crest cells. However, since only a very restricted number of neural crest derivatives are in fact abnormal, the abnormality (if one exists) in the neural crest could not extend to all neural crest cells. Mayer (1965) has suggested that an undue sensitivity to environmental factors may be involved. If so, the geographical restriction of the defective pigmentation or ganglion cell formation in the mice would point to a limited environmental defect as well.

The origin of enteric ganglia has not been ascertained until recently (in the chick; see below), and the actual cause of the aganglionosis remains unknown. Further consideration of this topic requires, first, a consideration of the derivation of the enteric ganglia. This follows:

III. THE EMBRYOLOGICAL ORIGIN OF MAMMALIAN ENTERIC GANGLION CELLS

The origin of enteric ganglion cells is still to some extent controversial. Early reports that the neurons of the gut were derived from mesoderm (Camus, 1921; Goormaghtigh, 1924; Tello, 1924; Keuning, 1944, 1948) or endoderm (Masson, 1923; Masson and Berger, 1923; Schack, 1932) have been disproved (Andrew, 1971), and it is now generally accepted that all neurons in the vertebrate enteric nervous system are of ectodermal, neural plate origin. However, investigators disagree about whether they are derived exclusively from neural crest (Van Campenhout, 1930a, 1931; Yntema and Hammond, 1945; Hammond and Yntema, 1947; Yntema and Hammond, 1947, 1952, 1954, 1955; Okamota and Ueda, 1967; Webster, 1973), neural tube (Jones, 1942; Kuntz, 1953), or both (Abel, 1909, 1912; Uchida, 1927; Andrew, 1969, 1970, 1971). Also at issue is the level of the neuraxis contributing presumptive neuroblasts to the enteric nervous system. Possible sources of enteric neuronal primordia which have all been considered are vagal neural crest (Yntema and Hammond, 1945; Hammond and Yntema, 1947; Yntema and Hammond, 1947, 1952, 1954, 1955; Okamoto and Ueda, 1967; Le Douarin and Teillet, 1973; Webster, 1973) and/or neural tube (Jones, 1942; Andrew, 1970), trunk neural crest and/or neural tube (Abel, 1909, 1912; Uchidida, 1927; Van Campenhout, 1930a, b, 1931, 1932; Jones, 1942; Dereymaeker, 1943; Kuntz, 1953; Andrew, 1963, 1964, 1969, 1970), and sacral neural crest (Abel, 1909; Jones, 1942; Cantino, 1970; Andrew, 1971; Le Douarin and Teillet, 1973) and/or tube (contributing ganglia to the more distal portions of the gut). Most of the available data in the literature have been obtained from morphological studies using silver impregnation techniques to recognize developing neurons or experiments involving the ablation of given parts of the neuraxis followed by a search, at later stages of development, for the presence or absence of neurons within the wall of the gut. However, for technical reasons, the majority of these experiments have been performed on birds or amphibia and not on mammals. Andrew, in her lengthy review of the data (Andrew, 1971), points out that many of the operations involving ablation, designed to remove the source of enteric ganglia from chick embryos, probably were performed after the commencement of neural crest migration or the arrival of progenitor neuroblasts in the intestine. Although most investigators agree that progenitor neuroblasts leave their site of origin in the neuraxis and migrate to the gut along preexisting vagal and/or pelvic nerves (Van Campenhout, 1931, 1932; Dereymaeker, 1943; Okamoto and Ueda, 1967; Cantino, 1970), this conclusion is based upon identifications made using nonspecific silver impregnation methods, which cannot be used to identify presumptive progenitor ganglion cells that may arrive in the gut before they are morphologically distinguishable as neurons. Furthermore, it is not known whether tissues which have been artificially neurogenically ablated are capable of receiving neuroblasts or pleuripotential cells that may migrate abnormally from other parts of the neuraxis (Andrew, 1971).

Thus, much of these older experimental data are difficult to interpret. More recent studies have relied upon the histochemical identification of acetylcholinesterase as a marker for neuroblasts (Cantino, 1970; Webster, 1973). Unfortunately, acetylcholinesterase is also a neuronal marker of doubtful specificity. It is present in cholinergic neurons, but it occurs in other cells as well (Schlaepfer, 1968; Eranko and Eranko, 1971). Moreover, its use would reveal only one of the multiple types of enteric neuron. Nevertheless, the histochemical demonstration of acetylcholinesterase was used by Webster to identify developing enteric neurons in normal and aganglionic (S^1 strain) mice (Webster, 1973). His results and those of Okamoto and Ueda (1967), who worked with normal human embryos, led to the idea that all enteric ganglia arise from vagal neural crest and migrate proximodistally through the gut itself. They propose that a defect leading to a slower rate of migration will cause ganglion cells to fail to reach the distal end of the developing gut and cause a terminal aganglionosis of the colon.

This interpretation is based on the observation that a proximodistal gradient occurs in the appearance of acetylcholinesterase-positive ganglion cells and that the rate of progression of this gradient is slower than normal in piebald mutant mice (S^1) that develop megacolon. However, three points are inconsistent with Webster's interpretation. One is the occurrence, although rare, of skip lesions in human megacolon, in which an aganglionic region is flanked by normal regions of the bowel that do contain ganglion cells (Kadair et al., 1977). The second point is that the proximodistal gradient in ganglion cell appearance that occurs in mice is not found in rabbits and rats (Cantino, 1970). In the rat, the midregions of the gut are filled in with cholinesterase-containing neurons from stomach and terminal intestine. The third and most important point is that the levels of the neuraxial precursors of enteric ganglia have finally been ascertained in recent experiments on birds. This work, by LeDouarin and Teillet (1973, 1974), used a biological marking technique involving the transplantation of quail neuraxis (the nuclei of quail cells can be recognized) into developing chicks. LeDouarin and Teillet demonstrated that both vagal and sacral levels of the neuraxis contribute neurons to the enteric ganglia. The sacral level supplies progenitors to the postumbilical gut, including the colon. Therefore, unless a different situation obtains in mammals (and the pattern of enteric ganglion cell appearance in rabbits and rats suggests that the situation is the same), it seems unlikely that slowing migration of vagally derived progenitor cells would produce megacolon. The lesion is usually in the distal colon, supplied with progenitors by the *sacral* as well as the vagal neural crest. Thus, the condition would be more likely to result either from a defect in the neural crest progenitors themselves or in the environment of the target tissue than from a defect in migration down the gut. Since the colon receives progenitors from two sources of neural crest, the absence of ganglion cells in the mature colon probably cannot be ascribed to a defect limited to the progenitors or migration of progenitors derived from either vagal or sacral levels alone. Moreover, since most of the gut does become ganglionated and skip lesions do occur, a global defect affecting the ability of neural crest precursors to form enteric ganglia would also seem to be excluded. Therefore, the simplest hypothesis consistent with the available data would be to attribute aganglionosis to a defect in the enteric microenvironment that renders the affected segments inhospitable to the differentiation and/or support of intrinsic enteric neurons. Recent studies have indicated that the microenvironment of the final tissue of residence powerfully affects the differentiation of neural crest progenitors (see below). Thus, it is reasonable to propose that the enteric microenvironment may significantly contribute to the pathogenesis of megacolon.

The distribution of enteric neurotransmitters in normal and aganglionic tissue supports a role for the microenvironment in the pathogenesis of megacolon. As noted earlier, in both humans and mice, the aganglionic segments of gut do become innervated by adrenergic and cholinergic axons (Kamijo et al., 1953; Adamo et al., 1960; Niemi et al., 1961; Ehrenpreis, 1966; Baumgarten, 1967; Gannon et al., 1969; Garret et al., 1969; Bolande and Towler, 1972; Webster, 1974; Wood, 1979). However, the enteric serotonergic axons fail to grow into these aganglionic regions (Rogawski et al., 1978; Goodrich and Gershon, 1977). In the human gut the serotonergic axons in the hypoganglionic transitional zone above the aganglionic segment appear to sprout, but the axons appear to form knots and remain sharply demarcated from the aganglionic zone (Figure 2). This evidence is not, of course, conclusive; but it does suggest that the environment of the aganglionic zone is inhospitable to the growth of serotonergic neurites. Earlier studies have also revealed the failure of nonadrenergic inhibitory neurons to innervate the aganglionic segments (Baumgarten et al., 1973b; Penninckx and Kerremans, 1975). Therefore, it is possible that the microenvironment of the gut contributes to the pathogenesis of congenital megacolon by being nonsupportive of intrinsic neuronal growth or differentiation.

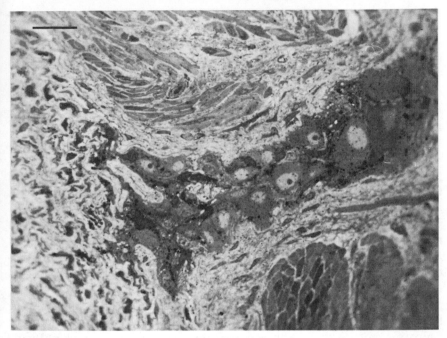

Figure 2. A radioautograph of the muscularis externa from a segment of human colon incubated with ³H-5-HT. The tissue was removed in treatment of Hirschsprung's disease. A ganglion of the myenteric plexus is shown at the border between the dilated gut and the transition to the aganglionic constricted segment. Note the intense labeling around ganglion cells, indicating the presence of ³H-5-HT in axons of the ganglionic neuropil. A number of axons have apparently sprouted and grown into the connective tissue in the transitional zone. Many of these have been labeled by ³H-5-HT. Therefore, serotonergic axons apparently are able to sprout. However, these serotonergic axons do not grow into the aganglionic segments. The marker (upper left) = 100 μm.

IV. MICROENVIRONMENTAL INFLUENCES ON NEURONAL DIFFERENTIATION

The question whether the definitive properties of peripheral neurons are predetermined in the neural crest, are acquired during migration of neural crest progenitors, or develop only within the tissue in which the mature cells ultimately reside has been the subject of considerable recent experimentation.

Most studies favor the view that the ultimate choice of cell type, as defined by neurotransmitter, has not been determined prior to the time that neuronal progenitor cells leave the neural crest. The notion that neurotransmitter choice is made by migrating precursor cells in response to cues they encounter as they move to their target tissues along a predetermined migratory pathway has been put forward by Weston and Butler (1966), Cohen (1972), and Norr (1973). Weston and Butler proposed that the environment through which progenitor cells migrate causes the cells to undergo changes in properties such as adhesiveness and motility. Based upon *in vitro* experiments in developing chick, Cohen concluded that contact of neural progenitors with the somitic mesoderm during migration was required in order for these cells to express adrenergic properties. This conclusion was supported by Norr, who further proposed that the ventral neural tube (and notochord [LeDouarin et al., 1978]) may secrete an inducing factor that acts upon the migrating progenitor cells. The importance of the notochord has been established by the observation that trunk neural crest can give rise to catecholamine-containing cells in the gut mesenchyme, providing that the notochord is present (LeDouarin et al., 1978). However, Cohen (1977) has recently shown that primary cultures of neural crest cells, grown in the absence of other cell types, can form adrenergic neurons. Therefore, although somitic mesoderm and ventral neural tube may act on neural crest progenitors to stimulate adrenergic neuron formation, a small population of neural crest cells may already be committed to neuron formation before migration begins. Neurotransmitter choice may be determined or become fixed at a later stage of development.

It now appears from the work of LeDouarin and her associates that the final destination is more important to the ultimate choice or fixation of neurotransmitter than is precommitment or the migratory pathway (LeDouarin and Teillet, 1973, 1974; LeDouarin et al., 1975; Smith, Cochard, and LeDouarin, 1977). These investigators, as noted earlier, placed isotopic and heterotopic grafts of quail neural crest into chick embryos (or the reverse) of similar developmental stages. They followed the subsequent migration of the cells of each species by identifying stable structural differences in the appearance of interphase nuclei of cells of the two species. The results of experiments in which quail neural anlage was isotopically transplanted into chick embryos revealed that truncal neural anlage between the eighth and twenty-fourth somites gives rise to CA-containing cells of the pre- and paravertebral ganglia (8 to 18) and adrenal medulla (18 to 24). On the other hand, enteric neurons originate from neural crest cells in the vagal (somites 1–7) and sacral (distal to twenty-eighth somite) regions. These enteric ganglia are not fluorescent for NE. However, many enteric ganglion cells contain acetylcholinesterase, and the innervated gut also has activity for choline acetyltransferase (CAT). Therefore, at least some enteric neurons are cholinergic (Smith et al., 1977). These results agree with earlier reports of Weston (1963, 1970) and Yntema and Hammond (1947, 1954) that cells in the neural crest migrate along specific predetermined pathways. However, heterotopic transplants made between the quail and the chick also showed that when neural crest cells from the vagal anlage, which if left alone would become cholinergic, are placed in the trunk, they migrate into the pre- and paravertebral ganglia and adrenal medulla and there develop into CA-containing cells. Alternatively, when trunk cells, which if left alone would become adrenergic, are placed in the vagal area, they migrate along predetermined pathways to the gut and differentiate there into nonfluorescent cholinergic cells. Thus, transmitter choice is not determined before progenitor cells leave the neural crest (LeDouarin and Teillet, 1974; LeDouarin et al., 1975).

Evidence that cells are influenced to choose their transmitter by the environment in which they differentiate has also been obtained by Smith et al. (1977). They showed that when neural anlage were placed directly into the gut wall prior to the gut's colonization by ganglionic precursors, and the migratory pathway was thereby eliminated, it did not matter whether the neural anlage was originally derived from the trunk or the vagal area; in each case nonfluorescent, cholinergic cells differentiated in the gut wall. An even more striking demonstration of the powerful effects mediated by the local environment has come from more recent work of LeDouarin et al. (1978). These investigators isolated a cholinergic ganglion from a quail embryo (4- to 6-day embryos were used) and grafted it into the dorsal trunk of a 2-day chick embryo at the adrenomedullary level of the neuraxis. The grafted cells were followed, and their subsequent differentiation was characterized by cytochemical and ultrastructural criteria. The ciliary ganglion and a portion of Remak's ganglion were used for these experiments. The grafted cholinergic cells migrated from their place of implantation and eventually came to rest in the same site as the host's own neural crest cells. Some of the grafted cells localized in adrenergic ganglia and the adrenal medulla. In these locations they synthesized catecholamines. However, cells that migrated into the gut wall did not become adrenergic. Thus, the final state of differentiation of autonomic neurons is dependent on tissue interactions even after ganglia form and even after biochemical differentiation has begun. At least for a time, therefore, young autonomic neurons are plastic and can express one or another phenotype, depending on the tissue environment to which the cells ultimately are subjected. Consequently, the neurotransmitter choice may be labile early in development and finally determined by factors in the microenvironment of the organs that the presumptive neurons populate.

An elegant demonstration of the influence of the microenvironment on neural differentiation can be seen in recent studies of the growth of dissociated cells derived from the superior cervical ganglia of new born rats in culture. Ninety-five percent of these cells normally exhibit adrenergic characteristics (Mains and Patterson, 1973a, b; Ko et al., 1976). However, if the culture conditions are changed to favor the growth of nonneuronal cells, or if medium conditioned by certain nonneuronal cells is added to the superior cervical ganglion neurons, they gradually change their transmitter from NE to ACh (Bunge, Johnson, and Ross, 1978; Patterson, 1978). This has been shown electrophysiologically (O'Lague et al., 1974, 1975; Ko et al., 1976), biochemically (Patterson and Chun, 1974, 1977a, b), and morphologically (Johnson et al., 1976; Landis, 1976). Interestingly, the change in transmitter from NE to ACh may not be associated with a change in properties of the plasma membrane. Waksull, Johnson, and Burton (1978) have reported that cultured neurons that have converted from adrenergic to cholinergic retain the amine uptake system that normally characterizes adrenergic neurons. The lability of the neurotransmitter choice is not a permanent characteristic of adrenergic neurons. Transmitter change occurs only in adrenergic cells removed for culture early in postnatal development (Ross, Johnson, and Bunge, 1977). As rats mature, the ability of sympathetic neurons to change transmitter in explants is apparently lost, and the transmitter choice becomes fixed.

The evidence supporting the hypothesis that the microenvironment is critical for selection and differentiation of a final transmitter has led Bunge et al. (1978) to propose that there are two separate stages in the ontogeny of peripheral neurons derived from the neural crest. During the first stage cells divide, migrate, and undergo axonal elongation but do not make a permanent decision about their choice of transmitter, ACh or NE. During the second stage the cells choose their definitive neurotransmitter under the influence of cues received from the microenvironment in which they find themselves. This transmitter choice is at first labile and can be changed. However, with time, it becomes fixed. This conclusion is well supported by the in vivo studies of LeDouarin et al. (1978), outlined above. However, the problem of the origin of enteric neuronal diversity is more complex than that of the origin of diversity in other autonomic ganglia. The transmitter choice is not limited to ACh or NE, as we have seen. A number of other transmitters, including 5-HT, neuropeptides, and probably ATP develop as well; and all these neurons develop within the enteric microenvironment. Thus, with respect to the gut, additional factors influencing the differentiation of neural crest emigres must be sought.

V. STUDIES OF THE DEVELOPMENT OF TRANSMITTER-SPECIFIC PROPERTIES OF ENTERIC NEURONS

Although a considerable amount of work has been done (see above) on the development of enteric neurons, relatively few studies have focused on the development of the various types of enteric neuron as identified by their neurotransmitter. Most studies that have looked at transmitters have considered only ACh or NE. Of those that have dealt with ACh, most have relied upon the histochemical demonstration of acetylcholinesterase, which, as has been noted above, cannot be accepted as a specific cholinergic marker. Therefore, very little is known in this area.

Probably the best studies with respect to the ontogeny of enteric cholinergic neurons are those of LeDouarin and her colleagues. Their studies used the CAT activity of developing gut as a marker (Smith et al., 1977) to supplement the acetylcholinesterase cytochemical methods. These investigators found measurable CAT activity appearing for the first time in the quail duodenum at 5 days and in the rectum at 7 days of incubation. In the chick CAT is first detectable in the duodenum of 6-day and the rectum of 8-day embryos. The activity increases exponentially (when measured in terms of total activity per organ) through the time of hatching. Coculture experiments, done on the chorioallantoic membrane of the chick, provided insight into the factors involved in cholinergic neuron differentiation. Neuraxial cells were found to differentiate into cholinergic ganglia when these cells were implanted into explants of gut removed prior to the gut's colonization by neuronal precursors. Therefore, neither cues from the migratory pathway nor preganglionic innervation are necessary for the differentiation of enteric cholinergic ganglia.

The development of adrenergic and serotonergic innervations of the chick intestine has recently been examined by using the specific uptake of the amines as markers (Epstein and Gershon, 1978). Serotonergic cells were identified by radioautography of tissues incubated with a low concentration of ^{3}H-5-HT in the presence of excess nonradioactive NE to prevent the nonspecific uptake of ^{3}H-5-HT by adrenergic axons. Controls included treatment with fluoxetine, a specific inhibitor of 5-HT uptake. Adrenergic axons were examined by histofluorescence with and without prior incubation with alpha-methyl NE. Little uptake of ^{3}H-5-HT could be detected prior to 9 days of incubation. At that time, and through day 13, ^{3}H-5-HT was found in cells surrounding enteric ganglia and within the ganglionic neuropil. After 13 days, ^{3}H-5-HT was confined to axons within the enteric plexuses. These observations suggest that cells able to take up 5-HT are present in the embryonic chick gut in 9-day embryos and migrate into the enteric plexuses between days 9 and 13. Within the plexuses, uptake was seen only in axons. In contrast, adrenergic neurites, which were rare at first, could be detected by histofluorescence only in tissue incubated with alpha-methyl NE, and not until days 11–12. This is similar to the findings of Bennett and Cobb (1969) in chick gizzard: endogenous NE was not detected before days 13–14. Enemar, Falck, and Hakanson (1965) found endogenous fluorescence in the mesentery of the chick gut at about this time but did not find NE in the myenteric plexus of the duodenum or rectum until days 16–18. Certainly, few adrenergic fibers exist prior to this late developmental stage. Therefore in the chick gut there seems to be a developmental sequence in which cholinergic neurons appear to differentiate first. Their appearance is followed by serotonergic neurons, and adrenergic axons do not appear until after the cholinergic and serotonergic innervations are present.

The mammalian gut has not been examined as completely as that of the chick from the point of view of cholinergic neuronal development. In rabbits, Gershon and Thompson (1973) found cholinergic function for the first time at day 17 (out of 31), the same time they were able to show nonadrenergic inhibition of the gut musculature. Therefore, the cholinergic innervation has been established by this time. However, function is a relatively complex parameter and probably follows by a significant period of time the earliest development in the tissue of a given type of neuron. Thus, in order for cholinergic excitation to occur, the cholinergic axons must be in place and sufficiently mature to release ACh; the muscle's muscarinic receptors must have developed and become coupled to the contractile machinery, and the muscle must be able to contract (based on mechanical activity measurements). Therefore, although a limit is set, the earliest time of appearance of cholinergic innervation in the rabbit remains unknown.

Radioautographic and biochemical studies have established that serotonergic innervation occurs at about the same time (16 days) as that at which cholinergic and nonadrenergic inhibitory function can be demonstrated (Rothman et al., 1976). The specific serotonin-binding protein (SBP) also appears in the developing rabbit gut at this time (Jonakait et al., 1977). In contrast, adrenergic innervation appears later and cannot be demonstrated until the twenty-first to the twenty-sixth day of gestation. Thus, the developmental sequence of formation of enteric neurons in the rabbit resembles that of the chick; and, as was found for the developing chick, development of adrenergic innervation trails the cholinergic and the serotonergic. However, the precise timing of cholinergic innervation in the rabbit still is uncertain, although it is likely that a more sensitive parameter, such as CAT activity or high-affinity choline uptake, would reveal it to be present at a time still earlier than 17 days.

Some observations have been made on the developing enteric innervation of guinea pigs (Gintzler and Gershon, unpublished observations). Guinea pigs are interesting because of their long period of gestation (approximately 72 days). This prolongs development and permits events to be distinguished that occur close to one another in time, and for this reason are difficult to resolve in animals with short periods of gestation. These studies are in progress, and the earliest appearance of the various neurons has not yet been ascertained. However, specific uptake of ^{3}H-5-HT was detected radioautographically in the guinea pig small intestine in 32-day embryos, and ^{3}H-ACh was found to be synthesized from ^{3}H-choline (1 μM) in 35-day embryos. Again, these times denote limits, and earlier times have not yet been examined. In contrast, the adrenergic innervation could not be detected until day 48 (by radioautography with ^{3}H-NE). Functional parameters, as expected, developed later than the time of detection of the various nerve fiber types. Stimulation of ganglia by 5-HT could be demonstrated at 42 days of gestation (5-HT produced a tetrodotoxin-sensitive relaxation); cholinergic enteric excitation appeared at 55 days of gestation. By day 55, but not before, the gut could also be relaxed by NE. Thus these preliminary studies again reveal the early development of the cholinergic and serotonergic innervations and the much later appearance of the adrenergic.

In human and rat embryos, the ingrowth of the cholinergic innervation once more appears to precede the ingrowth of the adrenergic innervation (Cantino, 1970; Read and Burnstock, 1970; Shvalev, Reidler, and Mingazova, 1972). In the rat the cholinergic innervation appears first in the stomach and terminal intestine and then merges to fill in the intervening areas. It should be pointed out again that this pattern is not compatible with the idea, referred to earlier (Okamoto and Ueda, 1967; Webster, 1973), of a proximodistal migration of ganglionic precursors derived exclusively from vagal neural crest. It is interesting that in rat and mouse intestines at day 12, a time when early cholinergic innervation is becoming established, adrenergic cells appear and then disappear at about day 15 from the gut wall (Cochard, Goldstein, and Black, 1978; Teitelman, Joh, and Reis, 1978). These cells contain tyrosine hydroxylase, dopamine beta-hydroxylase, and catecholamine. The mature pattern of adrenergic innervation is not seen in rat gut until after 18 days of gestation (Read and Burnstock, 1969; de Champlain et al., 1970).

In the mouse, in a strain similar to the lethal spotted mutant but lacking the gene for megacolon (Rothman and Gershon, unpublished observations), ^{3}H-ACh was synthesized from ^{3}H-choline (1 μM) in both small and large intestines of 14-day-old embryos. Earlier ages have not yet been examined. Following this early detection, ACh biosynthesis increased rapidly. The serotonergic innervation was detected by radioautography at day 14 in the small intestine but was questionable at this time in the colon.

In summary, a repeating sequential pattern of innervation appears to be emerging in which the enteric cholinergic and serotonergic neurons develop early and the adrenergic innervation appears late. This sequential pattern of development seems to be the same in a variety of animals. In the chick the cholinergic neurons definitely develop first. Which neuron develops first still needs to be established in mammals. It is interesting that the early development of the enteric serotonergic innervation is paralleled by the similarly early development of the serotonergic neurons of the CNS (Olson and Seiger, 1972; Lauder and Bloom, 1974).

The early ontogenetic development of the enteric serotonergic innervation is also reflected in the phylogenetic distribution of this system.

Serotonergic neurons have been detected in both classes of cyclostomes, lampreys (Baumgarten et al., 1973a), and hagfish (Goodrich and Gershon, 1978). They are also present in teleosts and amphibians (Goodrich et al., 1980), as well as birds and mammals. Therefore, the enteric serotonergic innervation appears to have arisen early in vertebrate evolution and to have been retained. This indicates that the serotonergic neurons are probably important to enteric function.

The peptidergic neurons appear to develop even later than the three types discussed above. In the mouse, immunoreactive nerves for substance P do not appear in the gut wall until 4 days after birth (Sundler et al., 1977). In the rat, substance P and VIP-immunoreactive nerves have been seen in the stomach for the first time 5–6 days after birth (Larsson, 1977), and substance P has been found 1–2 days after birth in the duodenum. Therefore it seems likely that the peptidergic neurons—which, like the cholinergic and serotonergic neurons, are intrinsic—nevertheless develop long after the cholinergic and serotonergic innervations have become established. It is of great interest that the peptidergic neurons can first be detected long after the migration of neural crest has been completed and long after recognizable neurons form enteric plexuses. This suggests either that nonrecognizable precursors are present in the gut at birth and develop into peptidergic neurons or that a preexisting neuron may change its transmitter or acquire a peptide in addition to its first transmitter substance. (Substance P has been found to coexist with 5-HT in CNS neurons [Chan-Palay, Jonsson, and Palay, 1978] and somatostatin to coexist with NE in peripheral sympathetic neurons [Hokfelt et al., 1977a]). In either case a role is implied for the enteric microenvironment in the differentiation of these neurons.

VI. NEURON AND TARGET INTERACTIONS DURING DEVELOPMENT

It seems clear from the work outlined above that the target tissue can have a profound effect on development, particularly the transmitter choice of neurons. However, very little is known about how this effect is mediated. Neuron–target tissue interactions other than those involved in neurotransmission are not well understood.

One observation that has excited several investigators has been the discovery of compounds that function as adult-animal neurotransmitters in early embryos prior to the development of the nervous system. Thus, for example, 5-HT and ACh have been found within early sea urchin embryos (Buznikov, Chudakova, and Zvezdina, 1964; Buznikov et al., 1968; Buznikov et al., 1972). This has suggested to some a role for these substances in early embryogenesis distinct from their role in neurotransmission (Buznikov et al., 1972; Gustafson and Toneby, 1970, 1971; Gustafson, Lundgren, and Treufeldt, 1972a; Gustafson, Ryberg, and Treufeldt, 1972b). In recent investigations of echinoderm embryos 5-HT has been found, and the occurrence of 5-HT correlates in time with the development of neurons (Toneby, 1977). Therefore, a role of neurotransmitters as growth factors (Ahmad and Zamenhof, 1978) has been sought. The evidence favoring such a role remains fragmentary at best, but intriguing suggestive information has emerged.

The early appearance of 5-HT, for example, in the embryos of prevertebrate species is complemented by the early appearance of 5-HT and catecholamines in vertebrate ontogeny. In the rat, catecholamines and 5-HT have been reported in the ovum prior to and during cleavage (Burden and Lawrence, 1973). In the chick brain, NE and dopamine have been reported at 8–10 days of incubation and 5-HT at days 7–13 (Bourne, 1965; Eiduson, 1966; Kellog, Vernadakis, and Rutledge, 1971; Suzuki, Nagose, and Yagi, 1975; Vernadakis, 1973). The pattern of early development of the monoamines and especially 5-HT is repeated in the rat brain. These studies have been reviewed by Lavier, Dunn, and Van Hartesveldt (1966). It seems clear that in a variety of species, neurotransmitter substances appear early in the life of the embryo. There appear to be two precocious phases of neurotransmitter substance development. One is a preneural phase found in very early embryos prior to organogenesis. The other is a preneurotransmission phase, occurring early in the life of developing neuroblasts.

Both of these phases have stimulated experimental work. However, the second phase has attracted the most attention from neurobiologists. The argument that neurotransmitters, synthesized and stored prior to the onset of neurotransmission, must have a function other than that of serving as the neurotransmitter has proven attractive. In particular, the presence of NE, DA, and 5-HT in the respective migrating neuroblasts in both central (Golden, 1973; Lauder, Krebs, and Bloom, 1974; Tennyson, Mytilneou, and Barrett, 1973) and peripheral nervous systems (Enemar et al., 1965; Rothman, Gershon, and Holtzer, 1978) has suggested a role for these substances in the establishment of neuronal connections. This role has never been proven, but the presence of the neurotransmitter substances is *compatible* with hypotheses that the substances contribute to the microenvironment of the regions in which the migratory neuroblasts ultimately come to reside.

Experimental work supporting these hypotheses is scant and recent, but some does exist. For example, 5-HT has been shown to be able to alter growth patterns of the brain in developing chick embryos. Ahmad and Zamenhof (1978) have reported that infusion of 5-HT, but not of DA or NE, into 7-day chick eggs increased cerebral weights and optic lobe weights as well as brain 5-HT. They also reported that increasing the temperature of incubation, a procedure that elevates brain 5-HT, has the same effect as infusing the amine. They concluded, "5-HT may be a growth promoting or regulating factor for embryonal brain."

The converse of these experiments, that is, the depletion of 5-HT from developing animals, has also been examined and found to affect brain embryogenesis. In this case, Lauder and Krebs (1978a, b) depleted 5-HT by injection of the inhibitor of 5-HT's biosynthesis, parachlorophenylalanine (PCPA), into pregnant rats. They found that PCPA altered the times when the neuroblasts in various brain regions ceased proliferating. Moreover, the regions affected were those that receive a 5-HT innervation. They therefore propose 5-HT as a "differentiation signal" and equate withdrawal of neuroblasts from the cell cycle with differentiation. These experiments, of course, are open to criticism because of the relative nonspecificity of the methods employed, injection of 5-HT into a mother, and administration of PCPA to pregnant rats, in which one might envisage a whole host of alternative explanations than the authors' for the observed findings. Nevertheless, the experiments are suggestive and do indicate that a role for the monoamines, such as 5-HT, in neuronal development merits continued exploration.

Considerable work has been done attempting to modify monoaminergic neurons at later stages of development, after the cessation of neuroblast division and migration and the extension of monoaminergic axons. This work, designed to evaluate the plasticity of young monoaminergic neurons in comparison to adult neurons, has used the selective neurotoxins 6-HD for catecholaminergic neurons and 5,7-DHT (in combination with desmethylimipramine) for serotonergic neurons (Sachs and Jonsson, 1975; Jonsson et al., 1978). These drugs have been given systemically to newborn animals when the blood-brain barrier to the compounds has not yet developed. The neurotoxins appear to be selectively concentrated in the respective neurons, and nonspecific cytotoxicity is avoided by such systemic administration. Under these conditions, the terminal arborizations of the monoaminergic neurons are destroyed, and this denervation of target areas seems permanent. However, a hyperinnervation by monoaminergic fibers ultimately develops in the regions of the cell bodies. This has been called a "pruning effect" (Schneider, 1973). These observations have led to the postulate that especially developing serotonergic neurons seem to be programmed to produce a certain quantity of terminal arborizations, which they "try" to conserve after injury to terminals, leading to the observed rearrangement of serotonergic axon terminals (Jonsson et al., 1978). Few effects were noted in these investigations with 5,7-DHT on other than serotonergic systems. However, the neurotoxins were administered relatively late in development, and sensitive techniques that might have revealed effects on neurons that depend on the 5-HT innervation were not used. Therefore, these experiments did not test a possible role for monoamines in early ontogeny.

Neurotransmitters might have a role in embryogenesis not only as indicated above, as growth factors, but in a more conventional sense as agents that contribute through their transmitter (or signalling) function to the stabilization of developing synapses. The formidable complexity of the vertebrate nervous system has indicated that "gene saving" mechanisms (Changeux and Danchin, 1976) must exist to govern the establishment of the adult patterns of connectivity. The number of connections seems to be too large for all the information to be coded in the genome. Several gene-saving theories of the development of neuronal connections exist. The theories attempt to explain development in ways that minimize the number of genes needed to govern specificity.

Sperry (1963) has proposed a chemoaffinity hypothesis in which growing nerve fibers bear chemical labels complementary to those of their neuronal target. This idea has been modified to include a graded affinity between axons and postsynaptic targets and a competition between ingrowing nerve terminals for targets (Gaze, 1974; Prestige, 1974). Temporal factors have also been shown to be important in establishing connections, making the timing of an axon's reaching its target a critical factor (Gaze, 1974; Jacobson, 1969). These ideas are all preformist (Changeux and Danchin, 1976) in that however they minimize the number of genes that are called into play, they assume that the neuronal network is specified before experience. The role of the environment would be limited to triggering preestablished programs and stabilizing the genetically specified synaptic organization.

An opposing view, that of empiricists (Changeux and Danchin, 1976), postulates that to a large extent the activity of a given neuronal system specifies its connectivity (Pettigrew, 1974; Rosenblatt, 1961). Changeux and Danchin (1976) have proposed a compromise view, which they call the selective stabilization hypothesis. They propose that the genetic program directs the proper interaction between main *categories* of neurons. However, during development within categories or sets of neurons, they conceive of a significant but limited redundancy or fluctuation of the connections—that is, several contacts may form at first but be lost. There may be an initial synaptic plasticity in which the early synapses are labile but become stable or regressed. The labile and stable states would transmit, but the regressed would not. An essential element of their theory is that the transitions from labile to stable or to regression are regulated by the *activity* of the postsynaptic cell, including the activity of the forming synapse. Therefore, the early role of monoamines in developing neurons could be in the selective stabilization process. The transmitter substances may develop precociously so that they can function in the critical period when a nerve terminal requires activity to become stable. If this hypothesis is correct, then it would follow that alteration of neurotransmitters or axons or the axon-target relationship early in development would profoundly affect the ultimate pattern of connections.

Certainly the establishment of connections is important in determining survival of presumptive neurons (Landmessar and Pilar, 1978). Critically timed interaction between neuron and target organ is necessary for full maturation and survival of presynaptic neurons. Cell death is an important feature of neuronal development and is increased by target organ removal (Cowan, 1973). Cell death does not occur because the dying neurons are grossly defective (Landmessar and Pilar, 1978), but rather appears to result from the failure of an interaction between the neuron and its peripheral target. The dying neurons appear to fail to compete effectively either for a limited number of synaptic sites or for a limited supply of a trophic factor. Therefore the precocious development of neurotransmitter substances, if these are important to synapse stabilization through activity, would be important to the final survival of the neuron.

In the sympathetic nervous system a trophic factor produced by target tissues has been identified: nerve growth factor (NGF). NGF can prevent the death of sympathetic ganglion cells (Hendry and Campbell, 1976) and can oppose some degenerative changes induced by axotomy (Hendry, 1975; Purves, 1976). Moreover, NGF is selectively taken up by sympathetic axon terminals and transported by retrograde transport to the sympathetic nerve cell body (Hendry, Stack, and Herrup, 1974; Stoekel and Thoenen, 1975).

Overproduction of presumptive neurons seems to be a common theme in vertebrate neural development (Landmessar and Pilar, 1978) and leads to a competition between neurons, discussed above, for specific targets. The function of this competition and all the factors that bring death to the losers have yet to be identified. However, the phenomenon must be considered in any study of neuronal development.

In addition to the above, the effect of presynaptic innervation in regulating the development of postsynaptic cells, an anterograde effect, must also be borne in mind as important to neuronal development. For example, transsynaptic regulation of the growth and development of adrenergic neurons has been elegantly demonstrated (Black, Hendry, and Iversen, 1971). In fact, the central nervous system participates through preganglionic activation in the regulation of sympathetic neuron development (Black, Bloom, and Hamill, 1976). Therefore, the activity of presynaptic neurons influences the development of the postsynaptic cells.

A. Sectional Summary

The interactions between neuron and target tissue in the development of each are not yet well understood. Monoamines and ACh appear early in embryological life, in some forms appearing before the development of the nervous system. Within neurons, they often appear before conventional neurotransmission is possible. Therefore, a role for these substances as growth factors has been sought. However, the precocious development of a neurotransmitter substance may also be related to the need for a neuron to compete effectively with other progenitor neurons. It is possible that early synapses must be active in order to avoid regression. In fact, early activity may be important to avoid cell death. In addition, the presynaptic innervation transynaptically influences the metabolism of developing postsynaptic cells. The early development of neurotransmitter substances may be related to this form of regulation. Certainly neuron-target interactions are vital in neuronal development. Neurotransmitter substances may be important and play a significant role in these interactions.

VII. SUMMARY AND CONCLUSION

We have developed the argument that the enteric nervous system merits a separate classification as a third autonomic division. Since many, if not most, of its intrinsic ganglion cells probably do not receive a preganglionic innervation from the craniosacral or thoracolumbar outflows that define the parasympathetic or sympathetic nervous systems, respectively; the enteric nervous system does not fall neatly into either of those well-recognized autonomic divisions. Moreover, the enteric nervous system also has numerous characteristics not found elsewhere in the PNS that serve to make it unique. These include an internal morphology that resembles the CNS; a barrier to the entrance into the system of small protein molecules; the presence of intrinsic primary afferent neurons, which permits the gut to manifest reflex activity *in vitro*; and an extraordinary degree of diversity in its intrinsic neurons and neurotransmitters. The origin in ontogeny of this last characteristic presents both a problem and an opportunity in developmental neurobiology. The problem is to explain how enteric neuronal diversity comes about. The opportunity is that it may be possible to do that.

Current ideas on the development of neurons, derived particularly from research on the ANS, including the enteric nervous system, emphasize the role of the microenvironment of the final site of neuronal residence in determining the ultimate neuronal choice of neurotransmitter. However, the neurotransmitter chosen by enteric neurons may be 5-HT, VIP, enkephalin, somatostatin, substance P, or even ATP, in addition to ACh. Therefore, the microenvironmental factors that induce a cholinergic neuron instead of an adrenergic neuron to form in the gut would not explain the full gamut of enteric neuronal diversity. Additional microenvironmental or other factors must be postulated to explain the formation of noncholinergic neurons. A clue to what these additional factors might be comes from emerging evidence suggesting that the various enteric neurons develop sequentially, with cholinergic and serotonergic neurons arising early in ontogeny and peptidergic and adrenergic innervation appearing late. This sequential formation, if it occurs, raises the possibility that neuronal interaction may be an important developmental determinant. A number of investigators have looked at neuronal interactions, neurotransmitters, and neuronal activity during development elsewhere in the nervous system; and these do appear to be important factors.

The gut has advantages for study. Developmental defects such as congenital aganglionosis may be studied and exploited. Moreover, enteric neurons are recognizable by their transmitter mechanisms, and the number of types of neuron is at least more limited in the gut than in the brain. Therefore, the enteric nervous system, the third autonomic division, may be a particularly valuable model system to use to study the development of a multiplicity of neurons from multipotential progenitor cells.

VIII. REFERENCES

Abel, W: The Development of the Autonomic Nerve Mechanism in the Alimentary Canal of the Chick. Proc R Soc Edinb 30(1909)327–247
Abel, W: Further Observations on the Development of the Sympathetic Nervous System in the Chick. J Anat 47(1912)35–72
Adamo, C.W.M.; Marples, E.A.; Trounce, J.R.: Achalasia of the Cardia and Hirschsprung's Disease: The Amount and Distribution of Cholinesterase. Clin Sci Mol Med (formerly Clin Sci) 19(1960)473–481
Adam-Vizi, V., Vizi, E.S.: Direct Evidence of Acetylcholine Releasing Effect of Serotonin in the Auerbach Plexus. J Neural Transm 42(1978)127–138
Aghajanian, G.K.; Asher, I.M.: Histochemical Fluorescence of Raphe Neurons: Selective Enhancement by Tryptophan. Science 172(1971)1159–1161
Aghajanian, G.K.; Kuhar, M.J.; Roth, R.H.: Serotonin Containing Neuronal Perikarya and Terminals: Differential Effects of p-Chlorophenylalamine. Brain Res 54(1973)85–101
Ahmad, G.; Zamenhof, S.: Serotonin as a Growth Factor for Chick Embryo Brain. Life Sci 22(1978)963–970
Albamus, L.: Central and Peripheral Effect of Anticholinergic Compounds. Acta Pharmacol Toxicol 28(1970)305–326
Aldridge, R.T.; Campbell, P.E.: Ganglion Cell Distribution in the Normal Rectum and Anal Canal. J Pediatr Surg 3(1968)475–490
Alexander, R.W.; Davis, J.N.; Lefkowitz, R.J.: Direct Identification and Characterization of B-Adrenergic Receptors in Rat Brain. Nature 258(1975)437–440
Andrew, A.: A Study of the Developmental Relationships between Enterochromaffin Cells and the Neural Crest. J Embryol Exp Morph 11(1963)307–324
Andrew, A.: The Origin of Intramural Ganglia. I. The Early Arrival of Precursor Cells in the Presumptive Gut of Chick Embryos. J Anat 98(1964)421–428
Andrew, A.: The Origin of Intramural Ganglia. II. The Trunk Neural Crest as a Source of Enteric Ganglia. J Anat 105(1969)89-101
Andrew, A.: The Origin of Intramural Ganglia. III. The 'Vagal' Source of Enteric Ganglion Cells. J Anat 107(1970)327–336
Andrew, A.: The Origin of Intramural Ganglia. IV. The Origin of Enteric Ganglia: a Critical Review and Discussion of the Present State of the Problem. J Anat 108(1971)169–184
Atlas, D.; Levitzki, A.: Probing B-Adrenergic Receptors by Novel Fluorescent B-Adrenergic Blockers. Proc Natl Acad Sci USA 74(1977)5290–5294
Atlas, D.; Segal, M.: Simultaneous Visualization of Noradrenergic Fibers and B-Adrenoceptors in Pre- and Postsynaptic Regions in the Rat Brain. Brain Res 135(1977)347–350

Baumgarten, H.G. Uber die Verteilung von Catecholaminen im darm des Menschen. Z Zellforsch Mikrosk Anat 83(1967)133–146

Baumgarten H.G.; Bjorklund, A.; Lachenmayer, L.; Nobin, A.; Rosengren, E.: Evidence for the Existence of Serotonin-, Dopamine- and Noradrenaline-Containing Neurons in the Gut of *Lampetra Fluviatilis*. *Z Zellforsch* Mikrosk Anat 141(1973a)33–54

Baumgarten, H.G.; Holstein, A.-F.; Owman, C.: Auerbach's Plexus of Mammals and Man: Electron Microscopic Identification of Three Different Types of Neuronal Processes in Myenteric Ganglia of the Large Intestine from Rhesus Monkeys, Guinea Pigs and Man. Z Zellforsch Mikrosk Anat 106(1970)376–397

Baumgarten, H.G.; Holstein, A.F.; Stelzner, F.: Nervous Elements in the Human Colon of Hirschsprung's Disease. (With Comparative Remarks on Neuronal Profiles in the Normal Human and Monkey Colon and Sphincter ani Internus). Virchows Arch Pathol Anat 358(1973b)113–136

Bayliss, W.M.; Starling, E.H.: The Movements and Innervation of the Small Intestine. J Physiol (Lond) 24(1899)99–143

Bayliss, W.M.; Starling, E.H.: The Movements and Innervation of the Large Intestine. J Physiol (Lond) 26(1900)107–118

Bayliss, W.M.; Starling, E.H.: The Movements and Innervation of the Small Intestine. J Physiol (Lond) 26(1901)125–138

Bennett, T., Cobb, J.L.S.: Studies on the Avian Gizzard: the Development of the Gizzard and Its Innervation. *Z Zellforsch* Mikrosk Anat 98(1969)599–621

Bianchi, C.; Beani, L.; Crema, C.: Effects of Metoclopramide on Isolated Guinea Pig Colon. 2) Interference with Ganglionic Stimulant Drugs. Eur J Pharmacol 12(1970)332–341

Bianchi, C.; Beani, L.; Frigo, G.M.; Crema, A.: Further Evidence for the Presence of Non-Adrenergic Inhibitory Structures in the Guinea Pig Colon. Eur J Pharmacol 4(1968)51–61

Bielschowsky, M.; Schofield, G.C.: Studies on the Inheritance and Neurohistology of Megacolon in Mice. Proc Univ Otago Med School 38(1960)14

Bielschowsky, M.; Schofield, G.C.: Studies of Megacolon in Piebald Mice. Austral J Exp Biol 40(1962)395–404

Black, I.B.; Bloom, E.M.; Hamill, R.W.: Central Regulation of Sympathetic Neuron Development. Proc Natl Acad Sci USA 73(1976)3575–3578

Black, I.B.; Hendry, I.A.; Iversen, L.L.: Trans-Synaptic Regulation of Growth and Development of Adrenergic Neurones in a Mouse Sympathetic Ganglion. Brain Res 34(1971) 229–240

Bloom, F.E.: Ultrastructural Identification of Catecholamine Containing Central Synaptic Terminals. J Histochem Cytochem 21(1973)333–348

Bloom, F.E., Battenberg, E.L.F.: A Rapid Simple and Sensitive Method for the Demonstration of Central Catecholamine-Containing Neurons and Axons by Glyoxylic Acid Induced Fluorescence. J Histochem Cytochem 24(1976)561–571

Bodian, M.: Chronic Constipation in Children, with Particular Reference to Hirschsprung's Disease. Practitioner 169(1952)517

Bodian, M.; Carter, C.O.: A Family Study of Hirschsprung's Disease. Ann Hum Genet 26(1963)261–277

Bodian, M.; Stephens, F.D.; Ward, B.C.H.: Hirschsprung's Disease and Idiopathic Megacolon. Lancet 1(1949)6–11

Bolande, R.P.: Animal Model of Human Disease. Hirschsprung's Disease, Aganglionic and Hypoganglionic Megacolon; Animal Model: Aganglionic Megacolon in Piebald and Spotted Mutant Mouse Strains. Am J Pathol 79(1975)189–192

Bolande, R.P.; Towler, W.F.: Ultrastructural and Histochemical Studies of Murine Megacolon. Am J Pathol 69(1972)139–154

Boley, S.J.: The Pathophysiology of Hirschsprung's Disease—a Continuing Search. J Pediatr Surg 10(1975)861–863

Bourne, B.B.: Metabolism of Amines in the Brain of the Chick During Embryonic Development. Life Sci 4(1965)583–591

Brown, E.M.; Aurbach, G.D.; Hauser, D.; Troxler, F.: B-Adrenergic Receptor Interactions: Characterization of Iodohydroxybenzylpindolol as a Specific Ligand. J Biol Chem 51(1976)1232–1238

Brownlee, G.; Johnson, E.S.: The Site of the 5-Hydroxytryptamine Receptor on the Intramural Nervous Plexus of the Guinea-Pig Isolated Ileum. Br J Pharmacol 21(1963)306–322

Bryant, M.D.; Polak, J.M.; Modlin, I.; Bloom, S.R.; Alburquerque, R.H.; Pearse, A.G.E.: Possible Dual Role of Vasoactive Intestinal Peptide as Gastrointestinal Hormone and Neurotransmitter Substance. Lancet 1(1976)991–993

Bulbring, E.; Crema, A.: Observations Concerning the Action of 5-Hydroxytryptamine on the Peristaltic Reflex. Br J Pharmacol Chemother 13(1958)444–457

Bulbring, E.; Gershon, M.D.: 5-Hydroxytryptamine Participation in the Vagal Inhibitory Innervation of the Stomach. J Physiol (Lond) 192(1967)823–846

Bulbring, E.; Lin, R.C.Y.: The Effect of Intraluminal Application of 5-Hydroxytryptamine and 5-Hydroxytryptophan on Peristalsis, the Local Production of 5-Hydroxytryptamine and Its Release in Relation to Intraluminal Pressure and Propulsive Activity. J Physiol (Lond) 140(1958)381–407

Bulbring, E.; Lin, R.C.Y.; Schofield, G.: An Investigation of the Peristaltic Reflex in Relation to Anatomical Observations. J Exp Physiol 43(1958)26–37

Bunge, R.; Johnson, M.; Ross, C.D.: Nature and Nurture in Development of the Autonomic Neuron. Science 199(1978)1409–1416

Burden, H.W.; Lawrence, I.E., Jr.: Presence of Biogenic Amines in Early Rat Development. Am J Anat 136(1973)251–257

Burn, J.H.: The Development of the Adrenergic Fibre. Br J Pharmacol 32(1968)575–582

Burnstock, G.: Purinergic Nerves. Pharmacol Rev 24(1972)509–581

Burnstock, G.; Campbell, G.; Rand, M.J.: The Inhibitory Innervation of the Taenia of the Guinea-Pig Caecum. J Physiol (Lond) 182(1966)504–526

Bursztajn, S.; Gershon, M.D.: Discrimination between Nicotine Receptors in Vertebrate Ganglia and Skeletal Muscle by Alpha-Bungarotoxin and Cobra Venoms. J Physiol (Lond) 269(1977)17–31

Buznikov, G.A.; Chudakova, I.V.; Berdysheva, L.V.; Vyazmina, N.M.: The Role of Neurohumours in Embryongenesis. II. Acetylcholine and Catecholamine Content in Developing Embryo of Sea Urchin. J Embryol Exp Morphol 20(1968)119–128

Buznikov, G.A.; Chudakova, I.V.; Zvezdina, N.D.: The Role of Neurohumours in Early Embryogenesis. I. Serotonin Content of Developing Embryos of Sea Urchin and Loach. J Embryol Exp Morphol 12(1964)563–573

Buznikov, G.A.; Sakharova, A.V.; Manukhin, B.N.; Markova, L.N.: The Role of Neurohumours in Early Embryogenesis. J Embryol Exp Morphol 27(1972)339–351

Bylund, D.B.; Charness, M.E.; Snyder, S.H.: Beta Adrenergic Receptor Labeling in Intact Animals with ^{125}I-Hydroxybenzylpinodol. J Pharmacol Exp Ther 201(1977)644–653

Campbell, G.: The Inhibitory Nerve Fibers in the Vagal Supply to the Guinea Pig Stomach. J Physiol (Lond) 185(1966)600–612

Campbell, G.: Autonomic Nervous System to Effector Tissues. In: Smooth Muscle, pp. 451–495, ed. by E. Bulbring, A. Brading, A. W. Jones, T. Tomita. London, Edward Arnold, 1970

Campbell, P.E.; Noblett, H.R.: Experience with Rectal Suction Biopsy in the Diagnosis of Hirschsprung's Disease. J Pediatr Surg 4(1969)410–415

Camus, R. Uber die Entwicklung des sympathischen Nervensystems beim Frosch. Arch Mikr Anat. Entw Mech 81(1921)1–52 (Quoted in: Van Campenhout, 1932)

Cannon, W.B. Law of Denervation. Am J Med Sci 198(1939)737–750

Cantino, D.: An Histochemical Study of the Nerve Supply to the Developing Alimentary Tract. Experientia 26(1970)766–767

Champlain, de, J.; Malmfors, T.; Olson, L.; Sachs, C.: Ontogenesis of Peripheral Adrenergic Neurons in the Rat: Pre and Postnatal Observations. Acta Physiol Scand 80(1970)276–288

Changeaux, J.-P., Danchin, A.: Selective Stabilisation of Developing Synapses as a Mechanism for the Specification of Neuronal Networks. Nature 264(1976)705–712

Chan-Palay, V. Fine Structure of Labelled Axons in the Cerebellar Cortex and Nuclei of Rodents and Primates after Intraventricular Infusions with Tritiated Serotonin. Anat Embryol 148(1975)235–265

Chan-Palay, V.; Jonsson, G.; Palay, S.L.: Serotonin and Substance P Coexist in Neurons of the Rat's Central Nervous System. Proc Natl Acad Sci USA 75(1978)1582–1586

Cobb, J.L.S.; Bennett, T.: An Electron Microscopic Examination of the Short Term Effects of

6-Hydroxydopamine on the Peripheral Adrenergic Nervous System. In: *6-Hydroxydopamine and Catecholamine Neurons*, pp. 33–45, ed. by T. Malmfors, H. Thoenen. American Elsevier, New York, 1971

Cochard, P.; Goldstein, M.; Black, I.B.: Ontogenetic Appearance and Disappearance of Tyrosine Hydroxylase and Catecholamines in the Rat Embryo. Proc Natl Acad Sci USA 75(1978)2986–2990

Cohen, A.M.: Factors Directing the Expression of Sympathetic Nerve Traits in Cells of Neural Crest Origin. J Exp Zool 179(1972)169–182

Cohen, A.M.: Independent Expression of the Adrenergic Phenotype by Neural Crest Cells in Vitro. Proc Natl Acad Sci USA 74(1977)2899–2903

Cook, R.D.; Burnstock, G.: The Ultrastructure of Auerbach's Plexus in the Guinea Pig. I. Neuronal Elements. J Neurocytol 5(1976a)171–194

Cook, R.D.; Burnstock, G.: The Ultrastructure of Auerbach's Plexus in the Guinea Pig. II. Non-Neuronal Elements. J Neurocytol 5(1976b)195–206

Cook, R.D.; and Peterson, E.R.: The Growth of Smooth Muscle and Sympathetic Ganglia in Organotypic Cultures. Light and electron microscopy. J Neurol Sci 22(1974)25–38

Costa, M.; and Gabella, G.: Adrenergic Innervation of the Alimentary Canal. Z Zellforsch Mikrosk Anat 122(1971)357–377

Cowan, W.M.: Neuronal Death as a Regulative Mechanism in Control of Cell Number in the Nervous System. In: *Development and Ageing in the Nervous System*, pp. 19–41, ed. by M. Rockstein. Academic, New York, 1973

Dajani, E.Z.; Roge, E.A.W.; Bertermann, R.E.: Effects of E Prostaglandins, Diphenoxylate and Morphine on Intestinal Motility in-vivo. Eur J Pharmacol 34(1975)105–113

Dale, H.H.: Acetylcholine as a Chemical Transmitter of the Effects of Nerve Impulses. I. History of Ideas and Evidence. Peripheral Autonomic Actions. Functional Nomenclature of Nerve Fibers. J Mt Sinai Hosp 4(1937a)401–415

Dale, H.H.: Acetylcholine as a Chemical Transmitter of the Effects of Nerve Impulses. II. Chemical Transmission at Ganglionic Synapses and Voluntary Motor Nerve Endings, Some General Considerations. J Mt Sinai Hosp 4(1937b)416–429

Dereymaeker, A.: Recherches Experimentales sur l'origine du système nerveux enterique chez l'embryon de poulet. Arch Biol (Paris) 54(1943)359–375

Derrick, E.H.; St. George-Grambauer, Megacolon in Mice. J Pathol (formerly J Pathol Bacteriol) 73(1957)569–571

Descarries, L.; Beaudet, A.; Watkins, K.C.: Serotonin Nerve Terminals in Adult Rat Neocortex. Brain Res., 100(1975)563–588

Dingledine, R.; Goldstein, A.; Kendig, V.: Effects of Narcotic Opiates and Serotonin on the Electrical Behavior of Neurons in the Guinea Pig Myenteric Plexus. Life Sci 14 (1974)2299–2309

Dobbins, W.O., III; Bill, A.H., Jr.: Diagnosis of Hirschsprung's Disease Excluded by Rectal Suction Biopsy. N Engl J Med 200(1965)990

Drakontides, A.B., Gershon, M.D.: Studies of the Interaction of 5-Hydroxytryptamine and the Perivascular Innervation of the Guinea Pig Caecum. Br J Pharmacol 45(1972)417–434

Dreyfus, C.F.; Bornstein, M.B.; Gershon, M.D.: Synthesis of Serotonin by Neurons of the Myenteric Plexus *in-situ* and in Organotypic Tissue Culture. Brain Res 128(1977a)125–139

Dreyfus, C.F.; Gershon, M.D.; Crain, S.M.: Innervation of Hippocampal Explants by Central Catecholaminergic Neurons in Co-Cultured Fetal Mouse Brain Stem Explants. Brain Res 168(1978)431–445

Dreyfus, C.F.; Sherman, D.L.; and Gershon, M.D.: Uptake of Serotonin by Intrinsic Neurons of the Myenteric Plexus Grown in Organotypic Tissue Culture. Brain Res 128(1977b)109–123

Ehrenpreis, T.: Some Newer Aspects of Hirschsprung's Disease. J Pediatr Surg 1(1966)329–337

Eiduson, S.: 5-Hydroxytryptamine in the Developing Chick Brain: Its Normal and Altered Development and Possible Control by End-Product Repression. J Neurochem 13(1966) 923–932

Elde, R.; Hokfelt, T.; Johansson, O.; Terenius, L.: Immunohistochemical Studies Using Antibodies to Leucine Enkephalin: Initial Observations on the Central Nervous System of the Rat. Neuroscience 1(1976)349–351

Enemar, A.; Falck, B.; Hakanson, R.: Observations on the Appearance of Norepinephrine in the Sympathetic Nervous System of the Chick Embryo. Dev Biol 11(1965)268–283

Epstein, M.L.; Gershon, M.D.: Development of Monoaminergic Neurons in the Enteric Nervous System of the Chick Embryo. Neurol Sci Abst 4(1978)271

Eranko, O.; Eranko, L.: Loss of Histochemically Demonstrable Catecholamine and Acetylcholinesterase from Sympathetic Nerve Fibers of the Pineal Body of the Rat after Chemical Sympathectomy with 6-Hydroxydopamine. Histochem J 3(1971)357–363

Erspamer, V.: Occurrence of Indolealkylamines in Nature. V. Erspamer, ed. In: *Handbuch der experimentellen Pharmakologie.* XIX. 5-Hydroxytryptamine and Related Indolealkylamines, pp. 132–181, ed. by V. Erspamer. Springer, New York, 1966

Falck, B.; Hillarp, N.-A.; Thieme, G.; Torp, A.: Fluorescence of Catecholamines and Related Compounds Condensed with Formaldehyde. J Histochem Cytochem 10(1962)348–354

Fonnum, F.: Radiochemical Microassays for the Determination of Choline Acetyltransferase and Acetylcholinesterase Activities. Biochem J 115(1969)465–472

Furness, J.B.; and Costa, M.: The Nervous Release and the Actions of Substances Which Affect Intestinal Muscle through neither Adrenoreceptors nor Cholinoreceptors. Philos Trans R Soc Lond (Biol) 265(1973)123–133

Fuxe, K.; Hokfelt, T.; Said, S.I.; Mutt, V.: Vasoactive Intestinal Polypeptide and the Nervous System: Immunohistochemical Evidence for Localization in Central and Peripheral Neurons, Particularly Intracortical Neurons of the Cerebral Cortex. Neurosci Lett 5(1977)241–246

Gabella, G.: Glial Cells in the Myenteric Plexus. Z Naturforsch 26B(1971)244–245

Gabella, G.: Fine Structure of the Myenteric Plexus in the Guinea Pig Ileum. J Anat 111(1972)69–97

Gaddum, J.H.: Tryptamine Receptors. J Physiol (Lond) 119(1953)363–368

Gaddum, J.H.; Picarelli, Z.P.: Two Kinds of Tryptamine Receptors. Br J Pharmacol 12(1957)323–328

Gannon, B.J.; Noblett, H.R.; Burnstock, G.: Adrenergic Innervation of Bowel in Hirschsprung's Disease. Br Med J 3(1969)338–340

Garret, J.R.; Howard, E.R.; Nixon, H.H.: Autonomic Nerves in Rectum and Colon in Hirschsprung's Disease. Arch Dis Child 44(1969)406–417

Gaze, R.M.: Neuronal specificity. In: Development and Regeneration in the Nervous System. Br Med Bull 30(1974)116–121

Gershon, M.D.: Effects of Tetrodotoxin on Innervated Smooth Muscle Preparations. Br J Pharmacol 29(1967a)259–279

Gershon, M.D.: Inhibition of Gastrointestinal Movement by Sympathetic Nerve Stimulation: The Site of Action. J Physiol (Lond) 189(1967b)317–327

Gershon, M.D.: Serotonin and the Motility of the Gastrointestinal Tract. Gastroenterology 54(1968)453–456

Gershon, M.D.; Altman, R.F.: An Analysis of the Uptake of 5-Hydroxytryptamine by the Myenteric Plexus of the Small Intestine of the Guinea Pig. J Pharmacol Exp Ther 179(1971)29–41

Gershon, M.D.; Bursztajn, S.: Properties of the Enteric Nervous System: Limitation of Access of Intravascular Macromolecules to the Myenteric Plexus and Muscularis Externa. J Comp Neurol 180(1978)467–487

Gershon, M.D.; Dreyfus, C.F.; Pickel, V.M.; Joh, T.H.; Reis, D.J.: Serotonergic Neurons in the Peripheral Nervous System: Identification in Gut by Immunohistochemical Localization of Tryptophan Hydroxylase. Proc Natl Acad Sci USA 74(1977)3086–3089

Gershon, M.D.; Vonakait, G.M.: Uptake and Release of 5-Hydroxytryptamine by Enteric 5-Hydroxytryptaminergic Neurones: Effects of Fluoxetine (Lilly 110140) and Chlorimipramine Br J Pharmacol 66(1979)7–9

Gershon, M.D.; Robinson, R.G.; Ross, L.L.: Serotonin Accumulation in the Guinea Pig's Myenteric Plexus: Ion Dependence, Structure Activity Relationship, and the Effect of Drugs. J Pharmacol Exp Ther 198(1976)548–561

Gershon, M.D.; Ross, L.L.: Radioisotopic studies of the binding, exchange, and distribution of 5-hydroxytryptamine synthesized from its radioactive precursor. J Physiol 186(1966a)451–476

Gershon, M.D.; Ross, L.L.: Location of sites of 5-hydroxytryptamine storage and metabolism by radioautography. J Physiol 186(1966b)477–492

Gershon, M.D.; Thompson, E.B.: The Maturation of Neuromuscular Function in a Multiply Innervated Structure: Development of the Longitudinal Smooth Muscle of the Foetal Mammalian Gut and Its Cholinergic Excitatory, Adrenergic Inhibitory, and Non-Adrenergic Inhibitory Innervation. J Physiol (Lond) 234(1973)257–278

Golden, S.F.: Prenatal Development of Biogenic Amine Systems of the Mouse Brain. Dev Biol 33(1973)300–311

Goodrich, J.T.; Bernd, P.; Sherman, D.; Gershon, M.D.: Phylogeny of Enteric Serotonergic Neurons. J. Comp. Neurol (1980) in press.

Goodrich, J.T.; Gershon, M.D.: Serotonergic Neurons in the Enteric Nervous System of Humans and Subhuman Primates. In: Proceedings of the International Union of Physiological Sciences, Vol. XIII, p. 2173. Paris, 1977

Goodrich, J.T.; Gershon, M.D.: Phylogeny of Enteric Serotonergic Neurons. Neurol Sci Abst 4(1978)99

Goormaghtigh, N.: L'origine du système nerveux sympathique des oiseaux. C R Ass Anat Strasbourg, 19e reunion, (1924)149–152 (Quoted in: Van Campenhout, 1932).

Gunn, M.: Cholinergic Mechanisms in the Gastrointestinal Tract. J Neuro-Visceral Relations 32(1971)224–240

Gustafson, T.; Lundgren, B.; Treufeld, R.: Serotonin and Contractile Activity in the Ecinopluteus. Acta Embryol Exp 2(1972a)115–139

Gustafson, T.; Ryberg, E.; Treufeldt, R.: Acetylcholine and Contractile Activity in the Echinopluteus. Acta Embryol Exp 2(1972b)199–223

Gustafson, T.; Toneby, M.: On the role of serotonin and acetylcholine in sea urchin morphogeneis. Exp Cell Res 62(1970)102–117

Gustafson, T.; Toneby, M.: How genes control morphogenesis. Am Scient 59(1971)452–462

Hammond, W.S.; Yntema, C.L.: Depletion of the Thoraco-Lumbar Sympathetic System Following Removal of Neural Crest in the Chick. J Comp Neurol 86(1947)237–265

Hendry, I.A.: The Response of Adrenergic Neurones to Axotomy and Nerve Growth Factor. Brain Res 94(1975)87–97

Hendry, I.A.; Campbell, J.: Morphometric Analysis of Rat Superior Cervical Ganglion after Axotomy and Nerve Growth Factor Treatment. J Neurocytol 5(1976)351–360

Hendry, I.A.; Stach, R.; Herrup, K.: Characteristics of the Retrograde Axonal Transport System for Nerve Growth Factor in the Sympathetic System. Brain Res 82(1974)117–128

Hirst, G.D.S.; and McKirdy, H.C.: Synaptic Potentials Recorded from Neurons of the Submucous Plexus of Guinea-Pig Small Intestine. J Physiol (Lond) 249(1975)369–385

Hirst, G.D.S.; Silinsky, E.M.: Some Effects of 5-Hydroxytryptamine, Dopamine and Noradrenaline on Neurons in the Submucous Plexus of Guinea-Pig Small Intestine. J Physiol (Lond) 251(1975)817–832

Hokfelt, T.: Ultrastructural Localization of Intraneuronal Monoamines. Some Aspects of Methodology. In: Progress in Brain Research. Vol. 34, Histochemistry of Nervous Transmission, pp. 213–222, ed. by O. Eranko. Elsevier, New York, 1971

Hokfelt, T.; Elfvin, L.-G.; Elde, R.; Schultzberg, M.; Goldstein, M.; Luft, R.: Occurrence of Somatostatin-Like Immunoreactivity in Some Peripheral Sympathetic Noradrenergic Neurons. Proc Natl Acad Sci USA 74(1977a)3587–3591

Hokfelt, T.; Johannson, O.; Efendic, S.; Luft, R.; and Arimura, A.: Are there Somatostatin-Containing Nerves in the Rat Gut? Immunohistochemical Evidence for a New Type of Peripheral Nerve. Experientia 31(1975)852–854

Hokfelt, T.; Johannson, O.; Kellerth, J.-O.; Ljungdahl, A.; Nilsson, G.; Nygards, A.; Pernow, B.: Immunohistochemical Distribution of Substance P. In: Substance P Nobel Symposium. Vol. 37, pp. 117–145, ed. by U.S. von Euler, B. Pernow. Raven, New York, 1977b

Hokfelt, T.; Kellerth, J.O.; Nelson, G.; Pernow, B.: Substance P: Localization in the Central Nervous System and in Some Primary Sensory Neurons. Science 190(1974)889–890

Hughes, J.: Isolation of an Endogenous Compound from the Brain with Pharmacological Properties Similar to Morphine. Brain Res 88(1975)295–308

Hukuhara, T.; Kotani, S.; Sato, G.: Effects of Destruction of Intramural Ganglion Cells on Colon Motility: Possible Genesis of Congenital Megacolon. Jpn J Physiol 11(1961)635–640

Huther, W.: Die Hirschsprung' sache Krankheit als Forge einer Entwicklungsstorung der intramuralen Ganglien. Beitr Pathol (formerly Beitr Pathol Anat) 114(1954)161–191

Imamura, K.; Yamamoto, M.; Sato, A.; Kashiki, Y.; Tokuro, K.: An Experimental Study on Agangliosis Produced by a New Method in the Rat. J Pediatr Surg 10(1975)865–873

Irwin, D.A.; The Anatomy of the Auerbach's Plexus. Am J Anat 49(1931)141–166

Jacobowitz, D.: Histochemical Studies of the Autonomic Innervation of the Gut. J Pharmacol Exp Ther 149(1965)358–364

Jacobson, M.: Development of Specific Neuronal Connections. Science 163(1969)543–547

Johnson, M.; Ross, D.; Meyers, M.; Rees, R.; and Bunge, R.: Synaptic Vesicle Cytochemistry Changes When Cultured Sympathetic Neurones Develop Cholinergic Interactions. Nature 262(1976)308–310

Jonakait, G.M.; Gershon, M.D.: Concentration of Serotonin and Tryptophan in Synaptosomes Derived from a Peripheral Serotonergic Neuron. Neurosci Abst 2(1976)467

Jonakait, G.M.; Gintzler, A.R.; and Gershon, M.D.: Isolation of Axonal Varicosities (Autonomic Synaptosomes) from the Enteric Nervous System. J Neurochem 32(1979)1387–1400

Jonakait, G.M.; Tamir, H.; Gintzler, A.R.; and Gershon, M.D.: Release of Serotonin and Its Binding Protein from Enteric Neurons. Int Cong Pharmacol Abst 7(1978)737

Jonakait, G.M.; Tamir, H.; Rapport, M.M.; and Gershon, M.D.: Detection of a Soluble Serotonin Binding Protein in the Mammalian Myenteric Plexus and Other Peripheral Sites of Serotonin Storage. J Neurochem 28(1977)277–284

Jones, D.S. The Origin of the Vagi and Parasympathetic Ganglion Cells of the Viscera of the Chick. Anat Rec 82(1942)185–197

Jonsson, G.; Pollare, T.; Hallman, H.; Sachs, Ch.: Developmental Plasticity of Central Serotonin Neurons after 5,7-Dihydroxytryptamine Treatment. In: Serotonin Neurotoxins, Annals of the New York Academy of Sciences, Vol. 305, pp. 328–345, ed. by J.H. Jacoby, L.D. Lytle. New York Acad. Sci. New York, 1978.

Kadair, R.G.; Sims, J.E.; Critchfield, C.F.: Zonal Colonic Hypoganglionosis. JAMA 238(1977)1838–1840

Kamijo, K.; Hiatt, R.B.; Koelle, G.B.: Congenital Megacolon. A Comparison of the Spastic and Hypertrophied Segments with Respect to Cholinesterase Activities and Sensitivities to Acetylcholine, DFP, and Barium Ion. Gastroenterology 24(1953)173–185

Kellog, C.; Vernadakis, A.; Rutledge, C.O.: Uptake and Metabolism of [^{3}H] norepinephrine in the Cerebral Hemispheres of Chick Embryos. J Neurochem 18(1971)1931–1938

Keuning, F.J.: The Development of the Intramural Nerve Elements of the Digestive Tract in Culture. Acta Neerl. Morph 5(1944)237–247

Keuning, F.J. Histogenesis and Origin of the Autonomic Nerve Plexus in the Upper Digestive Tube of the Chick. Acta Neerl Morph 6(1948)8–42

Ko, C.-P.; Burton, H.: Johnson, M.; Bunge, R.; Synaptic Transmission between Rat Superior Cervical Ganglion Neurons in Dissociated Cell Cultures. Brain Res 117(1976)461–485

Kosterlitz, H.W.; Lees, G.M.: Pharmacological Analysis of Intrinsic Intestinal Reflexes. Pharmacol Rev 16(1964)301–339

Kosterlitz, H.W.; Lydon, R.J.; and Watt, A.J.: The Effects of Adrenaline, Noradrenaline and Isoprenaline on Inhibitory A- and B-Adrenoceptors in the Longitudinal Muscle of the Guinea Pig Ileum. Br J Pharmacol 39(1970)398–413

Kottegoda, S.R.: An Analysis of Possible Nervous Mechanisms Involved in the Peristaltic Reflex. J Physiol (Lond) 200(1969)687–712

Kuhar, M.J.; Murrin, C.L.: Sodium-Dependent, High Affinity Choline Uptake. J Neurochem 301(1978)15–21

Kuntz, A.: In: The Autonomic Nervous System, pp. 117–134. Bailliere, Tindall, and Cox, London, 1953

Kyosola, K.; Veijola, L.; Rechardt, L.: Cholinergic Innervation of the Gastric Wall of the Cat. Histochem 44(1975)23–30

LaMont, T.J.; and Isselbacher, K.J.: Diseases of the Colon and Rectum. Thorn, G.W., Adams, R.D., Braunwald, E., Isselbacher, K.W. and Petersdorf, R.G., eds. In: Harrison's Principles of Internal Medicine, pp. 1547–1567, ed. by G.W. Thorn et al. McGraw-Hill, New York, 1977.

Landis, S.C.: Rat Sympathetic Neurons and Cardiac Myocytes Developing in Microcultures: Correlation of the Fine Structure of Endings with Neurotransmitter Function in Single Neurons. Proc Natl Acad Sci USA 73(1976)4220–4224

Landmesser, L. and Pilar, G. Interactions between Neurons and Their Targets During in vivo Synaptogenesis. Fed Proc 37(1978)2016–2022

Lane, P.W.: Association of Megacolon with Two Recessive Spotting Genes in the Mouse. J Hered 57(1966)29–31

Langley, J.N.: The Autonomic Nervous System, Part I. W. Heffer, Cambridge, 1921

Larsson, L.-I.: Ultrastructural Localization of a New Neuronal Peptide (VIP). Histochem 54(1977)173–176

Lauder, J.M.; Bloom, F.E.: Ontogeny of Monoamine Neurons in the Locus Coeruleus, Raphe Nuclei and Substantia Nigra of the Rat. I. Cell Differentiation. J Comp Neurol 155(1974)469–482

Lauder, J.M.; Krebs, H.: Serotonin and Early Neurogenesis. In: Maturation of Neurotransmission Satellite Symp. 6th Meeting International Society of Neurochemistry, pp. 171–180. Karger, Basel, 1978a

Lauder, J.M.; Krebs, H.: A role for Serotonin in Neuroembryogenesis. Anat Rec 190(1978b)455

Lauder, J.M.; Krebs, H.; Bloom, F.E.: Effects of PCPA on Differentiation of Serotonergic Receptive Cells During Embryogenesis. Trans Am Soc Neurochem 5(1974)155

Lavier, L.P.; Dunn, A.J.; Van Hartesvelt, C.: Development of Neurotransmitters and Their Function in Brain. In: Reviews of Neuroscience, Vol. 2, pp. 195–256, ed. by S. Ehrenpreis, I.J. Kopin. Raven, New York, 1976

LeDouarin, N.M.; Renaud, D.; Teillet, M.A.; LeDouarin, G.H.: Cholinergic Differentiation of Presumptive Adrenergic Neuroblasts in Interspecific Chimeras after Heterotypic Transplantations. Proc Nat Acad Sci USA 72(1975)728–732

LeDouarin, N.M.; Teillet, M.A.: The Migration of Neural Crest Cells to the Wall of the Digestive Tract in Avian Embryo. J Embryol Exp Morphol 30(1973)31–48

LeDouarin, N.M.; Teillet, M.A.: Experimental Analysis of the Migration and Differentiation of Neuroblasts of the Autonomic Nervous System and of Neuroectodermal Mesenchymal Derivatives, Using a Biological Cell Marking Technique. Dev Biol 41(1974)162–184

LeDouarin, N.M.; Teillet, M.A.; Ziller, C.; Smith, J.: Adrenergic Differentiation of Cells of the Cholinergic Ciliary and Remak Ganglia in Avian Embryo after in vitro Transplantation. Proc Natl Acad Sci USA 75(1978)2030–2034

Mains, R.E.; Patterson, P.H.: Primary Cultures of Dissociated Sympathetic Neurons. I. Establishment of Long-Term Growth in Culture and Studies of Differentiated Properties. J Cell Biol 59(1973a)329–345

Mains, R.E.; Patterson, P.H.: II. Initial Studies on Catecholamine Metabolisms. J Cell Biol 59(1973b)346–360

Manber, L.; and Gershon, M.D.: An Axo-Axonic Synapse between Adrenergic and Cholinergic Axons in the Mammalian Gut. Fed Proc 37(1978)227

Manber, L.M.; Gershon, M.D.: A Reciprocal Adrenergic-Cholinergic Axo-axonic Synapse in the Mammalian Gut. Am J Physiol 236(1979)E738–E745

Martinson, J.: Experimental Re-Investigation of the Concept of the Transmission Mechanism. Acta Physiol Scand 64(1965)453–462

Martinson, J.; Muren, A.: Excitatory and Inhibitory Effects of Vagus Stimulation on Gastric Motility in the Cat. Acta Physiol Scand 57(1963)309–316

Masson, P. Appendicite Neurogène et Carcinoides. Ann Anat Path Anat Norm Med-Chir 1(1923)3–59. (Quoted in: Masson and Berger, 1923)

Masson, P.; Berger, L.: Sur un nouveau mode de secretion interne: la neurocrinie. C R Acad Sci (D) (Paris) 176(1923)1748–1750

Mayer, C.J.; Wood, J.D.: Excitatory Action of Serotonin on Somal Membranes of Myenteric Neurons of Guinea Pig Small Bowel. Fed Proc 37(1978)227

Mayer, T.C.: The Development of Piebald Spotting in Mice. Dev Biol 11(1965)319–334

Mayer, T.C.; Maltby, E.L.: An Experimental Investigation of Pattern Development in Lethal Spotting and Belted Mouse Embryos. Dev Biol 9(1964)269–286

McElhannon, F.M.: Experimental Production of Megacolon Resembling Hirschsprung's Disease. Surg Forum 10(1960)218–221

Meier-Ruge, W.; Lutterbach, P.M.; Herzog, B.; Morger, R.; Maser, R.; Scharli, A.: Acetylcholinesterase Activity in Suction Biopsies of the Rectum in the Diagnosis of Hirschsprung's Disease. J Pediatr Surg 7(1972)11–17

Niemi, M.; Kouvalainen, K.; Hjelt, L.: Cholinesterase and Monoamine Oxidase in Congenital Megacolon. J Pathol 82(1961)363–366

Nilsson, G.; Larsson, L.-I.; Hakanson, R.; Brodin, E.; Sundler, F.; Pernow, B.: Localization of Substance P-Like Immunoreactivity in Mouse Gut. Histochem 43(1975)97–99

Norberg, K.-A.; Sjoqvist, F.: New Possibilities for Adrenergic Modulation of Ganglionic Transmission. Pharmacol Rev 18(1966)743–751

Norr, S.C.: In vitro Analysis of Sympathetic Neuron Differentiation from Chick Neural Crest Cells. Dev Biol 34(1973)16–38

Okamoto, E.; Ueda, T.: Embryogenesis of the Intramural Ganglia of the Gut and its Relation to Hirschsprung's Disease. J Pediatr Surg 2(1967)437–443

O'Lague, P.H.; MacLeish, P.R.; Nurse, C.A.; Claude, P.; Furshpan, E.J.; Potter, D.D.: Physiological and Morphological Studies on Developing Sympathetic Neurons in Dissociated Cell Culture. Cold Spring Harbor Symp Quant Biol 40(1975)399–407

O'Lague, P.H.; Obata, K.; Claude, P.; Furshpan, E.J.; Potter, D.D.: Evidence for Cholinergic Synapses between Dissociated Rat Sympathetic Neurons in Cell Culture. Proc Natl Acad Sci USA 71(1974)3602–3606

Olson, L.; Alund, M.; Norberg, K.-A.: Fluorescence-Microscopical Demonstration of a Population of Gastro-Intestinal Nerve Fibres with a Selective Affinity for Quinacrine. Cell Tissue Res 171(1976)407–423

Olson, L.; Seiger, A.: Early Prenatal Ontogeny of Central Monoamine Neurons in the Rat: Fluorescence Histochemical Observations. Z Anat Entwickl-Gesch 137(1972)301–316

Paton, W.D.M.; Vizi, E.S. The Inhibitory Effect of Noradrenaline and Adrenaline on Acetylcholine Output by Guinea Pig Ileum Longitudinal Muscle Strip. Br J Pharmacol 35(1969)10–28

Paton, W.D.M.; Zar, A.M.: The Origin of Acetylcholine Released from Guinea Pig Intestine and Longitudinal Muscle Strips. J Physiol (Lond) 194(1968)13–34

Patterson, P.H.: Environmental Determination of Autonomic Neurotransmitter Functions. Ann Rev Neurosci 1(1978)1–17

Patterson, P.H.; Chun, L.L.Y.: The Influence of Non-Neuronal Cells on Catecholamine and Acetylcholine Synthesis and Accumulation in Cultures of Dissociated Sympathetic Neurons. Proc Natl Acad Sci USA 9(1974)3607–3610

Patterson, P.H.; Chun, L.L.Y.: The induction of Acetylcholine Synthesis in Primary Cultures of Dissociated Rat Sympathetic Neurons. I. Effects of Conditioned Medium. Dev Biol 56(1977a)263–280

Patterson, P.H.; Chun, L.L.Y.: The Induction of Actylcholine Synthesis in Primary Cultures of Dissociated Rat Sympathetic Neurons. II. Developmental Aspects. Dev Biol 60(1977b)473–481

Penninckx, F., and Kerremans, R.: Pharmacological Characteristics of the Ganglionic and Aganglionic Colon in Hirschsprung's Disease. Life Sci 17(1975)1387–1394

Pert, C.B., and Snyder, S.H.: High Affinity Transport of Choline into the Myenteric Plexus of Guinea-Pig Intestine. J Pharmacol Exp Ther 191(1974)102–108

Pettigrew, J.D.: The Effect of Visual Experience on the Development of Stimulus Specificity by Kitten Cortical Neurons. J Physiol (Lond) 237(1974)49–74

Prestige, M.C.: Axon and Cell Numbers in the Developing Nervous System. In: Development and Regeneration in the Nervous System. Br Med Bull 30(1974)107–111

Purves, D.: Functional and Structural Changes in Mammalian Sympathetic Neurones Following Colchicine Application to Post-Ganglionic Nerves. J Physiol (Lond) 259(1976)159–175

Read, J.B.; Burnstock, G.: A Method for the Localization of Adrenergic Nerves During Early Development. Histochem 20(1969)197–200

Read, J.B.; Burnstock, G.: Development of the Adrenergic Innervation and Chromaffin Cells in the Human Fetal gut. Dev Biol 22(1970)513–534

Richards, J.G.; Tranzer, J.P.: Electron Microscopic Localization of 5-Hydroxydopamine a "False" Adrenergic Neurotransmitter in the Autonomic Nerve Endings of the Rat Pineal Gland. Experientia 25(1969)53–54

Richardson, J.: Pharmacologic Studies on a Murine Model of Hirschsprung's Disease. J Pediatr Surg 10(1975)875–883

Richter, J.A.; Marchbanks, R.M.: Synthesis of Radioactive Acetylcholine from ^{3}H-Choline and Its Release from Cerebral Cortex Slices in vitro. J Neurochem 18(1971)691–703

Rikimaru, A.: Contractile Properties of Organ-Cultured Intestinal Smooth Muscle. Tohoku J Exp Med 103(1971)317–329

Robinson, R.; Gershon, M.D.: Synthesis and Uptake of 5-Hydroxytryptamine by the Myenteric Plexus of the Small Intestine of the Guinea Pig. J Pharmacol Exp Ther 179(1971)29–41

Rogawski, M.A.; Goodrich, J.T.; Gershon, M.D.; Touloukian, R.J.: Hirschsprung's disease: Absence of Serotonergic Neurons in the Aganglionic Colon. J Pediatr Surg 13(1978)608–615

Rosenblatt, F.: Principles of Neurodynamics; Perceptions and the Theory of Brain Mechanisms. Spartan, Washington, 1962

Ross, D.; Johnson, M.; and Bunge, R.; Development of Cholinergic Characteristics in Adrenergic Neurons is Age Dependent. Nature (Lond) 267(1977)536–538

Rothman, T.P.; Gershon, M.D.; Holtzer, H.: The Relationship of Cell Division to the Acquisition of Adrenergic Characteristics by Developing Sympathetic Ganglion Cell Precursors. Dev Biol 65(1978)322–341

Rothman, T.P.; Ross, L.L.; Gershon, M.D.: Separately Developing Axonal Uptake of 5-Hydroxytryptamine and Norepinephrine in the Fetal Ileum of the Rabbit. Brain Res 115(1976)437–456

Sachs, Ch.; Jonsson, G.: Changes in the Development of Central Noradrenaline Neurons Following Neonatal 6-OH-DA Administration. In: Chemical tools in Catecholamine Research, Vol. I, pp. 163–171, ed. by G. Jonsson, T. Malmfors, Ch. Sachs. North Holland, Amsterdam, 1975

Schack, L.: Uber die gelben Zellen im menschlichen Wurmforstatz. Beitr Pathol 90(1932)441–478

Schlaepfer, W.W.: Acetylcholinesterase Activity of Motor and Sensory Nerve Fibers in Spinal Nerve Roots of Rat. Z Zellforsch Mikrosk Anat 88(1968)441–456

Schneider, G.E.: Early Lesions of Superior Colliculus: Factors Affecting the Formation of Abnormal Retinal Projections. Brain Behav Evol 8(1973)73–109

Schofield, G.C.: Anatomy of Muscular and Neural Tissues in the Alimentary Canal. In: Handbook of Physiology, Alimentary Canal, Sect. 6, IV, Motility, Chapter 80, pp. 1579–1627, ed. by C.F. Code. American Physiological Society, Washington, 1968

Schultzberg, M.; Dreyfus, C.F.; Gershon, M.D.; Hokfelt, T.; Elde, R.P.; Nilsson, G.; Said, S.; Goldstein, M.: VIP-, Enkephalin-, Substance P- and Somatostatin-Like Immunoreactivity in Neurons Intrinsic to the Intestine: Immunohistochemical Evidence from Organotypic Tissue Cultures. Brain Res 155(1978)239–248

Schulz, R.; Cartwright, C.: Effect of Morphine on Serotonin Release from the Myenteric Plexus of the Guinea Pig. J Pharmacol Exp Ther 190(1974)420–430

Shvelev, V.N.; Reidler, R.M.; Mingazova, I.V.: The Relationship between the Stages of Autonomic Nervous System Development and the Appearance of Its Chief Mediators During Embryogenesis (the Prenatal Development of the Choline- and Adrenergic Nerve Elements in Man and the Rabbit). Arkh Anat Gistol Embriol 63(1972)48–66

Smith, B.: Myenteric Plexus in Hirschsprung's Disease. Gut 8(1967)308–312

Smith, J.; Cochard, P.; LeDouarin, N.M.: Development of Choline Acetyl Transferase and Cholinesterase Activities in Enteric Ganglia Derived from Presumptive Adreneric and Cholinergic Levels of the Neural Crest. Cell Differ 6(1977)199–216

Spedding, M.; Sweetman, A.J.; and Weetman, D.F.: Antagonism of Adenosine 5-Triphosphate-Induced Relaxation by 2-2'-Pyridylisatogen in the Taenia of Guinea Pig Caecum. Br J Pharmacol 53(1975)575–583

Sperry, R.W.: Chemoaffinity in the Orderly Growth of Nerve Fiber Patterns and Connections. Proc Natl Acad Sci USA 50(1963)703–710

Stoeckel, K.; Thoenen, H.: Retrograde Axonal Transport of Nerve Growth Factor: Specificity and Biological Importance. Brain Res 85(1975)337–341

Sundler, F.; Hakanson, R.; Larsson, L.-I.; Brodin, E.; Nilsson, G.: Substance P in the Gut: An Immunochemical and Immunohistochemical Study of its Distribution and Development. In: Substance P, pp. 59–65, ed. by U.S. von Euler and B. Pernow. Raven, New York, 1977.

Suzuki, O.; Nagase, F.; Yagi, K.: Tryptophan Metabolism in Developing Chick Brain. Brain Res 93(1975)455–462

Swenson, O.: A New Surgical Treatment for Hirschsprung's Disease. Surgery 28(1950) 371–381

Swenson, O.: Congenital Defects in Pelvic Parasympathetic System. Arch Dis Child 30(1955)1–7

Swenson, O.; Bill, A.H., Jr.: Resection of Rectum and Rectosigmoid with Preservation of Sphincter for Benign Spastic Lesions Producing Megacolon; Experimental Study. Surgery 24(1948)212

Swenson, O.; Fisher, J.A.; MacMahon, H.E.: Rectal Biopsy as Aid in Diagnosis of Hirschsprung's Disease. N Engl J Med 253(1955)632

Tamir, H.; Huang, I.L.: Binding of Serotonin to Soluble Protein from Synaptosomes. Life Sci 17(1974)83–93

Tamir, H.; Kuhar, M.J.: Association of Serotonin-Binding Protein with Projections of the Midbrain Raphe Nuclei. Brain Res 83(1975)169–172

Teitelman, G.; Joh, T.H.; Reis, D.J.: Transient Expression of a Noreadrenergic Phenotype in Cells of the Rat Embryonic Gut. Brain Res 158(1978)229–234

Tello, J.F.: La précocité embryonnaire du plexus d'Auerbach et ses différences dans les intestines antérieurs et postérieurs. Trab Inst Cajal Invest Biol 22(1924)317–328 (Quoted in: Van Campenhout, 1932; and Yntema and Hammond, 1954)

Tennyson, V.M.; Mytilineou, C.; and Barrett, R.E.: Fluorescence and Electron Microscopy Studies of the Early Development of the Substantia Nigra and Area Ventralis Tegmenti in the Fetal Rabbit J Comp Neurol 149(1973)233–258

Thoenen, H.; Tranzer, J.P.: Chemical Sympathectomy by Selective Destruction of Adrenergic Nerve Endings with 6-Hydroxydopamine. Arch Exp Pathol Pharmacol (Naunyn-Schmiedeberg's) 261(1968)271–288

Tittel, K. Uber eine Angeborene Missbildung des Dickdarmes. Wien Klin Waschr 14(1901)903

Toneby, M.: Determination of 5-Hydroxytryptamine in Early Echinoderm Embryos. Comp Biochem Physiol 58C(1977)77–83

Tranzer, J.P.; and Richard, J.G.; The Effect of 6-Hydroxydopamine on the Peripheral Adrenergic Nerves. In: 6-Hydroxodopamine and Catecholamine Neurons pp. 15–31, ed. by T. Malmfors, H. Thoenen. American Elsevier, New York, 1971

Trendelenburg, P. Physiologische und pharmakologische Versoche uber die Dunndarm peristaltick. Arch Exp Pathol Pharmacol (Naunyn-Schmiedebergs) 81(1917)55–129

Uchida, S.: Uber die Entwicklung des sympathischen Nervensystems. Acta Sch Med Univ Kioto, 10(1927)63–136

U'Prichard, D.C.; Snyder, S.H.: Binding of ^{3}[H]Catecholamines to Alpha-Noradrenergic Receptor Sites in Calf Brain. J Biol Chem 252(1977)6450–6463

Van Campenhout, E.: Contribution to the Problem of the Development of the Sympathetic Nervous System. J Exp Zool 56(1930a)295–320

Van Campenhout, E.: Historical Survey of the Development of the Sympathetic Nervous System. Q Rev Biol 5(1930b)23–50, 217–234

Van Campenhout, E.: Le dévelopement du système nerveux sympathique chez le poulet. Arch Biol (Paris) 42(1931)479–507

Van Campenhout, E.: Further Experiments on the Origin of the Enteric Nervous System in the Chick. Physiol Zool 5(1932)333–353

Vernadakis, A.: Comparative Studies of Neurotransmitter Substances in the Maturing and Aging Central Nervous System of the Chicken. Prog Brain Res 40(1973)231–243

Wakshull, E.; Johnson, M.I.; Burton, H.: Persistence of an Amine Uptake System in Cultured Rat Sympathetic Neurons Which Use Acetylcholine as Their Transmitter. J Cell Biol 79(1978)121–131

Webster, W.: Embryogenesis of the enteric Ganglia in Normal Mice and in Mice That Develop Congenital Aganglionic Megacolon. J Embryol Exp Morphol 30(1973)573–585

Webster, W.: Aganglionic Megacolon in Piebald-Lethal mice. Arch Pathol Lab Med (formerly Arch Pathol) 97(1974)111–117

Weston, J.A.: A Radioautographic Analysis of the Migration and Localization of Trunk Neural Crest Cells in the Chick. Dev Biol 6(1963)279–310

Weston, J.A.: The Migration and Differentiation of Neural Crest Cells. In: Advances in Morphogenesis, Vol. 8, pp. 41–114, ed. by M. Abercrombie, J. Bracket, T.J. King. Academic, New York, 1970

Weston, J.A.; Butler, S.L.: Temporal Factors Affecting Localization of Neural Crest Cells in the Chick Embryo. Dev Biol 14(1966)246–266

Whitehouse, F.R.; Kernohan, J.W.: Myenteric Plexus in Congenital Megacolon. Arch Intern Med 82(1948)75-111

Williams, L.T.; Mullikin, D.; Lefkowitz, R.J.: Identification of Alpha-Adrenergic Receptors in Uterine Smooth Muscle Membranes by [³H] Dihydroergocryptine Binding. J Biol Chem 251(1976)6915-6923

Wong, W.T.; Horng, J.S.; Bymaster, F.P.; Houser, K.L.; Molloy, B.B.: A Selective Inhibitor of Serotonin Uptake: Lilly 110140, 3-(p-trifluormethylphenoxy)-N-methylphenylpropylamine. Life Sci 15(1974)471-479

Wood, J.D.: Congenital Megacolon: Hirschsprung's Disease. In: Alimentary Disease. Academic, New York, 1979, in press

Wood, J.D.; Mayer, C.J.: Intracellular Study of Electrical Behavior in Tonic Type Myenteric Neurons of Guinea Pig Small Bowel. Fed Proc 37(1978a)227

Wood, J.D.; Mayer, C.J.: Functional Significance of Slow EPSPs in Myenteric Ganglion Cells. Neurosci Abstr 4(1978b)586

Wood, J.D.; Mayer, C.J.: Intracellular Study of Tonic-Type Enteric Neurons in Guinea Pig Small Intestine. J Neurophysiol 42(1979a)569-581

Wood, J.D.; Mayer, C.J.: Serotonergic Activation of Tonic-Type Enteric Neurons in Guinea-Pig Small Bowel. J Neurophysiol 42(1979b)582-593

Yamamura, H.I.; Kuhar, M.J.; Snyder, S.H.: In vivo Identification of Muscarinic Cholinergic Receptor Binding in Rat Brain. Brain Res 80(1974)170-176

Yamamura, H.I.; Snyder, S.H.: Muscarinic Cholinergic Binding in Rat Brain. Proc Natl Acad Sci USA 71(1974a)1725-1729

Yamamura, H.I.; Snyder, S.H.: Muscarinic Cholinergic Receptor Binding in the Longitudinal Muscle of the Guinea Pig Ileum with [³H]-Quinuclidinyl benzylate. Mol Pharmacol 10(1974b)861-867

Yntema, C.L.; Hammond, W.S.: Depletions and Abnormalities in the Cervical Sympathetic System of the Chick Following Extirpation of the Neural Crest. J Exp Zool 100(1945)237-263

Yntema, C.L.; Hammond, W.S.: The Development of the Autonomic Nervous System. Biol Rev. 22(1947)344-359

Yntema, C.L.; Hammond, W.S.: Origin of Intrinsic Autonomic Ganglia of Trunk Viscera in the Chick Embryo. Anat Rec 112(1952)404

Yntema, C.L.; Hammond, W.S.: The Origin of Intrinsic Ganglia of Trunk Viscera from Vagal Neural Crest in the Chick Embryo. J Comp Neurol 101(1954)515-541

Yntema, C.L.; Hammond, W.S.: Experiments on the Origin and Development of the Sacral Autonomic Nerves in the Chick Embryo. J Exp Zool 129(1955)375-414

Yokoyama, S.; Ozaki, T.; Kajitsuka, T.: Excitation Conduction in Auerbach's Plexus of Rabbit Small Intestine. Am J Physiol 232(2)(1977)E100-E108

Zuelzer, W.W.; Wilson, J.L.: Functional Intestinal Obstruction on a Congenital Neurogenic Basis in Infancy. Am J Dis Child 75(1948)40-64

Nonadrenergic, Noncholinergic Transmission in the Autonomic Nervous System: Purinergic Nerves

Graeme Campbell and Ian L. Gibbins

I. INTRODUCTION

Langley's definitive monograph "The Autonomic Nervous System" (1921), based on about fifty years of pharmacological and anatomical research, provided a description of the autonomic nervous system (ANS) that is the basis of all modern work. The following features of the ANS were defined:

1. Autonomic pathways are efferent, with a nerve-nerve synapse lying outside the central nervous system (CNS).
2. The ANS has three divisions:
The *sympathetic*, arising from the thoracolumbar spinal cord, with ganglionic synapses usually remote from the target organ.

We wish to thank Jane Bird, Jenny Clevers, Brenda Grabsch, Chris Haller, Judy Morris, Lyn Ramsay, and Caroline Waid for their great help in preparing this manuscript.

The *parasympathetic*, arising from cranial or from sacral cord sources, with ganglionic synapses usually in or near the target organ.

The *enteric*, comprising the neuronal plexuses of the gut, uncertainly and only partially overlapping with the other two divisions (see Gershon, this volume).

3. The sympathetic and parasympathetic divisions were seen to have distinct, and often antagonistic, actions on their target organs.

The basis for sympathetic-parasympathetic antagonism became clear when it was realized that autonomic nerves could act by releasing either acetylcholine (cholinergic nerves) or adrenaline/noradrenaline (adrenergic nerves) (Dale, 1933). It was thought that adrenergic neurons were limited to the sympathetic postganglionic supply and that most parasympathetic postganglionic neurons were cholinergic. This conservative two-transmitter concept survived for about thirty years, with only minor arguments that other forms of transmission might occur (e.g., Henderson and Roepke, 1934; Euler, 1949).

During and since the 1960s, a number of what appear to be nonadrenergic, noncholinergic (NANC) autonomic transmissions were discovered. These examples have been revealed in three main ways. First, pharmacological experiments on the effects of autonomic nerve stimulation, using the wide range of cholinergic and adrenergic blocking drugs now available, have shown certain responses that appear to be mediated by neither cholinergic nor adrenergic nerves. Second, electron microscopic studies have shown that a number of tissues contain nerve fibers that do not have the appearance of adrenergic or cholinergic nerves. Third, histochemical techniques, comparable to those that have been so usefully applied to studies of adrenergic nerves, have been used to show that certain potential transmitter substances are in fact distributed with autonomic nerves.

One of the best documented examples of an NANC nerve supply in the ANS is the intrinsic inhibitory innervation of mammalian gut muscle. The reasons for claiming that the nerves are neither adrenergic nor cholinergic have been reviewed elsewhere (Campbell, 1970). Although a few later papers have claimed that the nerves might be adrenergic (e.g., Weisenthal et al., 1971), it seems that specific objections to the nerves' being NANC have been overcome (e.g., Gershon and Thompson, 1973). There is now general agreement that the nerves do exist and that they are NANC.

In 1970 it was postulated that the intrinsic inhibitory nerves in the gut cause smooth muscle relaxation by releasing adenosine triphosphate (ATP) or a related purine nucleotide (Burnstock et al., 1970). Burnstock (1971) proposed the name *purinergic* for such fibers and since then has reviewed the pharmacological evidence for purinergic transmission, the release of purines on nerve stimulation, the possible distribution of purinergic nerves, and the receptor pharmacology of purines (Burnstock, 1972; 1975a, b; 1978).

We intend to focus our discussion on the purinergic nerves, to show ways in which the ANS is being approached experimentally in the 1970s. Three areas of modern research—pharmacology, electron microscopy, and histochemical localization of transmitter substances—will be covered, and each will be related to the question of purinergic nerves. We use the term *purinergic* throughout for convenience, without implying devotion to the theory that the nerves act by releasing ATP.

II. PHARMACOLOGICAL STUDIES

Before we can comment on the pharmacology of purinergic nerves, we must state what NANC nerves we will take to be purinergic. There is no reason to believe that all NANC fibers are of the same class, and we do not wish to cloud the issue by including examples that may turn out not to be in the purinergic class. We have therefore adopted what we hope is a conservative attitude in determining the distribution of purinergic nerves, as outlined below.

A. The Distribution of Purinergic Nerves

The purinergic nerves were first identified physiologically as NANC fibres in the mammalian gut. Transmural stimulation of guinea-pig tenia ceci caused a neurogenic inhibition of the muscle that differed from sympathetic adrenergic effects in several ways: it was better developed at low frequencies of stimulation; it was resistant to adrenergic neuron-blocking drugs; it could be related to intrinsic ganglion cells; and it was accompanied by changes in the smooth muscle membrane potential, inhibitory junction potentials (IJPs), which were not seen on sympathetic nerve stimulation (Burnstock et al., 1963a, b, 1964; Burnstock, Campbell, and Rand, 1966; Bennett, Burnstock, and Holman, 1966; Campbell, 1970).

The IJP is a hyperpolarization of the smooth muscle membrane up to 25 mV in amplitude. It is produced in response to single stimuli, and individual IJPs summate on repeated stimulation at low frequency. It has a latency of about 50–100 ms, reaches a peak after about 150–300 ms, and lasts for up to about 1 s (Holman, 1970; Burnstock, 1972). The IJP interrupts spontaneous action potential firing in the smooth muscle, causing the muscle to relax. The presence of IJPs can be taken as a convenient indicator of the presence of purinergic nerves in particular gut regions. It has been shown that stimulation of intramural nerves in the mammalian gut produces IJPs in the *esophagus* (Diamant, 1973), the *stomach* (Kuriyama, Osa, and Tasaki, 1970; Beani, Bianchi, and Crema, 1971; Beck and Osa, 1971; Atanasova, Vladimirova, and Shuba, 1972), the *small intestine* (Kuriyama,

Osa, and Toida, 1967; Hidaka and Kuriyama, 1969; Hirst and McKirdy, 1974), the *cecum* (Bennett et al., 1966; Bülbring and Tomita, 1966; Tomita, 1972; Ito and Kuriyama, 1973; Jager and den Hartog, 1974), the *colon* (Furness, 1969; Julé and Gonella, 1972; Small, 1972) and the *internal anal sphincter* (Costa and Furness, 1973). The ubiquity of IJPs shows that the purinergic nerves are distributed throughout the mammalian gut. The presence of NANC neurogenic relaxation in all regions of the gut has been confirmed (Burnstock, 1972, 1975b). A similar inhibitory innervation has been found in certain regions of the gut of lower vertebrate animals (Burnstock, 1975b).

The purinergic nerves have their cell bodies in the gut wall, as can be seen from, for instance, the survival of purinergic responses in organ cultures of gut (Rikimaru, 1971). However, the neurons at either end of the gut receive an input from the central nervous system via parasympathetic pathways. Vagus nerve stimulation produces both purinergic relaxation and IJPs in the esophagus (Diamant, 1973) and the stomach (Martinson, 1965; Campbell, 1966; Bülbring and Gershon, 1967; Beani et al., 1971). The inhibitory fibers in the terminal rectum are activated by the pelvic nerves (Julé and Gonella, 1972; Costa and Furness, 1973). It is probable that the purinergic neurons in the intervening gut are not under extrinsic control, but take part in intrinsic gut reflexes. A considerable proportion of the vagal inhibition of the stomach is prevented by nicotinic ganglion-blocking drugs (Greef, Kasperat, and Osswald, 1962; Paton and Vane, 1963), which shows that the purinergic nerves are in fact autonomic and not, say, antidromically stimulated sensory fibers.

There have been a number of reports of NANC excitatory nerve effects on the gut of mammals (e.g., Fulgräff and Schmidt, 1964; Ambache and Freeman, 1968; Furness, 1970; Bennett and Fleshler, 1970; Furness and Costa, 1973). Burnstock (1972, 1975b) has left open the possibility that these nerves may be purinergic, as are the inhibitory nerves in the same segments of gut. We find it hard to credit that nerves releasing the same transmitter substance can simultaneously have two opposing actions on the same piece of intestinal muscle. It would be easier to accept the possibility if autonomic nerves made discrete endplatelike contacts with smooth muscle. However, the width of the synaptic cleft in gut muscle can be 100 nm or more (Bennett and Burnstock, 1968); therefore the excitatory and inhibitory nerves probably release their transmitter substances into a common extracellular space. This article rejects the possibility that NANC excitation in mammalian gut is mediated by purinergic nerves.

The participation of both cranial and sacral parasympathetic pathways in the purinergic innervation of the gut leads one to examine other organs supplied by these nerves. The vagal innervation of the lung comes to immediate notice, because there have been a number of reports of anomalous vagal effects dilating the airways (Widdicombe, 1963). Transmural stimulation of tracheobronchial muscle has now been shown to activate inhibitory NANC nerve fibers (Coleman, 1973; Coburn and Tomita, 1973; Coleman and Levy, 1974; Richardson and Bouchard, 1975; Kamikawa and Shimo, 1976b). Although it has not been shown in mammals that these inhibitory nerve fibers can be activated through the vagus nerves, the lung musculature in lower vertebrates receives an NANC inhibitory innervation from the vagi (Campbell, 1971; Robinson, McLean, and Burnstock, 1971; Berger, 1973). It seems highly likely that a similar vagal connection will eventually be shown in mammals. It is then a reasonable argument that the pulmonary inhibitory fibers, sharing common central connections with and having similar actions to the gut purinergic neurons, can also be regarded as purinergic. This is an important point to make, because a proposed ultrastructural identification of purinergic neurons has been based on studies of the amphibian lung (Robinson et al., 1971; also see below).

Although we are aware of other vagal effects that are resistant to adrenergic and cholinergic blockade—e.g., vagus-induce stimulation of pancreatic fluid and electrolytes in pig (Hickson, 1970)—too little is known of the effects to comment on their relationship to purinergic phenomena at this point.

When organs innervated by the pelvic nerves are considered, several examples of anomalous autonomic nerve effects are met (Gruber, 1933; Bell, 1972; Klinge and Sjöstrand, 1975). The most consistently documented responses to stimulation of the sacral autonomic outflow, apart from effects on the gut, are contraction of the urinary bladder, the production of at least partial penile erection by arterial and corpus cavernosum dilatation, and relaxation of the retractor penis muscle. A number of effects on the uterus, the vagina, the urethra, etc., and widespread vasodilator responses in the pelvic region have also been reported, but most of the observations are fifty or more years old. The most interesting recent studies on tissues from the pelvic area have been made on the anococcygeus muscles, which relax on sacral nerve stimulation (Gillespie and McGrath, 1973). The anococcygeus can be related to the retractor penis by the fact that they share a common insertion on the spinal column. Because of the limited information that exists on other organs, the next part of the discussion will concentrate on the innervation of the bladder, the anococcygeus, and the retractor penis muscles and the penile vasculature.

The *excitatory* effects of pelvic nerve stimulation on the urinary bladder are mimicked by acetylcholine and other muscarinic agonists (Gruber, 1933). But atropine, although it antagonizes muscarinic effects, fails to block the response to pelvic nerve stimulation (Langley and Anderson,

1895). Demonstrations of atropine resistance have been made repeatedly; and, largely because of this resistance, there have been numerous claims that transmission to the bladder is partly or wholly noncholinergic (Henderson and Roepke, 1934; Ambache and Zar, 1970; Dumsday, 1971; Burnstock, Dumsday, and Smythe, 1972; Taira, 1972; De Groat and Saum, 1976; Downie and Dean, 1977; Burnstock et al., 1978b). Recent papers have produced evidence that transmission is purinergic (Burnstock et al., 1972; 1978b, c; Dean and Downie, 1978), although this has been specifically denied (Ambache and Zar, 1970). Without claiming that the matter is resolved, there is sufficient doubt that transmission to the bladder is entirely cholinergic for us to include bladder innervation in the following discussion of purinergic nerves.

The *inhibitory* effects of pelvic nerve stimulation on the muscles and blood vessels of the male external genitalia and the anococcygeus can be treated together. It is now hard to see why pelvic nerve transmission to the penile system was ever regarded as cholinergic. Well before the end of the nineteenth century, it was shown that the erectile effects of the pelvic nerves (nervi erigentes) were not blocked by atropine (Klinge and Sjöstrand, 1975). Although there have been some reports that acetylcholine causes inhibition of genital muscles (Oppenheimer, 1938; Orlov, 1963; Hukovic and Bubic, 1967; Gillespie and McGrath, 1974), the great majority of workers have found that acetylcholine either excites or has no effect on them (Klinge and Sjöstrand, 1975, 1977; Gillespie, 1972). When each of the structures involved was subjected to *in vitro* study, it became clear that they received a strong NANC inhibitory innervation, see, for example, the *retractor penis* (Luduena and Grigas, 1966; Klinge and Sjöstrand, 1975, 1977), the *cavernous bodies* (Hukovic and Bubic, 1967; Klinge and Sjöstrand, 1977), the *penile artery* (Dorr and Brody, 1967; Klinge and Sjöstrand, 1975), and the *anococcygeus* (Gillespie, 1972; Gillespie and McGrath, 1974; Creed, Gillespie, and McCaffery, 1977). Electrophysiological studies of inhibitory innervation have shown that there is a marked similarity to the purinergic innervation of the gut: in both the retractor penis (Orlov, 1963) and the anococcygeus (rabbit but not rat [Creed and Gillespie, 1977]), stimulation of the intramural nerves with single pulses elicits IJPs, comparable in size and in time course to the IJPs of gut muscle. Evidence has now been found for the involvement of ATP in the responses of the anococcygeus (Burnstock, Cocks, and Crowe, 1978a). The similarities in central connections and in the mode of action on smooth muscle make it easy to concede that these inhibitory pelvic nerve supplies are of the same type as the gut purinergic system.

We emphasize that this delimitation of the distribution of purinergic nerves—to the gut, the lung, the urinary bladder, the anococcygeus muscle, and muscles associated with male external genitalia—is a conservative one.

It may well be that Burnstock's suggestions (1972, 1975b) of a wider distribution are correct.

B. Pharmacological Approaches to the Purinergic Theory

The process of nerve-effector transmission in adrenergic and cholinergic systems has been found to be susceptible to pharmacological intervention in a variety of ways. Established patterns of determining the nature of a nerve have grown on us. For instance, if it were claimed that the innervation of a particular organ was cholinergic, the *minimal* pharmacological evidence needed to support this contention would be, first, that acetylcholine should mimic the action of the nerve and second, that drugs like atropine, which prevent the action of acetylcholine, should also inhibit nervous transmission. Probably the next step would be to determine whether an anticholinesterase drug enhances both acetylcholine and nerve effects, and so on. The question is, to what extent can this type of approach be applied to test the purinergic theory on the postulated examples of purinergic transmission?

    1. ATP Mimicry of Nerve Effects   To mimic purinergic nerve action, ATP must cause contraction of the urinary bladder and relaxation of the gut, lung, and pelvic smooth muscle. To a considerable extent, this mimicry has already been shown. ATP has been found to contract the bladder of a number of species (Buchthal and Kahlson, 1944; Matsumura, Taira, and Hashimoto, 1968; Ambache and Zar, 1970; Dumsday, 1971; Burnstock et al., 1972; Burnstock et al., 1978b). Whereas the adenine nucleotides are excitatory, adenosine and adenine cause relaxation (Burnstock et al., 1972). It has been pointed out that the contraction caused by ATP has a comparable time course to the nerve-mediated contraction (Ambache and Zar, 1970). ·

    Adenine compounds have a widespread inhibitory effect on the mammalian gut (Drury and Szenty-Györgi, 1931; Barsoum and Gaddum, 1935; Ambache and Freeman, 1968; Axelsson and Holmberg, 1969; Burnstock et al., 1970; Weston, 1973b; Spedding and Weetman, 1976; Ohga and Taneike, 1977). The time course of relaxation is like that of responses to purinergic nerve stimulation (Brunstock et al., 1970). Perhaps more important, ATP causes hyperpolarization of the smooth muscle membrane (Imai and Takeda, 1967; Axelsson and Holmberg, 1969); it seems that the specific changes in membrane permeability that cause the hyperpolarization are the same as those produced by the transmitter substance mediating the IJP (Tomita and Watanabe, 1973; Jager, 1974).

    In a number of preparations, ATP also has excitatory actions on the gut muscle (Burnstock et al., 1970). In some of the preparations examined, the excitation is the dominant part of a biphasic response to ATP; and in at least one preparation, the longitudinal muscle of the rabbit rectum (Mackay and McKirdy, 1972), no inhibitory component at all could be found. Discrepancies of this type are discussed below.

There is agreement that adenine compounds cause relaxation of the smooth muscles of mammalian airways (Bennett and Drury, 1931; Bianchi, de Natale, and Giaquinto, 1963; Coleman and Levy, 1974; Coleman, 1976; Kamikawa and Shimo, 1976a, b). It has also been reported that ATP relaxes the musculature of the frog lung (Meves, 1953).

The response of the anococcygeus muscle varies with species. In the rat, ATP is excitatory (Gillespie, 1972; but see below), but in the cat and rabbit it causes relaxation (Gillespie and McGrath, 1974; Creed et al., 1977). The first reports of ATP effects on retractor penis indicated an excitatory action of ATP (dog: Luduena and Grigas, 1972; bull: Klinge and Sjöstrand, 1975), but inhibitory actions have been seen on the retractor and the corpus cavernosum of other mammals (Klinge and Sjöstrand, 1977). The penile artery of the bull is dilated by ATP (Klinge and Sjöstrand, 1975).

In this list of ATP effects, a lack of mimicry of nerve effects by ATP has been noted in relatively few preparations, any one of which may constitute a crucial test for the purinergic theory. The occurrence of mixed responses to ATP in a particular tissue does not disprove the purinergic theory, any more than the presence of both α- and β-adrenoceptors in a vascular bed disproves the adrenergic nature of the vasoconstrictor innervation. However, should one find a preparation in which ATP does not mimic the effects of nerve stimulation at all, as would seem to be the case in the rabbit rectal longitudinal muscle and some of the pelvic muscles, the purinergic theory would be strained. Unfortunately, life is not that simple.

The observed effects of ATP are subject to a number of interfering processes. First, there is evidence that ATP causes the production of prostaglandins from tissues (Needleman, Minkes, and Douglas, 1974). The prostaglandins may modify the response to ATP. These processes involving prostaglandins do not necessarily occur if ATP is released from nerve terminals, rather than added to an organ bath. It is therefore important to determine the effects of ATP without the influence of prostaglandins by treating the preparation with drugs that prevent either the synthesis (e.g., indomethacin) or the action (e.g., polyphloretin phosphate) of prostaglandins. This was done, with encouraging results for the purinergic theory, on one of the preparations in which ATP did not mimic nerve stimulation—the rat anococcygeus. Burnstock et al. (1978a) found that the excitatory effect of ATP was reversed to an inhibition, now mimicking nerve effects, after treatment with indomethacin. In the urinary bladder, mimicry was preserved when it was found that indomethacin antagonized both ATP and nerve effects (Johns and Paton, 1977; Dean and Downie, 1978). But, to balance the scales, discouraging results were obtained with tracheal muscle, in which both indomethacin and polyphloretin phosphate blocked the relaxing action of ATP without blocking the inhibitory effect of nerve stimulation (Kamikawa and Shimo, 1976a, b), thereby removing one of the examples of successful mimicry.

The second interfering factor is that when ATP is applied to a tissue, it is broken down largely to adenosine (e.g., Burnstock et al., 1970). The response to ATP will then be a result of the effect of ATP proper and that of adenosine, with changes in the proportion of the two agonists over time. Adenosine is actively taken up into tissues, and a number of drugs such as dipyridamole have been reported to inhibit adenosine uptake (dipyridamole: Pfleger, Volkmer, and Kolassa, 1969; Kolassa, Pfleger, and Rummel, 1970; hexobendine: Kraupp et al., 1966). Treatment with dipyridamole should therefore enhance the component of the effect of applied ATP that can be attributed to adenosine. Where ATP and adenosine are synergists, as in gut and trachea, dipyridamole usually enhances the effect of ATP (e.g., Satchell et al., 1972; Coleman and Levy, 1974); where they are antagonists, as in bladder, the effect of ATP is reduced (Burnstock et al., 1978b). It is worth noting that blockade of adenosine uptake can have profound effects on the apparent potency of ATP. Coleman and Levy (1974) found that ATP at concentrations up to 60 μmol/l had little effect on untreated tracheal muscle; after treatment with dipyridamole, concentrations of ATP as low as 0.6 μmol/l caused relaxation. Most workers have reported that when the response to ATP has been modified by dipyridamole, a comparable modification of purinergic nerve effects occurs (Satchell et al., 1972; Coleman and Levy, 1974; Burnstock et al., 1978b). However, Heazell (1975) found that ATP effects on rat stomach were enhanced by dipyridamole but purinergic nerve effects were often reduced, by a mechanism that was not determined.

When the question of nerve mimicry by ATP is being examined, it is important to control the above factors. Ideally, the breakdown of ATP should be prevented, but we know of no means by which this can be done. The effects of prostaglandins should be excluded. The response should be tested both with and without an adenosine uptake inhibitor. No experiments of this type are reported in the literature. Such an experiment has been carried out on the toad lung (Campbell and A. M. Rutherford, unpublished observation), in which the purinergic nerves are inhibitory. It was found that ATP caused contraction of the lung muscle, whether or not it had been treated with indomethacin or dipyridamole. This is the best way that these workers can devise to test the purinergic theory by mimicry. The failure to show mimicry gives them great concern about the validity of the theory.

2. Antagonism of ATP   There is a large literature on pharmacological actions of purine nucleosides and nucleotides. There are also scattered observations on modifications of the effects of ATP brought about by a rather random collection of drugs. But there is little sign as yet of an underlying rationale to explain purine actions and their antagonism. Burnstock (1978) has put forward an argument that there are two types of purine receptor. However, as he says, the proposal needs further experimentation before it can be evaluated. The fact remains that, at this moment, there are no commonly accepted specific antagonists of purine effects

The following drugs, which have blocking actions against ATP in some tissues, have been used to test the purinergic hypothesis: theophylline and other methylxanthines; imidazole; phentolamine and other imidazolines; quinidine; 2'-2'-pyridylisatogen (Burnstock, 1978). All these drugs have other actions. In perhaps the majority of cases reported, where a particular drug antagonized ATP effects, it also inhibited transmission from purinergic nerves—e.g., *bladder* (see Dean and Downie, 1978; Burnstock et al., 1972); *gut* (Burnstock et al., 1970; Satchell, Burnstock, and Dann, 1973; Tomita and Watanabe, 1973; Jager, 1974). However, there are reports that ATP effects on the gut can be antagonized without a concomitant inhibition of purinergic nerve effects (Rikimaru, Fukushi, and Suzuki, 1971; Spedding, Sweetman, and Weetman, 1975; Heazell, 1975).

An alternative to the use of antagonists is the induction of tachyphylaxis to ATP. It has been found that tachyphylactic desensitization of gut and bladder to ATP reduces the responses to purinergic nerve stimulation (Burnstock et al., 1970, 1972, 1978b; Dean and Downie, 1978). But contrary results have been reported for these tissues (Ambache and Zar, 1970; Weston, 1973a, b; Ohga and Taneike, 1977) and for the penile artery (Klinge and Sjöstrand, 1975).

In our opinion, little can be claimed for the data obtained to date with ATP antagonists. Although a number of treatments have been reported by some workers, producing differences between responses to ATP and to purinergic nerve stimulation, these experiments do not disprove the theory. It is only necessary to suggest in reply that the effects of endogenously released and of exogenously applied ATP may be achieved differently. This is exactly the argument used successfully for years by the defenders of atropine-resistant cholinergic transmissions, and it is quite respectable, if frustrating. However, only circumstantial evidence for the purinergic theory has been produced by these pharmacological experiments, for each of the antagonists has or is likely to have other actions. It is still worth searching for drugs that do have specific actions on purine receptors or on purinergic nerves, because, as always, the possible therapeutic uses of such drugs are highly interesting. However, it is unlikely that the purinergic theory will be proved or disproved by the use of ATP antagonists. It should be remembered that it was not the use of blocking drugs, but the isolation of transmitter substances released from nerves, that cemented the concepts of adrenergic and cholinergic transmission.

C. Alternative Transmitter Substances

There is considerable evidence for the release of ATP when purinergic nerves are activated. This is consistent with the purinergic theory and has been well reviewed by Burnstock (1972, 1975). The issue is clouded by the fact that other types of nerve also release ATP on stimulation. The argument for a special association of ATP release with purinergic transmission is therefore a quantitative one, difficult to carry out when dealing with the very loosely constructed autonomic nerve-muscle junction.

Throughout the modern literature there are scattered suggestions that the ATP released from purinergic nerves is not the real transmitter substance, but is simply released in association with it. This view is usually expressed by workers who have been unable to mimic purinergic nerve effects with applied ATP (e.g., Gillespie, 1972), and we belong to this group by virtue of our observations on the toad lung. If we are to disagree with the purinergic theory, we must comment on the nature of the real transmitter substance. Gillespie and McKnight (1976) have pointed out that certain peptides cause relaxation of the rat anococcygeus, which is not normally relaxed by ATP. They have therefore suggested that the inhibitory puri-nergic nerves might act by releasing a peptide—a proposal that is consistent with the electron microscopic identification of purinergic nerves (see below). It was therefore most interesting when Ambache, Killick, and Zar (1975) reported that a substance, apparently a peptide, could be extracted from a bull retractor penis which caused relaxation of that muscle. Gillespie and Martin (1978) have now confirmed the presence of the inhibitory peptide in the retractor penis. However, they, like others (A. M. Rutherford and G. Campbell, unpublished observation) have found that the material is distributed widely in tissues unlikely to have a purinergic innervation, such as skeletal muscle, umbilical artery, and heart. This distribution has discouraged Rutherford and Campbell, at least, from considering this inhibitory peptide a candidate transmitter for the purinergic nerves. The fact remains that, at least on electron microscopic evidence (see the next section), the transmitter could be a peptide. The possibility that the nerves are peptidergic will be further commented on in the third section.

II. ELECTRON MICROSCOPIC STUDIES

The essence of electron microscopic (EM) identification of autonomic nerves is the hypothesis, stated recently by Palay and Chan-Palay (1976), that "all nerve fibers and terminals arising from a particular group of nerve cells, or more precisely a particular nerve cell type, display similar axo-plasmic configurations despite variations in size and shape of the termination." The problem faced by early electron microscopists was to determine which of the features of nerve terminals gave the most appropriate information about the type of nerve fiber. A solution emerged twenty-five years ago.

At both the neuromuscular junction (Palade and Palay, 1954) and the interneuronal synapse (Palade and Palay, 1954; DeRobertis and Bennett, 1954), collections of small membrane-bound, spherical vesicles, 30–50 nm in diameter, were seen in the presynaptic element, often in close association with the terminal presynaptic membrane. Physiological studies at that time revealed that at the motor endplate, the nervous transmitter acetylcholine (ACh) was released in quanta. It seemed reasonable to suggest that the synaptic vesicles could be the subcellular organelles that were responsible for the storage and the all-or-none release of quantal "packets" of transmitter (Katz, 1966). Since transmission from autonomic nerve to smooth muscle is also a quantal process (Holman, 1970), it is only natural that the vesicles in axon terminals were examined for "similar axoplasmic configurations".

A. Adrenergic and Cholinergic Nerves

In tissues considered to receive a classical dual (i.e., cholinergic and adrenergic) autonomic innervation, such as heart and iris, two types of nerve profiles were seen in EM sections (e.g., Richardson, 1962, 1964; Yamauchi, 1969). One contained almost entirely small clear vesicles (SCV) of 30–60 nm diameter. The appearance of the terminals is therefore very like that of terminals of known cholinergic nerves at skeletal muscle endplates (Katz, 1966) and in autonomic ganglia (e.g., Pick, 1970), and the nerves were considered to be the cholinergic component of the innervation (Burnstock and Iwayama, 1971). It is worth adding that, if the problem is approached with a completely open mind, the observation of a typical cholinergic-type of nerve profile in the ANS does not necessarily mean that the nerve is cholinergic. A typical cholinergic appearance is seen in CNS nerve terminals thought to release γ-amino butyric acid (Bloom, 1972; Wood, McLaughlin, and Vaughn, 1976) and in invertebrate neuromuscular junctions, where glutamate may be the transmitter (e.g. Osborne, 1970; Holtzman, Freeman, and Kashner, 1971).

The second type of nerve contained numerous small vesicles, 30–60 nm in diameter, which contained small electron-dense granular cores. These small granular vesicles (SGV) were otherwise similar in size and shape to SCV. These nerves, by default, had to be the adrenergic nerve supply. The dense cores of SGV, by analogy with the dense-cored secretory granules of amine-containing adrenal medullary cells (DeRobertis and Pellegrino de Iraldi, 1961; DeRobertis, 1962), were therefore postulated to be the specific storage site of noradrenaline. Experiments with noradrenaline-depleting drugs, autoradiography following loading with ^{3}H-noradrenaline, and loading with electron-dense false transmitters have confirmed that noradrenaline is stored in the SGV (Bloom, 1972; Burnstock and Costa, 1975). It should be noted that there is considerable tissue and species variation in the ease with which the cores of SGV can be shown with routine fixatives (e.g., glu-taraldehyde followed by osmium tetroxide) (Grillo, 1966; Bloom, 1970; Fillenz and Pollard, 1976). This problem can usually be overcome by label-ing with false transmitters like 5-hydroxydopamine (5-OHDA) (Richards and Tranzer, 1970) or by using special fixatives (KMnO$_4$: Richardson, 1966; dichromate aldehyde: Woods, 1969; Richards and Tranzer, 1975; Tranzer and Richards, 1976). Although adrenergic, dopaminergic, and trypt-aminergic nerves can all contain SGV (Hökfelt, 1968; Zieher and Jaim Etcheverry, 1971; Lorez and Richards, 1975; Nojyo and Sano, 1978), they can be distinguished in a number of ways—e.g., specific enzymes involved in the formation of the different amines can be localized histochemically (Hartman, 1973; Pickel, Joh, and Reis, (1976).

Both adrenergic and cholinergic nerve profiles also contain large granular or dense-cored vesicles (LGV). These vesicles are usually round and 60–100 nm in diameter and contain a variably electron-dense core, usually surrounded by a relatively electron-lucent halo (Richardson, 1964; Grillo, 1966; Taxi, 1969; Uehara, Campbell, and Burnstock, 1976). Although generally in low numbers within cholinergic terminals, LGV are present in varying proportions in amine-containing nerves (Taxi, 1969; Bloom and Aghajanian, 1968; Hökfelt, 1969; Burnstock and Costa, 1975). Indeed, some adrenergic terminals in the gut (Baumgarten, Holstein, and Owman, 1970; Furness and Costa, 1974) have a clear predominance of LGV over SGV. Loading with the specific adrenergic false transmitter 5-OHDA (Tranzer and Thoenen, 1967) or using an aldehyde-chromate fixative (Tranzer et al., 1969; Tranzer and Richards, 1976) has shown that the adre-nergic LGV are different to LGV in cholinergic nerves in that only the former store amines (Burnstock and Costa, 1975).

B. Other Nerve Types

Early studies of the ANS disclosed various nerve profiles that in appearance conform neither to the typical adrenergic type (with many SGV and a varia-ble proportion of LGV), nor to the typical cholinergic type (with many SCV and some LGV) with respect to their vesicle populations. Most obvious of these were profiles containing an abundance of large vesicles, 80–200 nm in diameter, with a moderately but variably electron-dense core, often with a finely granular matrix almost completely filling the vesicle (Rogers and Burnstock, 1966; Robinson et al., 1971; Baumgarten et al., 1970; Gabella, 1970; Cook and Burnstock, 1976; Sporrong et al., 1977; Patent, Kechele, and Carrano, 1978). These vesicles have been termed large opaque vesicles (LOV) (Burnstock and Iwayama, 1971; Uehara et al., 1976). Mixed in among them are usually at least some SCV. There is generally much varia-bility between profiles in the relative proportion of LOV to SCV, as well as in the maximum size of the LOV (Gabella, 1970, 1972; Cook and

Burnstock, 1976). Because of this extreme variability, especially in the nerves of the enteric plexuses, the LOV have also been termed heterogeneous granular vesicles (Gabella, 1970). Nerve profiles containing large numbers of such vesicles will be discussed in the following sections.

Also within the enteric plexuses of mammals are profiles similar to typical cholinergic-type profiles containing occasional LGV and many SCV. But, unlike SCV in cholinergic-type profiles, these SCV are elliptical or flattened rather than round (Gabella, 1970, 1972; Cook and Burnstock, 1976). In the CNS (Uchizono, 1965) and in some invertebrate systems (Atwood, Lang, and Morin, 1972), these are very probably associated with inhibitory nerves using an unknown transmitter. Their function in the enteric plexuses is completely unknown. Similar profiles, but with relatively small (30–80 nm) flattened, dense-cored vesicles as well as flattened clear vesicles are seen in the enteric nerves of amphibians (Gibbins, unpublished observation). Too little is known about the latter two types for us to offer further comment.

By far the most confounding factor in the morphological classification of nerve profiles by their vesicle content is the tendency to extreme variability in vesicle populations. Classical cholinergic, adrenergic, and LOV-containing terminals do exist; and at their most typical, they are clearly distinguishable from each other (Burnstock and Iwayama, 1971). However, in many instances, it is extremely difficult with only routine fixation procedures to draw clear lines separating one nerve type from another. It has been claimed that because of variations of vesicle populations both between and within terminal varicosities, there is in fact no structural difference between cholinergic-type and LOV-containing profiles within the gut, there being all grades of vesicle distribution between the two extremes (Daniel et al., 1977). Despite this problem, Cook and Burnstock (1976) have classified eight morphological types of axon profiles from the enteric plexuses of guinea pigs, and Gabella (1972) decided that there were probably as many as six types in the same material. Similarly, at least six different nerve profile types can be distinguished in toad small intestine (Gibbins, unpublished observation). Even if all these types appear relatively distinct, they may not all necessarily represent different transmitters. For instance, within the gut, at least, it seems likely that there are two morphological classes of adrenergic nerves, one of typical adrenergic type, the other containing mainly LGV, as shown by uptake of 5-OHDA (Baumgarten et al., 1970; Furness and Costa, 1974).

C. Purinergic Nerves and p-Type Profiles

Nerve profiles containing LOV have been claimed to be the purinergic nerves (Burnstock, 1972). At various stages, similar profiles have been termed neurosecretory (e.g., in CNS: Szentágothai, 1970); peptidergic (in

CNS: Bargmann, Lindner, and Andres, 1967); sensory (Hoyes and Barber, 1976); p-type (Baumgarten et al., 1970).

Baumgarten et al. (1970) in fact chose the term *p-type* because of the similarity between LOV-containing profiles in the gut and the known peptidergic neurosecretory axons of the pituitary system (Bargmann et al., 1967). The neurosecretory axons are generally characterized by the presence of numerous 100-nm to 200-nm vesicles containing a moderately electron-dense homogeneous or finely granular core. These are the neurosecretory granules, which have been shown to contain the secreted peptide hormones (Dreifuss, 1975; Finlayson and Osborne, 1975; Normann, 1976; Morris, Nordmann, and Dyball, 1978). The endings also contain many 30-nm to 60-nm SCV. We will use the term *p-type* because it is sufficiently noncommittal to cover the possibilities that they are peptidergic or purinergic.

Although Pick (1967) had first suggested that the p-type profiles in gut might represent the NANC inhibitory nerves, Burnstock's (1972) identification of p-type profiles as purinergic nerves was largely derived from studies of the toad lung. It had been found physiologically that there is a purinergic vagal inhibitory innervation of the toad lung (Campbell, 1971). When Robinson et al. (1971) examined lung sections, they found profiles that were typically cholinergic and p-type profiles. They could not find typical adrenergic profiles, although the lung receives an adrenergic innervation; but they showed that the p-type profiles survived vagotomy and 6-OHDA treatment, both of which eliminated adrenergic fibers as seen by fluorescence histochemistry. It therefore seemed obvious that the purinergic nerve supply, which survives these treatments physiologically intact, coincided with the p-type profiles. Burnstock (1972) pointed out that the gut of vertebrates also contained both numerous p-type profiles and a purinergic innervation. The identification of p-type nerves as purinergic was completely acceptable until a few years ago.

In 1974, a paper by Gillespie and Lüllmann-Rauch on the ultrastructure of the rat anococcygeus muscle cast serious doubt on the correlation between nonadrenergic, noncholinergic nervous inhibition and the presence of LOV-containing nerves. The anococcygeus muscle has an adrenergic innervation and a powerful inhibitory innervation that may be classed as purinergic (see above). Yet following 5-hydroxydopamine loading and potassium permanganate fixation, which together would indicate any adrenergic nerves present, the only nonadrenergic nerve profiles present in the anococcygeus were reported to have an appearance identical to that accepted for cholinergic nerve endings. There is no physiological evidence for a functional cholinergic innervation. Therefore, the "cholinergic" profiles must in fact be the purinergic innervation.

This report, if correct, raised interesting possibilities. First, if the NANC inhibitory nerves of toad lung, vertebrate gut, and rat anococcygeus were in fact physiologically similar, they might be expected to have a common appearance. In that case, the only nerve profiles that could be identified with in toad lung, vertebrate gut, and rat anococcygeus were cholinergic-type profiles. In this case, all morphological identification of cholinergic nerves in the ANS would be suspect, and the p-type profiles in the toad lung would represent yet another class of nerve. Second, the nerves might be of the same physiological class but of different EM appearance. In this case, a categorical morphological definition of purinergic nerve fibers, especially in the gut, would be impossible. Third, the nerves might be of physiologically different classes with concomitant morphological differences. Evidence of physiological similarity between the nerves has been presented above.

The first possibility was tested on the toad lung (Campbell, Rogers, and Haller, 1978). When Robinson et al. (1971) denervated the lung, they carried out high vagosympathetic denervations that left both the cholinergic and the purinergic innervation of the lung intact (Wood and Burnstock, 1967); both cholinergic and p-type profiles remained in the lung. However, when the vagosympathetic nerve is sectioned at the lung root, the cholinergic supply is also lost, leaving only the purinergic innervation. After close denervation, the only fibers surviving in the lung were p-type (Campbell et al., 1978). At least in the lung, the purinergic nerves do not have the appearance of cholinergic nerves.

The innervation of the rat anococcygeus muscle has since been reinvestigated (Gibbins and Haller, 1979) by means of a sensitive chromaffin reaction for biogenic amines (Richards and Tranzer, 1975; Tranzer and Richards, 1976). Not two, but three morphologically distinct types of nerve profile were revealed. One of these, which was the most frequently encountered, conformed to the usual adrenergic type, with large numbers of SGV and a few LGV. Occasionally, typical cholinergic-type profiles full of homogeneous SCV and occasional LGV were seen. The third type of nerve profile, frequently encountered in nerve fiber bundles containing adrenergic fibers, was characterized by the presence of variable numbers of both SCV and LGV. The LGV, up to 120 nm in diameter (average about 100 nm), and chromaffin negative, often almost filled some varicosities. The SCV tended to be distributed through the varicosities, often being clustered in the middle of a varicosity or packed toward a portion of the axolemma, so that some sections might be confused with cholinergic profiles. However, serial and longitudinal sections through varicosities and nerve fibers indicated that the LGV-containing profiles and the typical cholinergic-appearing profiles do indeed represent discrete morphological populations (Fig. 1). Because of the predominance of the LGV and their similarity (apart from their small size) to the LOV in p-type nerves, we shall term these nerve profiles *small p-type* (sp-type).

There are so few cholinergic-type profiles in the anococcygeus that it is hard to credit that they can mediate the profound NANC inhibition occurring in this muscle. It therefore appears that, in the anococcygeus at least, purinergic nerves must be represented by sp-type profiles. A reconsideration of the toad lung material shows that the purinergic nerves there can also be classed as the sp-type. In the initial report on toad lung (Robinson et al., 1971), the large dense-core vesicles were reported to be 60–200 nm in diameter, i.e., larger than the LGV of the anococcygeus and covering the whole range of vesicle size in p-type fibers. However, in the recent study (Campbell et al., 1978) using the same fixation procedure as in the anococcygeus work, the maximum diameter of the filled vesicles was only about 140 nm. These observations suggest that purinergic neurons might be identified as sp-type profiles, not as profiles containing LOV of considerably greater maximal diameter (up to 200 nm).

If the purinergic nerves have sp-type profiles, such profiles should be found in all the organs defined in the preceding action as having a purinergic innervation, i.e., lung, gut, urinary tract, and smooth muscles of the male external genitalia, including anococcygeus.

D. The Occurrence of sp-Type Profiles in Tissues with Purinergic Innervation

1. Lung The presence of sp-type nerve profiles in the toad lung has been discussed above. Similar profiles, distinct from presumed cholinergic and adrenergic endings, have been described in the avian lung by Cook and King (1970).

The situation in mammals is not so clear. Almost certainly the mammalian airway smooth muscle has adrenergic endings characterized by the presence of relatively high numbers of LGV (70–120 nm in diamter) as well as SGV. These nerves degenerate after 6-OHDA treatment, leaving behind terminals with SCV and very variable numbers of LGV (70–120 nm in diameter), which were considered by the authors to be cholinergic. On the other hand, at least some of these remaining profiles could easily have been sp-type, as suggested by the relatively high proportions of LGV seen in their figures (cats: Silva and Ross, 1974). Similar terminals with numerous LGV (120 nm in diameter) that present a "neither typically adrenergic nor cholinergic appearance" have been reported in mouse pulmonary alveoli (Hung et al., 1972).

2. Urinary Tract Hoyes and his coworkers, in a series of papers (Hoyes, Bourne, and Martin, 1974, 1975c, 1976a, b; Hoyes, Barber, and Martin, 1975a, b; Hoyes and Barber, 1976) on the innervation of the mammalian ureter and bladder, have presented probably the most complete characterization to date of peripheral NANC nerve profiles. Although

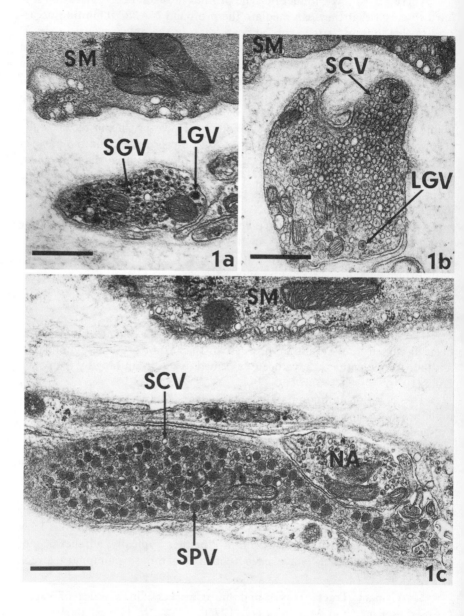

typical cholinergic and adrenergic profiles were present, most of the nerve profiles were conspicuous by their having variable mixtures of SCV and LGV. The LGV, 100–110 nm in diameter, were distributed throughout the varicosities and occasionally in axons. The proportion of SCV was variable. Often varicosities contained clusters of SCV, causing a corresponding variation in profile appearance that led to the possibility of confusion between these profiles and cholinergic ones. However, there were usually not nearly as many SCV in the NANC profiles as in presumed cholinergic endings, and the SCV of the former generally showed more differences in size and shape than did those of the latter. These LGV-containing terminals were unaffected by 6-OHDA. Although Hoyes et al. (1975c) recognized the morphological similarity of these terminals to those "defined by Burnstock as purinergic," they suggested that they represented sensory terminals (1975c, 1976a), despite the fact that only about 10% of nerve fibers degenerating in the cat bladder after afferent nerve section contain any vesicles at all (Uemura et al., 1973; Uemura, Fletcher, and Bradley, 1974). The detailed description of these NANC nerve types, however, corresponds very closely to that of similar profiles in the anococcygeus and lung; this fact suggests that these could once again be sp-type endings, corresponding in this case to the hyoscine-resistant, nonadrenergic nervous excitation observed in these tissues (see above). It is somewhat puzzling, therefore, that other workers have not reported such nerve types in their ultrastructural studies of the mammalian urinary tract (e.g., Dixon and Gosling, 1971; Gosling and Dixon, 1969, 1974). A possible explanation for this discrepancy will be discussed below.

3. **Gut** The most conspicuous gathering in the ANS of nerve profiles with prominent LGV of assorted sizes is in the enteric plexuses. On the basis of reported maximum vesicle sizes, it would seem there are probably two morphological classes of NANC nerve endings, although this has not

---

Figure 1. Representative nerve profiles from the rat anococcygeus muscle, fixed with chromate-dichromate–buffered formaldehyde-glutaraldehyde (Richards and Tranzer, 1975) and sections stained with alkaline lead citrate. Calibration bar in all electron micrographs represents 0.5 μm. (Micrographs courtesy of C. J. Haller.)

1a. Adrenergic profile showing a predominance of small granular vesicles (SGV) and some large granular vesicles (LGV). The cores of the vesicles have a very electron-dense chromaffin reaction product. Some vesicles are empty. The profile is near a smooth muscle cell (SM).

1b. A presumed cholinergic profile with many small clear vesicles (SCV). Some large granular vesicles (LGV) have slightly electron-dense cores, which are chromaffin negative. A smooth muscle cell (SM) is nearby.

1c. A small p-type (sp-type) profile containing large numbers of vesicles with moderately electron-dense cores almost filling them (SPV). Some small clear vesicles (SCV) are also present. Neither vesicle type is chromaffin positive (cf. the vesicles in the adrenergic profile, NA). SM, smooth muscle cell.

been recognized by all authors (e.g., Baumgarten et al., 1970; Gabella, 1972). One class contains vesicles of size range 80–100 nm to 120–140 nm; the other has vesicles ranging from 140–160 nm to 200 nm. Vesicles of both size classes have cores of variable density; and profiles with these vesicles can have varying proportions of SCV, which may have a somewhat pleomorphic appearance (Rogers and Burnstock, 1966; Cook and Burnstock, 1976; Feher, 1976; Yamamoto, 1977; see fig. 2). Neither group of terminals appears to take up ³H-noradrenaline actively (Taxi and Droz, 1967, 1969) or to be affected by 6-OHDA (Baumgarten et al., 1970; Feher, 1976). At least some LGV may take up 5-hydroxy-DOPA (Baumgarten et al., 1970). Another class of LGV-containing profiles in the gut has been shown to be adrenergic. Following loading with 5-OHDA, many of the LGV (90–130 nm) show an increase in electron density. These profiles, which occasionally also have SGV, degenerate after 6-OHDA treatment (Baumgarten et al., 1970). When fixed under conditions that do not optimally demonstrate adrenergic nerve endings, such profiles can easily be confused with some p-type profiles (e.g., Yamamoto, 1977).

Cook and Burnstock (1976) claimed that the NANC profiles with the smaller LGV (their type 5b) corresponded to the p-type endings of Baumgarten et al. (1970), although the maximum size of the large vesicles is significantly less than that reported by the latter workers (115 nm compared to 160 nm maximum sizes). Furthermore, they suggested that the profiles with the larger vesicles (their type 5c) were the purinergic nerves, these vesicles being similar to the LOV claimed by Burnstock (1972) to be characteristic of those nerves.

However, it seems from the above discussion that Cook and Burnstock's type 5b profiles are very similar to the sp-type profiles observed in the lung, the urinary tract, and the anococcygeus, and that these therefore are the gut purinergic nerves (fig. 2a; cf. fig. 1c). The type 5c profiles of Cook and Burnstock, on the other hand, seem restricted in mammals to the gut, where they are common, and to the myometrium, where they are rare (Silva, 1967; Hervonen, 1973; Sporrong et al., 1977). As such, they are unlikely to represent a widespread purinergic innervation. Since these profiles are distinguished by having large vesicles—up to 200 nm diameter, but with a lower size limit of about 140–160 nm—they represent only the upper portion of the range of sizes of LOV claimed by Burnstock to be typical of purinergic nerves (see above). The lower part of this range is taken by the vesicles of the sp-type profiles. Therefore, to avoid ambiguity, we suggest that p-type profiles with vesicles greater than 140–160 nm diameter be called *large p-type* (1p-type), as distinct from small p-type (sp-type) profiles, which are most likely to be the purinergic nerves; and that the term *large opaque vesicle* (LOV), as defined by Burnstock (1972) and

Burnstock and Iwayama (1971) be abandoned, or at least be restricted to synonomy with the large vesicles of lp-type endings.

4. **External Male Genitalia** The appearance of sp-type endings in the rat anococcygeus has been described above. However, it is still necessary to consider the discrepancies between our observations (three types of nerve profiles: adrenergic, cholinergic, and sp-type) and those of Gillespie and Lüllmann-Rauch (1974), who noted only adrenergic and cholinergic-type profiles in the same tissue. The most likely explanation is related to the use of different fixatives in each case. In their study of the effects of fixation on the appearance of sp-type terminals in the ureter, Hoyes and Barber (1976) found that when permanganate, osmium tetroxide, or paraformaldehyde alone was used as the primary fixative, most of the LGV in the p-type endings were not preserved, making it "difficult to differentiate vesicle containing areas of the [sp-type] axons from the terminals of cholinergic axons." (p. 118). Using veronal acetate as a buffer tended to increase the relative numbers of SCV, making it even harder to distinguish the two nerve types. With this result in hand, the discrepancy between the results of Hoyes and coworkers and Dixon and Gosling (see above) in their studies of ureter innervation becomes clearly explicable when it is realized that Gosling and Dixon (1969) and Dixon and Gosling (1971) used veronal-buffered osmium tetroxide and permanganate, respectively, as their primary fixatives. In all likelihood, the latter authors did not see any sp-type nerve endings simply because they did not preserve any. Presumably the same explanation holds true for the nerves of the anococcygeus muscle: Gillespie and Lüllman-Rauch (1974), using permanganate fixation, did not preserve the sp-type nerve endings sufficiently to recognize them. In their glutaraldehyde-fixed material, such terminals would often be very difficult to distinguish from adrenergic fibers in which the cores of SGV might not be preserved, and which can contain variable numbers of similar-sized LGV themselves.

If these conclusions are correct, very little reliability can be placed on the only paper concerning the morphological identification of nerve profile types in the retractor penis muscle, since permanganate was used as the primary fixative (Eränkö, Klinge, and Sjöstrand, 1976).

E. The Identification of Purinergic Nerve Endings

From the above discussion it may be concluded that the NANC nerve terminals originally classified by Burnstock (1972) as LOV-containing can in fact be split into two morphological groups: the lp-type, with vesicles of maximum size 200 nm; and the sp-type, with vesicles of maximum size up to 120–140 nm. A diagrammatic representation of both these types and of typical adrenergic and cholinergic profiles is shown in Figure 3. Only the sp-

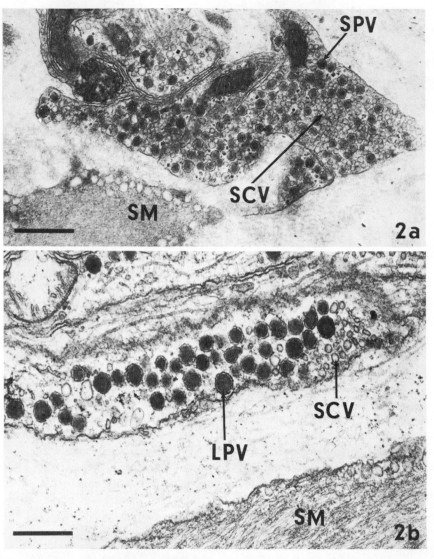

Figure 2. Representative p-type profiles in the amphibian gut. Scale bars represent 0.5 μm. (Gibbins, unpublished micrographs)

2a. A group of small p-type (sp-type) nerve profiles in frog small intestine circular muscle, fixed for the chromaffin reaction as in figure 1 and lead stained. Small clear vesicles (SCV) are abundant; there are also numerous larger vesicles with moderately electron-dense cores (SPV) typical of this nerve type. Neither vesicle type is chromaffin positive. Note close proximity of the nerves to a smooth muscle cell (SM).

2b. A large p-type (lp-type) nerve profile from toad stomach circular muscle fixed conventionally and stained with uranyl acetate and lead citrate to illustrate the variability of density and graininess of the large p-type vesicles (LPV), which are extraordinarily pale when fixed for the chromaffin reaction and stained only with lead. A clump of small clear vesicles is also present (SCV). SM, smooth muscle cell.

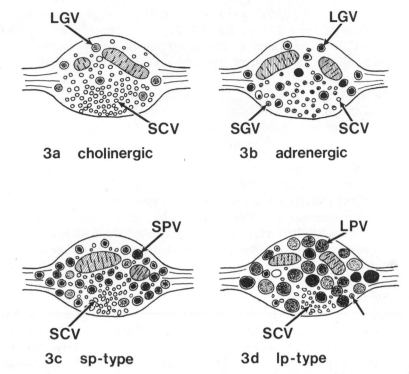

LGV
LGV

SCV
3a cholinergic

SGV **SCV**
3b adrenergic

SPV
SCV
3c sp-type

LPV
SCV
3d lp-type

Figure 3. Diagrammatic representations, to the same scale, of the typical appearance of cholinergic, adrenergic, sp-type, and lp-type nerve profiles after chromaffin fixation and light counter staining.

3a. Cholinergic: Small clear vesicles (SCV) are abundant, and large granular vesicles (LGV) with light to moderate electron-dense cores are occasionally encountered.

3b. Adrenergic: Both small clear (SCV) and small granular vesicles (SGV) are present. Large granular vesicles (LGV) often show variable degrees of filling. The chromaffin reaction product is extremely electron dense. The proportions of LGV and SGV can vary from tissue to tissue.

3c. sp-type: Although large vesicles with moderately electron-dense cores (SPV) are prominent, fairly high numbers of sometimes somewhat pleomorphic small clear vesicles (SCV) occur, often in clumps.

3d. lp-type: Very large vesicles with variably dense and grainy cores (LPV) nearly fill the varicosity. Some small clear vesicles (SCV) similar to those in the sp-type profiles are usually present, as are occasional smaller dense-cored vesicles (arrow).

type endings appear to conform to the distribution of purinergic nerves as determined by physiological studies.

The sp profiles can be characterised as follows:

Variable numbers of LGV exist, usually 90 to about 120 nm in diameter, with a somewhat variably dense core. These vesicles can almost completely fill the varicosity, be grouped at the ends of the varicosity, or be scattered throughout it.

Variable numbers of SCV exist, 30–60 nm in diameter, often showing more variation in size and shape than the SCV of cholinergic nerve endings. The SCV can be scattered throughout the varicosity, clumped in the middle of the varicosity, or aggregated towards the axolemma, especially at a synapse.

Both the LGV and the SCV are chromaffin negative, do not take up noradrenaline, and are unaffected by 5- or 6-OHDA.

The large vesicles in particular are labile in fixatives such as osmium tetroxide and especially in potassium permanganate.

Probably the most characteristic feature of these terminals is their variability with respect to the relative proportions of SCV and LGV, although similar variations in proportions of small vesicles to large vesicles exist in adrenergic nerves (Bisby and Fillenz, 1971; Fillenz and Pollard, 1976). This variability may at one extreme lead to confusion with cholinergic profiles; this confusion caused Daniel et al. (1977) to claim that it was in fact impossible to distinguish ultrastructurally NANC inhibitory nerves in the gut from cholinergic ones. The ease of distinction was probably not helped by their unusual fixation procedure (storage for at least 12 hours in glutaraldehyde). Nevertheless, in view of the overall constancy of appearance of known cholinergic endings (Uehara et al., 1976), it seems likely that a nonadrenergic nerve profile that does not clearly look like a typical cholinergic ending probably is not cholinergic at all, but rather of the sp-type. However, because of the tendency toward irregular distributions of the SCV in these nerve types, it is possible that a random section of an sp-type ending may produce a profile somewhat cholinergic in appearance. Only serial or longitudinal sections through the varicosity will solve any doubts raised in this way.

Without using specific marking methods, such as 5-OHDA loading or chromaffin reaction, it would also be possible to confuse the sp-type endings with those of LGV-containing adrenergic nerves, since the numbers and sizes of the LGV are similar. However, permanganate fixation to demonstrate adrenergic nerves, when NANC nerves are also thought to be present, should probably be avoided, since there is a good chance that the sp-type nerves will not be preserved in a recognizable state. It appears that sp-type endings, as well as being observed in the tissues discussed above as receiving a purinergic innervation, are in the pancreas (e.g., fish: Patent et al., 1978; bird: Watanabe and Yasuda, 1977; rodent: Kern, Hofmann, and Kern, 1971), and the adrenal gland (birds: Unsicker, 1973a, b). It may well be that the purinergic nerves are very widely distributed in the viscera, where their action, alas, remains unknown.

The implication in the term *p-type* is that nerves so labeled contain some kind of "peptidergic" transmitter, or transmitterlike substance. Certainly the large vesicles of the 1p-type endings show a remarkable similarity to the typical neurosecretory granules of known peptide-secreting nerves. Further, the organization of the 1p-type terminals themselves is very reminiscent of neurosecretory endings (Dreifuss, 1975; Finlayson and Osborn, 1975; Normann, 1976; Morris, 1976; Morris et al., 1978). Neurosecretory peptides have been shown to be stored in vesicles as small as 75–95 nm in diameter (Pelletier et al., 1974), so there is no intrinsic morphological reason why the sp-type nerves should not also be considered candidates for a peptidergic neurotransmission. These ultrastructural indications of possible peptide storage and release are all the more interesting for the observed distributions of peptides within nerves of at least some tissues with a purinergic innervation (discussed below).

IV. HISTOCHEMICAL STUDIES

The introduction of the formaldehyde-induced fluorescence technique for localizing catecholamines in adrenergic nerves (Falck and Torp, 1962; Falck, 1962) was a major advance in studies of the ANS. For the first time it was possible to visualize an autonomic transmitter substance directly. The light microscopic technique for showing adrenergic nerves has been supported by a number of EM techniques based on the chromaffin reaction (see above). One of the major trends in recent research has been the attempt to develop techniques for localizing other transmitter substances.

No comparable techniques for visualizing cholinergic nerves have yet been developed. Although there are good methods for localizing acetylcholinesterase (Koelle, 1963; Robinson, 1971), this enzyme is not a specific marker for cholinergic nerves (e.g., Robinson and Bell, 1967; Eränkö et al., 1970; Hervonen, Kanerva, and Rechardt, 1972; Barajas and Wang, 1975). Choline acetylase, which is probably a specific marker for cholinergic neurons, can be localized histochemically or immunohistochemically (Burt, 1970; Kasa, Mann, and Hebb, 1970; Kan, Chao, and Eng, 1978); but there are some doubts about the specificity of both methods (Burt and Silver, 1973; Rossier, 1975).

A. Histochemical Localization of Purinergic Nerves?

No technique has been developed for demonstrating the specific localization of ATP in tissue sections. However, there is some indication that purinergic nerves can be stained specifically by quinacrine, which can be localized by fluorescence microscopy. Olson, Ålund, and Norberg (1976) reported that incubation of surviving tissues in quinacrine-containing media stained certain neurons and axonal processes, as had been noted by Smith (1967). Quinacrine-positive cell bodies were found in Auerbach's plexus throughout the mouse intestine and in the urinary bladder. Stained nerve fibers were also found in the gut and bladder, but not in the iris. Olson et al. (1976) pointed out that, on the basis of distribution alone, the stainable nerves might be purinergic neurons. Burnstock et al. (1978b) have confirmed the presence of stained nerve fibers and cell bodies in the bladder and reported their absence from the iris and the vas deferens. Quinacrine-positive neurons and fibers, which survived treatment with 6-hydroxydopamine, were also found in the rat and rabbit anococcygeus muscles (Burnstock et al., 1978a).

It has been suggested (Burnstock et al., 1978a, b) that the ability of quinacrine to stain purinergic nerve fibers might be related to the chemical binding that occurs between quinacrine and ATP (Irvin and Irvin, 1954). However, the staining does not occur specifically unless the tissues are kept in a reasonably balanced medium at body temperature (Olson et al., 1976), which suggests that a specific uptake process in the nerve membrane may be involved.

If the fibers stained by quinacrine are indeed the purinergic nerves, it is interesting to note that chronic treatment with quinacrine can cause enteromegaly and damage to some fibers in the gut plexuses, with some signs of impairment of peristalsis (Keeler, Richardson, and Watson, 1966; Smith, 1967). Conceivably, quinacrine is concentrated in the purinergic neurons to levels that are generally or specifically cytotoxic. It may be that quinacrine can be used experimentally on the purinergic system in much the same way that 6-hydroxydopamine is used to produce adrenergic denervation.

B. Immunohistochemical Localization of Peptides

A number of peptides with considerable biological activity have been extracted from peripheral tissues (e.g., substance P: Euler and Gaddum, 1931) and have naturally been considered candidate transmitter substances. In the last few years the possibility that certain peptides are autonomic transmitters has come to the fore, because they have now been localized within autonomic neurons by immunohistochemical methods. The work was triggered in 1964, when Goodfriend, Levine, and Fasman showed that, when a small peptide was bound to proteins, the complex could be used as an antigen to raise antibodies showing specificity for the peptide. The natural peptide can then be shown in tissue sections, both light- and electron-microscopically, by treating the section with antibody labeled directly or indirectly with fluorescent or electron-dense markers. The potential value of these methods is enormous and is only now being realized.

Before peptide localizations are described, several limitations of immunochemistry will be indicated.

1. Antisera are mixtures of antibodies. For example, Swaab and Pool (1975) found that an antilysine vasopressin (LVP) combined equally well

with LVP or oxytocin and rather better with arginine vasopressin (AVP). The mixed antibodies can be separated: Swaab and Pool removed an oxytocin-reacting element from an AVP antiserum by adsorption onto oxytocin coupled to agarose beads. This type of contamination would not necessarily be detected by the commonly applied test of specificity, incubation of the antiserum with excess homologous antigen prior to its application to tissue sections.

2. Antibodies commonly react with only certain portions of an antigenic peptide and are selective either for a particular part of the peptide conformation or for the amino acid sequence. For instance, a radioimmunoassay for the 28-amino acid peptide, vasoactive intestinal peptide (Fahrenkrug and Schaffalitzky de Muckadell, 1977) gives 98% of full reactivity to sequence 7 to 28 and 13% to sequence 11 to 28. The same sequence or conformation in any other structure is likely to give a false positive reaction. The precaution can be taken, and regularly is taken, of checking for cross-reactivity with other known peptides. However, there will always be a possibility of cross-reaction with an unknown peptide or protein. These erroneous positive reactions will be prevented specifically by preincubation with homologous antigens.

In the following account we have adopted the common practice of referring to the localization of "immunoreactivity" (IR).

Four biologically active peptides have now been localized as IR in autonomic neurones: substance P, vasoactive intestinal peptide (VIP), enkephalin, and somatostatin. All are distributed in nerve fibers and neurons within the intestinal wall, but enkephalin-IR and somatostatin-IR fibers seem to be related mainly to the enteric plexuses and innervate gut muscle sparsely, if at all (Schultzberg et al., 1978).

Both substance P-IR and VIP-IR are found in nerve fibers distributed densely throughout gut muscle layers. Substance P causes contraction of all segments of the gut (Pernow, 1960), whereas VIP has inhibitory actions on gut muscle (see below). VIP, by its distribution and action, is therefore a candidate transmitter substance for purinergic nerves and we will discuss its histochemical distribution and physiological effects in detail.

C. Vasoactive Intestinal Peptide (VIP)

VIP was first identified as a novel vasodilator in secretin extracts of pig small intestine (Said and Mutt, 1970a, b; 1972). It is an octacosapeptide, and the amino acid sequence (Mutt and Said, 1974) is comparable to that of secretin or glucagon. An avian VIP, differing in only four amino acids, has been extracted from chicken intestine (Nilsson, 1974, 1975).

1. **Distribution of VIP in nerves** The distribution of VIP in the periphery has been studied by radioimmunoassay (Bloom, Bryant, and Polak, 1975; Larsson et al., 1976b; Said and Rosenberg, 1976; Larsson,

Fahrenkrug, and Schaffalitzky de Muckadell, 1977a, b; Yanaihara et al., 1977). VIP-IR has been found at high levels in both the muscularis and the submucosa-mucosa throughout the gastrointestinal tract and in many regions of the urinogenital tract; but little or none has been found in the heart, the liver, and the skeletal muscle. VIP-IR was found in peripheral neural tissue, specifically an unidentified sympathetic nerve (Said and Rosenberg, 1976).

With immunohistochemical techniques, nerve fibers showing VIP-IR have been found widely distributed in the periphery. The fibers often have the typical varicose appearance of terminal autonomic nerve fibers. Fibers have been found throughout the gastrointestinal tract (Bryant et al., 1976; Larsson et al., 1976b; Uddman et al., 1978), where they form a dense mesh-work in both the myenteric and the submucous plexus. They innervate the smooth muscle layers of the gut wall, but they are rare in the largely striated muscle of the rat esophagus. They are also distributed to the mucosa, especially in the intestine, where they make nets around crypts and in the core of small intestinal villi. VIP-IR fibers have been found in the wall of the gall bladder (Sundler et al., 1976) and around the acini of the pancreas (Bryant et al., 1976; Sundler et al., 1978; Larsson et al., 1978); throughout the urinogenital system, especially in the ureters and the trigonal bladder; the vagina and the uterine cervix; and the epididymis, the vas deferens, the prostate, the seminal vesicle, and the trabeculae of the penile corpora cavernosa (Alm et al., 1977; Larsson et al., 1977a, b). The heart contains no VIP-IR fibers (Larsson et al., 1976b), but the fibers appear to innervate muscular blood vessels in the above organs as well as cerebral vessels (Larsson, Edvinsson, and Fahrenkrug, 1976a). Fibers have also been seen forming baskets around sympathetic ganglion cells (Hökfelt et al., 1977b).

Larsson (1977) used peroxidase-antiperoxidase staining to localize VIP-IR electron-microscopically. In the cat colonic mucosa and submucosa he found nerve fiber profiles containing numerous LGV of 70–160 nm diameter in which VIP-IR was located. Although Larsson could not clearly distinguish different classes of p-type profiles in his material, his reported size range of VIP-IR LGV suggests that they could be in sp-type endings.

The source of VIP-IR fibers in the periphery is not particularly clear. The authors listed above have described neuron somata with VIP-IR scattered in both gut plexuses (see also Schultzberg et al., 1978), in the gall bladder wall, in the pancreas of dogs, and in bilateral ganglia near the urinary tract. In addition, Hökfelt et al. (1977b) have described a few VIP-IR cells in the coeliac-superior mesenteric ganglion of guinea pigs. There is considerable variation between species. For instance, no positive cells were found in pancreatic ganglia of pigs, cats, human beings, or mice (Larsson et al., 1978), or in the coeliac ganglion of rats (Hökfelt et al., 1977b). One is left with the impression that there are far too many nerve fibers to originate from the relatively few somata seen. This probably means, as is widely claimed in the literature, that peptide levels are low in the cell bodies of peptidergic neurons.

2. Actions of VIP   The autonomic actions of VIP have not been studied extensively. The list of actions given by Said (1975) will suffice, with a few additions:

Cardiovascular: Vasodilatation of pulmonary and systemic (including coronary) vessels; positive inotropic action on heart.

Respiratory: Relaxation of guinea pig trachea.

Metabolic: Stimulation of lipolysis and glycogenolysis; stimulation of endocrine pancreatic secretion of insulin and glucagon (Schebalin, Said, and Makhlouf, 1977).

Gastrointestinal secretion: Inhibition of gastric acid secretion; stimulation of exocrine pancreatic secretion of water and electrolytes (also Konturek, Pucher, and Radecki, 1976); stimulation of bile flow and relaxation of gall bladder muscle; stimulation of small-intestine secretion; production of Na^+ efflux into ileal lumen.

Gastrointestinal motility: Relaxation of muscle from many parts of the gut, including esophagus and lower esophageal sphincter (Domschke et al., 1978; Uddman et al., 1978). A crude extract of VIP from pig intestine, G2, caused relaxation of rat stomach, cat terminal ileum, and chick rectum and rectal cecum but did not affect guinea-pig ileum, cat jejunum, or rat colon or duodenum. A histamine impurity in this extract caused contraction of cat ileum (Piper, Said, and Vane, 1970). Pure VIP is reported to cause a contraction of human duodenum and ileum *in vitro* that is mediated by intrinsic nerves, since it is blocked by tetrodotoxin (Makhlouf and Said, 1975).

We have no information on the action of VIP on many of the other organs that are reported to contain VIP-IR nerves.

3. Release of VIP on nerve stimulation   In the calf, thoracic vagal stimulation causes the appearance of increased levels of VIP-IR in intestinal lymph, provided that the splanchnic nerves have been cut beforehand (Edwards et al., 1978). A similar phenomenon in the pig has been studied in greater detail by Fahrenkrug et al. (1978). They showed that vagal stimulation caused a release of VIP-IR into portal venous blood. The release was not antagonized by atropine but was prevented by hexamethonium treatment. Splanchnic nerve stimulation strongly antagonized vagal release of VIP-IR via an α-adrenergic mechanism, even after isolation of the adrenal glands. Close intra-arterial injections of acetylcholine caused a release of VIP-IR, but this was antagonized by atropine and not by hexamethonium.

Fahrenkrug et al. point out that this could hardly be a release of VIP from VIP-IR cells in the gut mucosa, since the antiserum to VIP used in this study did not react with mucosal cells in histochemical studies. No explanation of the effects of acetylcholine is apparent.

4. VIP and purinergic nerves Several features make VIP a strong contender as the transmitter substance for purinergic nerves. VIP-IR has been found in all of the organs that we have defined as having a purinergic innervation with the exception of lung, which has not been examined. It has been found in nerve cell bodies at points where synapses must exist in purinergic pathways. VIP-IR has been identified electron-microscopically in nerve profiles in the gut containing LGV of what may be the sp-type, which we have suggested are the purinergic nerves. The action of VIP on the gut is inhibitory. Unfortunately, its actions on other organs with purinergic innervation is not known. (We think we know why these observations are limited: a commercial preparation of VIP would cost $180,000,000 per gram in Australia!) Finally VIP-IR is released from the gut on vagus nerve stimulation in a way that is consistent with release from postganglionic neurons. As Fahrenkrug et al. (1978) have stated, VIP could mediate two of the known atropine-resistant effects of vagal stimulation in the pig, gastric relaxation and pancreatic secretion. We regard this evidence as strongly suggestive that VIP is the purinergic mediator.

One of the reported localizations of VIP-IR concerns us. VIP is apparently contained in many nerve fibers in the vas deferens. Although it has been suggested that excitatory transmission to the vas deferens is mediated by NANC nerves (Ambache and Zar, 1971), we are not convinced that the transmission is anything other than adrenergic. The EM studies of nerves in the vas deferens seem to have shown conclusively that the fibers are predominantly adrenergic, and no evidence for p-type fibers has been produced. On density alone of the VIP-IR fibers in the vas deferens, we can only think that VIP is here contained in adrenergic nerves and has no major transmitter function or that the reported localization is erroneous. Support for the first alternative comes from the localization of somatostatin-IR in peripheral, probably adrenergic, nerve cell bodies (Hökfelt et al., 1977a).

V. TRENDS IN RESEARCH

We have examined three areas of current research on the ANS: pharmacology, electron microscopy, and histochemistry. In each area, the concept that the ANS contains NANC nerves is strongly established, for what seem to be good reasons. In the future, we would expect work in the pharmacological area to center on screening potential antagonists for the many recently postulated NANC transmitter substances. In the morphological areas, there is no doubt that we are at the beginning of an explosion of immunochemical work. The versatility of immunohistochemistry is only now being realized: while much of the work to date has concentrated on large molecules, it has been found that antibodies can be produced with specificity to a substance as small as 5-hydroxytryptamine (Hökfelt et al., 1978). This could lead to immunochemical techniques for the localization of acetylcholine and ATP, which has proved so refractory.

A. The Purinergic Theory

Since this review has been written around purinergic nerves as established examples of NANC nerves, some summarizing comments on the purinergic theory must be made. The results of pharmacological experiments on purinergic nerves have by and large been consistent with purinergic theory. However, certain anomalous effects of ATP on purinergically innervated tissues have been reported. Since we have personal experience of such a preparation, we have a prejudice against the purinergic theory. The proposition that purinergic nerves appear electron-microscopically as p-type nerves with LOV of up to 200 nm is, we believe, an oversimplification. In fact, there seem to be at least two populations of p-type nerves in the ANS, and the purinergic nerves can be related to the population characterized by containing smaller (<140 nm) LOV. A reexamination of many tissues is called for. We do agree that purinergic nerves are p-type and, taking that name at face value, it is possible that the purinergic transmitter is a peptide. We are aware of pharmacological evidence against the involvement of many known peptides (e.g., substance P, bradykinin). However, VIP approximates a distribution in autonomic nerves and, as far as the limited information tells us, an action on effector organs that are appropriate to the purinergic transmitter.

REFERENCES

Alm, P.; Alumets, J.; Håkanson, R.; Sundler, F.: Peptidergic (Vasoactive Intestinal Peptide) Nerves in the Genitourinary Tract. Neuroscience 2(1977)751–754

Ambache, N.; Freeman, M.A.: Atropine-resistant Longitudinal Muscle Spasms Due to Excitation of Noncholinergic Neurons in Auerbach's Plexus. J Physiol (Lond) 199(1968)705–728

Ambache, N.; Killick, S.W.; Zar, M.A.: Extraction from Ox Retractor Penis of an Inhibitory Substance Which Mimics Its Atropine Resistant Neurogenic Relaxation. Br J Pharmacol 54(1975)409–410

Ambache, N.; Zar, M.A.: Non-Cholinergic Transmission by post-Ganglionic Motor Neurones in the Mammalian Bladder. J Physiol (Lond) 210(1970)761–783

Ambache, N.; Zar, M.A.: Evidence against Adrenergic Motor Transmission in the Guinea pig Vas Deferens. J Physiol (Lond) 216(1971)359–389

Atanasova, E.S.; Vladimirova, I.A.; Shuba, M.F.: Non-Adrenergic Inhibitory Postsynaptic Potentials of Stomach Smooth Muscle Cells. Neurophysiol (Russ) 4(1972)216–222

Atwood, H.L.; Lang, F.; Morin, W.A.: Synaptic Vesicles: Selective Depletion in Crayfish Excitatory and Inhibitory Neurons. Science 176(1972)1353

134 / Graeme Campbell and Ian L. Gibbins

Axelsson, J.; Holmberg, B.: The Effects of Extracellularly Applied ATP and Related Compounds on Electrical and Mechanical Activity of the Smooth Muscle Taenia Coli from the Guinea Pig. Acta Physiol Scand 75(1969)149-156.
Barajas, L.; Wang, P.: Demonstration of Acetylcholinesterase in the Adrenergic Nerves of the Renal Glomerular Arterioles. J Ultrastruct Res 53(1975)244-253
Bargmann, W.; Lindner, E.; Andres, K.: Über Synapsen an endokrinen Epithelzellen und die Definition sekretorischer Neuronen. Untersuchungen am Zwischenlappen der Katzenhypophyse. Z Zellforsch Mikr Anat 77(1967)282-298
Barsoum, G. S.; Gaddum, J.H.: The Pharmacological Estimation of Adenosine and Histamine in Blood. J Physiol (Lond) 85(1935)1-14
Baumgarten, H.G.; Holstein, A. F.; Owman, C.: Auerbach's Plexus of Mammals and Man: Electronmicroscopic Identification of Three Different Types of Neuronal Processes in Myenteric Ganglia of the Large Intestine from Rhesus Monkeys, Guinea-Pigs and Man. Z Zellforsch Mikr Anat 106(1970)376-397
Beani, L.; Bianchi, C.; Crema, A.: Vagal Non-Adrenergic Inhibition of Guinea-Pig Stomach. J Physiol (Lond) 217(1971)259-280
Beck, C. S.; Osa, T.: Membrane Activity in Guinea-Pig Gastric Sling Muscle: a Nerve-Dependent Phenomenon. Am J Physiol 220(1971)1397-1403
Bell, C.: Autonomic Nervous Control of Reproduction: Circulatory and Other Factors. Pharmacol Rev 24(1972)657-736
Bennett, A.; Fleshler, B.: Prostaglandins and the Gastrointestinal Tract. Gastroenterology 59(1970)790-800
Bennett, D.W.; Drury, A.N.: Further Observations Relating to the Physiological Activity of Adenine Compounds. J Physiol (Lond) 72(1931)288-320
Bennett, M.R.; Burnstock, G.: Electrophysiology of the Innervation of Intestinal Smooth Muscle. In: Handbook of Physiology. Section 6. Alimentary Canal IV Motility, pp. 1709-1732. American Physiological Society, Washington, 1968
Bennett, M.R.; Burnstock, G.; Holman, M.E.: Transmission from Intramural Inhibitory Nerves in the Smooth Muscle of the Guinea-Pig Taenia Coli. J Physiol (Lond) 182(1966)541-558
Berger, P.J.: Autonomic Innervation of the Visceral and Vascular Smooth Muscle of the Lizard Lung. Comp Gen Pharmacol 4(1973)1-10
Bianchi, A.; de Natale, G.; Giaquinto, S.: The Effects of Adenosine and its Phosphorylated Derivatives upon the Respiratory Apparatus. Arch Int Pharmacodyn Ther 145(1963)498-517
Bisby, M.A.; Fillenz, M.: The Storage of Endogenous Noradrenaline in Sympathetic Nerve Terminals. J Physiol (Lond) 215(1971)163-179
Bloom, F.E.: The Fine Structural Localization of Monoamines in Nervous Tissue. Int Rev Neurobiol 13(1970)27-66
Bloom, F.E.: Electron Microscopy of Catecholamine-Containing Structures. Handb Exp Pharmakol 33(1972)46-78
Bloom, F.E.; Aghajanian, G.K.: An Electron Microscope Analysis of Large Granular Synaptic Vesicles of the Brain in Relation to Monoamine Content. J Pharmacol Exp Ther 159(1968)261-273
Bloom, S.R.; Bryant, M.G.; Polak, J.M.: Distribution of Gut Hormones. Gut 16(1975)821
Bryant, M.G.; Bloom, S.R.; Polak, J.M.; Albuquerque, R.H.; Modlin, I.; Pearse, A.G.E.: Possible Dual Role for Vasoactive Intestinal Peptide as a Gastrointestinal Hormone and Neurotransmitter Substance. Lancet 1(1976)991-993
Buchthal, F.; Kahlson, G.: The Motor Effect of Adenosine Triphosphate and Allied Phosphorus Compounds on Smooth Mammalian Muscle. Acta Physiol Scand 8(1944)325-334
Bülbring, E.; Gershon, M.D.: 5-Hydroxytryptamine Participation in the Vagal Inhibitory Innervation of the Stomach. J Physiol (Lond) 192(1967)823-846
Bülbring, E.; Tomita, T.: Evidence Supporting the Assumption That the 'Inhibitory Potential' in the Taenia Coli of the Guinea-Pig Is a Post-Synaptic Potential Due to Nerve Stimulation. J Physiol (Lond) 185(1966)24-25P
Burnstock, G.: Neural Nomenclature. Nature 229(1971)282-283
Burnstock, G.: Purinergic Nerves. Pharmacol Rev 24(1972)509-581

Burnstock, G.: Purinergic Transmission. In: Handbook of Psychopharmacology, Vol. 5, pp. 131–194, ed. by L.L. Iversen, S.D. Iversen, S.H. Snyder. Plenum, New York, 1975a

Burnstock, G.: Comparative Studies of Purinergic Nerves. J Exp Zool 194(1975b)103–134

Burnstock, G.: Basis for Distinguishing Two Types of Purinergic Receptor. In: Cell Membrane Receptors for Drugs and Hormones: A Multidisciplinary Approach, pp. 107–118, ed. by L. Bolis, R.W. Straub, Raven, New York, 1978

Burnstock, G.; Campbell, G.; Bennett, M.; Holman, M.E.: Inhibition of the Smooth Muscle of the Taenia Coli. Nature 200(1963a)581–582

Burnstock, G.; Campbell, G.; Bennett, M.; Holman, M.E.: The Effects of Drugs on the Transmission of Inhibition from Autonomic Nerves to the Smooth Muscle of the Guinea-Pig Taenia Coli. Biochem Pharmacol 12 Suppl 134(1963b)

Burnstock, G., Campbell, G.; Bennett, M.; Holman, M.E.: Innervation of the Guinea-Pig Taenia Coli: Are There Intrinsic Inhibitory Nerves Which Are Distinct from Sympathetic nerves? Int J Neuropharmacol 3(1964)163–166

Burnstock, G.; Campbell, G.; Rand, M.J.: The Inhibitory Innervation of the Taenia of the Guinea-Pig Caecum. J Physiol (Lond) 182(1966)504–526

Burnstock, G.; Campbell, G.; Satchell, D.; Smythe, A.: Evidence That Adenosine Triphosphate or a Related Nucleotide is the Transmitter Substance Released by Non-Adrenergic Inhibitory Nerves in the Gut. Br J Pharmacol 40(1970)668–688

Burnstock, G.; Cocks, T.; Crowe, R.: Evidence For Purinergic Innervation of the Anococcygeus Muscle. Br J Pharmacol 64(1978a)13–20

Burnstock, G.; Cocks, T.; Crowe, R.; Kasakov, L.: Purinergic Innervation of the Guinea-Pig Urinary Bladder. Br J Pharmaol 63(1978b)125–138

Burnstock, G.; Cocks, T.; Kasakov, L.; Wong, H.K.: Direct Evidence For ATP Release from Non-Adrenergic, Non-Cholinergic ('Purinergic') Nerves in the Guinea-Pig Taenia Coli and Bladder. Eur J Pharmacol 49(1978c)145–149

Burnstock, G.; Costa, M.: Adrenergic Neurons. Their Organization, Function and Development in the Peripheral Nervous System. Chapman and Hall, London, 1975

Burnstock, G.; Dumsday, B.; Smythe, A.: Atropine-Resistant Excitation of the Urinary Bladder: the Possibility of Transmission via Nerves Releasing a Purine Nucleotide. Br J Pharmacol 44(1972)451–461

Burnstock, G.; Iwayama, T.: Fine Structural Identification of Autonomic Nerves and Their Relation to Smooth Muscle. Prog Brain Res 34(1971)389–404

Burt, A.M.: A Histochemical Procedure for the Localization of Choline Acetyltransferase Activity. J Histochem Cytochem 18(1970)408–415

Burt, A.M.; Silver, A.: Histochemistry of Choline Acetyltransferase: A Critical Analysis. Brain Res 62(1973)509–516

Campbell, G.: The Inhibitory Nerve Fibers in the Vagal Supply to the Guinea-Pig Stomach. J Physiol (Lond) 185(1966)600–612

Campbell, G.: Autonomic Nervous Supply to Effector Tissues. In: Smooth Muscle, pp. 451–495, ed. by E. Bülbring, A. Brading, A. Jones, T. Tomita. Edward Arnold, London, 1970

Campbell, G.: Autonomic Innervation of the Lung Musculature of the Toad (Bufo marinus). Comp Gen Pharmacol 2(1971)281–286

Campbell, G.; Haller, C.J.; Rogers, D.C.: Fine Structural and Cytochemical Study of the Innervation of Smooth Muscle in the Amphibian (Bufo marinus) Lung before and after Denervation. Cell Tissue Res, 194(1978)419–432

Coburn, R.F.; Tomita, T.: Evidence for Non-Adrenergic Inhibitory Nerves in the Guinea-Pig Trachealis Muscle. Am J Physiol 224(1973)1072–1080

Coleman, R.A.: Evidence for a Non-Adrenergic Inhibitory Nervous Pathway in Guinea-Pig Trachea. Br J Pharmacol 48(1973)360–361

Coleman, R.A.: Effects of Some Purine Derivatives on the Guinea-Pig Trachea and Their Interaction with Drugs That Block Adenosine Uptake. Br J Pharmacol 57(1976)51–57

Coleman, R.A.; Levy, G.P.: A Non-Adrenergic Inhibitory Nervous Pathway in Guinea-Pig Trachea. Br J Pharmacol 52(1974)167–174

Cook, R.D.; Burnstock, G.: The Ultrastructure of Auerbach's Plexus in the Guinea Pig. I. Neuronal elements. J Neurocytol 5(1976)171–194

Cook, R.D.; King, A.S.: Observations on the Ultrastructure of the Smooth Muscle and Its Innervation in the Avian Lung. J Anat 106(1970)273–283

Costa, M.; Furness, J.B.: The Innervation of the Internal Anal Sphincter in the Guinea-Pig. Rend Gastroenterologia 5(1973)37–38

Creed, K.E.; Gillespie, J.S.: Some Electrical Properties of the Rabbit Anococcygeus Muscle and a Comparison of the Effects of Inhibitory Nerve Stimulation in the Rat and Rabbit. J Physiol (Lond) 273(1977)137–153

Creed, K.E.; Gillespie, J.S.; McCaffery, H.: The Rabbit Anococcygeus and Its Response to Field Stimulation and to Some Drugs. J Physiol (Lond) 273(1977)121–135

Dale, H.H.: Nomenclature of Fibres in the Autonomic System and Their Effects. J Physiol (Lond) 80(1933)10P–11P

Daniel, E.E.; Taylor, G.S.; Daniel, V.P.; Holman, M.E.: Can Non-Adrenergic Inhibitory Varicosities Be Identified Structurally? Can J Physiol Pharmacol 55(1977)243–250

Dean, D.M.; Downie, J.W.: Interaction of Prostaglandin and Adenosine-5'-Triphosphate in the Noncholinergic Neurotransmission in Rabbit Detrusor. Prostaglandins 16(1978)245–251

De Groat, W.C.; Saum, W.R.: Synaptic Transmission in Parasympathetic Ganglia in the Urinary Bladder of the Cat. J Physiol (Lond) 256(1976)137–158

De Robertis, E.: Contribution of Electron Microscopy to Some Neuropharmacological Problems. Biochem Pharmacol 9(1962)49–59

De Robertis, E.; Bennett, H.S.: Submicroscopic Vesicular Component in the Synapse. Fed Proc 13(1954)35A

De Robertis, E.; Pellegrino de Iraldi, A.: A Plurivesicular Component in Adrenergic Nerve Endings. Anat Rec 139(1961)299A

Diamant, N.E.: Electrical Activity of the Cat Smooth Muscle Oesophagus *in Vitro*. Rend Gastroenterologia 5(1973)26–27

Dixon, J.S.; Gosling, J.A.: Histochemical and Electronmicroscopic Observations on the Innervation of the Upper Sector of the Mammalian Ureter. J Anat 110(1971)57–66

Domschke, W.; Lux, G.; Domschke, S.; Strunz, U.; Bloom, S.R.; Wünsch, E.: Effects of Vasoactive Intestinal Peptide on Resting and Pentagastrin Stimulated Lower Esophageal Sphincter Pressure. Gastroenterology 75(1978)9–12

Dorr, L.D.; Brody, M.J.: Haemodynamic Mechanisms of Erection in the Canine Penis. Am J Physiol 213(1967)1526–1531

Downie, J.W.; Dean, D.M.: The Contribution of Cholinergic Post-Ganglionic Neurotransmission to Contraction of Rabbit Detrusor. J Pharmacol Exp Ther 203(1977)417–425

Dreifuss, J.J.: A Review on Neurosecretory Granules: Their Contents and Mechanism of release. Ann NY Acad Sci 248(1975)184–201

Drury, A.N.; Szent-Györgi, A.: The Physiological Activity of Adenine Compounds with Especial Reference to Their Action upon the Mammalian Heart. J Physiol (Lond) 68(1936)213–237

Dumsday. B.H.: Atropine-Resistance of the Urinary Bladder. J Pharm Pharmacol 23(1971)222–225

Edwards, A.V.; Bircham, P.M.M.; Mitchell, S.J.; Bloom, S.R.: Changes in the Concentration of Vasoactive Intestinal Peptide in Intestinal Lymph in Response to Vagal Stimulation in the Calf. Experientia 34(1978)1186–1187

Eränkö, O.; Klinge, E.; Sjöstrand, N.O.: Different Types of Synaptic Vesicles in Axons of the Retractor Penis Muscle of the Bull. Experientia 32(1976)1335–1337

Eränkö, O.; Rechardt, L.; Eränkö, L.; Cunningham, A.: Light and Electron Microscopic Histochemical Observations on Cholinesterase Containing Sympathetic Nerve Fibers in the Pineal Body of the Rat. Histochem J 2(1970)479–489

Euler, U.S. von: Histamine as a Specific Constituent of Certain Autonomic Nerve Fibers. Acta Physiol Scand 19(1949)85–93

Euler, U.S. von; Gaddum, J.H.: An Unidentified Depressor Substance in Certain Tissue Extracts. J Physiol (Lond) 72(1931)74–87

Fahrenkrug, J.; Galbo, H.; Holst, J.J.; Schaffalitzky de Muckadell, O.B.: Influence of the Autonomic Nervous System on the Release of Vasoactive Intestinal Polypeptide from the Porcine Gastrointestinal Tract. J Physiol (Lond) 280(1978)405–422

Fahrenkrug, J.; Schaffalitzky de Muckadell, O.: Radioimmunoassay of Vasoactive Intestinal Polypeptide (VIP) in plasma. J Lab Clin Med 89(1977)1379-1388

Falck, B.: Observations on the Possibilities of the Cellular Localization of Monoamines by a Fluorescence Method. Acta Physiol Scand 56 Suppl 197(1962)1-25

Falck, B.; Torp, A.: New Evidence for the Localization of Noradrenaline in the Adrenergic Nerve Terminals. Med Exp (Basel) 6(1962)169-172

Feher, E.: Ultrastructural Study of Nerve Terminals in the Submucous Plexus and Mucous Membrane after Extirpation of the Myenteric Plexus. Acta Anat (Basel) 94(1976)74-88

Fillenz, M.; Pollard, R. M.: Quantitative Differences between Sympathetic Nerve Terminals. Brain Res 109(1976)443-454

Finlayson, L.H.; Osborne, M.P.: Secretory Activity of Neurons and Related Electrical Activity. Adv Comp Physiol Biochem 6(1975)165-258

Fülgraff, G.; Schmidt, L.: Untersuchungen über die atropinresistente Übertragung am Pelvicus-Colon-Präparat der Katze in vitro. Arch Int Pharmacodyn Ther 149(1964)552-559

Furness, J.B.: An Electrophysiological Study of the Innervation of the Smooth Muscle of the Colon. J Physiol (Lond) 205(1969)549-562

Furness, J.B.: An examination of Nerve-Mediated, Hyoscine-Resistant Excitation of the Guinea-Pig Colon. J Physiol (Lond) 207(1970)803-822

Furness, J.B.; Costa, M.: The Nervous Release and the Action of Substances Which Affect Intestinal Muscle through neither Adrenoceptors nor Cholinoceptors. Philos Trans R Soc Lond [Biol] 265(1973)123-133

Furness, J.B.; Costa, M.: Adrenergic Innervation of the Gastrointestinal Tract. Ergeb Physiol Biol Chem Exp Pharmakol 69(1974)1-51

Gabella, G.: Electron Microscopic Observations on the Innervation of the Intestinal Inner Muscle Layer. Experientia 26(1970)44-46

Gabella, G.: Fine Structure of the Myenteric Plexus in the Guinea-Pig Ileum. J Anat 111(1972)69-97

Gershon, M.D.; Thompson, G.B.: The Maturation of Neuromuscular Function in a Multiply Innervated Structure: Development of the Longitudinal Smooth Muscle of the Foetal Mammalian Gut and Its Cholinergic Excitatory, Adrenergic Inhibitory, and Non-Adrenergic Inhibitory Innervation. J Physiol (Lond) 234(1973)257-277

Gibbins, I.L.: Haller, C.J.: Ultrastructural Identification of Non-Adrenergic, Non-Cholinergic Nerves in the Rat Anococcygeus. Cell Tissue Res, in press

Gillespie, J.S.: The Rat Anococcygeus and Its Response to Nerve Stimulation and to Some Drugs. Br J Pharmacol 45(1972)404-416

Gillespie, J.S.; Lüllman-Rauch, R.: On the Ultrastructure of the Rat Anococcygeus Muscle. Cell Tissue Res 149(1974)91-104

Gillespie, J.S.; Martin, W.: A Smooth Muscle Inhibitory Material Extracted from the Bovine Retractor Penis and Rat Anococcygeus Muscles. J Physiol (Lond) 280(1978)45-46P

Gillespie, J.S.; McGrath, J.C.: The Spinal Origin of the Motor and Inhibitory Innervation of the Rat Anococcygeus Muscles. J Physiol (Lond) 230(1973)659-672

Gillespie, J.S.; McGrath, J.C.: The Response of the Cat Anococcygeus Muscle to Nerve or Drug Stimulation and a Comparison with the Rat Anococcygeus. Br J Pharmacol 50(1974)109-118

Gillespie, J.S.; McKnight, A.T.: The Action of Some Vasoactive Polypeptides and their Antagonists on the Anococcygeus Muscle. J Physiol (Lond) 260(1976)19-20P

Goodfriend, T.L.; Levine, L.: Fasman, G.D.: Antibodies to Bradykinin and Angiotensin: A Use of Carbodiimides in Immunology. Science 144(1964)1344-1346

Gosling, J.A.; Dixon, J.S.: The Fine Structure of the Vasa Recta and Associated Nerves in the Rabbit Kidney. Anat Rec 165(1969)503-514

Gosling, J.A.; Dixon, J.S.: Sensory Nerves in the Mammalian Urinary Tract. An Evaluation Using Light and Electron Microscopy, J Anat 117(1974)133-144

Greeff, K.; Kasperat, H.; Osswald, W.: Paradoxe Wirkungen der elekrischen Vagusreizung am isolierten Magen-und Herzvorhofpräparat des Meerschweinchens sowie deren Beeinflussung durch Ganglienblocker, Sympathicolytica, Reserpin und Cocain. Naunyn Schmiedebergs Arch Pharmakol 243(1962)528-545

Grillo, M.A.: Electronmicroscopy of Sympathetic Tissues. Pharmacol Rev 18(1966)387–399
Gruber, C.M.: The Autonomic Innervation of the Genito-Urinary System. Physiol Rev 13(1933)497–609
Hartman, B.K.: Immunofluorescence of Dopamine-β-Hydroxylase: Application of Improved Methodology to the Localization of the Peripheral and Central Noradrenergic Nervous System. J Histochem Cytochem 21(1973)312–332
Heazell, M.A.: Is ATP an Inhibitory Neurotransmitter in the Rat Stomach? Br J Pharmacol 55(1975)285–286P
Henderson, V. E.; Roepke, M. H.: The Role of Acetylcholine in Bladder Contractile Mechanisms and in Parasympathetic Ganglia. J Pharmacol Exp Ther 51(1934)97–111
Hervonen, A.: Large Vesicles of the Adrenergic Nerves of the Rabbit Uterus. Acta Physiol Scand 88(1973)430–432
Hervonen, A.; Kanerva, L.; Rechardt, L.: Localization of Catecholamines and Acetylcholinesterase in the Terminal Nerve Fibers of the Rabbit Myometrium. Histochemie 32(1972)89–93
Hickson, J.C.D.: The Secretion of Pancreatic Juice in Response to Stimulation of the Vagus Nerves in the Pig. J Physiol (Lond) 206(1970)275–297
Hidaka, T.; Kuriyama, H.: Responses of the Smooth Muscle Cell Membrane of the Guinea-Pig Jejunum to Field Stimulation. J Gen Physiol 53(1969)471–486
Hirst, G.D.S.; McKirdy, H.C.: A Nervous Mechanism for descending Inhibition in Guinea-Pig Small Intestine. J Physiol (Lond) 238(1974)129–143
Hökfelt, T.: In Vitro Studies on Central and Peripheral Monamine Neurons at the Ultrastructural Level. Z Zellforsch Mikr Anat 91(1968)1–74
Hökfelt, T.: Distribution of Noradrenaline Storing Particles in Peripheral Adrenergic Neurons As Revealed by Electron Microscopy. Acta Physiol Scand 76(1969)427–440
Hökfelt, T.; Elfvin, L.-G; Schultzberg, M.; Elde, R.; Goldstein, M.; Luft, R.: Occurrence of Somatostatin-Like Immunoreactivity in Some Peripheral Sympathetic Noradrenergic Neurons. Proc Natl Acad Sci USA 74(1977a)3587–3591
Hökfelt, T.; Elfvin, L.G.; Schultzberg, M.; Fuxe, K.; Said, S.I.; Mutt, V.; Goldstein, M.: Immunohistochemical Evidence of Vasoactive Intestinal Peptide-Containing Neurons and Nerve Fibers in Sympathetic Ganglia. Neuroscience 2(1977b)885–896
Hökfelt, T., Ljungdahl, Å.; Steinbusch, H.; Verhofstad, A.; Nilsson, G.; Brodin, E.; Pernow, B.; Goldstein, M.: Immunohistochemical Evidence of Substance P-Like Immunoreactivity in Some 5-Hydroxytryptamine-Containing Neurons in the Rat Central Nervous System. Neuroscience 3(1978)517–538
Holman, M.E.: Junction Potentials in Smooth Muscle. In: Smooth Muscle, pp. 244–288, ed. by E. Bülbring, A. Brading, A. Jones, T. Tomita. Edward Arnold, London, 1970
Holtzman, E.; Freeman, A.R.; Kashner, L.A.: Stimulation- Dependent Alterations in Peroxidase Uptake at Lobster Neuromuscular Junctions. Science 173(1971)733–736
Hoyes, A.D.; Barber, P.: Parameters of Fixation of the Putative Pain Afferents in the Ureter: Preservation of the Dense Cores of the Large Vesicles in the Axonal Terminals. J Anat 122(1976)113–120
Hoyes, A.D.; Barber, P.; Martin, B.G.H.: Comparative Ultrastructure of the Nerves Innervating the Muscle of the Body of the Bladder. Cell Tissue Res 164(1975a)133–144
Hoyes, A.D.; Barber, P.; Martin, B.G.H.: Comparative Ultrastructure of Ureteric Innervation. Cell Tissue Res 160(1975b)515–524
Hoyes, A.D.; Bourne, R.; Martin, B.G.H.: Ultrastructure and Distribution of the Subepithelial Nerves of the Rat Ureter. J Anat 117(1974)210A
Hoyes, A.D.; Bourne, R.; Martin, B.G.H.: Ultrastructure of the Sub-Mucous Nerves of the Rat Ureter. J Anat 119(1975c)123–132
Hoyes, A.D.; Bourne, R.; Martin, B.G.H.: Innervation of the Muscle of the Bladder in the Rat. Br J Urol 48(1976a)43–53
Hoyes, A.D.; Bourne, R.; Martin, B.G.H.: Ureteric Vascular and Muscle Coat Innervation in the Rat. A Quantitative Ultrastructural Study. Invest Urol 14(1976b)38–43
Hukovic, S.; Bubic, I.: Coeur et vaisseaux sanguins isolés avec leur nerfs comme moyen de recherche pharmacologique. Pathol et Biol 15(1967)153–157

Hung, K.S.; Hertweck, M.S.; Hardy, J.D.; Loosli, C.G.: Innervation of Pulmonary Alveoli of the Mouse Lung: an Electron Microscopic Study. Am J Anat 135(1972)477–496

Imai, S.; Takeda, K.: Effects of Vasodilators upon the Isolated Taenia Coli of the Guinea-Pig. J Pharmacol Exp Ther 156(1967)557–564

Irvin, J.L.; Irvin, E.M.: The Interaction of Quinacrine with Adenine Nucleotides. J Biol Chem 210(1954)45–56

Ito, Y.; Kuriyama, H.: Membrane Properties and Inhibitory Innervation of the Circular Muscle Cells of the Guinea-Pig Caecum. J Physiol (Lond) 231(1973)455–470

Jager, L.P.: The Effect of Catecholamines and ATP on the Smooth Muscle Cell Membrane of the Guinea-Pig Taenia Coli. Eur J Pharmacol 25(1974)372–382

Jager, L. P.; den Hartog, A.: Effect of Temperature on Transmitter Release from the 'Purinergic' Nerves in the Guinea-Pig Taenia Coli. Eur J Pharmacol 29(1974)201–205

Johns, A.; Paton, D.M.: Effect of Indomethacin on Atropine-Resistant Transmission in Rabbit and Monkey Urinary Bladder; Evidence for Involvement of Prostaglandins in Transmission. Prostaglandins 13(1977)245–255

Julé, Y.; Gonella, J.: Modifications de l'activité électrique du colon terminal de lapin par stimulation des fibres nerveuses pelviennes et sympathiques. J Physiol (Paris) 64 (1972)599–621

Kamikawa, Y.; Shimo, Y.: Mediation of Prostaglandin E_2 in the Biphasic Response to ATP of the Isolated Tracheal Muscle of Guinea-Pigs. J Pharm Pharmacol 28(1976a)294–297

Kamikawa, Y.; Shimo, Y.: Pharmacological Differences of Non-Adrenergic Inhibitory Response and of ATP-Induced Relaxation in Guinea-Pig Tracheal Strip Chains. J Pharm Pharmacol 28(1976b)854–855

Kan, K.K.S.; Chao, L.P.; Eng, L.F.: Immunohistochemical Localization of Choline Acetyltransferase in Rabbit Spinal Cord and Cerebellum. Brain Res 146(1978)221–229

Kasa, P.; Mann, S.P.; Hebb, C.: Localization of Choline acetyltransferase. Nature 226(1970)812–816

Katz, B.: Nerve, Muscle and Synapse, McGraw-Hill, New York, 1966

Keeler, R.; Richardson, H.; Watson, A.J.: Enteromegaly and Steatorrhea in the Rat Following Intraperitoneal Quinacrine (Atebrine). Lab Invest 15(1966)1253–1262.

Kern, H. F.; Hofmann, H.V.; Kern, D.: Licht-und elektronenmikroskopische Untersuchung der Langerhanschen Inseln von Nutria (*Myocastor coypus*), mit besonderer Berücksichtigung der neuroinsularen Komplexe. Z Zellforsch Mikr Anat 113(1971)216–229

Klinge, E.; Sjöstrand, N.O.: Contraction and Relaxation of the Retractor Penis Muscle and the Penile Artery of the Bull. Acta Physiol Scand Suppl 420(1975)1–88

Klinge, E.; Sjöstrand, N.O.: Comparative Study of Some Isolated Mammalian Smooth Muscle Effectors of Penile Erection. Acta Physiol Scand 100(1977)354–367

Koelle, G.B.: Cytological Distributions and Physiological Functions of Cholinesterases. Handb Exp Pharmakol 15(1963)187–198

Kolassa, N.; Pfleger, K.; Rummel, W.: Specificity of Adenosine Uptake into the Heart and Inhibition by Dipyridamole. Eur J Pharmacol 9(1970)265–268

Konturek, S.J.; Pucher, A.; Radecki, T.: Comparison of Vasointestinal Peptide and Secretin in Stimulation of Pancreatic Secretion. J Physiol (Lond) 255(1976)497–509

Kraupp, O.; Wolner, E.; Adler-Kastner, L.; Chirikdjian, J.J.; Polszczanski, B.; Tuisl, E.: Die Wirkung von Hexobendin auf Sauerstoffverbrauch, Energetik und Substratstoffwechsel des Herzens. Arzneim Forsch 16(1966)692–696

Kuriyama, H.; Osa, T.; Tasaki, H.: Electrophysiological Studies of the Antrum Muscle Fibers of the Guinea-Pig Stomach. J Gen Physiol 55(1970)48–62

Kuriyama, H.; Osa, T.; Toida, N.: Nervous Factors Influencing the Membrane Activity of Intestinal Smooth Muscle. J Physiol (Lond) 191(1967)257–270

Langley, J.N.: The Autonomic Nervous Sytem. Part 1. Heffer, Cambridge, 1921

Langley, J.N.; Anderson, H.K.: The Innervation of the Pelvic and Adjoining Viscera, Parts II-V. J Physiol (Lond) 19(1895)71–139

Larsson, L.I.: Ultrastructural Localization of a New Neuronal Peptide (VIP). Histochemistry 54(1977)173–176

Larsson, L.I.; Edvinsson, L.; Fahrenkrug, J.: Immunohistochemical Localization of a Vasodilatory Polypeptide (VIP) in Cerebrovascular Nerves. Brain Res 113(1976a)400–404

Larsson, L.I.; Fahrenkrug, J.; Holst, J.J.; Schaffalitzky de Muckadell, O.B.: Innervation of the Pancreas by Vasoactive Intestinal Peptide (VIP) Immunoreactive Nerves. Life Sci 22(1978)773–780

Larsson, L.I.; Fahrenkrug, J.; Schaffalitzky de Muckadell, O.B.: Vasoactive Intestinal Polypeptide Occurs in Nerves of the Female Genitourinary Tract. Science 197(1977a) 1374–1375

Larsson, L.I.; Fahrenkrug, J.; Schaffalitzky de Muckadell, O.B.: Occurrence of Nerves Containing Vasoactive Intestinal Polypeptide Immunoreactivity in the Male Genital Tract. Life Sci 21(1977b)503–508

Larsson, L.I.; Fahrenkrug, J.; Schaffalitzky de Muckadell, O.B.; Sundler, F.; Håkanson, R.; Rehfeld, J.F.: Localization of Vasoactive Intestinal Polypeptide (VIP) to Central and Peripheral Neurones. Proc Natl Acad Sci USA 73(1976b)3197–3200

Lorez, H.P.; Richards, J.G.: 5-HT Nerve Terminals in the Fourth Ventricle of the Rat Brain: Their Identification and Distribution Studied by Fluorescence Histochemistry and Electron Microscopy. Cell Tissue Res 165(1975)37–48

Luduena, F.P.; Grigas, E.O.: Pharmacological Study of Autonomic Innervation of Dog Retractor Penis. Am J Physiol 210(1966)435–445

Luduena, F.P.; Grigas, E.O.: Effect of Some Biological Substances on the Dog Retractor Penis in Vitro. Arch Int Pharmacodyn Ther 196(1972)269–274.

MacKay, D.; McKirdy, H.C.: Effect of Vasopressin and of Adenosine Triphosphate on the Flat Preparation of Rabbit Rectum. Br J Pharmacol 44(1972)366–367P

Makhlouf, G.M.: Said, S.I.: The Effect of Vasoactive Intestinal Peptide (VIP) on Digestive and Hormonal Function. In: Gastrointestinal Hormones, pp. 599–610, ed. by C.J. Thompson. Univ Texas Press, Austin, 1975

Martinson, J.: Vagal Relaxation of the Stomach. Experimental Re-Investigation of the Concept of the Transmission Mechanism. Acta Physiol Scand 64(1965)453–462

Matsumura, S.; Taira, N.; Hashimoto, K.: The Pharmacological Behaviour of the Urinary Bladder and Its Vasculature of the Dog. Tohoku J Exp Med 96(1968)247–258

Meves, H.: Die Wirkung von Adrenalin and Adrenalinverwandten auf Gefässe und Muskulatur der Froschlunge. Pfluegers Arch 258(1953)200–210

Morris, J.F.: Distribution of Neurosecretory Granules among the Anatomical Compartments of the Neurosecretory Processes of the Pituitary Gland: A Quantitative Ultrastructural Approach to Hormone Storage in the Neural Lobe. J Endocrinol 68(1976)225–234

Morris, J.F.; Nordmann, J.J.; Dyball, R.E.J.: Structure-Function Correlation in Mammalian Neurosecretion. Int Rev Exp Pathol 18(1978)2–96

Mutt, V.; Said, S.I.: Structure of the Porcine Vasoactive Intestinal Octacosapeptide. The Amino Acid Sequence. Use of Kallikrein in Its Determination. Eur J Biochem 42(1974)581–589

Needleman, P.; Minkes, M.S.; Douglas, J.R.: Stimulation of Prostaglandin Biosynthesis by Adenine Nucleotides. Cir Res 34 (1974) 455–460

Nilsson, A.: Isolation, Amino Acid Composition and Terminal Amino Acid Residues of the Vasoactive Octacosapeptide from Chicken Intestine. Partial Purification of Chicken Secretin. FEBS Lett 47(1974)284–289

Nilsson, A.: Structure of the Vasoactive Intestinal Octacosapeptide from Chicken Intestine. The Amino Acid Sequence. FEBS Lett 60(1975)322–326

Nojyo, Y.; Sano, Y.: Ultrastructure of the Serotonergic Nerve Terminals in the Suprachiasmic and Interpeduncular Nuclei of Rat Brains. Brain Res 149(1978)482–488

Normann, T.C.: Neurosecretion by Exocytosis. Int Rev Cytol 46(1976)1–77

Ohga, A.; Taneike, T.: Dissimilarity between the Responses to Adenosine Triphosphate or Its Related Compounds and Non-Adrenergic Inhibitory Nerve Stimulation in the Longitudinal Muscle of Pig Stomach. Br J Pharmacol 60(1977)221–231

Olson, L.; Ålund, M.; Norberg, K.A.: Fluorescence Microscopical Demonstration of a Population of Gastro-Intestinal Nerve Fibres with a Selective Affinity for Quinacrine. Cell Tissue Res 171(1976)407–423

Oppenheimer, M.J.: Autonomic Control of the Retractor Penis in the Cat. Am J Physiol 122(1938)745–752

Orlov, R.S.: Transmission of Inhibitory Impulses from Nerve to Smooth Muscle. Fiziol Zh 49(1963)575–582

Osborne, M.P.: Structure and Function of Neuromuscular Junctions and Stretch Receptors. Symp R Ent Soc (Lond) 5(1970)77–100

Palade, G.E.; Palay, S.L.: Electron Microscope Observations of Inter-Neuronal and Neuromuscular Synapses. Anat Rec 118(1954)335–336

Palay, S.L.; Chan-Palay, V.: A Guide to the Synaptic Analysis of the Neuropil. Cold Springs Harbor Symp Quart Biol 40(1976)1–16

Patent, G.J.; Kechele, P.O.; Carrano, V.T.: Non-Conventional Innervation of the Pancreatic Islets of the Teleost fish. *Gillichthys mirabilis*. Cell Tissue Res 191(1978)305–315

Paton, W.D.M.; Vane, J.R.: An Analysis of the Responses of the Isolated Stomach to Electrical Stimulation and to Drugs. J Physiol (Lond) 165(1963)10–46

Pelletier, G.; Labrie, F.; Arimura, A.; Schally, A.V.: Electron Microscopic Immunohistochemical Localization of Growth Hormone-Release Inhibiting Hormone (Somatostatin) in the Rat Median Eminence. Am J Anat 140(1974)445–450

Pernow, B.: Effect of Substance P on Smooth Muscle. In: Polypeptides Which Affect Smooth Muscles and Blood Vessels, pp. 171–178, ed. M. Schachter. Pergamon, Oxford, 1960

Pfleger, K.; Volkmer, I.; Kolassa, N.: Hemmung der Aufnahme von Adenosin und Verstarkung seiner Wirkung am isolierten Warmbluterherzen durch Coronarwirksame Substanzen. Arzneim Forsch 19(1969)1972–1974

Pick, J.: Fine Structure of Nerve Terminals in the Human Gut. Anat Rec 159(1967)131–146

Pick, J.: The Autonomic Nervous System. Lippincott, Philadelphia, Toronto, 1970

Pickel, V.M.; Joh, T.H.; Reis, D.J.: Monoamine-Synthesizing Enzymes in Central Dopaminergic, Noradrenergic and Serotonergic Neurons. Immunocytochemical Localization by Light and Electron Microscopy. J Histochem Cytochem 24(1976)792–796

Piper, P.J.; Said, S.I.; Vane, J.R.: Effects on Smooth Muscle Preparations of Unidentified Vasoactive Peptides from Intestine and Lung. Nature 225(1970)1144–1146

Richards, J.G.; Tranzer, J.P.: The Ultrastructural Localization of Amine Storage Sites in the Central Nervous System with the Aid of a Specific Marker: 5-hydroxydopamine. Brain Res 17(1970)463–469

Richards, J.G.; Tranzer, J.P.: Localization of Amine Storage Sites in the Adrenergic Cell Body. A Study of the Superior Cervical Ganglion of the Rat by Fine Structural Cytochemistry. J Ultrastruct Res 53(1975)204–216

Richardson, J.B.; Bouchard, T.: Demonstration of a Nonadrenergic Inhibitory Nervous System in the Trachea of the Guinea Pig. J Allergy Clin Immunol 56(1975)473–480

Richardson, K.C.: The Fine Structure of Autonomic Nerve Endings in Smooth Muscle of the Rat Vas Deferens. J Anat 96(1962)427–442

Richardson, K.C.: The Fine Structure of Albino Rabbit Iris with Special Reference to the Identification of Adrenergic and Cholinergic Nerves and Nerve Endings in the Intrinsic Muscles. Am J Anat 114(1964)173–205

Richardson, K.C.: Electron Microscopic Identification of Autonomic Nerve Endings. Nature 210(1966)756

Rikimaru, A.: Contractile Properties of Organ-cultured Intestinal Smooth Muscle. Tohoku J Exp Med 103(1971)317–329

Rikimaru, A.; Fukushi, Y.; Suzuki, T.: Effects of Imidazole and Phentolamine on the Relaxant Responses of Guinea-Pig Taenia Coli to Transmural Stimulation and to Adenosine Triphosphate. Tohoku J Exp Med 105(1971)199–200

Robinson, P.M.: The Demonstration of Acetylcholinesterase in Autonomic Axons with the Electron Microscope. Prog Brain Res 34(1971)357–370

Robinson, P.M.; Bell, C.: The Localization of Acetylcholinesterase at the Autonomic Neuromuscular Junction. J Cell Biol 33(1967)93–102

Robinson, P.M.; McLean, J.R.; Burnstock, G.: Ultrastructural Identification of Non-Adrenergic Inhibitory nerve Fibers. J Pharmacol Exp Ther 179(1971)149–160

Rogers, D.C.; Burnstock, G.: Multiaxonal Autonomic Junctions in Intestinal Smooth Muscle of the Toad (*Bufo marinus*). J Comp Neurol 126(1966)625–652

Rossier, J.: Immunohistochemical Localization of Choline Acetyltransferase: Real or Artefact? Brain Res 98(1975)619–622

Said, S.I.: Vasoactive Intestinal Peptide (VIP): Current Status. In: Gastrointestinal Hormones, pp. 591–597, ed. by J.C. Thompson. Univ Texas Press, Austin, 1975

Said, S.I.; Mutt, V.: Polypeptide with Broad Biological Activity: Isolation from Small Intestine. Science 169(1970a)1217–1218

Said, S.I.; Mutt, V.: Potent Peripheral and Splanchnic Vasodilator Peptide from Normal Gut. Nature 225(1970b)863–864

Said, S.I.; Mutt, V.: Isolation from Porcine Intestinal Wall of a Vasoactive Octacosapeptide Related to Secreton and Glucagon. Eur J Biochem 28(1972)199–204

Said, S.I.; Rosenberg, R.N.: Vasoactive Intestinal Peptide: Abundant Immunoreactivity in Neural Cell Lines and Normal Nervous Tissue. Science 192(1976)907–908

Satchell, D.; Burnstock, G.; Dann, P.: Antagonism of the Effects of Purinergic Nerve Stimulation and Exogenously Applied ATP on the Guinea-Pig Taenia Coli by 2-Substituted Imidazolines and Related Compounds. Eur J Pharmacol 23(1973)264–269

Satchell, D.G.; Lynch, A.; Bourke, P.M.; Burnstock, G.: Potentiation of the Effects of Exogenously Applied ATP and Purinergic Nerve Stimulation on the Guinea-Pig Taenia Coli by Dipyridamole and Hexobendine. Eur J Pharmacol 19(1972)343–350

Schebalin, M.; Said, S.I.; Makhlouf, G.M.: Stimulation of Insulin and Glucagon Secretion by Vasoactive Intestinal Peptide. Am J Physiol 232(1977)E197–E200

Schultzberg, M.; Dreyfus, C.F.; Gershon, M.D.; Hökfelt, T.; Elde, R.P.; Nilsson, G.; Said, S.; Goldstein, M.: VIP-, Enkephalin-, Substance P-, and Somatostatin-Like Immunoreactivity in Neurons Intrinsic to the Intestine: Immunohistochemical Evidence from Organotypic Organ Cultures. Brain Res 155(1978)239–248

Silva, D.G.: The Ultrastructure of the Myometrium of the Rat with Special Reference to the Innervation. Anat Rec 158(1967)21–33

Silva, D.G.; Ross, G.: Ultrastructure and Fluorescence Histochemical Studies on the Innervation of the Tracheo-Bronchial Muscle of Normal Cats and Cats Treated with 6-Hydroxydopamine. J Ultrastruct Res 47(1974)310–328

Small, R.C.: Transmission from Intramural Inhibitory Neurones to Circular Smooth Muscle of the Rabbit Caecum and the Effects of Catecholamines. Br J Pharmacol 45(1972)149–150P

Smith, B.: The Myenteric Plexus in Drug-Induced Neuropathy. J Neurol Neurosurg Psychiatry 30(1967)506–510

Spedding, M.; Sweetman, A.J.; Weetman, D.F.: Antagonism of Adenosine-5'-Triphosphate-induced Relaxations by 2-2'-Pyridylisatogen in the Taenia of Guinea-Pig Caecum. Br J Pharmacol 53(1975)575–583

Spedding, M.; Weetman, D.F.: Identification of Separate Receptors for Adenosine and Adenosine-5'-Triphosphate in Causing Relaxation of the Isolated Taenia of the Guinea-Pig Caecum. Br J Pharmacol 57(1976)305–310

Sporrong, B.; Clase, L.; Owman, c.; Sjöberg, N.: Electron Microscopy of Adrenergic, Cholinergic and 'p-Type' Nerves in the Myometrium, and a Special Kind of Synaptic Contact with the Smooth Muscle Cells. Am J Obstet Gynecol 127(1977)811–817

Sundler, F.; Alumets, J.; Håkanson, R.; Fahrenkrug, J; Schaffalitzky de Muckadell, O.B.: Peptidergic (VIP) Nerves in the Pancreas. Histochemistry 55(1978)173–176

Sundler, F.; Alumets, J.; Håkanson, R.; Ingemansson, S.; Fahrenkrug, J.; Schaffalitzky de Muckadell, O.: VIP Innervation of the Gallbladder. Gastroenterology 72(1976)1375–1377

Swaab, D.F.; Pool, C.W.: Specificity of Oxytocin and Vasopressin Immunofluorescence. J Endocrinol 66(1975)263–272

Szentágothai, J.: The Morphological Identification of the Active Synaptic Region: Aspects of General Arrangement of Geometry and Topology. In: Excitatory Synaptic mechanisms, pp. 9–26, ed. by P. Andersen, J.K.S. Jansen. Universitetsforlaget, Oslo, 1970

Taira, N.: The Autonomic Pharmacology of the Bladder. Annu Rev Pharmacol 12 (1972)197–208

Taxi, J.: Morphological and Cytochemical Studies on the Synapses in the Autonomic Nervous System. Prog Brain Res 31(1969)5–20

Taxi, J.; Droz, B.: Localization d'amines biogènes dans le système neurovégétatif périphérique. Étude radioautographique en microscopie électronique après injection de noradrenaline-^{3}H et de 5-hydroxytryptophane-³H. In: Neurosecretion, pp. 191–202, ed. by F. Stutinsky. Springer, Berlin-Heidelberg-New York, 1967

Taxi, J.; Droz, B.: Radioautographic Study of the Accumulation of Some Biogenic Amines in the Autonomic Nervous System. In: Cellular Dynamics of the Neuron, pp. 175–190, ed. by S.H. Barondes. Academic Press, New York, 1969

Tomita, T.: Conductance Change During the Inhibitory Potential in the Guinea-Pig Taenia Coli. J Physiol (Lond) 225(1972)693–704

Tomita, T.; Watanabe, H.: A Comparison of the Effects of Adenosine Triphosphate with Noradrenaline and with the Inhibitory Potential of the Guinea-Pig Taenia Coli. J Physiol (Lond) 231(1973)167–177

Tranzer, J.P.; Richards, J.G.: Ultrastructural Cytochemistry of Biogenic Amines in Nervous Tissue: Methodologic Improvements. J Histochem Cytochem 24(1976)1178–1193

Tranzer, J.P.; Thoenen, N.: Electronmicroscopic Localization of 5-hydroxydopamine (3,4,5-trihydroxy-phenylethylamine), a New 'False' Sympathetic Transmitter. Experientia 23(1967)743–745

Tranzer, J.P.; Thoenen, H.; Snipes, R.L.; Richards, J.G.: Recent Developments on the Ultrastructural Aspects of Adrenergic Nerve Endings in Various Experimental Conditions. Prog Brain Res 31(1969)33–46

Uchizono, K.: Characteristics of Excitatory and Inhibitory Synapses in the Central Nervous System of the Cat. Nature 207(1965)642–643

Uddman, R.; Alumets, J.; Edvinsson, L.; Hakanson, R.; Sundler, F: Peptidergic (VIP) Innervation of the Oesophagus. Gastroenterology 75(1978)5–8

Uehara, Y.; Campbell, G.R.; Burnstock, G.: Muscle and Its Innervation: An Atlas of Fine Structure. Edward Arnold, London, 1976

Uemura, E.; Fletcher, T.F.; Bradley, W.E.: Distribution of Lumbar Afferent Axons in Muscle Coat of Cat Urinary Bladder. Am J Anat 139(1974)389–398

Uemura, E.; Fletcher, T.F.; Dirks, V.A.; Bradley, W.E.: Distribution of Sacral Afferent Axons in Cat Urinary Bladder. Am J Anat 136(1973)305–313

Unsicker, K.: Fine Structure and Innervation of the Avian Adrenal Gland. III Non-Cholinergic Nerve Fibers. Z Zellforsch Mikr Anat 145(1973a)557–575

Unsicker, K.: Fine Structure and Innervation of the Avian Adrenal Gland. V. Innervation of Interrenal Cells. Z Zellforsch Mikr Anat 146(1973b)403–416

Watanabe, T.; Yasuda, M.: Electron Microscopic Study on the Innervation of the Pancreas in the Domestic Fowl. Cell Tissue Res 180(1977)453–465

Weisenthal, L.M.; Hug, C.C.; Weisbrudt, N.W.; Bass, P.: Adrenergic Mechanisms in the Relaxation of Guinea-Pig Taenia Coli in vitro. J Pharmacol Exp Ther 178(1971)497–508

Weston, A.H.: The Effect of Desensitization to Adenosine Triphosphate on the Peristaltic Reflex in the Guinea-Pig Ileum. Br J Pharmacol 47(1973a)606–608

Weston, A.H.: Nerve-Mediated Inhibition of Mechanical Activity in Rabbit Duodenum and the Effects of Desensitization of Adenosine and Several of Its Derivatives. Br J Pharmacol 48(1973b)302–308

Widdicombe, J.G.: Regulation of Tracheobronchial Smooth Muscle. Physiol Rev 43(1963)1–37

Wood, J.G.; McLaughlin, B.J.; Vaughn, J.E.: Immunocytochemical localization of GAD in electronmicroscopic Preparations of Rodent CNS. In: GABA in Neurosystem Function, pp. 133–148, ed. by E. Roberts, T. N. Chase, D.B. Tower. Raven Press, New York, 1976

Wood, M.J.; Burnstock, G.: Innervation of the Lungs of the Toad (Bufo marinus) 1. Physiology and pharmacology. Comp Biochem Physiol 22(1967)755–766

Woods, R.I.: Acrylic Aldehyde in Sodium Dichromate as a Fixative for Identifying Catecholamine Storage Sites with the Electron Microscope. J Physiol (Lond) 203(1969)35P-36P

Yamamoto, M.: Electron Microscopic Studies on the Innervation of the Smooth Muscle and the Interstitial Cells of Cajal in the Small Intestine of the Mouse and Bat. Arch Histol Jpn 40(1977)171–201

Yamauchi, A.: Innervation of the Vertebrate Heart as Studied with the Electron Microscope. Arch Histol Jpn 31(1969)83–117

Yanaihara, N.; Sakagami, M.; Sato, H.; Yamamoto, K; Hashimoto, T.; Yanaihara, C.; Ito,

Z.; Yamaguchi, K.; Abe, K.: Immunological Aspects of Secretin, Substance P and VIP. Gastroenterology 72(1977)803–810

Zieher, L.M.; Jaim Etcheverry, G.: Ultrastructural Cytochemistry and Pharmacology of 5-Hydroxytryptamine in Adrenergic nerve endings. II. Accumulation of 5-Hydroxytryptamine in Nerve Vesicles Containing Norepinephrine in Rat Vas Deferens. J Pharmacol Exp Ther 178(1971)30–41

Cholinergic Mechanisms in Adrenergic Function

John Fozard

I. INTRODUCTION

This article is to be published exactly 75 years after the historic note from T.R. Elliott appeared in the *Journal of Physiology* suggesting, with reference to sympathetic nervous transmission, that "(adrenalin) . . . might then be the chemical stimulant liberated on each occasion when the impulse arrives at the periphery" (Elliott, 1904). Since that time peripheral adrenergic mechanisms have been a popular field of research endeavor, attracting highly talented investigators and being the subject of regular and competent review. The specific subject of this essay is no exception to this generalization, there being several accounts of cholinergic influences on adrenergic mechanisms in the recent literature (Starke, 1977; Vanhoutte, 1977; Westfall, 1977; Löffelholz, 1979; Muscholl, 1979). A mere representation of the recent findings in this area, therefore, cannot be justified as the content of this essay. Rather, in accordance with the aims of this volume, an attempt has been made to appraise certain concepts of the role of acetylcholine (ACh) in adrenergic transmission. Two general headings serve as the framework for this purpose: first, the postsynaptic actions of

ACh at the ganglion are discussed. These are not only important per se; they also, since the sympathetic terminals are but the furthest extension to the periphery of the ganglion cell, provide a reference for the mechanisms encountered at the nerve endings. Second, the effects of acetylcholine at the terminals will be considered, including the hypothesis of a cholinergic link in the sympathetic transmission process (Burn and Rand, 1959) and the counterpart of this, the muscarinic "inhibitory" mechanisms of ACh (Lindmar, Löffelholz, and Muscholl, 1968). For each heading, the associated concepts will be placed in historical context, their development to the present time reviewed, their current standing appraised, and their relevance and value as the basis for future investigations assessed.

II. THE POSTSYNAPTIC ACTIONS OF ACETYLCHOLINE IN SYMPATHETIC GANGLIA

The classical view of the mechanism by which impulses are transmitted from pre- to postganglionic neurons has ACh playing the primary transmitter role. The arrival of an action potential at the preganglionic terminals leads to an accelerated release of ACh which through interaction with specific receptors initiates an action potential in the postganglionic cell. This interpretation evolved logically from neuroanatomical studies showing large postganglionic neurons with which the preganglionic nerves formed synapses (De Castro, 1965), complemented by the pioneer physiological and pharmacological studies (fascinatingly reviewed by Bacq, 1975), which led to the demonstration of the key role for chemical transmission and for ACh at the ganglionic synapse. Basically, this concept remains as valid today as formerly. Inevitably, however, as experimental techniques have advanced, so have the subtleties of the ganglionic transmission process been increasingly revealed.

In particular, the improvements in electrophysiological technology, through primarily extracellular recording studies (reviewed by Volle, 1966) to sophisticated intracellular ones (Haefely, 1972) have revealed postsynaptic potentials of low intensity but of remarkably slow onset and duration and apparently unconnected to the primary transmission process. Such advances were paralleled by equally significant developments in the field of histochemical fluorescence microscopy following the discovery that primary amines form fluorescent condensation products with formaldehyde (Falck et al., 1962). Such techniques facilitated the demonstration within sympathetic ganglia of small intensely fluorescent, or SIF, cells (Eränkö and Härkönen, 1965), now considered of fundamental importance to our understanding of cholinergic mechanisms in the ganglion. Also evolving in recent years has been the case for cyclic nucleotides, in particular cyclic

3′,5′-adenosine monophosphate (cyclic AMP) and cyclic guanosine 3′,5′-monophosphate (cyclic GMP) as intermediaries in the postsynaptic events following preganglionic stimulation (Greengard, 1976). Information accumulated from all three of these general areas has added extra dimensions to our concept of the role of ACh in the sympathetic ganglion.

A. The Cholinergic Postsynaptic Potentials

Haefely (1972) has set out full details of the different terminologies used to describe membrane potential changes obtained either by extracellular or intracellular recording techniques. For clarity, the terminology appropriate to data obtained by intracellular methodology will be used throughout, although details of the recording technique will be specified in most instances.

Under favorable conditions, most vertebrate postganglionic cells respond to a weak preganglionic stimulus, or to stimulation during partial nicotinic receptor blockade, with potential changes that can be differentiated both temporally and pharmacologically into three components. First, there is a depolarization of short duration, designated the fast excitatory postsynaptic potential, or fast EPSP, which on reaching a critical threshold triggers an action potential. This is succeeded by two slow potentials: the first, a phase of hyperpolarization, which is slow in onset (35 ms) and lasts up to 500 ms, is labeled the slow inhibitory postsynaptic potential, or slow IPSP. The second, a phase of depolarization, which can persist for many seconds, is called the slow excitatory postsynaptic potential, or slow EPSP (see extensive reviews of original work by Volle, 1966; Haefely, 1972). The fast EPSP is abolished selectively by nicotine receptor blocking agents; both slow postsynaptic potentials are inhibited by atropine (e.g., Eccles and Libet, 1961; Libet and Tosaka, 1969; Haefely, 1974a).

These potentials are indisputably postsynaptic, since they can be detected by intracellular recording from single ganglion cells (Libet and Tosaka, 1969). They also derive from the action of acetylcholine released from the preganglionic nerves, since they are reduced if transmitter release is prevented by botulinus toxin (Eccles and Libet, 1961) or an adverse Ca^{++}/Mg^{++} ratio (Libet, 1970), enhanced by eserine (Haefely, 1974b) and mimicked by acetylcholine applied exogenously (Takeshige and Volle, 1964). There is general agreement that the fast EPSP is generated directly through a combination of acetylcholine with the nicotine receptors on the subsynaptic membrane and that no intermediary mechanism is involved (Haefely, 1972; Greengard, 1976). This is not the case for the slow potentials mediated through the muscarinic sites.

B. Intermediary Mechanisms in the Genesis of Cholinergic Slow Postsynaptic Potentials

1. Dopamine, cyclic AMP, and the slow IPSP In the past, there has been no satisfactory method for isolating either a "pure" slow IPSP or a "pure" slow EPSP to facilitate their separate analysis, although exclusively slow EPSP responses are claimed to occur in ganglia treated with bethanechol (Libet, Kobayashi, and Tanaka, 1975; Kobayashi, Hashiguchi, and Ushiyama, 1978). Thus, interpretation of the majority of the available data is subject to the difficulties attendant on the accurate identification of the mechanism(s) underlying changes in the individual components of a multiphasic event. Nevertheless, most of the important observations that have led to definition of the slow potentials are clear-cut and conclusive (see, for example, the effects of cholinoceptor antagonists, Eccles and Libet, 1961; Libet and Tosaka, 1969; Haefely, 1974b). One of the more difficult problems of interpretation concerned the evidence adduced in support of the first suggestion of a specific association between endogenous catecholamines and the slow IPSP. Eccles and Libet, using extracellular wire electrodes, observed that the slow IPSP obtained from rabbit superior cervical ganglion (scg) was reduced more than either the fast or the slow EPSP by dibenamine. On this basis, the authors hypothesized that secretion of "an adrenaline-like substance . . . . by the chromaffin cells in response to preganglionic volleys after diffusion to appropriate sites on the postganglionic neurone would initiate a hyperpolarizing response." This interpretation of the original data has been repeatedly criticized (e.g., Volle, 1966; Tauc, 1967; Haefely, 1972), mainly on the grounds that dibenamine is not a specific antagonist and that other potent α-adrenoceptor antagonists such as dihydroergotamine (Eccles and Libet, 1961) or phentolamine (Libet and Tosaka, 1970) were ineffective. Certainly, dibenamine blocks muscarine receptors at concentrations equivalent to those used to inhibit the slow IPSP (Burgen and Spero, 1968), whereas dihydroergotamine and phentolamine, even at high concentrations (10^{-4}M), do not (Shibata, Carrier, and Frankenheim, 1968). Thus it is clearly possible that muscarinic receptor blockade is a major factor in the blocking activity of dibenamine toward the slow IPSP; and this would accord with the associated, though less dramatic, reduction in the EPSP after this drug is administered (Eccles and Libet, 1961).

Despite these criticisms, evidence consistent with a catecholaminergic component in the action of acetylcholine at the sympathetic ganglion has continued to accumulate. A fundamental change of emphasis came in 1970 when Libet and Tosaka proposed dopamine as the intermediary catecholamine involved in the rabbit scg and specified the SIF cells as the source of this amine. The evidence for this was reviewed by Libet and

Tosaka (1970) and by Libet (1977) and may be summarized under three headings.

a. *Presence and Localization of Dopamine in Sympathetic Ganglia* The cells considered to contain the catecholamine thought to mediate in ganglion transmission are the SIF cells, first described by Eränkö and Härkönen (1963) in rat superior cervical ganglia and subsequently identified in ganglia at several sites and in many species (Eränkö, 1978). Elegant and systematic histological studies have shown certain of the SIF cells to be true interneurons, receiving an afferent input through synapses containing "empty" vesicles that degenerate after preganglionic nerve section (Taxi, Gautron, and L'Hermite, 1969; Matthews and Ostberg, 1973), and themselves synapsing with perikarya and dendrites of postganglionic neurons (Williams and Palay, 1969; Matthews and Nash, 1970; Black et al., 1978). These were defined as type I SIF cells by Chiba and Williams (1975). Type II SIF cells were suggested to occur in clusters and to be more closely related to blood vessels than to postganglionic cells (Chiba and Williams, 1975).

SIF cells were shown by microspectrofluorimetry to contain a primary catecholamine (Norberg, Ritzen, and Ungerstedt, 1966), subsequently identified as dopamine, in superior cervical ganglia of cat, rat, rabbit, pig, and cow (for extensive bibliography, see Eränkö, 1978). Thus the presence of a catecholamine, principally dopamine, in the SIF cell interneurons of the ganglia of the major species used in electrophysiological and biochemical studies seems not to be in doubt. Nor is the fact in doubt that the processes of type I SIF cells ramify widely within the ganglion (Jacobowitz, 1970; Dail and Evan, 1978); this certainty allows speculation that the majority of ganglion cells receive an SIF cell input (Matthews and Raisman, 1969; Libet, 1977).

b. *A Functional Release of Dopamine?* The paper of Libet and Owman (1974) provides the principal direct evidence for a functional release of dopamine during orthodromic stimulation and for its causal relationship to the generation of the slow IPSP. Changes in the dopamine content of the SIF cells of rabbit scg were studied by cytospectrofluorimetry and related to changes in the slow IPSP measured by extracellular techniques. Procedures that produced a loss of dopamine fluorescence (prolonged orthodromic stimulation or treatment with the muscarinic agonist bethanethol) resulted in reduction of the slow IPSP. Significantly, temporary exposure to dopamine plus a monoamine oxidase inhibitor restored both the fluorescence of the SIF cells and the slow IPSP in ganglia subjected either to nerve stimulation or to bethanechol (Libet and Owman, 1974). In contrast, neither adrenaline nor noradrenaline restored the slow IPSP when depressed by bethanechol (Libet and Tosaka, 1970). Although there are some inconsistencies in the paper of Libet and Owman (1974)—for instance, a decrease in slow IPSP could occur with no apparent change in fluorescence intensity, they should be considered in the context of the undoubted difficulties in the quantitative interpretation of both the histochemical and the electrophysiological data (discussed in detail by Libet and Owman, 1974). It is significant that the observations with bethanechol have recently been confirmed for the rat scg by Tsevdos, Humbertson, and Gardier (1978), who also demonstrated that presumed blockade of the muscarinic sites on the SIF cell with gallamine or pancuronium (Gardier, Tsevdos, and Jackson, 1978a; Gardier et al., 1978b) prevented the decrease in fluorescence due to bethanechol. These results are clearly in accord with a release of dopamine during nerve stimulation linked functionally to generation of the slow IPSP.

Additional evidence recently obtained directly supports this conclusion. In rabbit scg treated with d-tubocuramine, iontophoretic application of either ACh or dopamine produced hyperpolarization of individual ganglion cells (Dun, Kaibara, and Karczmar, 1977b; Dun and Karczmar, 1978). Dopamine-induced hyperpolarization was blocked by haloperidol (Dun et al., 1977b) and that induced by ACh by both atropine and haloperidol (Dun and Karczmar, 1978). Most significantly, blockade of transmitter release by treatment with solutions either depleted of calcium or containing tetrodotoxin effectively and reversibly inhibited acetylcholine-induced hyperpolarization (Dun and Karczmar, 1978). Hyperpolarizing responses to dopamine had earlier been shown to be unaffected in low-calcium solutions (Libet, 1970). Taken together, the data suggest that in the rabbit scg, the slow IPSP elicited by orthodromic stimulation involves the release by acetylcholine of a second transmitter, probably dopamine, from an interneuron positioned between the preganglionic terminals and the ganglion cells.

A circumstantial association between SIF cell catecholamine release and the slow IPSP can also be inferred from consideration of data obtained from the scg of the guinea pig. In this tissue, the SIF cells contain noradrenaline rather than dopamine (Wamsley et al., 1978) and make few, if any, synaptic contacts with the postganglionic neurons (Elfvin, Hökfelt, and Goldstein, 1975; Wamsley et al., 1978). Significantly, exogenously applied noradrenaline does not cause hyperpolarization in the guniea pig scg (Dun and Karczmar, 1977b), and slow IPSP responses cannot be elicited by preganglionic stimulation (Libet, 1970; Dun and Karczmar, 1977b).

Despite the above suggestive evidence, there is a disappointing lack of corroborative evidence for a release of dopamine from the superior cervical ganglion by orthodromic stimulation. For instance, it might be expected that manipulation of the intraganglionic stores of dopamine would influence the postsynaptic events. Yet neither administration of reserpine (0.2 mg/kg) daily to rabbits for 10 days (Libet and Tosaka, unpublished observations, quoted in Libet, 1970) nor complete blockade of monoamine oxidase with pargyline (Henderson, 1971) produced data supporting an intermediary role for dopamine in the genesis of the slow IPSP. However, in neither study was biochemical information on the changes in ganglion monoamine content presented, and the results must therefore be regarded as inconclusive.

More direct attempts to demonstrate dopamine release from ganglia by orthodromic nerve stimulation have similarly not been successful. Libet et al. (unpublished observations, 1970, quoted in Libet, 1977, p. 543) failed to detect a release of amine from rabbit superior cervical ganglion prelabeled with ^{3}H-dopamine following preganglionic stimulation. Further, Noon, McAfee, and Roth (1975) could not detect ^{3}H-dopamine or its metabolite 3-methoxytyramine in the superfusate from stimulated rabbit superior cervical ganglion preincubated in ^{3}H-tyrosine, despite the fact that 14% of the newly synthesized catecholamine was ^{3}H-dopamine. Similarly, in rat superior cervical ganglion in vitro, no release of stored ^{14}C-dopamine could be detected in the bathing fluid after incubation with ^{14}C-tyrosine and following preganglionic nerve stimulation (Steinberg and Keller, 1978). These negative findings may simply reflect the release of extremely small amounts of dopamine, which the methods used could not detect. Alternatively, the release of labeled material after accumulation of exogenous amine or following de novo synthesis may not reflect the behavior of the endogenous transmitter pool. In this context, there is sound experimental evidence for profound changes in endogenous dopamine metabolism in response to orthodromic stimulation or treatment with muscarinic agonists.

For example, Pearson and Sharman (1974) detected significant concentrations of the two acid metabolites of dopamine, 3,4-dihydroxyphenylacetic acid (DOPAC) and homovanillic acid (HVA) in ganglia from monkey, dog, and pig. Moreover, preganglionic nerve stimulation to the superior cervical ganglion of the pig resulted in marked increases in the concentrations of DOPAC and HVA. The authors concluded that dopamine was "released to a site where it can be metabolized when nerve impulses arrive at the ganglion" (Pearson and Sharman, 1974). Data essentially complementary to these findings were obtained in the superior cervical ganglion of the rat by Karoum et al. (1977). These authors estimated dopamine metabolism of the ganglion both from the decline in DOPAC concentrations following inhibition of monoamine oxidase with pargyline and from the decline in dopamine after giving α-methyltyrosine. They observed a rapid rate of dopamine metabolism in the normal ganglion that was reduced after decentralization. Furthermore, stimulation of muscarinic receptors enhanced dopamine formation, whereas stimulation of nicotine receptors diminished dopamine metabolism. They concluded that "dopamine plays an essential role in the function of the ganglion" and that "cholinergic activity may be essential for regulating phasic changes of dopamine metabolism" (Karoum et al., 1977). Thus a clear association between orthodromic stimulation, activation of cholinoceptors, and modulation of dopamine mechanisms in the ganglion can be demonstrated if changes in endogenous dopamine metabolism *in vivo* (Pearson and Sharman, 1974; Karoum et al., 1977), rather than the release of amine newly synthesized from tyrosine (Noon et al., 1975; Steinberg and Keller, 1978) are monitored. The findings clearly complement the reports of Libet and Owman (1974) and Dun and Karczmar (1978) that either preganglionic stimulation or application of acetylcholine releases dopamine from SIF cells.

   c. Postsynaptic Actions of Dopamine and Their Blockade Hyperpolarization of the postsynaptic membrane by dopamine has been demonstrated both by extracellular techniques (Libet, 1970; McAfee and Greengard, 1972; Caulfield, 1978) and by intracellular ones (Dun and Nishi, 1974; Dun et al., 1977b). The response mimics closely the slow IPSP elicited by preganglionic nerve stimulation (Libet, 1970; Dun et al., 1977b) and can be abolished by phenoxybenzamine, 10^{-5}M (Dun and Nishi, 1974) or the dopamine receptor antagonist, haloperidol, 10^{-7}M (Dun et al., 1977b) although not by phentolamine, 10^{-6}M (Caulfield, 1978). When Libet and Tosaka (1970) specified dopamine as the mediator of the slow IPSP, they also demonstrated phenoxybenzamine to be an effective antagonist of the response. However, phenoxybenzamine, like dibenamine, has muscarinic receptor blocking activity (Shibata et al., 1968; Cook, 1971), and a positive dissociation of muscarinic from catecholaminergic effects cannot be easily made with this drug. On the other hand, the observation of Dun et al. (1977b) that dopamine-induced hyperpolarization can be abolished selectively by haloperidol is of considerable significance. If dopamine truly mediates the slow IPSP, it too should be blocked selectively by haloperidol—or, indeed, by other dopamine receptor antagonists. In practice, few data appear to be available on this point; and the results are equivocal. Gardier et al. (1978a, b) measured cat scg surface potentials *in vivo* and observed *enhanced* slow IPSP responses following haloperidol, 0.5 mg/kg—a dose normally adequate to block dopamine receptors in many experimental situations (see, for example, Møller Nielsen et al., 1973). Their suggestion, that haloperidol might enhance the hyperpolarization by preferentially blocking presynaptic autoinhibitory receptors for dopamine (Carlsson, 1977), is plausible, although direct evidence for the presence of such sites on SIF cells is lacking. In preliminary experiments with rabbit scg, haloperidol was found to block both the slow IPSP and the slow EPSP nonspecifically (Dun, personal communication). However, the possibility that in these experiments haloperidol was blocking preganglionic transmission, possibly though inhibition of sodium currents (Pencek, Schauf, and Davis, 1978) could not be discounted.

d.   An Intermediary Role for Cyclic AMP?   An extra dimension to the proposed role of dopamine as the mediator of the slow IPSP (Libet and Tosaka, 1970) came from the results presented in two papers in *Science* in 1971. McAfee, Schorderet, and Greengard (1971) observed that brief periods of stimulation of the preganglionic nerve fibers produced a several-fold increase in the concentration of cyclic AMP in the postsynaptic cells of the rabbit scg. Kebabian and Greengard (1971) demonstrated the remarkable potency of dopamine as an activator of the adenylate cyclase from bovine scg. The data in the two articles were interpreted by McAfee et al. (1971) as consistent with the hypothesis of "dopamine-containing internuncial cells, which when activated by acetylcholine released from preganglionic nerve endings secrete dopamine; the dopamine activates a dopamine-sensitive adenylcyclase in the postganglionic neurons leading to the formation of cyclic AMP; and the newly formed cyclic AMP, in turn, causes the slow hyperpolarization of these ganglion cells." The hypothesis was given apparently sound support by subsequent experimentation.

First, the increase in cyclic AMP following nerve stimulation was conclusively shown to be mediated through the muscarinic actions of acetylcholine (Kalix et al., 1974). Second—a finding that fulfilled an important criterion—exogenous cyclic AMP applied to the rabbit scg caused hyperpolarization of the postganglionic neurons (McAfee and Greengard, 1972), thus mimicking the response to orthodromic stimulation (Eccles and Libet, 1961) or application of dopamine (McAfee and Greengard, 1972; Dun and Nishi, 1974; Dun et al., 1977b). Third, phenoxybenzamine inhibited both the rise in cyclic AMP and the slow hyperpolarization following either dopamine administration or preganglionic stimulation (Libet and Tosaka, 1970; Dun and Nishi, 1974; Kalix et al., 1974). Finally, phosphodiesterase inhibitors applied to the ganglion increased the elevation of cyclic AMP seen after preganglionic stimulation (Kalix et al., 1974) or after dopamine (Kebabian, Steiner, and Greengard, 1975b) and enhanced both the physiological slow IPSP and the hyperpolarization seen after dopamine (McAfee and Greengard, 1972). Taken together, these observations provide strong support for an association between intracellular cyclic AMP and a physiological slow IPSP mediated through dopamine (Greengard and Kebabian, 1974; Greengard, 1976; Kebabian, 1977). There are, however, observations in the literature that fit less readily with this interpretation of events.

For example, the rabbit scg is the tissue from which most electrophysiological data have been obtained and that responds regularly to orthodromic stimulation and to dopamine with hyperpolarization. Yet, unlike the bovine scg, it responds poorly with an increase in cyclic AMP to preganglionic stimulation, and especially to dopamine, where the increase even with 100 μM did not exceed 16% of the control value (Kalix et al.,

1974). Lack of penetration or metabolic factors seem unlikely to explain the discrepancy, since lower doses of dopamine applied under similar conditions gave prominent hyperpolarizing responses (McAfee and Greengard, 1972). In a similar context, dopamine is the principal amine found in the SIF cells of the rat scg (Björklund et al., 1970), and exogenous dopamine produces hyperpolarization in this tissue with an EC50 of 17 μM (Caulfield, 1978). Further, slow IPSP responses can be regularly recorded after stimulation of the preganglionic nerves (Dunant and Dolivo, 1967). Yet even at the high concentration of 1 mM, dopamine failed to increase cyclic AMP levels of the rat scg, despite the presence of an inhibitor of phosphodiesterase (Lindl and Cramer, 1975).

Furthermore, although some consistency is apparent when phenoxybenzamine is used as an α-adrenoceptor antagonist to block cyclic AMP changes and electrophysiological events, the use of compounds with greater selectivity of action reveals anomalies. For instance, phentolamine (28–100 μM) inhibits the rise in ganglionic cyclic AMP after dopamine (Kebabian and Greengard, 1971; Tomasi et al., 1977), preganglionic stimulation, or the muscarinic agonist, carbachol (Kalix et al., 1974); yet it has no selective action on the slow IPSP after preganglionic stimulation (Libet and Tosaka, 1970). Similarly, the potent α-adrenoceptor antagonist, dihydroergotamine, has little effect on the physiological slow IPSP of rabbit scg at concentrations up to 30 μM (Eccles and Libet, 1961; Libet and Tosaka, 1970). In contrast, the dopamine receptor antagonist, haloperidol, which has only weak blocking activity against the rise in cyclic AMP caused by dopamine in rabbit or bovine scg (Kalix et al., 1974), proved an effective antagonist of dopamine hyperpolarization elicited directly (Dun et al., 1977b) or indirectly through acetylcholine (Dun and Karczmar, 1978).

Recent experimental data justify reappraisal of the enhancing effects of theophylline on the physiological slow IPSP and the hyperpolarizing response to dopamine (McAfee and Greengard, 1972). Dun and Karczmar (1977a) used similar extracellular recording techniques and confirmed the enhancement of the physiological slow IPSP by theophylline on rabbit scg. However, by using a second inhibitor of phosphodiesterase that was several times more potent than theophylline, 3-isobutyl-1-methyl-xanthine, they observed a dissociation between potency to inhibit phosphodiesterase and capacity to enhance the slow IPSP. For this reason, and because the effects of theophylline could not be mimicked by dibutyryl cyclic AMP, they concluded that enhancement of the slow IPSP by theophylline "probably involves mechanisms other than inhibition of phosphodiesterase."

Finally, the crucial evidence that cyclic AMP or its butyryl derivatives cause a membrane hyperpolarization similar to that seen after dopamine or preganglionic nerve stimulation (McAfee and Greengard, 1972) must be reconsidered. Although the observation was initially confirmed by using the cat scg in situ (Machová and Krištofová, 1973), subsequent experiments using both extracellular recording techniques (Dun and Karczmar, 1977a; Busis, Weight, and Smith, 1978b) and intracellular ones (Kuba and Nishi, 1976; Dun et al., 1977b; Gallagher and Shinnick-Gallagher, 1977; Busis et al., 1978a; Hsu and McIsaac, 1978; Kobayashi et al., 1978; Weight, Smith, and Schulman, 1978) have yielded negative results. It should be emphasized that membrane effects of dibutyryl cyclic AMP could not be elicited in postganglionic neurons of the rabbit scg despite the presence of a phosphodiesterase inhibitor and the same cells' responding to dopamine with hyperpolarization (Dun and Karczmar, 1977b).

e. Conclusion The principal experimental data supporting an intermediary role for dopamine and/or cyclic AMP in the genesis of the physiological slow IPSP is set out in Table 1.

The evidence for a disynaptic pathway in which dopamine is the mediator of the physiological slow IPSP can be summarized as follows. Ganglia in which the slow IPSP can regularly be elicited (rabbit, rat, and, to some extent, cat scg) contain specialized cells suited anatomically and biochemically to serve as interneurons. These SIF cells have muscarinic receptors and store chiefly dopamine. Exogenously applied acetylcholine and dopamine mimic closely the physiological slow IPSP; only responses to acetylcholine are abolished by procedures that inhibit transmitter release. The endogenous dopamine metabolism of ganglia from several species is rapid and can be radically altered through cholinergic mechanisms and by preganglionic stimulation. Changes in SIF cell dopamine content can be correlated with the magnitude of the slow IPSP in rabbit scg.

However, the pharmacological analysis of the mechanism is as yet incomplete. Thus, although selective blockade of postsynaptic inhibitory responses to exogenously applied and endogenously released dopamine has been achieved with haloperidol, a corresponding inhibition of the physiological IPSP remains to be demonstrated. Willems (1973) used haloperidol, pimozide, and chlorpromazine in his experiments in dog paravertebral ganglia *in situ* and successfully differentiated a specific receptor mediating dopamine-induced inhibition of the ganglion transmission process. A similar approach applied to the elucidation of the slow IPSP must be counted an important priority in any future research effort. There are now available a large number of antagonists of dopamine with varying degrees of selectivity and potency at different sites in the body (Goldberg, Volkman, and Kohli, 1978; Kebabian, 1978). Data from such experiments would not only contribute to the definition of the receptor mechanism of the slow IPSP; since antagonists are available to discriminate between receptors linked to adenylate cyclase and those not so linked (Kebabian, 1978), such data might also help clarify the putative link with cyclic AMP (see below).

It is important to emphasize at this point that the concept of a dopaminergic link in the sympathetic ganglion transmission process cannot be considered either a general or, indeed, a necessary phenomenon. Thus,

Table 1. Relationship between SIF cell interneurons, the dopamine-receptor–adenylate-cyclase complex, and the slow IPSP in superior cervical ganglia from various mammalian species

	Animals from which superior cervical ganglia were used				
	Rabbit	Rat	Cow	Cat	Guinea pig
N° of SIF cells/mg tissue[1]	6.9	280	5.2	6.7	76
% "type I" SIF cells[2] (presumed interneurons)	75	Mixed clusters*	24	0.5	Mixed clusters*[17]
SIF cell monoamine[3]	Dopamine	Dopamine	Dopamine	Dopamine	Noradrenaline
Dopamine-sensitive adenylate cyclase	Yes[4]	No[5]	Yes[6]	Weak[2]	No[7]
Increased cyclic AMP on preganglionic stimulation	Weak[4]	Yes[5]	?	Yes[8]	?
Slow IPSP present on preganglionic stimulation	Yes[9]	Yes[10]	?	Yes[11]	No[15]
Hyperpolarization to dopamine/noradrenaline	Yes[12]	Yes[13]	?	Yes[14]	No[15]
Hyperpolarization to cyclic AMP or analogues	Yes/No†	No[16]	?	Yes[14]	?

Adapted from Black et al. (1978).
* Both type I and type II SIF cells are present, but their occurrence in clusters precludes accurate quantification.
† "No" is the majority opinion; see text.
? Signifies effect not established.

[1] Williams et al. (1977).
[2] Black et al. (1978).
[3] Eränkö (1978).
[4] Kalix et al. (1974).
[5] Lindl and Cramer (1975).
[6] Kebabian and Greengard (1971).

[7] Black et al. (1976).
[8] Chatzkell et al. (1974).
[9] Eccles and Libet (1961).
[10] Dunant and Dolivo (1967).
[11] Haefely (1974b).
[12] Libet (1970).
[13] Caulfield (1978).
[14] Machová and Kristofová (1973).
[15] Dun and Karczmar (1977b).
[16] Gallagher and Shinnick-Gallagher (1977).
[17] Wamsley et al. (1978).

although there is sound histochemical evidence for SIF cell interneurons in a large number of sympathetic and some parasympathetic ganglia from several species (Eränkö, 1978), meaningful evidence for their *functional* role in transmission is limited to the relatively few scg listed in Table 1. Furthermore, dopamine is only one of the catecholamines that have been found in SIF cells. In certain ganglia of the rat, and particularly in the guinea pig, noradrenaline and/or adrenaline appear to the quantitatively the more important. The fact that SIF cells of the guniea pig scg contain noradrenaline yet do not respond with a slow IPSP either to preganglionic stimulation or to added noradrenaline suggests caution in inferring functional relationships from histological findings. It further suggests that ganglion transmission can operate apparently satisfactorily in the absence of the capacity to generate the slow IPSP. Finally, in this context, it seems important to stress that neither dopamine, or indeed other catecholamines need be considered critical to the production of a slow IPSP by ACh. Thus, in the parasympathetic cardiac ganglion of the mudpuppy, *Necturus maculosus*, there are dopamine interneurons analogous to those of mammalian sympathetic ganglia (McMahan and Purves, 1976; Criss Hartzell et al., 1977). Yet ACh released from the vagal preganglionic fibers induces a slow IPSP by an action directly on the muscarine receptors of the postsynaptic membrane of the principal cells (Criss Hartzell et al., 1977).

The further possibility that cyclic AMP functions as a "second messenger" in the generation of the slow IPSP is not convincingly supported by the evidence available. In particular, there is a generally poor correlation between the occurrence of dopamine-sensitive adenylate cyclase, the effects of preganglionic stimulation, and the generation of the slow IPSP (Table 1). Further, the repeated failure to demonstrate a direct hyperpolarizing response of a single ganglion cell to cyclic AMP or its analogues remains a serious obstacle to acceptance of the proposed second messenger role for cyclic AMP in the genesis of the slow IPSP. However, the possibility of there being other functional roles for cyclic AMP formed during orthodromic stimulation, perhaps related to enhancement of the slow EPSP (see below), remains open and a subject for further investigation.

2. **Dopamine, cyclic nucleotides, and the slow EPSP**

a. *Facilitation of Muscarinic Depolarization by Dopamine* The genesis of the slow EPSP, it is generally accepted, results from direct activation of muscarinic receptors on the principal ganglion cells by ACh released from preganglionic fibers (Volle, 1966; Libet, 1970; Dun and Karczmar, 1978). However, a role for dopamine in this response was suggested by Libet and Tosaka (1970) on the basis of an "extraordinary" facilitating effect lasting several hours on the slow depolarization produced by the muscarinic agonist, methacholine. The effect was selective in that depolarization through activation of the nicotinic sites was unaltered and adrenaline and noradrenaline were considerably less effective than dopamine in producing the effect (Libet and Tosaka, 1970). The phenomenon was confirmed by Libet, Kobayashi, and Tanaka (1975) and shown to be mimicked by cAMP applied either extracellularly (Libet et al., 1975) or intracellularly (Kobayashi et al., 1978) and by repetitive preganglionic stimulation (Kobayashi et al., 1978).

The phenomenon is clearly of considerable pharmacological interest, especially since it links the action of dopamine to that of cyclic AMP in the ganglion. Its physiological significance, however, remains to be established. The original suggestion (Libet and Tosaka, 1970) that the synaptic release of dopamine was "a necessary condition for the generation of any slow EPSP" seems not to be supported by recent data. Thus, apparently unaltered slow EPSP responses can be evoked by stimulation of ganglia in which the functional release of dopamine was prevented by treatment with bethanechol (Kobayashi et al., 1978). Similarly, iontophoretically applied ACh produced normal slow depolarizing responses when transmitter release was prevented by low-calcium solutions or tetrodotoxin or when dopamine receptors were blocked by haloperidol (Dun and Karczmar, 1978). The very real possibility that the phenomenon assumes significance following repetitive ganglion stimulation, which releases dopamine intraganglionically (Libet and Owman, 1974; Karoum et al., 1977) and raises the cyclic AMP concentrations (Kalix et al., 1974), is considered in the following section.

b. Cyclic GMP, Cyclic AMP, and the Slow EPSP McAfee and Greengard (1972) demonstrated by means of the sucrose-gap technique that dibutyryl cGMP causes a small transient hyperpolarization of rabbit scg followed by prolonged depolarization. They suggested that "conceivably cyclic GMP may mediate the slow EPSP and thereby increase the responsiveness of the postganglionic neurons to subsequent excitatory input." Subsequently, Kebabian et al. (1975b) showed low doses of ACh or bethanechol to increase the level of cyclic GMP in postganglionic neurons (Kebabian et al., 1975a) of bovine superior cervical ganglion—responses that were blocked by atropine but not by hexamethonium. Further, Weight, Petzold, and Greengard (1974) produced evidence for a link with orthodromic transmission when they demonstrated an increase in cyclic GMP after preganglionic nerve stimulation, again blocked by atropine.

However, data are available that are not entirely consistent with the hypothesis. Thus it is somewhat anomalous that whereas the increase in cyclic GMP induced by ACh in bovine scg is dependent on calcium (Kebabian et al., 1975b), the muscarinic slow depolarization of postganglionic neurons from rabbit scg (Dun and Karczmar, 1978) or frog paravertebral ganglia (Busis et al., 1978a) is not. Further, there have been several recent reports that the membrane changes induced by cyclic GMP differ from those accompanying the slow EPSP itself. For example, Dun, Kaibara, and

Karczmar (1977a) recorded potential changes from individual neurons of rabbit scg and observed that the initial depolarization with cyclic GMP was followed by a prolonged hyperpolarization. In contrast, the muscarinic depolarizing effect of ACh is not succeeded by hyperpolarization (Dun et al., 1978; Hashiguchi et al., 1978). Further—a finding of considerable significance—there appear to be differences in the electrogenesis of the two phenomena. Thus, muscarinic depolarization and the physiological slow EPSP were associated either with no change or with an increase in membrane resistance (Libet, 1970; Dun et al., 1978; Hashiguchi et al., 1978), whereas dibutyryl cyclic-GMP–induced hyperpolarization was followed by a marked decrease in membrane resistance (Gallagher and Shinnick-Gallagher, 1977; Dun et al., 1978; Hashiguchi et al., 1978). It should, however, be pointed out that Hashiguchi et al. (1978) consistently observed a distinct range of lower concentrations within which cyclic GMP resembled the slow EPSP in causing depolarization without a change in membrane resistance. The finding provides at least partial support for the hypothesis, but it has to be qualified by the observations that the membrane change after dibutyryl cyclic AMP is often biphasic (Dun et al., 1977a) and that the decrease in membrane resistance evident at higher concentrations of dibutyryl cyclic GMP is not seen after high concentrations of muscarinic agonists or repetitive preganglionic stimulation (Libet, 1970; Dun et al., 1978; Hashiguchi et al., 1978; Kobayashi et al., 1978).

Cyclic AMP has also been implicated in the mechanisms of production of the slow EPSP (Libet et al., 1975) on the basis of its mimicking the facilitatory effects of dopamine on muscarinic depolarization (Libet and Tosaka, 1970) (see section IIB2a above). Although enhancement of the slow EPSP by cyclic AMP was not observed by Dun and Karczmar (1977a) when the sucrose-gap technique was used, apparently convincing confirmation of the original observations was recently obtained with intracellular recording methods (Kobayashi et al., 1978). In the latter study, the physiological slow EPSP of individual neurons of rabbit scg was enhanced by intracellular injection of dibutyryl cAMP as well as by repetitive stimulation of the preganglionic nerves in a manner known to release dopamine from SIF cells (Libet and Owman, 1974) and generate cyclic AMP (Kalix et al., 1974). There was no significant change in resting membrane potential or resistance during enhanced slow EPSP, suggesting an actual modulatory change in the intraneuronal mechanisms generating the response to acetylcholine. Thus, the concept of Libet and Tosaka (1970) that "modulation of the slow EPSP . . . by dopamine . . . appears to consist of a long-lasting metabolic and/or structural change in the postsynaptic neurone" may have as its basis the intracellular production of cyclic AMP.

  c. *Conclusion* A role for cyclic GMP as the mediator of the muscarinic slow EPSP cannot be advanced with confidence, principally because the fundamental condition that the nucleotide should mimic closely the membrane effects of the physiological slow EPSP has not been satisfactorily met. On the other hand, there appears to be no serious objection to the concept of a dopamine–cyclic-AMP link leading to enhanced responses of the muscarinic slow EPSP, at least for rabbit scg. For reasons outlined above (section IIB2a), the phenomenon seems not to be a significant feature of the slow EPSP unless dopamine, cyclic AMP, or prolonged repetitive preganglionic stimulation is applied. Under certain conditions, however, there may be important effects on the ganglion excitation and transmission process. For example, it has been suggested that the atropine-sensitive facilitation of transmission through the rat scg seen after treatment with theophylline may reflect inhibition of phosphodiesterase of the ganglion cells, leading to enhanced muscarinic transmission (Hsu and McIsaac, 1978). It may also be noted that the usual preconditioning stimuli for enhancing orthodromic transmission through muscarinic sites (treatment with eserine or repetitive preganglionic stimulation [see section below]) are precisely the conditions under which generation of cyclic AMP through activation of a dopamine-sensitive adenylate cyclase would be expected to occur (McAfee et al., 1971; Chatzkell, Zimmerman, and Berg, 1974; Kalix et al., 1974). A similar mechanism may be a relevant factor in the prolonged sensitization to nonnicotinic ganglion stimulants produced by repetitive preganglionic stimulation (Trendelenburg, 1967), for which there is no satisfactory explanation (Haefely, 1972).

Finally, it should be pointed out that cyclic GMP has the capacity to disrupt the enhancement of muscarinic depolarization produced either by dopamine or by cyclic AMP (Libet et al., 1975). Thus, despite the unlikelihood of cyclic AMP and cyclic GMP having definitive roles as second messengers in the generation of the slow IPSP and slow EPSP respectively, they may both be important in the long-term modulation of ganglion excitability. The value of this concept and its wider significance, particularly to mechanisms of transmitter function in the CNS (Nishi, Karczmar, and Dun, 1978), including mechanisms of learning and memory (Libet et al., 1975), remains a fascinating area for future experimental development.

C. The Significance of Cholinergic Slow Synaptic Potentials to the Ganglion Transmission Process

Volle (1969) has pointed out that "the procedures for activation of the atropine sensitive sites have been relatively complicated. Obviously, the question of a physiological role for the several sites is clouded by the technique used." It is certainly true that the responsiveness of ganglion muscarinic receptors can best be demonstrated after a variety of conditioning procedures, including desensitization of nicotinic receptors, treatment with anticholinesterases, and repetitive preganglionic nerve stimulation (Haefely,

1974b, and references therein). However, the important finding that slow synaptic potentials are generated in ganglia in which nicotinic transmission is intact (Libet, 1964) suggests that they may be of physiological significance. Two principal possibilities are recognized in this respect: first, modulation of transmission resulting from previous activity at the ganglion synapse; second, direct participation in the transmission process.

Modulation of transmission through muscarinic sites can readily be demonstrated by using exogenously applied cholinoceptor agonists as inhibition during the phase of hyperpolarization or enhancement through mediation of the slow EPSP (Takeshige et al., 1963; Jaramillo and Volle, 1967; Schulman and Weight, 1976). Blockade by atropine of the same effects produced through endogenous transmitter action would theoretically lead to facilitation or inhibition of the primary transmission process, respectively; and this can in fact be demonstrated (Libet, 1964; Dunant and Dolivo, 1967; Brimble and Wallis, 1974). The question whether such modulation occurs as a normal feature of the physiological transmission process cannot be answered with certainty, although the available data would suggest that the level of excitability of ganglion cells can be effectively determined by the slow synaptic potentials, and particularly the slow EPSP (Schulman and Weight, 1976; Hsu and McIsaac, 1978), produced by the preceding preganglionic activity (Haefely, 1972).

The physiological relevance of muscarinic mechanisms participating directly in ganglion transmission seems more certain. There are many reports of transmission of preganglionic impulses through muscarinic receptors after blockade of the primary nicotinic pathway (e.g., Trendelenburg, 1966; Brown, 1967; Flacke and Gillis, 1968; Chinn and Hilton, 1976), and there is little doubt that the muscarinic pathway of ganglionic transmission operates through the slow EPSP (Haefely, 1974b; McIsaac, 1977). The studies of Hilton and Steinberg (1966) and Henderson and Ungar (1978) are especially interesting, since in both cases natural stimulation of the ganglion was used. Hilton and Steinberg (1966) found that complete blockade of the reflex vasoconstriction following raised intracranial pressure in the dog could be achieved only by combined nicotinic and muscarinic receptor blockade. In the study by Henderson and Ungar (1978), although the reflex vasoconstrictor response to lowering the pressure in the carotid sinuses was conventionally nicotinic, the response to carotid body chemoreceptor stimulation by hypoxia was almost entirely mediated through muscarinic sites. This interesting observation serves to illustrate the marked differences that have been demonstrated in the capacity of different ganglia to transmit impulses through the muscarinic pathway (e.g., Flacke and Gillis, 1968; Holman et al., 1971; Haefely, 1974b; Chinn and Hilton, 1976). It serves also to stimulate speculation that a reflex discharge of preganglionic fibers in response to sudden, strong afferent stimuli appears to provide the conditions under which transmission through muscarinic mechanisms can occur physiologically.

III. THE ROLE OF ACh IN POSTGANGLIONIC SYMPATHETIC TRANSMISSION

Two distinct actions of acetylcholine are now recognized at the majority of terminal sympathetic fibers, each of which has provided the basis of a postulated role for ACh in peripheral adrenergic transmission. Thus, nicotinic excitation was a key observation in the genesis of the hypothesis of a cholinergic link in the terminal sympathetic transmission process (Burn and Rand, 1959). Conversely, the discovery of muscarinic inhibition (Löffelholz, Lindmar, and Muscholl, 1967; Lindmar et al., 1968) led directly to the concept of a modulatory inhibitory role for ACh in adrenergic transmission (Löffelholz and Muscholl, 1969, 1970; Muscholl, 1970). Despite their basic dissimilarities, each of these hypotheses has in common the requirement that ACh should be normally available at or near the terminal sympathetic fibers. The evidence relevant to this point is considered first in the section that follows.

A. Cholinergic Fibers in Mammalian Sympathetic Nerves

Early indications of the presence of cholinergic fibers within postganglionic sympathetic nerve trunks came from pharmacological experiments demonstrating that muscarinic blocking agents inhibited and anticholinesterases enhanced responses to sympathetic nerve stimulation. In several tissues, a release of ACh from organs as a result of sympathetic stimulation was shown. By means of such methods evidence was obtained for a cholinergic component in the sympathetic supply to many tissues from all the common laboratory species (for extensive bibliography of the early literature, see Burn & Rand, 1962, 1965; Campbell, 1970; Kosterlitz and Lees, 1972). For technical reasons, there has been no unequivocal demonstration of acetylcholine itself within adrenergic fibers. Burn (1963) suggested that the small, agranular vesicles often seen in adrenergic nerve endings might contain ACh and represent the morphological correlate of the cholinergic link. However, results from experiments in which adrenergic nerves were loaded with noradrenaline or 5-hydroxydopamine showed that such vesicles were empty granular vesicles and very likely the consequence of the poor preservation of noradrenaline during fixation (Tranzer et al., 1969). On the other hand, a close association between acetylcholinesterase and adrenergic axons has been demonstrated in a number of tissues, including rat pineal gland (Eränkö et al., 1970); vasa deferentia from rat (Mottram et al., 1973), mouse (Jones and Spriggs, 1975), and guinea pig (Jacobowitz and Koelle, 1965); rabbit ear artery (Waterson, Hume, and De La Lande, 1970); rabbit nictitating membrane; and cat uterus and fallopian tube (Jacobowitz and Koelle, 1965). The association could not, however, be demonstrated in other tissues, notably cat nictitating membrane (Jacobowitz and Koelle, 1965; Esterhuizen et al., 1968) vas deferens (Jacobowitz and Koelle, 1965; but see also Lever et al., 1970) and pancreatic arterioles (Graham, Lever, and Spriggs, 1968b) of the cat. The interpretation of these data in terms of the precise localization of ACh is difficult (Jacobowitz and Koelle, 1965; Graham et al., 1968b), not least because acetylcholinesterase is widely distributed both inside and outside the nervous system without necessarily being related to cholinergic transmission (Robinson, 1971).

The situation has been clarified in recent years by consistent electron microscopic evidence of a close apposition between cholinergic and adrenergic axons, often without the intervention of insulating Schwann cell processes, and, in some cases with the appearance of a potentially synaptic relationship. Such data have been obtained for vasa deferentia of cat, rat, mouse, and guinea pig (Thoenen et al., 1966; Thoenen and Tranzer, 1968; Jones and Spriggs, 1975); for rat atrium and iris (Ehinger and Falck, 1966; Ehinger, Falck, and Sporrong, 1970b); for cat iris (Ehinger et al., 1970a), nictitating membrane (Esterhuizen et al., 1968), and pancreatic arterioles (Graham et al., 1968b); and for cerebral arterioles from cat and rat (Iwayama, Furness, and Burnstock, 1970; Nielsen, Owman, and Sporrong, 1971; Edvinsson et al., 1972). Neither chemical nor surgical sympathectomy caused any decrease in the ACh content of cat iris (Ehinger et al., 1970a; Consolo et al., 1972), and in several tissues sympathetic denervation has been shown to leave cholinergic terminals morphologically unchanged (Tranzer et al., 1969; Ehinger et al., 1970a; Iwayama et al., 1970).

The observations suggest that the ACh likely to influence sympathetic transmission is contained within discrete cholinergic axons. In most cases they represent parasympathetic fibers mixed with the sympathetic nerve supply, but the existence of separate cholinergic sympathetic fibers cannot be excluded (Campbell, 1970). The anatomical evidence thus favors an interaction between ACh released from cholinergic axons and the adjacent sympathetic terminals rather than a cholinergic mechanism within the adrenergic neurons themselves. This conclusion would be compatible with the observations that sympathetic responses in tissues from newborn animals change from predominantly cholinergic to adrenergic during ontogeny (Boatman et al., 1965; Burn, 1968; Gulati and Panchal, 1978) if, as seems likely (Pappano, 1977), there is a temporal delay in the development of adrenergic compared with cholinergic nerves.

B. Stimulant Effects of ACh on Sympathetic Nerves

1. **Release of transmitter through activation of nicotine receptors** The sympathomimetic effects of nicotine or ACh in the presence of atropine have been known for many years. Initially, they were ascribed to stimula-

tion of intramural sympathetic ganglia (Dixon, 1924; Kottegoda, 1953); but it was soon demonstrated that similar effects could be produced on tissues devoid of sympathetic ganglia (Middleton et al., 1956; Lee and Shideman, 1959), and the possibility of a release of transmitter directly from the terminals was suggested. In the intervening years, this concept has become firmly established. The principal evidence adduced in its support is that nicotinic activity is manifested consistently on tissues free of sympathetic ganglia (Daly and Scott, 1961; Bevan and Su, 1964; Lindmar et al., 1968; Furchgott, Steinsland, and Wakade, 1975), that acetylcholine and nicotine induce firing in the terminal parts of postganglionic adrenergic fibers (see below), and that sympathomimetic effects can be abolished by selective destruction of the terminal sympathetic neurons with 6-hydroxydopamine (Westfall and Brasted, 1972; Fozard and Mwaluko, 1976). Further, the original observations of Hoffman et al. (1945) showing the release of an adrenalinelike substance from isolated organs under the influence of nicotinic agonists have been repeatedly confirmed by using both fluorimetric assay techniques and estimations of radioactivity release following labeling of the endogenous transmitter stores (for detailed bibliography, see Muscholl, 1970; Westfall, 1977; Löffelholz, 1979).

Acetylcholine acting through nicotinic receptors can excite the terminals of a variety of mammalian neurons (Ferry, 1966), and in particular initiate spike activity in postganglionic sympathetic fibers (Ferry, 1963; Cabrera, Torrance, and Viveros, 1966; Concha and Norris, 1968; Davey, Hayden, and Scholfield, 1968; Haeusler et al., 1968, 1969b; Bevan and Haeusler, 1975). The associated transmitter release mechanism is dependent on the presence of extracellular calcium (Lindmar, Löffelholz, and Muscholl, 1967; Haeusler et al., 1968; Westfall and Brasted, 1972; Fozard and Mwaluko, 1976). These observations are consistent with the following sequence; nicotine receptor stimulation—membrane depolarization—increased calcium influx—transmitter release, probably by exocytosis (Smith and Winkler, 1972; Thoa et al., 1975). The important question whether generation of action potentials is fundamental to the release process has been explored in a number of tissues, chiefly by the use of tetrodotoxin, which inhibits spike activity by blocking the entry of sodium into the cell (Kao, 1966).

In practice, tetrodotoxin, used in concentrations demonstrably able to inhibit responses to electrical stimulation of the sympathetic nerves, had little or no effect on transmitter release and/or the sympathomimetic response to nicotinic agonists in hearts from rabbit (Fozard and Mwaluko, 1976) or guinea pig (Westfall and Brasted, 1972), in cat spleen (Jayasundar and Vohra, 1978), in mouse vas deferens (Lindamood, Johnson, and Fleming, 1978), and in a number of isolated blood vessels (Su and Bevan, 1970; Toda, 1975; Furchgott et al., 1975). In direct contrast to these observations,

Bell (1968) found tetrodotoxin to abolish the effects of both sympathetic stimulation and nicotine on atria and taenia coli from guinea pig, on rabbit ear artery, and on rat vas deferens. Although Bell's observations on atria and vas deferens have not subsequently been confirmed (Pappano and Rembish, 1971; Jayasundar and Vohra, 1978), a possible explanation why variable results might be obtained with tetrodotoxin is suggested by the data of Furchgott et al. (1975). Using rabbit ear artery and guinea pig atria, these authors demonstrated that whereas tetrodotoxin blocked low doses of nicotinic agonists almost completely, at higher doses the block was minimal. Their proposal—that action potentials are primarily responsible for release only with low doses of agonist—is appropriate to their data, although it may not be generally applicable. Thus, on the rabbit heart, tetrodotoxin displayed no inhibitory activity despite the use of a full range of agonist doses (Fozard and Mwaluko, 1976).

There is additional direct evidence for a dissociation between spike activity and transmitter release evoked by nicotinic agonists. Thus tetrodotoxin was found to abolish antidromic discharges evoked by ACh in the nerves supplying cat heart (Haeusler et al., 1969b) and spleen (Krauss et al., 1970), although transmitter release remained unaffected. Conversely, Haeusler et al. (1968) noted inhibition of transmitter release with minimal effects on spike discharge when the extracellular calcium-ion concentration was reduced. Finally, bretylium was found to block transmitter release from cat heart before any change in firing was apparent (Haeusler, Haefely, and Huerlimann, 1969a).

Thus, although activation of nicotine receptors affects both local depolarization and generation of action potentials in the terminal postganglionic sympathetic nerves, in most instances local depolarization is the principal stimulus to transmitter release. In this respect the mechanism differs fundamentally from that involved when the sympathetic fibers are stimulated electrically where transmitter release is closely linked to the generation of action potentials (Kao, 1966; Smith and Winkler, 1972).

In contrast to continuous electrical stimulation of the postganglionic sympathetic nerves (Fuder and Muscholl, 1974; Steinsland and Furchgott, 1975b), prolonged exposure to nicotine receptor stimulant drugs evokes an initial, "explosive" release of transmitter, which then declines despite the continuing presence of the angonist (Löffelholz, 1970a; Steinsland and Furchgott, 1975b; Nedergaard and Schrold, 1973, 1977). The phenomenon probably represents the counterpart at the terminals of the selective desensitization of nicotine receptors that occurs in ganglion cells, despite return of the membrane potential to normal levels (Trendelenburg, 1967; Haefely, 1972, 1974a). Thus, at both sites, essentially normal responses to depolarizing stimuli can be observed despite the cells' being completely refractory to stimulation through nicotinic receptors (Trendelenburg, 1967;

Löffelholz, 1970b; Haefely, 1972; Steinsland and Furchgott, 1975b). The rapid autoinhibition characteristically seen during exposure to nicotinic agonists should be contrasted with the generally well-sustained responses following electrical stimulation of the sympathetic nerves (Fuder and Muscholl, 1974; Steinsland and Furchgott, 1975b).

2. The facilitatory effects of ACh on sympathetic transmission   Malik and Ling (1969) first demonstrated an enhancing effect of very low concentrations (5–50 pg/ml) of ACh on sympathetic transmission in the rat mesenteric artery perfused at 22°C. The response was inconsistent and rather small, the optimal effect being less than a 10% increase over control values at 50 pg/ml.

A similar small enhancement of sympathetic stimulation after low concentrations of ACh was reported for the rabbit ear artery by Rand and Varma (1970). The effect was confirmed by Allen et al. (1975), who, in addition, demonstrated an associated increase in the overflow of radioactivity from arteries whose transmitter stores were labeled with ^{3}H-noradrenaline. Facilitation could not be ascribed to either a nicotinic or a muscarinic mechanism, since neither atropine nor hexamethonium abolished the effect (Allan et al., 1975). The phenomenon was, however, highly sensitive to changes in extracellular calcium ion concentration (Hope et al., 1978). On the negative side, it should be noted that other workers have not been successful in demonstrating the low-concentration facilitation of transmission in rabbit ear artery (Hume, De La Lande, and Waterson, 1972). Further, some reservation would be justified in attaching general significance to the phenomenon, since the effect has been sought but not found in rabbit pulmonary artery (Rand, McCulloch, and Story, 1975; Endo et al., 1977), in rabbit heart (Muscholl, 1973), in guinea pig atria (Story et al., 1975), and in several blood vessels from the dog (Vanhoutte, 1977).

C. Inhibition of Sympathetic Transmission Through Muscarine Receptors

Despite the fact that muscarine receptors had long been known to exist on sympathetic ganglion cells (Volle, 1966; Trendelenburg, 1967), it was not until 1967 that the first clear evidence of their presence on the terminal fibers was presented (Löffelholz et al., 1967). To be sure, inhibition of sympathetic stimulation by ACh had been demonstrated on a variety of tissues (Brücke, 1935; Huković, 1959; Burn and Rand, 1960; Comer and Di Palma, 1961; Hellmann, 1963). However, the prevailing opinion attributed the mechanism of this effect to nicotine receptor desensitization (Burn and Rand, 1965; Ferry, 1966) despite, in some instances, partial reversal of the effects by atropine (Huković, 1959; Hellmann, 1963).

Profiting from an accidental observation that omission of atropine from solutions perfusing isolated rabbit hearts results in a *decrease* in the noradrenaline-releasing effects of ACh, Muscholl and his colleagues subsequently established the presence of muscarinic sites functionally able to inhibit transmitter release evoked by nicotine receptor activation (Löffelholz et al., 1967; Lindmar et al., 1968), sympathetic nerve stimulation (Löffelholz and Muscholl, 1969; Fozard and Muscholl, 1972), and raised extracellular potassium ion (Muscholl, 1973; Dubey, Muscholl, and Pfeiffer, 1973).

The majority of experiments of the Muscholl group were carried out on isolated rabbit hearts. There is now abundant evidence for the existence of the muscarinic inhibitory mechanism in many other tissues. Transmitter release studies have revealed such a mechanism in hearts from cat (Haeusler et al., 1968), guinea pig (Lindmar et al., 1968; Westfall and Hunter, 1974; Langley and Gardier, 1977), dog (Levy and Blattberg, 1976; Lavallée et al., 1978), and chicken (Engel and Löffelholz, 1976). Similar experiments have established the phenomenon in cat spleen (Kirpekar et al., 1972; Kirpekar, Prat, and Wakade, 1975); in rabbit lung (Mathé, Tong, and Tisher, 1977), pulmonary artery (Endo et al., 1977), and ear artery (Steinsland, Furchgott, and Kirpekar, 1973; Allen et al., 1975); in guinea pig vas deferens (Stjärne, 1975; Leighton and Westfall, 1976); and in several blood vessels from the dog, including saphenous vein (Vanhoutte, Lorenz, and Tyce, 1973) and mesenteric vein and pulmonary artery (Vanhoutte, 1974). There is additional indirect evidence for the muscarinic inhibitory mechanism, based on a greater inhibition of responses to nerve stimulation than exogenously added noradrenaline, for the rat mesenteric artery bed (Leach and Zumani, 1969; Malik and Ling, 1969) and isolated strips of dog femoral and muscle veins and femoral, mesenteric, muscle, tibial, and gastric arteries (Vanhoutte, 1974; Van Hee and Vanhoutte, 1978).

In general, the inhibitory effects of ACh in the tissues listed above were attributed to activation of muscarine receptors, because atropine blocked the responses, whereas hexamethonium or other nicotinic antagonist drugs were without effect. The nature of the receptor sites has been further defined in some tissues by quantitative estimations of agonist and antagonist activities. In the experiments of Fozard and Muscholl (1972) the potencies of nine compounds with different muscarinic affinities were compared both as inhibitors of evoked noradrenaline release and in their ability to decrease atrial tension development and ventricular rate. There was good agreement between the compounds with respect to their relative potencies on each parameter tested. All the effects were abolished by low concentrations of atropine; this was unequivocal evidence that the receptors mediating inhibition of cardiac performance and evoked transmitter release were muscarinic and closely similar, if not identical. The relative potencies obtained on the heart with ACh, carbachol, and methacholine are in good agreement with those presented by Steinsland et al. (1973) for inhibition of transmitter release from rabbit ear artery and for contraction of stomach strip (Table 2). The data obtained with the use of antagonists confirm the similarity between pre- and postsynaptic muscarinic receptors. Thus, the dissociation constant of the receptor-atropine complex was 8×10^{-10}M for inhibition of transmission in the rabbit ear artery (Steinsland et al., 1973) and 4.5×10^{-10}M for the same phenomenon in guinea pig vas deferens (Leighton and Westfall, 1976), both values being similar to published values obtained for recognized muscarinic sites elsewhere (Steinsland et al., 1973).

Recently, a direct biochemical demonstration of the localization of muscarinic receptors on the sympathetic nerve endings of rat cardiac muscle has been made. Sharma and Banerjee (1977, 1978) measured the specific binding of ^{3}H-quinuclididyl benzilate to particulate fractions from rat heart and found a 45–70% reduction in hearts from animals whose sympathetic nerves had been destroyed by treatment with 6-hydroxydopamine. In confirmation of the pharmacological data, the pre- and postsynaptic cardiac receptors were found to be only "slightly different" in terms of their kinetic properties (Sharma and Banerjee, 1977).

Activation of the muscarinic receptor results in inhibition of transmitter release evoked by electrical nerve stimulation (see references above), nicotinic agonists (Lindmar et al., 1968; Fozard and Muscholl, 1972; Westfall and Hunter, 1974; Engel and Löffelholz, 1976), and raised extracellular potassium ion concentrations (Muscholl, 1973; Dubey et al., 1975; Vanhoutte and Verbeuren, 1976; Verbeuren and Vanhoutte, 1976; Vanhoutte, 1977), but not that evoked by tyramine (Löffelholz and Muscholl, 1969; Vanhoutte et al., 1973; Vanhoutte, 1974) or by solutions depleted of sodium ion (Dubey et al., 1975; Göthert, 1977; Muscholl,

Table 2. Comparison of potency between acetylcholine, carbachol, and methacholine at pre- and postsynaptic muscarine receptors

	Presynaptic			Postsynaptic	
	Rabbit heart* Inhibition of transmitter release by		Rabbit ear artery†	Rabbit atrium* (Inhibition of tension)	Rabbit stomach† (Contraction)
	SNS[a]	DMPP[b]	SNS		
Acetylcholine	1[c]	1	1 [1][d]	1	[1]
Carbachol	0.17	0.25	0.25 [0.12]	0.46	[0.18]
Methacholine	0.39	0.31	0.25 [0.18]	0.52	[0.30]

* Fozard and Muscholl (1972).

† Steinsland et al. (1973).

[a] SNS = electrical stimulation of the postganglionic sympathetic nerves.

[b] DMPP = perfusion with the nicotinic agonist, dimethylphenylpiperazinium.

[c] The numerals not enclosed in brackets are the molar ratios of potency.

[d] The numerals in brackets were obtained in the presence of an inhibitor of cholinesterase.

Ritzel, and Rössler, 1979). Since release by tyramine and low-sodium solutions are known to occur independently of extracellular calcium ion, the mechanism of muscarinic inhibition seems likely to involve an interference with the availability of calcium for the exocytotic mechanism triggered by a depolarizing stimulus. This conclusion is given strong support by the observations that muscarinic inhibition is enhanced by lowering the extracellular calcium-ion concentration (Dubey et al., 1975; Leighton and Westfall, 1976) and inhibited when calcium is raised (Leighton and Westfall, 1976; Hope et al., 1978), although the dog saphenous vein is a notable exception to this generalization (Vanhoutte, Verbeuren, and Collis, 1977). Further, ACh inhibited both transmitter release and the accompanying dopamine-β-hydroxylase evoked by electrical stimulation of the sympathetic nerves to the guinea pig heart (Langley and Gardier, 1977) and vas deferens (Leighton and Westfall, 1976).

Despite the obvious link with calcium, the precise mechanism by which muscarinic agonists inhibit release remains unknown. At the ganglion cell body, ACh acts at muscarinic sites to cause hyperpolarization (see section above); and evidence that similar hyperpolarizing receptors are present on the terminal fibers has been obtained (Fozard and Muscholl, 1972). Hyperpolarization would theoretically oppose a depolarizing stimulus, and this concept has been repeatedly suggested as an explanation of muscarinic inhibition (Haeusler et al., 1968; Vanhoutte and Verbeuren, 1976; Vanhoutte, 1977; Shepherd et al., 1978). Yet it is hard to visualize how such a mechanism could oppose the depolarizing effects of a large increase in extracellular potassium. Further, it has been argued that release arising from action potential generation would be enhanced if the terminals were hyperpolarized (Haefely, 1972). Finally, hyperpolarization is unlikely to be relevant to the atropine-sensitive mechanism by which methacholine inhibits transmitter release evoked by introduction of calcium to rabbit hearts fully depolarized by perfusion with high-potassium Tyrode solution (Göthert, 1977).

D. A Physiological Role for ACh Based on Nicotinic Excitation: The Cholinergic Link Hypothesis

In 1969, J. H. Burn, referring to his belated conversion to the view that sympathetic denervation supersensitivity was not causally related to changes in monoamineoxidase activity, wrote, "If a scientific worker can once make a mistake like that, and even give lectures about it, then any other ingenious ideas he may put forward must be eyed with the suspicion which is then due". Certainly, his subsequent "ingenious idea" of a cholinergic link in the sympathetic transmission process, originally proposed by Burn with Rand, in 1959, seems to have attracted from the outset more than its share of suspicion. Nevertheless, or possibly as a result, the hypothesis generated tremendous interest at the time and has since stimulated an extraordinary amount of research effort devoted to its elucidation. The status of the hypothesis has been regularly and critically reviewed (Ferry, 1966; Campbell, 1970; Kosterlitz and Lees, 1972; Westfall, 1977) and equally regularly championed and defended with enthusiasm by its chief advocates (for example Burn, 1961; Burn and Rand, 1962; Burn, 1963; Burn and Rand, 1965; Burn, 1967; 1971; 1977a; Burn and Rand, 1978).

1. Conception As originally conceived, the cholinergic link hypothesis stated that ACh liberated from cholinergic fibers present in the postganglionic sympathetic supply might liberate noradrenaline from its peripheral storage sites by a nicotinelike action (Burn and Rand, 1959, 1960). The hypothesis arose from three observations: cholinergic fibers were present in many postganglionic nerve supplies; ACh, through its nicotinic action, could evoke both a tissue response and a release of transmitter similar to the effect of stimulation of the sympathetic nerves; large doses of ACh could abolish the effects of postganglionic nerve stimulation. As is clear from sections IIIA and B1 above, cholinergic fibers are present in many mammalian sympathetic nerve trunks, and ACh can stimulate the sympathetic fibers to release noradrenaline through its action on nicotinic sites. These observations are fundamental in that they provide the essential framework within which a cholinergic link in adrenergic transmission can exist. They provide no evidence for a direct role for ACh in the release process. In contrast, the fact that ACh in high doses blocks both its own sympathomimetic action *and* the effects of postganglionic nerve stimulation is direct evidence for a functional role for ACh in transmitter release. It will therefore be considered in detail along with the principal other evidence that can be used specifically to implicate ACh in the sympathetic transmission process.

1. Nicotine receptor blockade and postganglionic sympathetic transmission At the time the cholinergic link hypothesis was advanced, the evidence that ACh could inhibit postganglionic sympathetic transmission came from two sources. Brücke (1935) had shown that a high dose of ACh injected at the base of a tuft of hair on a cat's tail prevented the piloerection produced by stimulation of the lumbar sympathetic chain. Burn and Rand (1960) confirmed Brücke's observation and in addition demonstrated inhibition of nerve stimulation to the rabbit ear by ACh, 2.5 to 20 μg/ml. The evidence for these preliminary, but key, observations in the genesis of the cholinergic link hypothesis being manifested through nicotinic receptors is surprisingly weak. Thus, although Brücke stated, "dass sich diese Wirkung durch Atropin nicht beheben lässt," it is not clear to which of his several experimental results he was referring. Further, since no experimental details were given, the validity of the claim cannot be assessed. Burn and Rand

(1960) did not demonstrate atropine resistance of the ACh-inhibitory effect on either the cat tail or the rabbit ear. With hindsight, the probability is that the muscarinic inhibitory effect of ACh was a contributory factor in the two experimental situations. The possibility is rendered more likely by the fact that inhibition of sympathetic transmission in the rabbit ear artery by ACh has been conclusively shown to be muscarinic in nature (Rand and Varma, 1970; Hume et al., 1972; Steinsland et al., 1973) and that complete blockade of nicotine receptors either by an excess of agonist (Steinsland and Furchgott, 1975a) or by competitive antagonists (Steinsland and Furchgott, 1975b) leaves responses of the ear artery to electrical nerve stimulation unaffected. Similarly, the pilomotor response of the cat tail to sympathetic stimulation could not be abolished by complete nicotine receptor blockade following either hexamethonium (Hellmann, 1963; Wolner, 1965) or an excess of agonist (Hellmann, 1963). On the other hand, the inhibitory effects of ACh on the pilomotor response to electrical stimulation could be "slightly reversed" by a low concentration of atropine (Hellman, 1963).

There are now many examples of normal or even enhanced responses to stimulation of postganglionic sympathetic nerves during complete blockade of nicotine receptors either by an excess of agonist or by the classical competitive antagonists (for example, Blakeley, Brown, and Ferry, 1963; Hertting and Widhalm, 1965; Nedergaard and Bevan, 1969; Fozard and Muscholl, 1972; Furchgott et al., 1975; Toda, 1975; Nedergaard and Schrold, 1977). Since it was recognized that such observations lent no support to an intermediary role for nicotine receptors in the sympathetic transmission process, the original hypothesis was modified and extended. First, the site of the interaction between ACh and the receptor was emphasized to be within the nerve, and thus relatively inaccessible to poorly penetrating, fully ionized compounds such as hexamethonium (Burn and Gibbons, 1964). Second, the adrenergic neuron-blocking agents, in particular bretylium, were suggested to be antagonists at the putative receptors for ACh, mediating sympathetic transmitter release in an analogous way to atropine acting at the parasympathetic neuroeffector junction, tubocurarine at the neuromuscular junction, and hexamethonium at autonomic ganglia (Burn, 1961). In the face of the anatomical evidence for distinct cholinergic and adrenergic terminals (see section III A) and inconsistencies in the tissue penetration theory when a number of nicotinic agonists and antagonists was used (see Nedergaard and Bevan, 1969; Steinsland and Furchgott, 1975a), the former suggestion is no longer seriously entertained (Burn, 1967; Burn, 1977a). The case for bretylium as an antagonist at ACh receptors is considered below.

3. **The mode of action of bretylium**   That bretylium might interfere with the release of noradrenaline by ACh was first suggested on the basis of

the observations of Huković (1960) that xylocholine and bretylium blocked both the effects of sympathetic nerve stimulation and the nicotinic actions of ACh in rabbit ears and atria (Burn, 1961). This dual blocking effect of *high* concentrations of bretylium has been repeatedly observed (Boyd, Chang, and Rand, 1961; Burn and Gibbons, 1964; Hertting and Widhalm, 1965; Davey et al., 1968; Krauss et al., 1970; Su and Bevan, 1970; Toda, 1975), and is entirely consistent with the proposed role for bretylium in the cholinergic link hypothesis. On the other hand, there are observations that fit less readily with the concept of a single intermediary receptor. Thus, depression of the nicotinic response to ACh could be easily reversed by washing, whereas the effects on sympathetic stimulation could not (Huković, 1960). Further, with *low* concentrations of bretylium (< 10 μg/ml) blockade of sympathetic stimulation can be consistently obtained with little or no associated blockade of responses to nicotinic agonists (Hertting and Widhalm, 1965; Wolner, 1965; Fischer, Weise, and Kopin, 1966; Davey et al., 1968; Krauss et al., 1970; Su and Bevan, 1970).

Further evidence adduced in support of an interaction of bretylium with ACh at a specific receptor site is that bretylium has structural similarities to ACh and proven capacity to block cholinoceptors at other sites (for references see Boura and Green, 1965; Lederer, Rand, and Wilson, 1970). A concerted attempt by Rand and his colleagues to define the receptor suggested to mediate in adrenergic transmission, by establishing the structure-activity relationships of a series of derivatives of choline and guanidine, revealed similarities between requirements for cholinoceptor blockade and for adrenergic blocking activity (Rand and Wilson, 1967a, b, c; Lederer et al., 1970). However, interpretation of these data solely in terms of the structural requirements for the hypothetical ACh receptor seems unduly restrictive. Thus, differences between the various compounds might also reflect differences in their local anesthetic properties and/or their affinities for the adrenergic terminals. Furthermore, differences in their intraneuronal localization and in various additional actions on intraneuronal structures might also contribute to the estimates of potency obtained. The data available do not allow these alternative interpretations to be eliminated with confidence.

Last, the fact that bretylium and other adrenergic neuron-blocking agents themselves cause transmitter release (Bhagat and Shideman, 1963; Kirpekar and Furchgott, 1964; Boura and Green, 1965) has been taken to indicate a partial agonist effect on the ACh receptor (Green, 1962; Rand and Wilson, 1967b; Burn, 1971). Yet, in contrast to ACh, bretylium does not evoke antidromic firing in adrenergic fibers (Cabrera et al., 1966; Haeusler et al., 1969a). Further, its sympathomimetic effects are resistant to blockade by nicotine receptor blocking agents (Kirpekar and Furchgott, 1964; Boura and Green, 1965) although readily eliminated by cocaine, which blocks the access of bretylium to the transmitter store (Kirpekar and Furchgott, 1964; Garcia and Sanchez-Garcia, 1975).

In summary, therefore, the case for bretylium, or any adrenergic neuron-blocking agent acting through interference with a cholinergic link in adrenergic transmission cannot be considered strong. It is further weakened by the availability of an alternative and entirely plausible explanation for its mechanism of action. This suggests that bretylium, although nominally a weak local anesthetic (Boyd et al., 1961), by virtue of its selective accumulation in adrenergic neurons (Garcia and Sanchez-Garcia, 1975; Ross and Gosztonyi, 1975), achieves concentrations adequate to block nervous transmission (Boura and Green, 1965; Haeusler et al., 1969a). There may also be depletion of a small but functionally important transmitter pool in the adrenergic nerve endings (Abbs and Robertson, 1970; Abbs and Pycock, 1973; Abbs and Pycock, 1974). Such a mechanism would provide a perfectly satisfactory explanation for the blockade by bretylium of the classical direct-release mechanism for noradrenaline and obviate the need to invoke a cholinergic link in the transmission process.

4. Drugs that interfere with cholinergic transmission

a. Hemicholinium The hemicholinium designated N°3 (HC3) has been shown to block ACh synthesis, and, as a result, cholinergic transmission, by interfering with choline transport to the intraneuronal site of synthesis (Schueler, 1960; Long, 1961; MacIntosh, 1961). Conceptually, therefore, it suggested a means of differentiating a mechanism involving ACh from a direct release of noradrenaline. Chang and Rand (1960) carried out experiments to investigate whether postganglionic sympathetic transmission was affected by HC3 in preparations of guinea pig vas deferens; cat atria and pilomotor muscles; and rabbit ear, colon, and uterus. Without exception, responses diminished greatly over the period of contact with HC3 (2 to 6 h). Similar qualitative observations were made on cat spleen (Brandon and Rand, 1961); on rabbit nictitating membrane (Jacobowitz and Koelle, 1965); and, somewhat less consistently, on guinea pig colon and rabbit ileum (Rand and Ridehalgh, 1964). In several instances, addition of choline chloride to the tissues induced at least partial reversal of the depressed responses. The observations are considered important evidence for the cholinergic link hypothesis (Chang and Rand, 1960; Burn and Rand, 1965; Ferry, 1966; Burn, 1977b).

There are, however, other observations with HC3 that lend no support to the concept of an intermediary role for acetylcholine in the sympathetic transmission process. For instance, although Leaders and Pan (1967) showed that HC3 abolished both parasympathetic and sympathetic stimulation of dog salivary glands *in situ*, the significance of the observation is lessened by the fact that atropine produced a qualitatively identical result.

Further, the observation that HC3 attenuated the renal vasoconstrictor response to sympathetic stimulation in the dog (McGiff, Burns, and Blumenthal, 1967) could not be confirmed by Takeuchi et al. (1971). More significantly, HC3 has been shown definitely not to influence postganglionic sympathetic transmission to the cat nictitating membrane either *in vivo* (Wilson and Long, 1959; Mirkin and Cervoni, 1962; Jacobowitz et al., 1965) or *in vitro* (Gardiner and Thompson, 1961), to the perfused rabbit ear *in vivo* (Rogers and Leaders, 1966), to the perfused dog hindlimb (Takeuchi et al., 1971), or to the rabbit pulmonary artery (Bevan and Su, 1964) or ileum (Bentley, 1962) *in vitro*. Perhaps of most significance, there are several investigations where HC3 has been demonstrated to have no effect on postganglionic sympathetic stimulation *at a time when cholinergic nerve stimulation had been abolished*. Such data are available for the cat atria, stimulated either through the dissected nerves (Leaders and Long, 1962; Leaders, 1963) or by selective field stimulation (Vincenzi and West, 1965); for the field-stimulated rabbit atria (Vincenzi and West, 1965; Appel and Vincenzi, 1970); for the coaxially stimulated chick rectal cecum (Everett, 1968); for guinea pig and rat vas deferens, stimulated pre- and postganglionically (Bentley and Sabine, 1963; Graham, Al Katib, and Spriggs, 1968a; Westwood and Whaler, 1968); and for the perfused dog or rat hindlimb *in situ* (Leaders, 1965; Fray and Leaders, 1967). Further, Leaders and Dayrit (1965) showed the isolated dog spleen responds normally to splenic nerve stimulation despite abolition by HC3 of the small associated release of ACh.

Burn (1967, 1971, 1977b) has suggested that where negative results were obtained with HC3, the time of exposure to the drug might not have been long enough. Yet, as noted above, there are many examples of the obtaining of normal responses to sympathetic stimulation after exposure times adequate to insure complete blockade of the cholinergic component. Further, exposure to HC3 for periods similar to those which had been shown to yield positive results (4 h) failed to interfere with postganglionic sympathetic transmission in either nictitating membrane (Mirkin and Cervoni, 1962) or cat and rabbit atria (Vincenzi and West, 1965).

It should be pointed out that in several of the experiments in which positive results with HC3 were obtained, specific controls to demonstrate the changes occurring as a result of repeated nerve stimulation for the lengthy time periods involved were not included. Thus, the possibility of a progressive deterioration with time being a factor in the decline in response following HC3 cannot be ruled out for experiments carried out on cat atria; rabbit ear, uterus, and colon (Chang and Rand, 1960); cat spleen (Brandon and Rand, 1961); or rabbit colon (Rand and Ridehalgh, 1964). That this is unlikely to be merely of theoretical significance is illustrated by the fact that although HC3 was found to depress the response to sympathetic stimulation of cat nictitating membrane (Mirkin and Cervoni, 1962), rat atria (Chiang and Leaders, 1965), and guinea pig vas deferens (Bevan and Su, 1964), it was in each case found not to exceed the change that occurred over the same period in the absence of HC3.

Reversal of the depressed responses after treatment with HC3 by choline has been considered as strong evidence for a selective effect on a cholinergic mechanism (Rand and Ridehalgh, 1964; Burn, 1966). Yet failure of nerve-mediated responses of guinea pig vas deferens after exposure to HC3 could be reversed by a number of compounds whose common property is stimulation of the smooth muscle cells (Bentley, 1962; Bentley and Sabine, 1963). The fact that choline depolarizes smooth muscle cells and enhances responses of the untreated vas deferens both to nerve stimulation and to added noradrenaline (Bell, 1967; Graham et al., 1968a) suggests that choline would produce at least partial restoration of responses reduced by HC3 by a postsynaptic mechanism, regardless of whether the reduction was due to a specific or a nonspecific mechanism.

In summary, the significance of much of the evidence supporting a cholinergic link arising from the use of HC3 is lessened by interpretational difficulties arising from poor experimental design and, in some instances, failure of the observations to be confirmed. When considered with the many negative findings that have also been reported, the evidence cannot be used actively to support the cholinergic link hypothesis. The one exception to this generalization is the rabbit nictitating membrane, where responses to sympathetic stimulation were rapidly blocked by HC3 (Jacobowitz et al., 1965) in a dose, and with a time course, similar to its effect on cholinergic transmission (Wilson and Long, 1959).

b. Triethylcholine This compound is reported to inhibit ACh synthesis (Hemsworth and Bosmann, 1971) and has been used in a few instances to investigate the role of ACh in adrenergic transmission. Rand and Ridehalgh (1964) demonstrated inhibition of sympathetic stimulation to guinea pig colon and rabbit colon and ileum during exposure to 100 to 400 μg/ml of triethylcholine. However, the small reduction in responses of rabbit ileum observed after 50 m exposure to 400 μg/ml triethylcholine was not subsequently confirmed by Alkondon et al. (1978), who incubated tissues with up to 600 μg/ml for 2 h. The latter workers also failed to observe inhibition of postganglionic sympathetic transmission in rat and guinea pig vas deferens, despite the fact that preganglionic transmission and cholinergic responses of the urinary bladder were markedly inhibited under considerably less rigorous treatment conditions. The experiments with triethylcholine thus provide no consistent support for the cholinergic link hypothesis.

c. Botulinus Toxin As Ferry (1966) has pointed out, blockade of postganglionic sympathetic neurotransmission by botulinus toxin can be taken as strong evidence for a direct role for ACh because the toxin is considered to inhibit selectively the cholinergic transmitter release process. Rand and Whaler (1965) showed that botulinus toxin type D inhibited responses to stimulation of the guinea pig vas deferens through the hypogastric nerve, of the rabbit ileum through the periarterial sympathetic nerves, and of the cat pilomotor muscles through the fibers leaving the lumbar sympathetic chain. In general, high concentrations (20,000–50,000 mouse LD_{50}/ml) applied for a long time (2–5 h) were necessary. The observations with vas deferens were confirmed by Westwood and Whaler (1968), who also demonstrated, using a smaller concentration of the toxin (12,000 LD_{50}/ml), that preganglionic stimulation was more easily blocked than postganglionic stimulation. These data contrast with the earlier results of Ambache (1951), which showed for cat and rabbit pupillodilator fibers and for rabbit and guinea pig ileum that transmission from adrenergic nerves to the smooth muscle cells was little affected by the toxin. Further, Vincenzi (1967) showed that whereas cholinergic responses to field stimulation of the rabbit sinoatrial node were abolished by exposure to 850 LD_{50}/ml of botulinus toxin type E for 80 m, the sympathetic component resisted 240 m perfusion with a fourfold higher concentration.

The difference between these positive and negative findings with botulinus toxin is not easy to explain, since different conditions, tissues, and toxin types have been used. Nevertheless, since the value of the toxin in this context rests entirely with the assumption of specificity for the ACh release mechanism, the report by Vincenzi (1967) that high concentrations (17,000 LD_{50}/ml) of the toxin had neuronal depressant effects apparently unconnected to depression of a cholinergic mechanism is of interest. Such a mechanism would certainly help clarify the puzzling differences that exist between the actions of botulinus toxin and HC3 at some sympathetic neuroeffector junctions. For example, although botulinus toxin inhibited postganglionic stimulation to the vas deferens, the same response was resistant to HC3, 200 μg/ml, applied for 60 m (Westwood and Whaler, 1968). Similarly, sympathetic stimulation of the rabbit ileum could be blocked by the toxin (Rand and Whaler, 1965), although it was barely affected by either HC3 (Bentley, 1962; Rand and Ridehalgh, 1964) or triethylcholine (Alkondon et al., 1978; but see also Rand and Ridehalgh, 1964). Finally, although botulinus toxin abolished the pilomotor response of the cat tail to sympathetic stimulation (Rand and Whaler, 1965), a large dose of HC3 did not prevent a maximum elevation of the tufts (Chang and Rand, 1960).

In summary, in three tissues—the guinea pig vas deferens, the rabbit ileum, and the cat pilomotor muscles—botulinus toxin has been shown to inhibit sympathetic postganglionic stimulation. This observation is consistent with an essential role for ACh in the sympathetic transmitter release process. However, this conclusion should be qualified by the possibility that a nonspecific neuronal inhibition may operate at the high concentrations of toxin required to obtain positive data. Further, there remains for satisfactory explanation the fact that botulinus toxin and HC3, which nominally affect the same transmitter mechanism, have disparate effects on the sympathetic transmission process in the three tissues.

5. Inhibitors of cholinesterase and postganglionic sympathetic transmission The fact that inhibitors of acetylcholinesterase enhance the responses to postganglionic sympathetic stimulation in certain tissues has been used as evidence in support of a functional role for ACh in adrenergic transmission. There can be no doubt that inhibitors of cholinesterase, particularly physostigmine and neostigmine, enhance responses to postganglionic nerve stimulation to the rat mesenteric vessels (Malik, 1970), the rabbit isolated heart (Huković, 1966), the guinea pig vas deferens (Burn and Weetman, 1963) and tenia coli (Ng, 1966), and both the femoral artery (Bernard and De Schaepedryver, 1964) and retractor penis (Armitage and Burn, 1967) of the dog *in situ*. On the other hand, the clear enhancement of responses to nerve stimulation to the cat nictitating membrane obtained by Burn, Rand, and Wien (1963) were not observed in the experiments of Mirkin and Cervoni (1962); Gardiner, Hellmann, and Thompson (1962); or Bowman, Callingham, and Cuthbert (1964). Further, inhibition of cholinesterase was found not to enhance responses of cat spleen (Blakeley et al., 1963; Thoenen et al., 1966), rabbit ear artery (Hume et al., 1972), and rabbit pulmonary artery (Bevan and Su, 1964) to sympathetic stimulation. In isolated cat tail (Hellmann, 1963); dog gastric artery (Van Hee and Vanhoutte, 1978); and cat, horse, elk, ram, and goat retractor penis muscles (Klinge and Sjöstrand, 1977), responses to postganglionic sympathetic stimulation were actually reduced in the presence of inhibitors of cholinesterase. The obvious point to be made from these data is that experiments with inhibitors of cholinesterase provide no support for a generalized functional role for ACh in adrenergic transmission. Further, even in tissues where enhanced responses to SNS were seen, for the observation to provide active support for the cholinergic link hypothesis, it would be necessary to establish, first, that the response truly reflected an increased transmitter release; and second, that such an increase resulted from inhibition of cholinesterase.

In fact, in all cases where enhanced responses to sympathetic stimulation have been demonstrated, the response of the effector tissue has been measured and not the release of noradrenaline. As Starke (1977) has pointed out, such measurements reflect not only the release of the transmitter, but also the activity of inactivation mechanisms, and especially the sensitivity of the postsynaptic cells. The latter is particularly important where both ACh and noradrenaline have the same qualitative effects on the effector organ. For example, ACh was found to decrease the efflux of transmitter resulting from sympathetic stimulation in dog mesenteric and saphenous veins (Vanhoutte, 1974; Shepherd et al., 1978) and guinea pig vas deferens (Stjärne, 1975); yet in each case, the tension changes were increased through the direct effects of ACh on the smooth muscle. Moreover, the use of exogenous noradrenaline is not necessarily a reliable indicator of postsynaptic sensitivity changes. For the assumption is made that distribution and inactivation mechanisms are identical and that a similar population of receptors is involved in the effector response to added noradrenaline and to the released transmitter, and this need not be the case (Hotta, 1969; Bevan and Su, 1971; Brandão and Guimarães, 1974).

In practice, in nearly all the experiments showing increased effector responses to sympathetic stimulation after cholinesterase inhibitors, muscarinic antagonist drugs were given to exclude the direct effects of ACh on the effector organ. With hindsight, the obvious disadvantage to this approach is that any effect of the preserved ACh on the muscarinic receptors of the terminals would be excluded and the true presynaptic interaction distorted. There are, nevertheless, several examples of the enhancement of responses to sympathetic nerve stimulation by anticholinesterases in the absence of anticholinergic drugs, among which the experiments of Malik (1970) using rat mesenteric artery bed are particularly impressive. Yet, even here, proof is lacking that the striking enhancement of responses to sympathetic stimulation is actually a consequence of inhibition of cholinesterase. The concentrations of inhibitors used by Malik were probably higher than those required to inhibit the enzyme (Hume et al., 1972), and it is known that enhancement of effector responses can occur that are unconnected either to an inhibition of cholinesterase or to an increase in transmitter release (Thoenen et al., 1966; Hume et al., 1972).

The positive indications obtained when effector response measurements are made should be contrasted with the data obtained in experiments where transmitter release has been monitored. In perfused cat spleen, neither Blakeley et al. (1963)—who applied stimuli at 10 Hz to atropinized preparations—nor Thoenen et al. (1966)—who used 2–6 Hz but no atropine—could demonstrate enhanced transmitter release after treatment with inhibitors of cholinesterase. These results occurred in spite of strong pharmacological indications of effective inhibition of the enzyme in each case. In field-stimulated vas deferens, physostigmine did not alter transmitter release evoked by stimulation at 1 Hz (Stjärne, 1975); and in rabbit atria and dog retractor penis, transmitter efflux after field stimulation was significantly *reduced* by physostigmine (Story et al., 1975; Klinge and Sjöstrand, 1977).

Thus, the evidence for the cholinergic link hypothesis arising from the use of inhibitors of cholinesterase comes solely from experiments in which effector cell responses have been used as the index of transmitter release and where the interpretational difficulties discussed above assume most significance. When data from the more reliable transmitter release studies are considered, it is clear that no evidence supporting an essential role for ACh in adrenergic transmission has been obtained.

6. Conclusion It is evident from the foregoing sections that there is no unequivocal evidence that can be used to support a general role for ACh as the link in the peripheral adrenergic transmitter release mechanism. As originally suggested by Ferry (1966), the effects of drugs interfering with cholinergic transmitter mechanisms ought to provide the strongest evidence in support of the hypothesis. Yet, in practice, the available data reveal numerous examples of adrenergic neuroeffector junctions that are resistant to blockade by hemicholinium (HC3) or by triethylcholine. Moreover, there are inconsistencies between the effects observed with botulinus toxin and HC3, introducing doubts whether the positive effects obtained truly reflect an interference with the cholinergic release mechanism. Moreover, proponents of the hypothesis have to account for a formidable series of observations and anomalies apparently irreconcilable with the proposed mechanism. For instance, the mechanism of transmitter release evoked by nicotinic agonists appears to differ fundamentally from that of postganglionic sympathetic stimulation in being largely independent of the generation of action potentials. Further, it is difficult to envisage how the comparatively well sustained responses to nerve stimulation could be mediated through receptors that when stimulated by agonists result in an explosive initial transmitter release which rapidly ceases because of autoinhibition. Related to this is the fact that complete blockade/densensitization of nicotine receptors does not affect the sympathetic transmission process. This observation is surely incompatible with the proposed role for ACh if, as the anatomical evidence suggests, it reaches the outer surface of the sympathetic neuronal membrane after being released from the adjacent cholinergic nerves. Further, there are at least two tissues where the presence of excitatory nicotine receptors on the terminal sympathetic fibers have not been demonstrated (chicken heart: Engel and Löffelholz, 1976; rat heart: Westfall and Saunders, 1977), yet where sympathetic transmission appears to take place normally (Katz and Kopin, 1969; Engel & Löffelholz, 1976). Finally, it is difficult to accept a physiological role for the nicotinic excitatory responses when muscarinic inhibition occurs at consistently lower concentrations (Muscholl, 1973; Starke, 1977; Muscholl, 1979).

E. A Physiological Role for ACh Based on Muscarinic Inhibition

Muscarinic inhibitory receptors have been found in all tissues where they have been sought with the single exception of guinea pig atria (Story et al., 1975), although it should be emphasized that they can be readily demonstrated in the whole guinea pig heart (Westfall and Hunter, 1974; Langley and Gardier, 1977). Their physiological significance is indicated beyond reasonable doubt by the demonstration of an inhibitory interaction between ACh released from parasympathetic nerve endings and the terminal sympathetic release mechanism in four different tissues by five separate research groups.

In the experiments of Löffelholz and Muscholl (1970), supramaximal stimulation at 20 Hz of the vagus nerve supplying perfused rabbit atria was found to decrease the noradrenaline output evoked by concurrent stimulation of the right postganglionic sympathetic nerves at 10 Hz. Similar observations were made by Mathé et al. (1977) on the perfused rabbit lung. They observed that transmitter release following sympathetic stimulation at 10 Hz was inhibited by concurrent vagal stimulation at 10 Hz. These data were confirmed by two *in vivo* studies carried out in open-chest dogs. Levy and Blattberg (1976) observed that supramaximal vagal stimulation at 15 Hz inhibited both the increase in ventricular tension and the overflow of noradrenaline into the coronary sinus blood resulting from sympathetic stimulation at 2 and 4 Hz. The effects were abolished by atropine. In the experiments of Lavallée et al. (1978), the inhibitory effect of vagal stimulation and its susceptibility to blockade by atropine were confirmed. Of considerable additional significance was the demonstration that vagal inhibition of noradrenaline release was frequency dependent, that the phenomenon was present under conditions of low-frequency vagal stimulation, and that the degree of inhibition could be correlated with a decrease in ventricular contractility. Taken together, the evidence strongly supports a functional vagal inhibition of sympathetic transmitter liberation, with evidence—for the left ventricle of the dog, at least—for the phenomenon contributing to the physiological control of ventricular performance. One further site for a functional interaction between the vagus and sympathetic nerve transmission may be in the blood vessels of the dog stomach. Van Hee and Vanhoutte (1978) demonstrated that vagal stimulation, through an atropine-sensitive mechanism, inhibited the vasoconstrictor response to stimulation of the coeliac plexus more than that to infused noradrenaline. It should be emphasized, however, that transmitter release was not monitored in this study and alternative explanations for the observation are possible (see section III D 5 above).

Evidence that is less direct, but supportive, comes from observations made in several tissues that atropine augments, whereas anticholinesterases depress, transmitter efflux arising from field stimulation of tissues receiving dual cholinergic and adrenergic innervation. Thus, Story et al. (1975) reported that atropine enhanced the stimulation-evoked overflow of ^{3}H derived from ^{3}H-noradrenaline from the rabbit atria, whereas physostigmine decreased the overflow. Similar data have been reported for guinea pig vas deferens (Stjärne, 1975) and dog retractor penis (Klinge and Sjöstrand, 1977).

In summary, the evidence for a functional interaction between opposing branches of the autonomic nervous system involving an inhibitory effect of ACh on sympathetic transmitter release is strong for rabbit and dog heart and suggestive for blood vessels of dog stomach. However, it can be considered only a theoretical possibility for guinea pig vas deferens and dog retractor penis. This is true, first, because interpretation of the data assumes specific activities of the cholinergic antagonists/anticholinesterases used, and this may not necessarily be the case; Second, and more important, because of the method of stimulation employed. Thus field stimulation implies a simultaneous activation of all types of nerves within the tissue, a situation unlikely to be typical of normal physiological function.

F. Final Comments

The morphological evidence for the role for ACh in peripheral sympathetic transmission is strong in many tissues and is consistent with a release of ACh from cholinergic axons and subsequent action on the outer surface of the sympathetic terminals. This action will result, in most tissues, in *modulation* of sympathetic transmission by inhibition of noradrenaline release through a muscarinic mechanism. (The possible exceptions are rabbit ear artery and cat pial arteries [Edvinsson, Falck, and Owman, 1977].) This modulation raises the possibility that in tissues receiving both an adrenergic and a cholinergic innervation, the fine control of the tissues' responsiveness may depend not only on the postsynaptic interaction of the respective transmitters but also on the presynaptic suppression of sympathetic transmitter release by ACh. In this context, the possible reciprocal influence arising from α-adrenoceptor-mediated inhibition of ACh release may also be important (Kosterlitz and Lees, 1972; Starke, 1977).

In a purely pharmacological context, the inhibitory effects of ACh on adrenergic nerve endings would be expected greatly to reinforce its direct smooth muscle relaxant activity on tissues in which there is sympathetic neurogenic tone. This has been proposed as the reason for the potent vasodilator effect of the drug in the intact organism, in contrast to its weak effect on vascular smooth muscle *in vitro* (Vanhoutte, 1977; Westfall, 1977). The concept of muscarinic inhibition has also been invoked to explain a well-known clinical finding for which no satisfactory explanation is available. Thus, Van Hee and Vanhoutte (1978) have proposed that at least part of the beneficial effects of vagotomy on diffuse gastric bleeding might result from withdrawal of the inhibitory effect of the cholinergic transmitter on the local adrenergic vasomotor control.

In contrast to the proposed modulatory role for ACh, the evidence for its *essential* role as the link in adrenergic transmission is negligible; and speculation about its relevance, therefore, is pointless. Nevertheless, credit must go to Burn and his colleagues for formulating a hypothesis which, by Burn's own definition, should "have its main value in stimulating investigations and in challenging assumptions which have been accepted without question" (Burn, 1969). It certainly did that. Moreover, by focusing the interests of students of the autonomic nervous system on the concept of presynaptic receptor mechanisms, it could arguably be said to have been the true forerunner of the many subsequent exciting developments in the area of transmitter release control through presynaptic receptors.

IV. REFERENCES

Abbs, E.T.; Pycock, C.J.: The Effect of Bretylium on the Subcellular Distribution of Noradrenaline and on Adrenergic Nerve Function in Rat Heart. Br J Pharmacol 49(1973)11–22

Abbs, E.T.; Pycock, C.J.: The Effect of Bretylium on Endogenous and Newly-Synthesized Noradrenaline in the Microsomal Fraction of Rat Heart. Br J Pharmacol 50(1974)606–608

Abbs, E.T.; Robertson, M.I.: Selective Depletion of Noradrenaline: a Proposed Mechanism of the Adrenergic Neurone-Blocking Action of Bretylium. Br J Pharmacol 38(1970)776–791

Alkondon, M.; Vedasiromoni, J.R.; Mukherjee, P.K.; Ganguly, D.K.: Influence of triethylcholine on Autonomic Transmission in vitro. Arch Int Pharmacodyn Ther 231(1978)63–69

Allen, G.S.; Glover, A.B.; McCulloch, M.W.; Rand, M.J.; Story, D.F.: Modulation by Acetylcholine of Adrenergic Transmission in the Rabbit Ear Artery. Br J Pharmacol 54(1975)49–53

Ambache, N.: A Further Study of the Action of Clostridium Botulinum Toxin on Different Types of Autonomic Nerve Fibre. J Physiol (Lond) 113(1951)1–17

Appel, W.C.; Vincenzi, F.F.: Effects of Hemicholinium and Bretylium on the Release of Autonomic Transmitters in the Isolated Sino-atrial Node. Br J Pharmacol 40(1970)268–274

Armitage, A.K.; Burn, J.H.: Effect of Physostigmine on the Contraction of the Retractor Penis of the Dog in Response to Sympathetic Stimulation. Br J Pharmacol 29(1967)218–229

Bacq, Z.M.: Chemical Transmission of Nerve Impulses. A Historical Sketch. Pergamon, Oxford, 1975

Bell, C.: Effects of Exogenous Choline on Adrenergic Responses of the Guinea-Pig Vas Deferens. Br J Pharmacol 29(1967)436–444

Bell, C.: Differential Effects of Tetrodotoxin on Sympathomimetic Actions of Nicotine and Tyramine. Br J Pharmacol 32(1968)96–103

Bentley, G.A.: Studies on Sympathetic Mechanisms in Isolated Intestinal and Vas Deferens Preparations. Br J Pharmacol 19(1962)85–98

Bentley, G.A.; Sabine, J.R.: The Effects of Ganglion Blocking and Postganglionic Sympatholytic Drugs on Preparations of the Guinea Pig Vas Deferens. Br J Pharmacol 21(1963)190–201

Bernard, P.J.; De Schaepedryver, A.F.: Adrenergic Mechanisms in the Dog Hindleg. Arch Int Pharmacodyn Ther 148(1964)301–305

Bevan, J.A.; Haeusler, G.: Electrical Events Associated with the Action of Nicotine at the Adrenergic Nerve Terminal. Arch Int Pharmacodyn Ther 218(1975)84–95

Bevan, J.A.; Su, C.: The Sympathetic Mechanism in the Isolated Pulmonary Artery of the Rabbit. Br J Pharmacol 22(1964)176

Bevan, J.A.; Su, C.: Distribution Theory of Resistance of Neurogenic Vasoconstriction to Alpha Receptor Blockade in the Rabbit. Circ Res 28(1971)179–187

Bhagat, B.; Shideman, F.E.: Mechanism of the Positive Inotropic Responses to Bretylium and Guanethidine. Br J Pharmacol 20(1963)56–62

Björklund, A.; Cegrell, L.; Falck, B.; Ritzen, M.; Rosengren, E.: Dopamine-Containing Cells in Sympathetic Ganglia. Acta Physiol Scand 78(1970)334–338

Black, A.C., Jr.; Chiba, J.; Wamsley, J.K.; Bhalla, R.C.; Williams, T.H.: Interneurons of

Sympathetic Ganglia: Divergent Cyclic AMP Responses and Morphology in Cat and Cow. Brain Res 148(1978)389–398

Black, A.C.; Chiba, T.; Wamsley, J.K.; Williams, T.H.: Adenylate Cyclase Responsiveness to Catecholamines in the Superior Cervical Ganglion of Various Species. Neuroscience Abs 2 Part 1 (1976)577

Blakeley, A.G.H.; Brown, G.L.; Ferry, C.B.: Pharmacological Experiments on the Release of the Sympathetic Transmitter. J Physiol (Lond) 167(1963)504–514

Boatman, D.L.; Shaffer, R.A.; Dixon, R.L.; Brody, M.J.: Function of Vascular Smooth Muscle and its Sympathetic Innervation in the New Born Dog. J Clin Invest 44(1965)241–246

Boura, A.L.A.; Green, A.F.: Adrenergic Neurone Blocking Agents. Ann Rev Pharmacol 5(1965)183–212

Bowman, W.C.; Callingham, B.A.; Cuthbert, A.W.: The Effects of Physostigmine on the Mechanical and Electrical Responses of the Cat Nictitating Membrane. Br J Pharmacol 22(1964)558–576

Boyd, H.; Chang, V.; Rand, M.J.: The Local Anaesthetic Activity of Bretylium in Relation to its Action in Blocking Sympathetic Responses. Arch Int Pharmacodyn Ther 131(1961)10–23

Brandão, F.; Guimarães, S.: Inactivation of Endogenous Noradrenaline Released by Electrical Stimulation in vitro of Dog Saphenous Vein. Blood vessels II(1974)45–54

Brandon, K.W.; Rand, M.J.: Acetylcholine and the Sympathetic Innervation of the Spleen. J Physiol (Lond) 157(1961)18–32

Brimble, M.J.; Wallis, D.I.: The Role of Muscarinic Receptors in Synaptic Transmission and Its Modulation in the Rabbit Superior Cervical Ganglion. Eur J Pharmacol 29(1974) 117–132

Brown, A.M.: Cardiac Sympathetic Adrenergic Pathways in Which Synaptic Transmission is Blocked by Atropine Sulphate. J Physiol (Lond) 191(1967)271–288

Brücke, F.T.: Über die Wirkung von Acetylcholin auf die Pilomotoren. Klin Wochenschr 14(1935)7–9

Burgen, A.S.V.; Spero, L.: The Action of Acetylcholine and Other Drugs on the Efflux of Potassium and Rubidium from Smooth Muscle of the Guinea-Pig Intestine. Br J Pharmacol 34(1968)99–115

Burn, J.H.: A New View of Adrenergic Nerve Fibres, Explaining the Action of Reserpine, Bretylium, and Guanethidine. Br Med J 1(1961)1623–1627

Burn, J.H.: The release of norepinephrine from the sympathetic postganglionic fibre. Bull. Johns Hopkins Hosp. 112(1963)167–182

Burn, J.H.: Introductory Remarks, Section V Adrenergic Transmission. Pharmacol Rev 18(1966)459–470

Burn, J.H.: Release of Noradrenaline from the Sympathetic Postganglionic Fibre. Br Med J 2(1967)197–201

Burn, J.H.: The Development of the Adrenergic Fibres. Br J Pharmacol 32(1968)575–582

Burn, J.H.: Essential Pharmacology. Ann Rev Pharmacol 9(1969)1–20

Burn, J.H.: Release of Noradrenaline from Sympathetic Nerve Endings. Nature 231 (1971)237–240

Burn, J.H.: Evidence that Acetylcholine Releases Noradrenaline in the Sympathetic Fibre. J. Pharm Pharmacol 29(1977a)325–329

Burn, J.H.: The Function of Acetylcholine Released from Sympathetic Fibres. Clin Exp Pharmacol Physiol 4(1977b)59–100

Burn, J.H.; Gibbons, W.R.: The Sympathetic Postganglionic Fibre and the Block by Bretylium; the Block Prevented by Hexamethonium and Imitated by Mecamylamine. Br J Pharmacol 22(1964)549–557

Burn, J.H.; Rand, M.J.: Sympathetic Postganglionic Mechanism. Nature 184(1959)163–165

Burn, J.H.; Rand, M.J.: Sympathetic Postganglionic Cholinergic Fibres. Br J Pharmacol 15(1960)56–66

Burn, J.H.; Rand, M.J.: A New Interpretation of the Adrenergic Nerve Fiber. Ad Pharmacol Chemother 1(1962)1–30

Burn, J.H.; Rand, M.J.: Acetylcholine in Adrenergic Transmission. Ann Rev Pharmacol 5(1965)163–182

184 / John Fozard

Burn, J.H.; Rand, M.J.: The Cholinergic Link in Sympathetic Fibres. In: Proceedings of the Seventh International Congress on Pharmacology, Paris, 1978. Abstract 216.

Burn, J.H.; Rand, M.J.; Wien, R.: The adrenergic Mechanism in the Nictitating Membrane. Br J Pharmacol 20(1963)83–94

Burn, J.H.; Weetman, D.F.: The Effect of Eserine on the Response of the Vas Deferens to Hypogastric Nerve Stimulation. Br J Pharmacol 20(1963)74–81

Busis, N.A.; Schulman, J.A.; Smith, P.A.; Weight, F.F.: Do Cyclic Nucleotides Mediate Slow Postsynaptic Potentials in Sympathetic Ganglia? Br J Pharmacol 62(1978a)378P–379P

Busis, N.A.; Weight, F.F.; Smith, P.A.: Synaptic Potentials in Sympathetic Ganglia: Are They Mediated by Cyclic Nucleotides? Science 200(1978b)1079–1081

Cabrera, R.; Torrance, R.W.; Viveros, H.: The Action of Acetylcholine and Other Drugs upon the Terminal Parts of the Postganglionic Sympathetic Fibre Br J Pharmacol 27(1966)51–63

Campbell, G.: Autonomic Nervous Supply to Effector Tissues. In: Smooth Muscle, pp. 451–495, ed. by E. Bülbring, A.F. Brading, A.W. Jones, T. Tomita. Arnold, London, 1970

Carlsson, A.: Dopaminergic Autoreceptors: Background and Implications. Adv Biochem Psychopharmacol 16(1977)439–441

Caulfield, M.P.: Receptors Mediating Hyperpolarizing Responses to Catecholamines in Rat Superior Cervical Ganglia. Br J Pharmacol 62(1978)377P–378P

Chang, V.; Rand, M.J.: Transmission Failure in Sympathetic Nerves produced by Hemicholinium. Br J Pharmacol 15(1960)588–600

Chatzkel, S.; Zimmerman, I.; Berg, A.: Modulation of Cyclic AMP Synthesis in the Cat Superior Cervical Ganglion by Short Term Presynaptic Stimulation. Brain Res 80(1974)523–526

Chiang, T.S.; Leaders, F.E.: Mechanism for Nicotine and DMPP on the Isolated Rat Atria-Vagus Nerve Preparation. J Pharmacol Exp Ther 149(1965)225–232

Chiba, T.; Williams, T.H.: Histofluorescence Characteristics and Quantification of Small Intensely Fluorescent (SIF) Cells in Sympathetic Ganglia of Several Species. Cell Tissue Res 162(1975)331–341

Chinn, C.; Hilton, J.G.: Selective Activation of Nicotinic and Muscarinic Transmission in Cardiac Sympathetic Ganglia of the Dog. Eur J Pharmacol 40(1976)77–82

Comer, M.S.; Di Palma, J.R.: TM 10 Activity in Cholinergic Compounds. Arch Int Pharmacodyn Ther 131(1961)368–377

Concha, J.; Norris, B.: Studies on Renal Vasomotion. Br J Pharmacol 34(1968)277–290

Consolo, S.; Garattini, S.; Ladinsky, H.; Thoenen, H.: Effect of Chemical Sympathectomy on the Content of Acetylcholine, Choline and Choline Acetyltransferase Activity in the Cat Spleen and Iris. J Physiol (Lond) 220(1972)639–646

Cook, D.A.: Blockade by Phenoxybenzamine of the Contractor Response Produced by Agonists in the Isolated Ileum of the Guinea Pig. Br J Pharmacol 43(1971)197–209

Criss Hartzell, H.; Kuffler, S.W.; Stickgold, R.; Yoshikami, D.: Synaptic Excitation and Inhibition Resulting from Direct Action of Acetylcholine on Two types of Chemoreceptors on Individual Amphibian Parasympathetic Neurones. J Physiol (Lond) 271(1977)817–846

Dail, W.G.; Evan, A.P.: Ultrastructure of Adrenergic Terminals and SIF Cells in the Superior Cervical Ganglion of the Rabbit. Brain Res 148(1978)469–477

Daly, M. de B.; Scott, M.J.: The Effects of Acetylcholine on the Volume and Vascular Resistance of the Dog's Spleen. J Physiol (Lond) 156(1961)246–259

Davey, M.J.; Hayden, M.L.; Scholfield, P.C.: The Effects of Bretylium on C Fibre Excitation and Noradrenaline Release by Acetylcholine and Electrical Stimulation. Br J Pharmacol 34(1968)377–387

De Castro, F.: Sympathetic Ganglia, Normal and Pathological. In: Cytology and Cellular Pathology of the Nervous System, pp. 356–359, ed. by W. Penfield. Haefner, New York, 1965

Dixon, W.E.: Nicotin, Coniin, Piperidin, Lupetidin, Ceytisin, Lobelin, Spartein, Gelsemin. Mittel, welche auf bestimmte Nervenzellen wirken. Heffter-Heubners Handb Exp Pharmak 2(1924)656–736

Dubey, M.P.; Muscholl, E.; Pfeiffer, A.: Muscarinic Inhibition of Potassium-Induced Noradrenaline Release and Its Dependence on the Calcium Concentration. Naunyn-Schmiedebergs Arch Pharmacol 278(1975)179–194

Dun, N.J.; Kaibara, K.; Karczmar, A.G.: Direct Postsynaptic Membrane Effect of Dibutyryl Cyclic GMP on Mammalian Sympathetic Neurons. Neuropharmacology 16(1977a)715–717

Dun, N.J.; Kaibara, K.; Karczmar, A.G.: Dopamine and Adenosine 3',5'-Monophosphate Responses of Single mammalian sympathetic neurons. Science 197(1977b)778–780

Dun, N.J.; Kaibara, K.; Karczmar, A.G.: Muscarinic and cGMP Induced Membrane Potential Changes: Differences in Electrogenic Mechanisms. Brain Res 150(1978)658–661

Dun, N.J.; Karczmar, A.G.: A Comparison of the Effect of Theophylline and Cyclic Adenosine 3':5'-Monophosphate on the Superior Cervical Ganglion of the Rabbit by Means of the Sucrose-Gap Method. J Pharmacol Exp Ther 202(1977a)89–96

Dun, N.; Karczmar, A.G.: The Presynaptic Site of Action of Norepinephrine in the Superior Cervical Ganglion of the Guinea Pig. J Pharmacol Exp Ther 200(1977b)328–335

Dun, N.J.; Karczmar, A.G.: Involvement of an Interneuron in the Generation of the Slow Inhibitory Postsynaptic Potential in Mammalian Sympathetic Ganglia. Proc Natl Acad Sci USA 75(1978)4029–4032

Dun, N.J.; Nishi, S.: Effects of Dopamine on the Superior Cervical Ganglion of the Rabbit. J Physiol (Lond) 239(1974)155–164

Dunant, Y.; Dolivo, M.: Relations entre les potentiels synaptiques lents et l'excitabilité du ganglion sympathique chez le rat. J Physiol (Paris) 59(1967)281–294

Eccles, R.M.; Libet, B.: Origin and Blockade of the Synaptic Responses of Curarised Sympathetic Ganglia. J Physiol (Lond) 157(1961)484–503

Edvinsson, L.; Falck, B.; Owman, C.: Possibilities for a Cholinergic Action on Smooth Musculature and on Sympathetic Axons in Brain Vessels Mediated by Muscarinic and Nicotinic Receptors. J Pharmacol Exp Ther 200(1977)117–126

Edvinsson, L.; Nielsen, K.C.; Owman, Ch.; Sporrong, B.: Cholinergic Mechanisms in Pial Vessels. Histochemistry, Electron Microscopy and Pharmacology. Z Zellforsch 134 (1972)311–325

Ehinger, B.; Falck, B.: Concomitant Adrenergic and Parasympathetic Fibres in the Rat Iris. Acta Physiol Scand 67(1966)201–207

Ehinger, B.; Falck, B.; Persson, H.; Rosengren, A-M.; Sporrong, B.: Acetylcholine in Adrenergic Terminals of the Cat Iris. J Physiol 209(1970a)557–565

Ehinger, B.; Falck, B.; Sporrong, B.: Possible Axo-Axonal Synapses between Adrenergic and Cholinergic Nerve Terminals. Z Zellforsch 107(1970b)508–521

Elfvin, L.G.; Hókfelt, T.; Goldstein, M.: Fluorescence Microscopical, Immunohistochemical and Ultrastructural Studies on Sympathetic Ganglia of the Guinea Pig, with Special Reference to the SIF Cells and Their Catecholamine Content. J Ultrastruct Res 51(1975)377–396

Elliott, T.R.: On the Action of Adrenalin. J Physiol (Lond) 31(1904)XX–XXI

Endo, T.; Starke, K.; Bangerter, A.; Taube, H.D.: Presynaptic Receptor Systems on the Noradrenergic Neurones of the Rabbit Pulmonary Artery. Naunyn-Schmiedebergs Arch Pharmacol 269(1977)229–247

Engel, V.; Löffelholz, K.: Presence of Muscarinic Inhibitory and Absence of Nicotinic Excitatory Receptors at the Terminal Sympathetic Nerves of Chicken Hearts. Naunyn-Schmiedebergs Arch Pharmacol 295(1976)225–230

Eränkö, O.: Small Intensely Fluorescent (SIF) Cells and Nervous Transmission in Sympathetic Ganglia. Ann Rev Pharmacol Toxicol 18(1978)417–430

Eränkö, O.; Härkönen, M.: Histochemical Demonstration of Fluorogenic Amines in the Cytoplasm of Sympathetic Ganglion Cells of the Rat. Acta Physiol Scand 58(1963)285–286

Eränkö, O.; Härkönen, M.: Monoamine-Containing Small Cells in the Superior Cervical Ganglion of the Rat and an Organ Composed of Them. Acta Physiol Scand 63 (1965)511–512

Eränkö, O.: Rechardt, L.; Eränkö, L.; Cunningham, A.: Light and Electron-Microscopic Histochemical Observations on Cholinesterase-Containing Sympathetic Nerve Fibres in the Pineal Body of the Rat. Histochem J 2(1970)479–489

Esterhuizen, A.C.; Graham, J.D.P.; Lever, J.D.; Spriggs, T.L.B.: Catecholamine and Acetylcholinesterase Distribution in Relation to Noradrenaline Release. An Enzyme Histochemical and Autoradiographic Study on the Innervation of the Cat Nictitating Membrane. Br J Pharmacol 32(1968)46–56

Everett, S.D.: Pharmacological Responses of the Isolated Innervated Intestine and Rectal Caecum of the Chick. Br J Pharmacol 33(1968)342–356

186 / John Fozard

Falck, B.; Hillarp, N.-Å.; Thieme, G.; Torp, A.: Fluorescence of Catecholamines and Related Compounds Condensed with Formaldehyde. J Histochem Cytochem 10(1962)348–354

Ferry, C.B.: The Sympathetic Effect of Acetylcholine on the Spleen of the Cat. J Physiol (Lond) 167(1963)487–504

Ferry, C.B.: Cholinergic Link Hypothesis in Adrenergic Neuroeffector Transmission. Physiol Rev 46(1966)420–456

Fischer, J.E.; Weise, V.K.; Kopin, I.J.: Interactions of Bretylium and Acetylcholine at Sympathetic Nerve Endings. J Pharmacol Exp Ther 153(1966)523–529

Flacke, W.; Gillis, R.A.: Impulse Transmission via Nicotinic and Muscarinic Pathways in the Stellate Ganglion of the Dog. J Pharmacol Exp Ther 163(1968)266–276

Fozard, J.R.; Muscholl, E.: Effects of Several Muscarinic Agonists on Cardiac Performance and the Release of Noradrenaline from Sympathetic Nerves of the Perfused Rabbit Heart. Br J Pharmacol 42(1972)616–629

Fozard, J.R.; Mwaluko, G.M.P.: Mechanism of the Indirect Sympathomimetic Effect of 5-Hydroxytryptamine on the Isolated Heart of the rabbit. Br J Pharmacol 57(1976)115–125

Fray, R.; Leaders, F.E.: Demonstration of Separate Adrenergic and Cholinergic Fibres to the Vessels of the Rear Quarters of the Rat by Hemicholinium and a Proposed Role in Peripheral Vascular Regulation. Br J Pharmacol 30(1967)265–273

Fuder, H.; Muscholl, E.: The Effect of Methacholine on Noradrenaline Release from the Rabbit Heart Perfused with Indometacin. Naunyn-Schmiedebergs Arch Pharmacol 285(1974)127–132

Furchgott, R.F.; Steinsland, O.S.; Wakade, T.D.: Studies on Prejunctional Muscarinic and Nicotinic Receptors. In: Chemical Tools in Catecholamine Research, pp. 167–174, ed. by O. Almgren, A. Carlsson, J. Engel. North-Holland, Amsterdam, 1975

Gallagher, J.P.; Shinnick-Gallager, P.: Cyclic Nucleotides Injected Intracellularly into Rat Superior Cervical Ganglion Cells. Science 198(1977)851–852

Garcia, A.G.; Sanchez-Garcia, P.: Influence of Cocaine and Sodium on Bretylium Uptake by Reserpine-Treated Guinea-Pig Left Atrium. Br J Pharmacol 53(1975)247–255

Gardier, R.W.; Tsevdos, E.J.; Jackson, D.B.: The Effect of Pancuronium and Gallamine on Muscarinic Transmission in the Superior Cervical Ganglion. J Pharmacol Exp Ther 204(1978a)46–53

Gardier, R.W.; Tsevdos, E.J.; Jackson, D.B.; Delaunois, A.L.: Distinct Muscarinic Mediation of Suspected Dopaminergic Activity in Sympathetic Ganglions. Fed Proc 37(1978b) 2422–2428

Gardiner, J.E.; Hellmann, K.; Thompson, J.W.: The Nature of the Innervation of the Smooth Muscle, Harderian Gland and Blood Vessels of the Cat's Nictitating Membrane. J Physiol (Lond) 163(1962)436–456

Gardiner, J.E.; Thompson, J.W.: Lack of Evidence for a Cholinergic Mechanism in Sympathetic Transmission. Nature 191(1961)86

Goldberg, L.I.; Volkman, P.H.; Kohli, J.D.: A Comparison of the Vascular Dopamine Receptor with Other Dopamine Receptors. Ann Rev Pharmacol Toxicol 18(1978)57–79

Göthert, M.: Effects of Presynaptic Modulators on Ca^{2+}-Induced Noradrenaline Release from Cardiac Sympathetic Nerves. Naunyn-Schmiedebergs Arch Pharmacol 300(1977)267–272

Graham, J.D.P.; Al Katib, H.; Spriggs, T.L.B.: The Isolated Hypogastric Nerve-Vas Deferens Preparation of the Rat. Br J Pharmacol 32(1968a)34–45

Graham, J.D.P.; Lever, J.D.; Spriggs, T.L.B.: An Examination of Adrenergic Axons around Pancreatic Arterioles of the Cat for the Presence of Acetylcholinesterase by High Resolution Autoradiographic and Histochemical Methods. Br J Pharmacol 33(1968b)15–20

Green, A.F.: Antihypertensive Drugs. Ad Pharmacol Chemother 1(1962)161–225

Greengard, P.: Possible Role for Cyclic Nucleotides and Phosphorylated Membrane Proteins in Postsynaptic Actions of Neurotransmitters. Nature 260(1976)101–108

Greengard, P.; Kebabian, J.W.: Role of Cyclic AMP in Synaptic Transmission in the Mammalian Peripheral Nervous System. Fed Proc 33(1974)1059–1067

Gulati, O.D.; Panchal, D.I.: Some Observations on the Development of Adrenergic Innervation in Rabbit Intestine. Br J Pharmacol 64(1978)247–251

Haefely, W.: Electrophysiology of the Adrenergic Neurone. In: Catecholamines, pp. 661–725, ed. by H. Blaschko, E. Muscholl. Springer, Berlin, Heidelberg, New York, 1972

Haefely, W.: The Effects of Various "Nicotine-Like" Agents in the Cat Superior Cervical Ganglion in Situ. Naunyn-Schmiedebergs Arch Pharmacol 281(1974a)93–117
Haefely, W.: Muscarinic Postsynaptic Events in the Cat Superior Cervical Ganglion in Situ. Naunyn-Schmiedebergs Arch Pharmacol 281(1974b)119–143
Haeusler, G.; Haefely, W.; Huerlimann, A.: On the Mechanism of the Adrenergic Nerve Blocking Action of Bretylium. Naunyn-Schmiedebergs Arch Pharmacol 265(1969a)260–277
Haeusler, G.; Thoenen, H.; Haefely, W.; Huerlimann, A.: Electrical Events in Cardiac Adrenergic Nerves and Noradrenaline Release from the Heart Induced by Acetylcholine and KCl. Naunyn-Schmiedebergs Arch Pharmacol 261(1968)389–411
Haeusler, G.; Thoenen, H.; Haefely, W.; Huerlimann, A.: Electrosekretorische Koppelung bei der Noradrenalin-Freisetzung aus adrenergen Nervenfasern durch nicotinartig wirkende Substanzen. Naunyn-Schmiedebergs Arch Pharmacol 263(1969b)217–218
Hashiguchi, T.; Ushiyama, N.S.; Kobayashi, H.; Libet, B.: Does Cyclic GMP Mediate the Slow Excitatory Synaptic Potential in Sympathetic Ganglia? Nature 271(1978)267–268
Hellmann, K.: The Isolated Pilomotor Muscles as an in Vitro Preparation. J Physiol (Lond) 123(1963)289–300
Hemsworth, B.A.; Bosmann, H.B.: The Incorporation of Triethylcholine into Isolated Guinea Pig Cerebral Cortex Synaptosomal and Synaptic Vesicle Fractions. Eur J Pharmacol 16(1971)164–170
Henderson, G.: Effect of Monoamine Oxidase (MAO) inhibition Upon the N, P and LN Potentials of the Rabbit Superior Cervical Ganglia. Br J Pharmacol 43(1971)436P
Henderson, C.G., Ungar, A.: Effect of Cholinergic antagonists on Sympathetic Ganglionic Transmission of Vasomotor Reflexes from the Carotid Baroreceptors and Chemoreceptors of the Dog. J Physiol (Lond) 277(1978)379–385
Hertting, G.; Widhalm, S.: Über den Mechanismus der Noradrenalin-Freisetzung aus sympathischen Nervendigungen. Arch Exp Path Pharmak 250(1965)257–258
Hilton, J.G.; Steinberg, M.: Effects of Ganglion- and Parasympathetic-blocking Drugs upon the Pressor Response Elicited by Elevation of the Intracranial Fluid Pressure. J Pharmacol Exp Ther 153(1966)285–291
Hoffmann, F.; Hoffmann, E.J.; Middleton, S.; Talesnik, J.: The Stimulating Effect of Acetylcholine on the Mammalian Heart and the Liberation of an Epinephrine-Like Substance by the Isolated Heart. Am J Physiol 144(1945)189–198
Holman, M.E.; Muir, T.C.; Szurszewski, J.H.; Yonemura, K.: Effect of Iontophoretic Application of Cholinergic Agonists and Their Antagonists to Guinea-Pig Pelvic Ganglia. Br J Pharmacol 41(1971)26–40
Hope, W.; McCulloch, M.W.; Rand, M.J.; Story, D.F.: The Effect of Calcium on the Interaction between acetylcholine and Noradrenergic Transmission in the Rabbit Ear Artery. Clin Exp Pharmacol Physiol 5(1978)290
Hotta, Y.: Some Properties of the Junctional and Extrajunctional Receptors in the Vas Deferens of the Guinea Pig. Agents Actions 1(1969)69–77
Hsu, S.Y.; McIsaac, R.J.: Effects of Theophylline and N^6,O^2-Dibutyryl Adenosine $3':5'$-Monophosphate on Sympathetic Ganglionic Transmission in Rats. J Pharmacol Exp Ther 205(1978)91–103
Huković, S.: Isolated Rabbit Atria with Sympathetic Nerve Supply. Br J Pharmacol 14(1959)372–376
Huković, S.: The Action of Sympathetic Blocking Agents on Isolated and Innervated Atria and Vessels. Br J Pharmacol 15(1960)117–121
Huković, S.: The Effect of Anticholinesterases on the Increase in rate of the Isolated Heart in Response to Sympathetic Stimulation. Br J Pharmacol 28(1966)273–281
Hume, W.R.; De La Lande, I.S.; Waterson, J.G.: Effect of Acetylcholine on the Response of the Isolated Rabbit Ear Artery to Stimulation of the Peri-vascular Sympathetic Nerves. Eur J Pharmacol 17(1972)227–233
Iwayama, T.; Furness, J.B.; Burnstock, G.: Dual Adrenergic and Cholinergic Innervation of the Cerebral Arteries of the Rat: An Ultrastructural Study. Circ Res 26(1970)635–646
Jacobowitz, D.: Catecholamine fluorescence Studies of Adrenergic Neurons and Chromaffin Cells in Sympathetic Ganglia. Fed Proc 29(1970)1929–1944
Jacobowitz, D.; Johnson, P.; Kitchner, I.; Koelle, G.B.: The Effect of Hemicholinium (HC-3)

188 / John Fozard

on Sympathetic Transmission at the Nictitating Membrane of the Rabbit. Br J Pharmacol 25(1965)527-533
Jacobowitz, D.; Koelle, G.B.: Histochemical Correlations of Acetylcholinesterase and Cate-cholamines in Postganglionic Autonomic Nerves of the Cat, Rabbit and Guinea-Pig. J Pharmacol Exp Ther 148(1965)225-237
Jaramillo, J.; Volle, R.L.: Ganglion Blockade by Muscarine, Oxotremorine and AHR-602. J Pharmacol Exp Ther 158(1967)80-88
Jayasundar, S.; Vohra, M.M.: Mechanism of Nicotine-Induced Release of norepinephrine from Adrenergic Nerve Endings: Is Generation and Propagation of Impulses Necessary? Arch Int Pharmacodyn Ther 232(1978)202-210
Jones, M.E.L.; Spriggs, T.L.B.: An Inhibitory Effect of Atropine on Responses of the Vas Deferens of the Mouse to Field Stimulation. Br J Pharmacol 54(1975)339-349
Kalix, P.; McAfee, D.A.; Schorderet, M.; Greengard, P.: Pharmacological Analysis of Synaptically Mediated Increase in Cyclic Adenosine Monophosphate in Rabbit Superior Cervical Ganglion. J Pharamcol Exp Ther 188(1974)676-687
Kao, C.Y.: Tetrodotoxin, Saxitoxin and Their Significance in the Study of Excitation Phenomena. Pharmacol Rev 18(1966)997-1049
Karoum, F.; Garrison, C.K.; Neff, N.; Wyatt, R.J.: Trans-Synaptic Modulation of Dopamine Metabolism in the Rat Superior Cervical Ganglion. J Pharmacol Exp Ther 201(1977) 654-661
Katz, R.I.; Kopin, I.J.: Electrical Field-Stimulated Release of Norepinephrine-^{3}H from Rat Atrium: Effects of Ions and Drugs. J Pharmacol Exp Ther 169(1969)229-236
Kebabian, J.W.: Cyclic Nucleotides and Synaptic Transmission in Sympathetic Ganglia. Adv Biochem Psychopharmacol 16(1977)533-539
Kebabian, J.W.: Multiple Classes of Dopamine Receptors in Mammalian Nervous System: The Involvement of Dopamine Sensitive Adenylyl Cyclase. Life Sci 23(1978)479-484
Kebabian, J.W.; Bloom, F.E.; Steiner, A.L.; Greengard, P.: Neurotransmitters Increase Cyclic Nucleotides in Postganglionic Neurones: Immunocytochemical Demonstration. Science 190(1975a)157-159
Kebabian, J.W.; Greengard, P.: Dopamine Sensitive Adenyl Cyclase: Possible Role in Synaptic Transmission. Science 174(1971)1346-1349
Kebabian, J.W.; Steiner, A.L.; Greengard, P.: Muscarinic Cholinergic Regulation of Cyclic Guanosine 3',5'-Monophosphate in Autonomic Ganglia: Possible Role in Synaptic Trans-mission. J Pharmacol Exp Ther 193(1975b)474-488
Kirpekar, S.M.; Furchgott, R.F.: The Sympathomimetic Action of Bretylium on Isolated Atria and Aortic Smooth Muscle. J Pharmacol Exp Ther 143(1964)64-76
Kirpekar, S.M.; Prat, J.C.; Puig, M.; Wakade, A.R.: Modification of the Evoked Release of Noradrenaline from the Perfused Cat Spleen by Various Ions and Agents. J Physiol (Lond) 221(1972)601-615
Kirpekar, S.M.; Prat, J.C.; Wakade, A.R.: Effect of Calcium on the Relationship between Frequency of Stimulation and Release of Noradrenaline from the Perfused Spleen of the Cat. Naunyn-Schmiedebergs Arch Pharmacol 287(1975)205-212
Klinge, E.; Sjöstrand, N.O.: Suppression of the Excitatory Adrenergic Neurotransmission; a Possible Role of Cholinergic Nerves in the Retractor Penis Muscle. Acta Physiol Scand 100(1977)368-376
Kobayashi, H.; Hashiguchi, T.; Ushiyama, N.S.: Postsynaptic Modulation of Excitatory Process in Sympathetic Ganglia by Cyclic AMP. Nature 271(1978)268-270
Kosterlitz, H.W.; Lees, G.M.: Interrelationships between Adrenergic and Cholinergic Mechanisms. In: Catecholamines. Handbuch der experimentellen Pharmakologie, Vol 33, pp. 762-812, ed. by H. Blaschko, E. Muscholl. Springer, Berlin-Heidelberg-New York, 1972
Kottegoda, S.R.: Stimulation of Isolated Rabbit Auricles by Substances Which Stimulate Ganglia. Br J Pharmacol 8(1953)83-86
Krauss, K.R.; Carpenter, D.O.; Kopin, I.J.: Acetylcholine-Induced Release of Norepinephrine in the Presence of Tetrodotoxin. J Pharmacol Exp Ther 173(1970)416-421
Kuba, K.; Nishi, S.: Rhythmic Hyperpolarisations and Depolarisations of Sympathetic Gang-lion Cells Induced by caffeine. J Neurophysiol 39(1976)547-563
Langley, A.E.; Gardier, R.W.: Effect of Atropine and Acetylcholine on Nerve Stimulated

Output of Noradrenaline and Dopamine-Beta-Hydroxylase from Isolated Rabbit and Guinea Pig Hearts. Naunyn-Schmiedebergs Arch Pharmacol 297(1977)251–256

Lavallée, M.; De Champlain, J.; Nadeau, R.A.; Yamaguchi, N.: Muscarinic Inhibition of Endogenous Myocardial Catecholamine Liberation in the dog. Can J Physiol Pharmacol 56(1978)642–649

Leach, G.D.H.; Zumani, E.C.: The Effects of Some Changes in the Perfusion Solution on the Vasoconstrictor Responses of the Isolated Rat Mesentery Preparation. Br J Pharmacol 36(1969)209–210

Leaders, F.E.: Local Cholinergic-Adrenergic Interaction: Mechanism for the Biphasic Chronotropic Response to Nerve Stimulation. J Pharmacol Exp Ther 142(1963)31–38

Leaders, F.E.: Separation of Adrenergic and Cholinergic Fibers in Sympathetic Nerves to the Hind Limb of the Dog by Hemicholinium (HC-3). J Pharmacol Exp Ther 148(1965)238–246

Leaders, F.E.; Dayrit, C.: The Cholinergic Component in the Sympathetic Innervation to the Spleen. J Pharmacol Exp Ther 147(1965)145–152

Leaders, F.E.; Long, J.P.: Mechanism of the Positive Chronotropic Response to Nicotine. J Pharmacol Exp Ther 137(1962)206–212

Leaders, F.E.; Pan, P.J.: Local Cholinergic-Adrenergic Interaction in the Dog Salivary Gland Preparation. Arch Int Pharmacodyn Ther 165(1967)71–80

Lederer, E.; Rand, M.J.; Wilson, J.: Evidence for the Participation of a Cholinergic Receptor in Adrenergic Transmission. Arch Int Pharmacodyn Ther 185(1970)105–120

Lee, W.C.; Shideman, F.E.: Mechanism of the Positive Inotropic Response to Certain Ganglionic Stimulants. J Pharmacol Exp Ther 126(1959)239–249

Leighton, H.J.; Westfall, T.C.: Role of Impulse Flow in the Muscarinic Inhibitory Control of ^{3}H-Norepinephrine Release from Guinea-Pig Vasa Deferentia. Fed Proc 35(1976)406

Lever, J.D.; Spriggs, T.L.B.; Graham, J.D.P.; Ivens, C.: The Distribution of ^{3}H-Noradrenaline and Acetylcholinesterase Proximal to Constrictions of Hypogastric and Splenic Nerves in the Cat. J Anat 107(1970)407–419

Levy, M.N.; Blattberg, B.: Effect of Vagal Stimulation on the Overflow of Norepinephrine into the Coronary Sinus during Cardiac Sympathetic Nerve Stimulation in the Dog. Circ Res 38(1976)81–85

Libet, B.: Slow Synaptic Responses and Excitatory Changes in Sympathetic Ganglia. J Physiol (Lond) 174(1964)1–25

Libet, B.: Generation of Slow Inhibitory and Excitatory Postsynaptic Potentials. Fed Proc 29(1970)1945–1956

Libet, B.: The Role SIF Cells Play in Ganglionic Transmission. Adv Biochem Psychopharmacol 16(1977)541–546

Libet, B.; Barchas, J.; Ciaranello, R.; Tosaka, T.: Unpublished observations (1970) quoted in Libet (1977) p. 543

Libet, B.; Kobayashi, H.; Tanaka, T.: Synaptic Coupling into the Production and Storage of a Neuronal Memory Trace. Nature 158(1975)155–157

Libet, B.; Owman, Ch.: Concomitant Changes in Formaldehyde-Induced Fluorescence of Dopamine Interneurones and in Slow Inhibitory Postsynaptic Potentials of the Rabbit Superior Cervical Ganglion, Induced by Stimulation of the Preganglionic Nerve or by a Muscarinic Agent. J Physiol (Lond) 237(1974)635–662

Libet, B.; Tosaka, T.: Slow Inhibitory and Excitatory Postsynaptic Responses in Single Cells of Mammalian Sympathetic Ganglia. J Neurophysiol 32(1969)43–50

Libet, B.; Tosaka, T.: Dopamine as a Synaptic Transmitter and Modulator in Sympathetic Ganglia: A Different Mode of Synaptic Action. Proc Natl Acad Sci USA 67(1970)667–673

Lindamood, C.; Johnson, S.M.; Fleming, W.W.: Dual Excitatory Effect of Acetylcholine in the Mouse Vas Deferens. Proc Soc Exp Biol Med 157(1978)200–201

Lindl, T.; Cramer, H.: Evidence against Dopamine as the Mediator of the Rise of Cyclic AMP in the Superior Cervical Ganglion of the Rat. Biochem Biophys Res Commun 65(1975)731–739

Lindmar, R.; Löffelholz, K.; Muscholl, E.: Unterschiede zwischen Tyramin und Dimethylphenyl piperazinium in der Ca^{++} -Abhängigkeit und im zeitlichen Verlauf der Noradrenalin-Freisetzung am isolierten Kaninchenherzen. Experientia (Basel) 23(1967)933–934

Lindmar, R.; Löffelholz, K.; Muscholl, E.: A Muscarinic Mechanism Inhibiting the Release of

190 / John Fozard

Noradrenaline from Peripheral Adrenergic Nerve Fibres by Nicotinic Agents. Br J Pharmacol 32(1968)280-294

Löffelholz, K.: Autoinhibition of Nicotinic Release of Noradrenaline from Postganglionic sympathetic Nerves. Naunyn-Schmiedebergs Arch Pharmacol 267(1970a)49-63

Löffelholz, K.: Nicotinic Drugs and Postganglionic Sympathetic Transmission. Naunyn-Schmiedebergs Arch Pharmacol 267(1970b)64-73

Löffelholz, K.: Release Induced by Nicotinic Agonists. In the Release of Catecholamines from Adrenergic Neurones, pp. 275-301, ed. by D.M. Paton. Pergamon, Oxford-New York, 1979

Löffelholz, K.; Lindmar, R.; Muscholl, E.: Der Einfluss von Atropin auf die Noradrenalin-Freisetzung durch Acetylcholin. Naunyn-Schmiedebergs Arch Pharmacol 257(1967)308

Löffelholz, K.; Muscholl, E.: A Muscarinic Inhibition of the Noradrenaline Release Evoked by Postganglionic Sympathetic Nerve Stimulation. Naunyn-Schmiedebergs Arch Pharmacol 265(1969)1-15

Löffelholz, K.; Muscholl, E.: Inhibition by Parasympathetic Nerve Stimulation of the Release of the Adrenergic Transmitter. Naunyn-Schmiedebergs Arch Pharmacol 267(1970)181-184

Long, J.P.: Hemicholiniums: Structure Activity Relationships and Actions on the Peripheral Nervous System. Fed Proc 20(1961)583-586

McAfee, D.A.; Greengard, P.: Adenosine 3',5'-Monophosphate: Electrophysiological Evidence for a Role in Synaptic Transmission. Science 178(1972)310-312

McAfee, D.A.; Schorderet, M.; Greengard, P.: Adenosine 3',5'-Monophosphate in Nervous Tissue: Increase Associated with Synaptic Transmission. Science 171(1971)1156-1158

McGiff, J.C.; Burns, R.B.P.; Blumenthal, M.R.: Role of Acetylcholine in the renal Vasoconstrictor Response to Sympathetic Nerve Stimulation of the Dog. Circ Res 20 (1967)616-629

Machová, J.; Krištofová, A.: The Effect of Dibutyryl Cyclic AMP, Dopamine and Aminophylline on Ganglionic surface Potential and Transmission. Life Sci 13(1973)525-535

MacIntosh, F.C.: Effect of HC-3 on Acetylcholine Turnover. Fed Proc 20(1961)562-568

MacIsaac, R.J.: Afterdischarge on Postganglionic Sympathetic Nerves Following Repetitive Stimulation of the Preganglionic Nerve to the Rat Superior Cervical Ganglion in vivo. J Pharmacol Exp Ther 200(1977)107-116

McMahan, U.J.; Purves, D.: Visual Identification of Two Types of Nerve Cells and Their Synaptic Contacts in a Living Autonomic Ganglion of the Mudpuppy (Necturus maculosus). J Physiol (Lond) 254(1976)405-425

Malik, K.U.: Potentiation by Anticholinesterases of the Response of Rat Mesenteric Arteries to Sympathetic Postganglionic Nerve Stimulation. Circ Res 27(1970)647-655

Malik, K.U.; Ling, G.M.: Modification by Acetylcholine of the Response of Rat Mesenteric Arteries to Sympathetic Stimulation. Cir Res (1969)1-9

Mathé, A.A.; Tong, E.Y.; Tisher, P.W.: Norepinephrine Release from the Lung by Sympathetic Nerve Stimulation Inhibition by Vagus and Methacholine. Life Sci 20(1977) 1425-1430

Matthews, M.R.; Nash, J.R.G.: An Efferent Synapse from a Small Granule-Containing Cell to a Principal Neurone in the Superior Cervical Ganglion. J Physiol (Lond) 210(1970) 11P-14P

Matthews, M.R.; Ostberg, A.: Effects of Preganglionic Nerve Section upon the Afferent Innervation of the Small Granule-Containing Cells in the Rat Superior Cervical Ganglion. Acta Physiol Pol 24(1973)215-223

Matthews, M.R.; Raisman, G.: The Ultrastructure and Somatic Efferent Synapses of Small Granule-Containing Cells in the Superior Cervical Ganglion. J Anat 105(1969)255-282

Middleton, S.; Oberti, C.; Prager, R.; Middleton, H.H.: Stimulating effect of Acetylcholine on the Papillary Mycardium. Acta Physiol Lat Am 6(1956)82-89

Mirkin, B.L.; Cervoni, P.: The Adrenergic Nature of Neurohumoral Transmission in the Cat Nictitating Membrane Following Treatment with Reserpine. J Pharmacol Exp Ther 138(1962)301-308

Møller Nielsen, I.; Pedersen, V.; Nymark, M.; Franck, K.F.; Boeck, V.; Fjalland, B.; Christensen, A.V.: The Comparative Pharmacology of Flupenthixol and some Reference Neuroleptics. Acta Pharmacol Toxicol 33(1973)353-362

Mottram, D.R.; Ivens, C.; Lever, J.D.; Presley, R.: A Fine Structural and Enzyme Histochemical Study of Muscle Innervation in the Normal and 6-Hydroxydopamine Treated Rat Vas Deferens Including a Numerical Assessment of Axonal Changes Within 48h of a Single Injection of the Drug. Neuropharmacology 12(1973)583-595

Muscholl, E.: Cholinomimetic Drugs and Release of the Adrenergic Transmitter. In: New Aspects of Storage and Release Mechanisms of Catecholamines, pp. 168-186, ed. by H.J. Schümann, G. Kroneberg. Springer, Berlin-Heidelberg-New York, 1970

Muscholl, E.: Muscarinic Inhibition of the Norepinephrine Release from Peripheral Sympathetic Fibres. In: Pharmacology and the Future of Man, Proc 5th Int Congr Pharmacol. Vol. 4, pp. 440-457. Karger, Basel, 1973

Muscholl, E.: Presynaptic Muscarine Receptors and Inhibition of Release. In: The Release of Catecholamines from Adrenergic Neurones, pp. 87-110, ed. by D.M. Paton. Pergamon, Oxford-New York, 1979

Muscholl, E.; Ritzel, H.; Rössler, K.: Presynaptic Muscarinic Control of Neuronal Noradrenaline Release. In: Symposium on Presynaptic Receptors, pp. 287-291, ed. S.Z. Langer. Pergamon, Oxford-New York, 1979

Nedergaard, O.A.; Bevan, J.A.: Effects of Nicotine, Dimethylphenylpiperazinium and Cholinergic Blocking Agents at Adrenergic Nerve Endings of the Rabbit Pulmonary Artery. J Pharmacol Exp Ther 168(1969)127-136

Nedergaard, O.A.; Schrold, J.: Release of ³H-Noradrenaline from Incubated and Superfused Rabbit Pulmonary Artery. Acta Physiol Scand 89(1973)296

Nedergaard, O.A.; Schrold, J.: The Mechanism of Action of Nicotine on Vascular Adrenergic Neuroeffector Transmission. Eur J Pharmacol 42(1977)315-330

Ng, K.K.F.: The Effect of Some Anticholinesterases on the Response of the Taenia to Sympathetic Nerve Stimulation. J Physiol (Lond) 182(1966)233-243

Nielson, K.C.; Owman, Ch.; Sporrong, B.: Ultrastructure of the Autonomic Innervation Apparatus in the Main Pial Arteries of Rats and Cats. Brain Res 27(1971)25-32

Nishi, S.; Karczmar, A.G.; Dun, N.J.: Physiology and Pharmacology of Ganglionic Synapses as Models for Central Transmission. In: Adv. in Pharmacology and Therapeutics, Vol. 2, pp. 63-86, Pergamon, Oxford-New York, 1978.

Noon, J.P.; McAfee, D.A.; Roth, R.H.: Norepinephrine Release from Nerve Terminals within the Rabbit Superior Cervical Ganglion. Naunyn-Schmiedebergs Arch Pharmacol 291(1975)139-162

Norberg, K.A.; Ritzen, M.; Ungerstedt, U.: Histochemical Studies on a Special Catecholamine Containing Cell Type in Sympathetic Ganglia. Acta Physiol Scand 67 (1966)260-270

Pappano, A.J.: Ontogenetic Development of Autonomic Neuroeffector Transmission and Transmitter Reactivity in Embryonic and Fetal Hearts. Pharmacol Rev 29(1977)3-33

Pappano, A.J.; Rembish, R.A.: Negative Chronotropic Effects of McN A-343 and Nicotine in Isolated Guinea-Pig Atria; Insensitivity to Blockade by Tetrodotoxin. J Pharmacol Exp Ther 177(1971)40-47

Pearson, J.D.M.; Sharman, D.F.: Increased Concentrations of Acidic Metabolites of Dopamine in the superior Cervical Ganglion Following Preganglionic Stimulation in vivo. J Neurochem 22(1974)547-550

Pencek, T.L.; Schauf, C.L.; Davis, F.A.: The Effect of Haloperidol on the Ionic Currents in the Voltage-Clamped Mode of Ranvier. J Pharmacol Exp Ther 204(1978)400-405

Rand, M.J.; McCulloch, M.W.; Story, D.F.: Pre-Junctional Modulation of Noradrenergic Transmission by Noradrenaline, Dopamine and Acetylcholine. In: Central Action of Drugs in Blood Pressure Regulation, pp. 94-132, ed. by D.S. Davies, J.L. Reid. Pitman Medical, London, 1975

Rand, M.J.; Ridehalgh, A.: Actions of Hemicholinium and Triethylcholine on Responses of Guinea-Pig Colon to Stimulation of Autonomic Nerves. J Pharm Pharmacol 17(1964) 144-155

Rand, M.J.; Varma, B.: The Effects of Cholinomimetic Drugs on Responses to Sympathetic Nerve Stimulation and Noradrenaline in the Rabbit Ear Artery. Br J Pharmacol 38(1970)758-770

Rand, M.J.; Whaler, B.C.: Impairment of Sympathetic Transmission by Botulinum Toxin. Nature 206(1965)588-591

Rand, M.J.; Wilson, J.: The Actions of Some Adrenergic Neurone Blocking Drugs at Cholinergic Junctions. Eur J Pharmacol (1967a)210–221

Rand, M.J.; Wilson, J.: Receptor Site of Adrenergic Neuron Blocking Drugs. Circ Res Suppl III 20 and 21(1967b)89–99

Rand, M.J.; Wilson, J.: The Relationship between Adrenergic Neurone Blocking Activity and Local Anaesthetic Activity in a Series of Guanidine Derivatives. Eur J Pharmacol 1(1967c)200–209

Robinson, P.M.: The Demonstration of Acetylcholinesterase in Autonomic Axons with the Electron Microscope. Prog Brain Res 34(1971)357–370

Rogers, D.K.; Leaders, F.E.: Search for a Cholinergic Component in the Sympathetic Nerves to the Perfused Rabbit Ear. Arch Int Pharmacodyn Ther 163(1966)20–27

Ross, S.B.; Gosztonyi, T.: On the Mechanism of the Accumulation of ^{3}H-Bretylium in Peripheral Sympathetic Nerves. Naunyn-Schmiedebergs Arch Pharmacol 228(1975)283–293

Schueler, F.W.: The Mechanism of Action of the Hemicholiniums. In: Int Rev Neurobiol. Vol. 2, pp. 77–97, ed. by C.C. Pfeiffer, J.R. Smythies. Academic, New York, 1960

Schulman, J.A.; Weight, F.F.: Synaptic Transmission: Long-Lasting Potentiation by a Postsynaptic Mechanism. Science 194(1976)1437–1439

Sharma, V.K.; Banerjee, S.P.: Presynaptic Muscarinic Cholinergic Receptors in Rat Heart Sympathetic Nerves. Eur J Pharmacol 46(1977)75–76

Sharma, V.K.; Banerjee, S.P.: Presynaptic Muscarinic Cholinergic Receptors. Nature 272 (1978)276–278

Shepherd, J.T.; Lorenz, R.R.; Tyce, G.M.; Vanhoutte, P.M.: Acetylcholine-Inhibition of Transmitter Release from Adrenergic Nerve Terminals Mediated by Muscarinic Receptors. Fed Proc 37(1978)191–194

Shibata, S.; Carrier, O., Jr.; Frankenheim, J.: Effect of Chlorpromazine, Dibenamine and Phenoxybenzamine on the Contractile Response of Taenia Coli to Potassium, Acetylcholine, Angiotensin and Barium. J Pharmacol Exp Ther 160(1968)106–111

Smith, A.D.; Winkler, H.: Fundamental Mechanisms in the Release of Catecholamines. In: Catecholamines, pp. 538–617, ed. by H. Blaschko, E. Muscholl. Springer, Berlin-Heidelberg-New York, 1972

Starke, K.: Regulation of Noradrenaline Release by Presynaptic Receptor Systems. Rev Physiol Biochem Pharmacol 77(1977)1–124

Steinberg, M.I.; Keller, C.E.: Enhanced Catecholamine Synthesis in Isolated Rat Superior Cervical Ganglia Caused by Nerve Stimulation: Dissociation between Ganglionic Transmission and Catecholamine synthesis. J Pharmacol Exp Ther 204(1978)384–399

Steinsland, O.S.; Furchgott, R.F.: Desensitisation of the Adrenergic Neurones of the Isolated Rabbit Ear Artery to Nicotinic Agonists. J Pharmacol Exp Ther 193(1975a)138–148

Steinsland, O.S.; Furchgott, R.F.: Vasoconstriction of the Isolated Rabbit Ear Artery Caused by Nicotinic Agonists Acting on Adrenergic Neurons. J Pharmacol Exp Ther 193 (1975b)128–137

Steinsland, O.S.; Furchgott, R.F.; Kirpekar, S.M.: Inhibition of Adrenergic Neurotransmission by Parasympathomimetics in the Rabbit Ear Artery. J Pharmacol Exp Ther 184(1973)346–356

Stjärne, L.: Pre-and Post-Junctional Receptor-Mediated Cholinergic Interactions with Adrenergic Transmission in the Guinea-Pig Vas Deferens. Naunyn-Schmiedebergs Arch Pharmacol 288(1975)305–310

Story, D.F.; Allen, G.S.; Glover, A.B.; Hope, W.; McCulloch, M.W.; Rand, M.J.; Sarantos, C.: Modulation of Adrenergic Transmission by Acetylcholine. Clin Exp Pharmacol Physiol Suppl 2(1975)27–33

Su, C.; Bevan, J.A.: Blockade of the Nicotine-Induced Norepinephrine Release by Cocaine, Phenoxybenzamine and Desipramine. J Pharmacol Exp Ther 175(1970)533–540

Takeshige, C.; Pappano, A.J.; De Groat, W.C.; Volle, R.L.: Ganglionic Blockade Produced in Sympathetic Ganglia by Cholinomimetic Drugs. J Pharmacol Exp Ther 141(1963)333–342

Takeshige, C.; Volle, R.L.: Modification of Ganglionic Responses to Cholinomimetic Drugs Following Preganglionic Stimulation, Anticholinesterase Agents and Pilocarpine. J Pharmacol Exp Ther 146(1964)335–343

Takeuchi, J.; Aoki, S.; Nomura, G.; Mizumura, Y.; Shimizu, H.; Kubo, T.: Nervous Control of Renal Circulation—on the Existence of Sympathetic Cholinergic Fibres. J Appl Physiol 31(1971)686–692

Tauc, L.: Transmission in Invertebrate and Vertebrate Ganglia. Physiol Rev 47(1967)521–593

Taxi, J; Gautron, J.; L'Hermite, P.: Données ultrastructurales sur une éventuelle modulation adrénergique de l'activité du ganglion cervical supérieur du rat. CR Acad Sci 269(1969)1281–1284

Thoa, N.B.; Wooten, F.G.; Axelrod, J.; Kopin, I.J.: On the Mechanism of Release of Norepinephrine from Sympathetic Nerves Induced by Depolarizing Agents and Sympathomimetic Drugs. Mol Pharmacol 11(1975)10–18

Thoenen, H.; Tranzer, J.P.: Chemical Sympathectomy by Selective Destruction of Adrenergic Nerve Endings with 6-Hydroxydopamine. Naunyn-Schmiedebergs Arch Pharmacol 261(1968)271–288

Thoenen, H.; Tranzer, J.P.; Hürlimann, A.; Haefely, W.: Untersuchungen zur Frage eines cholinergischen Gliedes in der postganglionären sympathischen Transmission. Helv Physiol Acta 24(1966)229–246

Toda, N.: Nicotine-Induced Relaxation in Isolated Canine Cerebral Arteries. J Pharmacol Exp Ther 193(1975)376–384

Tomasi, V.; Biondi, C.; Trevisani, A.; Martini, M.; Perri, V.: Modulation of Cyclic AMP Levels in the Bovine Superior Cervical Ganglion by Prostaglandin E_1 and Dopamine. J Neurochem 28(1977)1289–1297

Tranzer, J.P.; Thoenen, H.; Snipes, R.L.; Richards, J.G.: Recent Developments on the Ultrastructural Aspect of Adrenergic Nerve Endings in Various Experimental Conditions. Prog Brain Res 31(1969)33–46

Trendelenburg, U.: Transmission of Preganglionic Impulses through the Muscarinic Receptors of the Superior Cervical Ganglion of the Cat. J Pharmacol Exp Ther 154(1966)426–440

Trendelenburg, U.: Some Aspects of the Pharmacology of Autonomic Ganglion Cells. Ergebn Physiol 59(1967)1–85

Tsevdos, E.J.; Humbertson, A.O.; Gardier, A.W.: Surface Potential and Histofluorescence Studies Demonstrating Selective Blockade of a Ganglionic Inhibitory Pathway. Abs 328, Proc 7th Int Cong Pharmacol Paris 1978

VanHee, R.H.; Vanhoutte, P.M.: Cholinergic Inhibition of Adrenergic Neurotransmission in the Canine Gastric Artery. Gastroenterology 74(1978)1266–1270

Vanhoutte, P.M.: Inhibition by Acetylcholine of Adrenergic Neurotransmission in Vascular Smooth Muscle. Cir Res 34(1974)317–326

Vanhoutte, P.M.: Cholinergic Inhibition of Adrenergic Transmission. Fed Proc 36 (1977)2444–2449

Vanhoutte, P.M.; Lorenz, R.R.; Tyce, G.M.: Inhibition of Norepinephrine-^{3}H release from Sympathetic Nerve Endings in Veins by Acetylcholine. J Pharmacol Exp Ther 185(1973)386–394

Vanhoutte, P.M.; Verbeuren, T.J.: Inhibition Evoked by Acetylcholine of the Norepinephrine Release Evoked by Potassium in Canine Saphenous Veins. Circ Res 39(1976)263–269

Vanhoutte, P.M.; Verbeuren, T.J.; Collis, M.G.: Muscarinic Inhibition of Adrenergic Neurotransmission Is Not Due to a Decrease of Ca^{++} Entry in the Adrenergic Nerve Endings. J Pharmacol (Paris 8(1977)556–557

Verbeuren, T.J.; Vanhoutte, P.M.: Acetylcholine Inhibits Potassium Evoked Release of ^{3}H-Norepinephrine in Different Blood Vessels of the Dog. Arch Int Pharmacodyn Ther 221(1976)347–350

Vincenzi, F.F.: Effect of Botulinum Toxin on Autonomic Nerves in a Dually Innervated Tissue. Nature 213(1967)394–395

Vincenzi, F.F.; West, T.C.: Effect of Hemicholinium on the Release of Autonomic Mediators in the Sinoatrial Node. Br J Pharmacol 24(1965)773–780

Volle, R.L.: Modification by Drugs of Synaptic Mechanisms in Autonomic Ganglia. Pharmacol Rev 18(1966)839–869

Volle, R.L.: Ganglionic Transmission. Ann Rev Pharmacol 9(1969)135–146

Wamsley, J.K.; Black, A.C.; Redick, J.R.; West, J.R.; Williams, T.H.: SIF Cells, Cyclic AMP

Responses, and Catecholamines of the Guinea Pig Superior Cervical Ganglion Brain Res 156(1978)75–82

Waterson, J.G.; Hume, W.R.; De La Lande, I.S.: The Distribution of Cholinesterase in the Rabbit Ear Artery. J Histochem Cytochem 18(1970)211–216

Weight, F.F.; Petzold, G.; Greengard, P.: Guanosine 3',5'-Monophosphate in Sympathetic Ganglia: Increase Associated with Synaptic Transmission. Science 186(1974)942–944

Weight, F.F.; Smith, P.A.; Schulman, J.A. Postsynaptic Potential Generation Appears Independent of Synaptic Elevation of Cyclic Nucleotides in Sympathetic Neurones. Brain Res 158(1978)197–202

Westfall, T.C.: Local Regulation of Adrenergic Neurotransmission. Physiol Rev 57(1977) 659–728

Westfall, T.C.; Brasted, M.: The Mechanism of Action of Nicotine on the Adrenergic Neurones in the Perfused Guinea-Pig Heart. J Pharmacol Exp Ther 182(1972)409–418

Westfall, T.C.; Hunter, P.E.: Effect of Muscarinic Agonists on the Release of (^{3}H) Noradrenaline from the Guinea Pig Perfused Heart. J Pharm Pharmacol 26(1974)458–460

Westfall, T.C.; Saunders, J.: Absence of Nicotinic Receptors Mediating the Release of Norepinephrine from Adrenergic Neurons in the Rat Heart. Proc Soc Exp Biol Med 156(1977)476–479

Westwood, D.A.; Whaler, B.C.: Postganglionic Paralysis of the Guinea-Pig Hypogastric Nerve-Vas Deferens Preparation by *Clostridium botulinum* Type D Toxin. Br J Pharmacol 33(1968)21–30

Willems, J.L.: Dopamine Induced Inhibition of Synaptic Transmission in Lumbar Paravertebral Ganglia of the Dog. Naunyn Schmiedeberg Arch Pharmacol 279(1973)115–126

Williams, T.H.; Black, A.C. Jr.; Chiba, T.; Jew, J.Y.: Species Differences in Mammalian SIF Cells. Adv Biochem Psychopharmacol 16(1977)505–511

Williams, T.H.; Palay, S.L.: Ultrastructure of the Small Neuron in the Superior Cervical Ganglion. Brain Res 15(1969)17–34

Wilson, H.; Long, J.P.: The Effect of Hemicholinium (HC-3) at Various Peripheral Cholinergic Transmitting Sites. Arch Int Pharmacodyn Ther 70(1959)343–352

Wolner, E.: Versuche über die Innervation der Pilomotoren. Naunyn-Schmiedebergs Arch Pharmacol 250(1965)437–450

Exocytosis as a Mechanism of Noradrenergic Transmitter Release

José M. Trifaró and Luigi Cubeddu X.

I. INTRODUCTION

As early as 1905, Scott advanced the hypothesis that neurons were something more than a system of conducting paths. They were true secreting

Original studies in the authors' laboratories were supported by grants from the Medical Research Council of Canada to J.M.T. and from the Consejo Nacional de Investigaciones Scientíficas y Technológicas of Venezuela to L.C.X.

cells that acted upon one another and upon the cells of other tissues by a passage of a chemical substance from the first to the second cell (Scott, 1905).

In adrenergic neurons, the idea of chemical transmission was also developed early. The similarities between the effects of sympathetic nerve stimulation and the actions of directly applied adrenaline led to the suggestion that the transmitter released from sympathetic nerves was adrenaline (Langley, 1901; Elliott, 1905). Later on, Barger and Dale (1910) demonstrated that the effects of noradrenaline were more closely related to those of sympathetic nerve stimulation. These observations led to the suggestion that noradrenaline might be the sympathetic transmitter (Barger and Dale, 1910; Bacq, 1933; Melville, 1937), and this was demonstrated by von Euler (1946). However, Loewi's (1921) original hypothesis that adrenaline was the transmitter released from the sympathetic nerves of the frog heart was correct, because this catecholamine is the neurotransmitter in sympathetic nerves of most amphibians.

Since all these early observations, our knowledge about the functions of neurons has moved forward quickly, because of the development of powerful electrophysiological, histochemical, electron microscopic, and biochemical techniques.

There are few investigators now who doubt that in sympathetic neurons transmitter substances are stored in membrane-bound vesicles. However, there are quite a few who, although recognizing this form of storage and its advantages, have doubts about exocytosis as the mechanism of transmitter release.

The purpose of this review is to analyze and discuss the series of findings that led to the advance of the concept of exocytosis as the mechanism of release from sympathetic neurons. Special emphasis will also be placed on the mechanisms that may control and modulate the exocytotic release of the noradrenergic transmitter. Furthermore, some findings in other secretory systems, which are known to release by exocytosis, will be discussed here because of the possible functional implications of these observations for the sympathetic neuron.

II. TRANSMITTER STORAGE

One of the properties of the adrenergic neuron is its ability to store noradrenaline (NA). The transmitter, however, is not evenly distributed throughout the neuron, but is localized mostly in the varicosities of terminal axons. Indirect estimates of the intensity of observed fluorescence indicate that the NA concentration in the cell body and axon is about 10–100 μg $\times$ g^{-1}, whereas in the varicosities of the axon terminals it is about 10,000 μg $\times$ g^{-1} (Norberg and Hamberger, 1964; Geffen and Livett, 1971). Electron microscopic observations have revealed that adrenergic nerves contain vesicles (Bloom, 1972), and biochemical observations have indicated that these vesicles contain NA (Geffen and Livett, 1971; Smith and Winkler, 1972).

A. Why Does the Nerve Have the Ability to Store NA in Vesicles?

We know that the nerve can synthesize NA at a very fast rate, so it can be argued that the release of NA could simply occur by a sudden increase in the rate of synthesis of the transmitter. This type of process is known to occur in endocrine tissues (e.g., adrenal cortex, ovary, testes), which do not store the hormone they secrete, but instead store the hormone precursor (for review, see Trifaró, 1977). In order to answer the above question, three important functions of the noradrenergic vesicles should be considered:

1. The vesicles allow the nerve to reuse the NA that has been taken up (uptake$_1$) from the extracellular environment (for review, see Iversen, 1967).
2. The NA storage vesicles are directly involved in the synthesis of NA (see below).
3. The NA storage vesicles are involved in the release of NA, as will be discussed later.

Our knowledge of these vesicle functions is largely the result of applying to adrenergic tissues subcellular fractionation techniques followed by biochemical studies on the composition and properties of the adrenergic vesicles.

B. Types of Noradrenergic Vesicles

Von Euler and Hillarp (1956) first demonstrated that part of the NA present in homogenates of sympathetic nerves was particle bound. Since this original observation, many studies, using various centrifugation techniques, have been carried out (for reviews, see Geffen and Livett, 1971; De Potter, Chubb, and De Schaepdryver, 1972). These studies showed that when the homogenates of tissues rich in adrenergic innervation were subjected to sucrose density-gradient centrifugation, NA was distributed in a bimodal fashion with one peak at the approximate density of 0.4–0.6 M sucrose and another peak at the density of 1.1–1.2 M sucrose (Glassman, Angelakos, and McNary, 1965; Chubb, De Potter, and De Schaepdryver, 1970; Bisby and Fillenz, 1971). The NA-containing particles of these fractions have been called "light" and "heavy" particles or vesicles (Geffen and Livett, 1971). The presence of these two types of particles has been clearly demonstrated in homogenates of the spleen (Chubb et al., 1970; De Potter et al., 1972). However, the homogenates of the nonterminal axons of the splenic nerve contained only one kind of noradrenergic vesicle, which had the same sedimentation properties as heavy (or "large") vesicles of spleen homogenates (Chubb et al., 1970; De Potter et al., 1972). To prove that the light vesicles were indeed part of the splenic nerve terminals, Chubb et al. (1970) showed that both types of vesicles were absent from the homogenates of spleens chronically denervated.

To validate these biochemical findings, a correlation with morphological observations should be found. Three types of vesicles have been observed in the varicosities: large dense-cored vesicles (LDCV) (750–1000 Å), small dense-cored vesicles (SDCV) (450–500 Å) and small electron-translucent vesicles (450–500 Å) (Grillo, 1966; Tranzer et al., 1969; Bisby and Fillenz, 1971; Hökfelt, 1973). Furthermore, histochemical methods have demonstrated that both types of dense-cored vesicles contain catecholamines (Fillenz, 1971) and that the small translucent vesicles can take up and store amines (Tranzer et al., 1969; Tranzer, 1973). In contrast to the morphological observation on the varicosities, the nonterminal axons showed only the large type of vesicles (Smith, 1972). The percentage of each vesicle type was not the same in all nerve terminals examined. In fact, LDCV represented 20%–25% of the vesicle population found in splenic nerve terminals, whereas they constituted only 4%–5% of the vesicle population in the terminals of adrenergic nerves innervating the vas deferens, iris, and heart (Hökfelt, 1969; Bisby and Fillenz, 1971; Tranzer, 1973; Fillenz and West, 1974). These observations on the distribution of LDCV and SDCV were reflected in differences in the subcellular distribution of NA. In the vas deferens, only a low-density peak (SDCV) was observed, whereas in the spleen a clear bimodal distribution of NA was obtained (Bisby and Fillenz, 1971).

In addition to the determination of NA, as a soluble vesicular component in density-gradient centrifugation studies, dopamine beta-hydroxylase (DBH) has been used as a marker for the vesicle membrane. DBH is an enzyme present in a soluble and in a membrane-bound form, not only in LDCV, but also in chromaffin granules (Trifaró, 1970; Lagercrantz, 1976). Thus, when the distribution of DBH was measured after density-gradient centrifugation of vas deferens homogenates, two peaks of DBH activity were found (Bisby, Fillenz, and Smith, 1973). With dog spleen homogenates, only one DBH peak, which corresponded to the position of LDCV, was observed (Chubb et al., 1970; De Potter and Chubb, 1977). On the other hand, subcellular fractionation of homogenates from dog spleens which had been electrically stimulated showed a second DBH peak, which corresponded to the position of the light peak of NA distribution (De Potter and Chubb, 1977). This observation contrasts with the results published by Nelson and Molinoff (1976), who found a bimodal distribution of DBH after centrifugation of dog spleen homogenates. If the increase in sympathetic activity brings about an increase in the number of small vesicles containing DBH, as De Potter and Chubb (1977) have suggested, it is possible that dogs sacrificed under different conditions and degrees of sympathetic stimulation would show percentage differences in the distribution of DBH between light and heavy regions of the density gradients.

Most of the workers agreed on the presence of LDCV in the cell body, axon, and varicosities of the adrenergic neuron; and, as in the case of chromaffin granules (Trifaró, Duerr, and Pinto, 1976), on the origin of LDCV in the Golgi apparatus of the cell (Kapeller and Mayor, 1967; Akert et al., 1972; Stelzner, 1971; Iijima and Awazi, 1973). However, there is not complete agreement on the types or on the origin of the small vesicles present in the varicosities. It is possible that two types of small vesicles exist in the varicosities. One is devoid of DBH but has the capacity to store NA. This type of vesicle probably has its origin in the "tubular reticulum-like structure" (smooth endoplasmic reticulum) described by Tranzer (1972, 1973). In this regard, an origin for the cholinergic synaptic vesicles in the agranular endoplasmic reticulum of the nerve terminals has also been suggested (Droz, Rambourg, and Koenig, 1975). The other type of small vesicle present in the adrenergic nerve varicosities contains DBH, has the capacity of storing NA, and is probably formed by the membrane retrieval process that follows exocytosis of the LDCV (De Potter and Chubb, 1977). A similar mechanism of formation has been proposed for the small vesicles observed in the vasopressin- and oxytocin-containing neurons of the neurohypophysis (Nagasawa, Douglas, and Schulz, 1970).

C. Composition of the Vesicles

Fractions of LDCV of a high degree of purity were prepared by Lagercrantz (1976) and their chemical compositions determined and compared to those of chromaffin granules (CG). The LDCV, being smaller than CG, released less soluble protein upon hypoosmotic shock. Twenty-five percent of LDCV proteins were solubilized by this treatment (Lagercrantz and Thureson-Klein, 1975), whereas, in CG, 63%–75% of the protein was found to be soluble (Trifaró, 1970; Stjärne, 1972). As with CG (Trifaró, 1970; Stjärne, 1972), chromogranin A and DBH have been detected among the soluble components of LDCV (Stjärne, Roth, and Lishajko, 1967; Hörtnagl, Hörtnagl, and Winkler, 1969; De Potter, Smith, and De Schaepdryver, 1970; Helle, Lagercrantz, and Stjärne, 1971; Lagercrantz, Kirksey, and Klein, 1974). Eight percent to 18% of the total DBH of LDCV could be released by freeze-thawing or hypotonic shock (Hörtnagl et al., 1969; De Potter et al., 1970; Lagercrantz et al., 1974), whereas a similar treatment released about 50% of the DBH of CG prepared from medullae of several animal species (Trifaró, 1970; Winkler, 1976; Barbella et al., 1978). Chromogranin A, which is a major component of CG-soluble proteins (Trifaró; 1970; Winkler, 1976), is present only in trace amounts in LDCV. Thus, DBH is the major soluble component of the LDCV. This is reflected in DBH:chromogranin A ratios of 298:1 to 472:1 found in LDCV, which are significantly greater than those found in CG (Bartlett, Lagercrantz, and Smith, 1976).

Among the membrane-bound proteins of LDCV, Mg-ATPase, DBH, cytochrome b_{561}, and chromomembrin B have been detected (Lagercrantz, 1976). The membranes of the LDCV contain more phospholipid than those of CG, a difference due to the fact that the membranes of the LDCV form a larger proportion of the mass of the particles than they do in CG (Smith, 1972). The distribution of the individual phospholipids is very similar between LDCV and CG, with one exception: the LDCV contain only 0%–3% of lysolecithin (Lagercrantz, 1971, 1976), whereas CG contain 13%–17% of the same lipid (Douglas, Poisner, and Trifaró, 1966; Blaschko et al., 1967; Trifaró, 1973; Trifaró et al., 1976).

The other two components of the LDCV that deserve further consideration are ATP and, of course, NA. These two components are present in CG in a catecholamine:ATP molar ratio of 4:1 (Trifaró and Dworkind, 1970; Winkler, 1976). In contrast, NA:ATP molar ratios of 6.8:1 to 12:1 have been obtained from the analysis of LDCV (De Potter et al., 1970; Lagercrantz and Stjärne, 1974; Yen et al., 1975). Determinations of the NA:ATP ratio in LDCV prepared from different axon segments showed that this ratio was greater in the distal than in the proximal portions of the axons while the ratio of ATP to protein remained constant (Lagercrantz, 1976). The NA:protein and NA:DBH ratios were also found to be greater in the distal than in the proximal part of the axons (De Potter et al., 1972; Lagercrantz, 1976). The increase in the NA:ATP ratio from the proximal to the distal part of the axon is an indication that the LDCV is acquiring its full storage capacity during axonal transport. This process of maturation is also reflected in the observed increase in the buoyant density during axonal transport (De Potter et al., 1972). Klein (1973) has also shown that there are two pools of NA in adrenergic vesicles: a slowly depletable pool with a half-life of 28–42 m and a rapidly depletable pool with a half-life of 4–4.5 m. Klein found that this latter pool increases during axonal transport, since the rapidly depletable pool, which in the proximal segments of the axon makes up 9% of the amine pool, represents in the distal segment 40% of that pool. Therefore, this rapidly depletable pool is probably the dominating storage form in the distal nerve vesicles, and recent studies suggest that this pool probably stores the newly synthesized NA (Klein and Harden, 1975).

All the above findings raise another question which may be of importance in the understanding of the release mechanism; it is discussed below.

D.   How Is NA Stored in the Noradrenergic Vesicles?

The presence of slowly and rapidly depletable pools in noradrenergic vesicles suggests that NA is probably stored in at least two different forms. The slowly depletable pool of transmitter seems to have characteristics similar to the amine storage pool of CG (Taugner, 1971; Slotkin, 1973). However, there are differences between these two types of storage particles: a) the loss of catecholamines from isolated CG is slow when compared to that of LDCV (Stjärne, 1964); b) only about 20% of the endogenous amine pool of CG is exchangeable with labeled catecholamines (Taugner and Hasselbach, 1966), whereas in LDCV the entire amine pool is exchangeable (Lagercrantz, 1976); and c) the larger ratios of NA:ATP and NA:chromogranin A found in LDCV suggest that the formation of a storage complex, as in CG (Berneis, Pletscher, and Da Prada, 1971), is perhaps not the main form of storage.

The kinetic properties of the NA pools together with the presence of insufficient concentrations of chromogranin A and nucleotides for amine binding, therefore, suggest that other mechanisms might be responsible for the storage of NA. The active amine uptake pump is probably one of the principal mechanisms for maintaining the vesicular storage of NA (Lagercrantz, 1976).

In addition to the three important functions of the vesicular storage of NA mentioned at the beginning of this section, other advantages of this type of storage should be considered here: a) the transmitter can reach high concentrations within the vesicles (that is, up to 0.15 M and 0.5 M in LDCV and CG respectively), and consequently the capacity for transmitter storage is very high; b) the transmitter is protected from enzyme inactivation or catabolism (monoamine oxidase and aldehyde reductase in this case); c) each vesicle can provide a certain amount (quantum) of transmitter to be released; and d) the vesicles facilitate the intracellular and axonal transport of large quantities of transmitter.

This section would not be complete without discussing the possibility of an extravesicular compartment storing *free* amines. Early subcellular fractionation studies have suggested the presence of an extravesicular compartment, with a size depending on the tissue studied (Iversen, 1967; von Euler, 1966). The results obtained with subcellular fractionation procedures could, in part, be due to artifacts of preparation—e.g., rupture of vesicles during homogenization (Hillarp, Lagerstedt, and Nilson, 1953) or postmortem delay in the homogenization of tissue samples (Hillarp et al., 1953; Klein, 1973). Moreover, it has been recently assumed that in terminal varicosities, most of the NA is stored in vesicles (Geffen and Livett, 1971; De Potter et al., 1972). The presence of small concentrations of free amines in the cytosol might, however, be the result of the active uptake process (uptake$_1$) of NA, although this process is generally followed by vesicle storage or metabolism (Iversen, 1967). Furthermore, the possible role of the free amine pool in the regulation of NA synthesis through end product feedback inhibition has been extensively considered (Weiner, 1970). The possibility that a *free* amine pool might be involved in the release process will be discussed below.

III. EXOCYTOSIS

Exocytosis was first proved to be the mechanism of release of catecholamines from the adrenal medulla. This was the result of the work of several laboratories (for review see Smith and Winkler, 1972; Douglas, 1975; Trifaró, 1977), which by applying different analytical techniques provided biochemical evidence for the morphological observations of De Robertis and Vaz Ferreira (1957). These authors suggested that secretion in the adrenal medulla was by *reverse pinocytosis* (exocytosis), a mechanism whereby the membrane of the secretory granule fuses with the plasma membrane, allowing the escape of the content of the granules to the cell exterior. Thus, because of these morphological and biochemical observations, the early theories proposed as mechanisms of release were discarded (Trifaró, 1970, 1977). These early hypotheses were as follows: a) release by extrusion of intact secretory granules to the cell exterior (Cramer, 1918); b) release from a *free* amine pool (Hillarp, 1960); c) release by diffusion of amines out of the granules and into the cytoplasm (Blaschko and Welch, 1953); or d) release by dissolution of the granule membrane in the cytoplasm (Lever and Findlay, 1966). The final common path proposed for the last three mechanisms was the diffusion of the catecholamines from the cytoplasmic sap across the plasma membrane to the cell exterior. If the disadvantages of all other forms of release are considered, it is immediately obvious that exocytosis is the simplest, most economical, and most efficient mechanism for releasing not only catecholamines but also hormones and enzymes from endocrine and exocrine glands respectively (Trifaró, 1977). If catecholamines were released from the granules into the cytosol, they would diffuse in all directions, large quantities of amines would be destroyed by enzymes present in the cytoplasm (MAO in mitochondria and aldehyde dehydrogenase and reductase in the cytosol), and only a fraction of the catecholamines would reach the cell exterior (Trifaró, 1977). Furthermore, the catecholamines would have to cross at least two membranes, that of the granule and that of the cell. Finally, if release were not by exocytosis, special transport mechanisms through these membranes would have to exist, since the molecular size of the components stored in granules varies from very simple molecules like adrenaline to more complex ones like DBH and chromogranin A (see section on storage and sections following it).

Chromaffin cells and sympathetic neurons have the same ancestral origin, the neural crest. Therefore, to study the secretory process of the adrenergic neuron, Smith et al. (1970) adopted a similar approach to that previously undertaken for the adrenal medulla. In this case, however, the interpretation of the results was more difficult, because there were differences in morphology (two types of vesicles; see storage section), anatomy (release into effector organ rather than direct secretion into blood), and function (uptake and metabolism of NA). Effector organ responses, electrophysiological recordings, and measurements of NA overflow have been employed to assess the amount of NA released from sympathetic nerves. The term of endogenous or exogenous radioactive NA overflow has been employed to indicate the fraction of transmitter, which, after being released by nerve stimulation, escapes unchanged to the incubation or perfusion medium. It probably represents the difference between the amount of NA secreted and the amount recaptured and metabolized. Therefore, NA overflow could be modified by drugs or procedures which affect neuronal and/or extraneuronal uptake and metabolism without changing the release process per se (Iversen, 1967; von Euler, 1972). In studies of the tissues labeled with radioactive NA, measurements of the overflow of total radioactivity have usually been employed to estimate NA release, since they take into account the metabolism of the released transmitter. In addition, measurements of total radioactivity have been performed in the presence of inhibitors of the neuronal and extraneuronal uptake processes. However, the results obtained with the use of these agents must be accepted with caution, since the agents could have important effects on the secretion of NA. In fact, local anesthetic properties (e.g., cocaine), direct activation of alpha receptors (e.g., normetanephrine), and alpha receptor antagonistic effects (e.g., desipramine) have been observed for drugs commonly employed in studies on NA overflow.

The following is an analysis of how the ideas about exocytosis developed and why and how the experiments were conducted.

As early as 1956, von Euler and Hillarp reported that some of the NA present in the homogenates of sympathetic nerves was particle bound. During the years that followed this discovery, as with the adrenal medulla, many theories about the possible mechanisms of release were advanced (Figure 1).

A. NA Is Not Released
from Extragranular Stores during Nerve Stimulation

Even ten years after von Euler and Hillarp's observation, some investigators still believed that NA was released from an extragranular store (Fig. 1e;

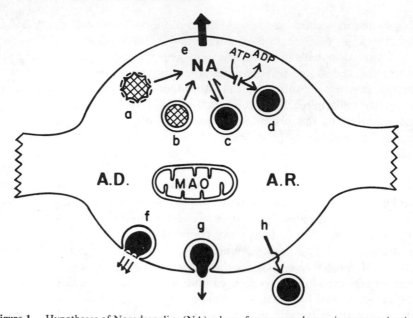

Figure 1. Hypotheses of Noradrenaline (NA) release from a noradrenergic nerve varicosity.

a) Dissolution of the membrane vesicle, allowing NA to diffuse into the cytosol.

b) Dissociation of the storage complex.

c) Release of NA from the vesicle into the cytosol due to a previous decrease in the concentration of NA in cytosol.

d) Inhibition of NA uptake pump of the vesicle.

e) Release of NA from the cytosol ("free" pool).

f) Release of NA through an increased permeability at the site of fusion ("tight" or "gap" junction).

g) Exocytosis.

h) Extrusion of the intact vesicle

MAO: Monoamine oxidase

A.R.: Aldehyde reductase

A.D.: Aldehyde dehydrogenase

Stjärne, 1966). In order to show that the noradrenergic vesicle was the site of the release of NA, it became necessary to rule out the cytosol as the origin of the NA found in the effluents from organs during adrenergic nerve stimulation. One of the ways of testing this was to induce the accumulation of NA in the cytosol. This was achieved by interfering with vesicle storage (fig. 1d), as for example by using reserpine. This treatment, when accompanied by the use of MAO inhibitors, resulted in the accumulation of intact NA in the cytosol. Under these conditions, sympathetic nerves can take up and store NA. This type of cytosol storage can be demonstrated by a smooth distribution of fluorescence in the neuron (Malmfors, 1965); by subcellular fractionation studies, which have shown that most of the NA taken up is not sedimentable (Iversen, Glowinski, and Axelrod, 1965; Potter, 1967; Lundborg, 1967); and by radioautography, which shows that the cytoplasm of the neuron and not the vesicles becomes labeled (Taxi, 1969). When, under these conditions, the sympathetic nerves were stimulated, no

NA was released into the extracellular space (Van Orden, Bensch, and Giarman, 1967; Potter, 1967; Häggendal and Malmfors, 1969a; Farnebo and Hamberger, 1970b). Therefore, from these experiments it was concluded that when amine metabolism and the vesicle pump were inhibited—conditions leading to an accumulation of NA in extragranular sites (fig. 1d)—no release of the amine was observed upon nerve stimulation. Experiments with false transmitters discussed below also seem to rule out release from extragranular stores.

B. The Vesicle Is the Origin Of the NA Released during Nerve Stimulation

The experiments discussed in the preceding section have been taken as evidence against the hypotheses (a) to (e), as shown in figure 1, which were developed to explain the mechanisms of transmitter release from adrenergic neurons and at the same time suggest the vesicle (Figs. 1f, g, and h) as the immediate site of origin of the released transmitter. Among the approaches followed in order to study this aspect of the release process, three will be discussed here.

1. Electrophysiological studies on smooth muscle Excitatory spontaneous junction potentials (ESJPs) have been detected by intracellular recording in smooth muscle cells innervated by sympathetic nerves (Holman, 1970; Bennett, 1973a, b; Burnstock and Costa, 1975). In the vas deferens the frequency of the ESJPs increased following stimulation of the hypogastric nerve and decreased following administration of reserpine (Holman, 1970). In the dog retractor penis, the ESJPs were abolished by denervation (Holman, 1970). These observations suggested that the transmitter was released in packages. It was not possible to conclude, however, whether such packages were of uniform size (quantal). This might have been due to some of the following reasons: 1) The relationship between varicosities and smooth muscle is extremely variable. The cleft width between these two structures varies from 10 nm in the rat vas deferens to 100 nm in the tenia coli of the guinea pig (Burnstock and Costa, 1975). 2) There is more than one type of vesicle in the varicosity (see storage of NA). 3) There is a possibility that the transmitter could be released from successive varicosities of the same adrenergic nerve. 4) There is electrical coupling of neighboring muscle cells (Burnstock and Costa, 1975). In spite of all these anatomical and morphological differences, the evidence accumulated so far seems to be in favor of quantal release of NA rather than molecule-by-molecule release (for review see Burnstock and Costa, 1975).

2. False transmitters There is a lack of specificity in some of the important functions of the sympathetic neuron such as uptake, vesicle storage, and β-hydroxylation (Kaufman and Friedman, 1965; Potter, 1966; Iversen, 1967). Thus, in addition to NA, many phenylethylamine derivatives can be taken up, stored in vesicles, become β-hydroxylated, and be released upon nerve stimulation (Muscholl and Maître, 1963; Muscholl, 1972; Fisher, Horst, and Kopin, 1965). Inhibition of vesicle retention (i.e., after reserpine) makes these false transmitters unavailable for release (Muscholl, 1972). Another piece of evidence in favor of release from vesicles is that (with the exception of dopamine and α-methyldopamine) the output of non-β-hydroxylated amines (tyramine, α-methyltyramine, phenylethylamine, amphetamine, etc.) is not increased by nerve stimulation. However, the output of their β-OH derivatives is increased (Musacchio, Kopin, and Weise, 1965; Muscholl, 1972). These results suggest that in order to be released from an adrenergic terminal, a substance must first be stored in a vesicle; and this implies that the vesicles are directly involved in the transmitter release mechanism.

    3. Release of proteins The discovery that two vesicle proteins, DBH and chromogranin A, were found together with NA in the effluents escaping from perfused spleens suggested that the adrenergic vesicle was involved in the release process (De Potter et al. 1969a, b; Smith et al., 1970; Gewirtz and Kopin, 1970; Weinshilboum et al., 1971; Cubeddu et al., 1974a; Cubeddu, Barnes, and Weiner, 1974b). First, however, it was necessary to answer the following question: Were these proteins released from the nerve? It had already been demonstrated that stimulation of the splenic nerve increased the overflow of not only NA but also acetylcholine (Leaders and Dayrit, 1965). Therefore, it was possible that during nerve stimulation, the released acetylcholine was acting on chromaffin cells which might be present in the spleens. This possibility was ruled out by the following results of experiments: (a) the addition of atropine and hexamethonium to the fluid during perfusion of the spleen did not block the release of DBH and chromogranin A during the stimulation of the splenic nerve (Smith et al., 1970); (b) there was no histochemical evidence for the presence of chrom-affin cells in the spleen; (c) there was no evidence of the presence of chromaffin granules in spleen homogenates (Smith and Winkler, 1972).

    Another possibility which was considered was that there was blood containing these proteins pooled in the sinuses of the spleen and that during nerve stimulation the released NA induced the contraction of the spleen with the consequent squeeze of blood into the venous effluent. However, the following pieces of evidence negated this possibility: (a) injection of exogenous NA produced spleen contraction but failed to increase the over-flow of DBH, and (b) introduction of the alpha-blocker phenoxybenzamine abolished the contraction of the spleen but increased the release of proteins upon nerve stimulation (De Potter et al., 1971; Cubeddu et al., 1974a, c). Furthermore, DBH has been released into the incubation medium from another organ, the vas deferens, during stimulation of the hypogastric nerve

(Weinshilboum et al., 1971). In this case, the possibility of blood contamination was low.

All these experiments indicate that dopamine-β-hydroxylase and chromogranin A are released from nerves and therefore from the adrenergic vesicles, since these two proteins are components of the vesicles (see section on storage).

C. How Is NA Released from the Vesicles?

The evidence discussed so far is compatible with the release of transmitter from vesicles by any of the mechanisms described in figure 1 as f, g, or h. However, before describing the findings in adrenergic nerves, it would be useful to discuss briefly the findings in the adrenal medulla. As a result of numerous morphological (Diner, 1967; Malamed et al., 1968; Smith et al., 1973) and biochemical studies it has been concluded that exocytosis (fig. 1g) is the mechanism of catecholamine release from the adrenal medulla. These studies have shown that catecholamines are released from the adrenal medulla during stimulation, along with other soluble chromaffin granule components, such as ATP (Douglas, Poisner, and Rubin, 1965; Lastowecka and Trifaró, 1974), chromogranin A (Banks and Helle, 1965), and DBH (Viveros, Arqueros, and Kirshner, 1968). These soluble granule substances are quantitatively recovered in the effluents escaping from stimulated glands (Douglas et al., 1965; Banks and Helle, 1965; Viveros et al., 1968; Lastowecka and Trifaró, 1974). Furthermore, subcellular fractionation studies carried out on stimulated glands have shown that membrane-bound components of the granules are not released into the perfusates but are retained in the gland (Trifaró, Poisner, and Douglas, 1967; Poisner, Trifaró, and Douglas, 1967; Schneider, Smith, and Winkler, 1967; Viveros et al., 1969a, b; Trifaró, 1973). In addition, release from the adrenal medulla seems to be an all-or-none process (Viveros, Arqueros, and Kirshner, 1969c). Although large molecules such as DBH (290,000 mw), leave the gland during stimulation, no cytoplasmic markers, such as lactate dehydrogenase (Schneider et al., 1967; Lastowecka and Trifaró, 1974) or phenylethanolamine-N-methyltransferase (Kirshner et al., 1966), are detected in the effluents escaping from the gland.

Exocytosis also seems to be the mechanism of secretion in endocrine glands, which share with the adrenal medulla the property of storing hormones in subcellular granules (for review see Trifaró, 1977).

In 1968, Geffen and Livett demonstrated that the rate of axonal transport of ^{14}C-labeled proteins and ^{3}H-amines was the same (0.5 cm/h) in splenic nerves of cats injected previously in the celiac ganglion with ^{14}C-leucine and ^{3}H-NA. It was suggested from these studies that these rapidly transported proteins might be components of adrenergic vesicles (Livett, Geffen, and Austin, 1968), since the stimulation of these nerves produced the release of not only ^{3}H-NA but also ^{14}C-proteins (Geffen and Livett, 1968). Immunohistochemical methods proved that these transported proteins were indeed vesicle proteins. Thus, by the use of antibodies against DBH and chromogranin A, it was possible to demonstrate qualitatively that not only were these proteins present in the axons; they were also released upon splenic nerve stimulation (Geffen, Livett, and Rush, 1969, 1970). About the same time, although independently, other preliminary but more quantitative results were reported about the release of chromogranins during the stimulation of the sympathetic nerves to dog and calf spleens (De Potter et al., 1969a, b). These observations were followed by more extensive studies (Smith et al., 1970) showing that the release of DBH and chromogranin A from the stimulated splenic nerves (30 Hz) of calves and dogs—similar to protein release from the adrenal medulla—required the presence of Ca^{++} in the extracellular environment. It was also shown that cat splenic nerves released NA together with DBH during stimulation at higher (30 Hz) (Gewirtz and Kopin, 1970) and at lower (5–20 Hz) and more physiological frequencies (De Potter et al., 1971; Cubeddu and Weiner, 1975a). Furthermore, stimulation (25 Hz) of the hypogastric nerves of the guinea pig vas deferens, as well as the addition to the incubation medium of depolarizing concentrations of veratridine and KCl, resulted in a concomitant release of both NA and DBH (Weinshilboum et al., 1971; Thoa et al., 1975). Moreover, highly significant correlations were found between the amounts of DBH and chromogranin A and the amounts of NA during the stimulation of the splenic nerve at high (30 Hz) and low (5 Hz) frequencies (Smith et al., 1970; Cubeddu et al., 1974a). A similar correlation between DBH and NA was also found in the incubation medium after stimulation of the sympathetic nerves to the vas deferens of the guinea pig (Weinshilboum et al., 1971) or after exposure of the preparation to depolarizing concentrations of either veratridine or KCl (Thoa et al., 1975). The proportional release during stimulation of NA and soluble-vesicle proteins, together with the lack of release of tyrosine hydroxylase and dopa decarboxylase (enzymes which are free in the cytosol of the nerve) suggested that DBH and chromogranin A were not released, first, from the vesicle into the cytosol, and second, to the cell exterior, since this latter step would imply the presence of specific carriers, not only for protein but also for NA (De Potter et al., 1969a, b). The absence in the perfusates of dopa decarboxylase, a protein of smaller molecular weight and hydrodynamic ratio than DBH, also ruled out an increase in the permeability of the plasma membrane during release. The release through a "tight" or "gap" junction (fig. 1f) also seems improbable, because DBH and chromogranin A are large molecules, with diameters greater than 7 nm. Only proteins with this dimension or less can cross gap junctions (Kanno and Loewenstein, 1966). Therefore, the evidence discussed so far indicates that the possible mechanism of release is either exocytosis (fig. 1g) or extrusion of the intact vesicle to the cell exterior (fig. 1h). This latter mechanism was discarded in the adrenal medulla following experiments which showed quantitative recovery of granule membranes after secretion (Poisner et al., 1967; Viveros et al., 1969b). Somewhat similar results have been obtained with sympathetic nerves. In fact, De Potter and Chubb (1977), in experiments using gradient differential centrifugation techniques, were able to show that membrane-bound DBH lost from LDCV upon stimulation was quantitatively recovered in the small noradrenergic vesicles. Furthermore, addition of Triton X-100 to spleen effluents failed to increase the activity of DBH released by nerve stimulation (Cubeddu and Weiner, unpublished results, 1974). These two observations deny the idea of extrusion of the intact vesicle to the cell exterior (fig. 1h) as a mechanism of transmitter release.

Therefore, after all the evidence presented and discussed above, it should be concluded that exocytosis is the most probable mechanism of transmitter release from sympathetic neurons. Whether all the vesicles or only the large dense-core vesicles (LDCV) release their contents by exocytosis is considered next.

D. Release from One Or More Than One Type of Vesicle

In initial studies the ratios of the overflow of DBH to NA and chromogranin A to NA in the perfusates were smaller than those measured in the soluble content of LDCV isolated from nonterminal axons (Smith et al., 1970; Gewirtz and Kopin, 1970). This suggested that proteins were released from the LDCV, whereas NA was released from both large and small vesicles (Smith et al., 1970). It was found subsequently that the LDCV of terminal axons contained at least 10 times more NA per unit of DBH activity than those of LDCV isolated from preterminal axons (De Potter et al., 1972; see also section on storage). This centrifugal decrease in the DBH:NA ratio was due not to the loss of protein from the vesicle but to the gain of NA (see storage section). When these observations were taken into consideration in the calculations, the ratios in the perfusates of DBH to NA were 33% (dog), 64% (calf), and 68% (cat) of those calculated from the soluble contents of LDCV and that of chromogranin A to NA was 8.5% (calf) (Smith and Winkler, 1972). It was then assumed that the released NA comes equally from two populations of vesicles, large and small, since there is approximately an equal distribution of both types of vesicles in the splenic nerve terminal (Smith and Winkler, 1972). On this assumption, the above percentages should be doubled (66%–146% for DBH and 17% for chromogranin A). Furthermore, Weinshilboum et al. (1971) compared the ratios of DBH to NA found in the incubation media of stimulated vas deferens to the ratios obtained from the soluble extract of the frozen tissue. The ratios in the media were 54%–57% of those found in soluble tissue extracts.

Many things could have accounted for these lower ratios:

1. All the released protein might not have reached the organ effluents or incubation solutions because of the following: (a) Part of the protein could have been lost by adsorption to the tissue surface. The lower levels of chromogranin A recovered with the effluents, in comparison to the levels of DBH, might have been due to the more acidic nature and different hydrodynamic properties of chromogranin A, which made this protein more readily bound to tissues (Smith et al., 1970). (b) Part of the released protein could have been taken up by an endocytotic process, possibly followed by retrograde transport. Nerve uptake and retrograde transport of horseradish peroxidase, tetanus toxin, nerve growth factor, and antibodies against DBH have been demonstrated (Kristensson, Olsson, and Sjöstrand, 1971; Schwab and Thoenen, 1977; Jacobowitz, Ziegler, and Thomas, 1975; Ziegler, Thomas, and Jacobowitz, 1976; Fillenz et al., 1976). However, no evidence for uptake of DBH or chromogranin A is available. (c) Part of the protein (DBH and chromogranin A) might have been trapped in the extracellular space, even in organs perfused in vitro; and part of the DBH might have reached the general circulation through the lymphatic system and not been detected in organ effluents. Electrical stimulation of the stellate ganglion of the dog or administration of dimethylphenylpiperazinium iodide (DMPP), a ganglionic stimulant, in cats, produced an increase in the output of DBH in the thoracic lymph duct (Ngai et al., 1974; Ross, Eriksson, and Hellström, 1974). Similarly, some of the DBH released from the adrenal medulla during hemorrhagic hypotension in dogs was found in the lymph of the thoracic duct (Cubeddu et al., 1978).

2. There may have been problems related to the determination of DBH in tissue and fluid samples. Many variables can be involved in measurements of this enzyme, and these variables must be taken into account: (a) DBH's instability in low-protein or protein-free solutions and its sensitivity to peroxide necessitate the addition of serum albumin and catalase to the buffer solutions to preserve the enzyme's activity (Weinshilboum et al., 1971; Goldstein and Cubeddu, 1976). (b) To obtain the optimal DBH activity the enzyme assays are generally performed with several dilutions of the sample and at different concentrations of $CuSO_4$. This is probably made necessary by the presence of inhibitors of enzyme activity (probably acting through copper chelation). Addition of a DBH internal standard of a known enzyme activity has been used to correct for remaining inhibitory activity (Molinoff, Weinshilboum, and Axelrod, 1971). (c) The use of sensitive radioenzymatic assays (Molinoff et al., 1971; Goldstein, Freedman, and Bonnay 1971) has been required for detecting changes

in the overflow of enzyme activity after short periods of stimulation. These assays employ substrate concentrations around the Km value. Therefore, changes in enzyme activity can be related to the presence of inhibitors and/or activators and are not necessarily always due to an increase in the amount of DBH released. (d) The composition of the saline *physiological* solutions employed for incubation or organ perfusion have often been adjusted for salt and buffer concentrations. The enzyme phenyleth-anolamine N-methyl transferase, employed in the second step of the two-step DBH assays, is very sensitive to changes in ionic strength and pH (Cubeddu and Vargas, 1977). In addition, because of the pH requirements of the first enzymatic step (DBH step), strong buffers should be used to keep the pH between 5 and 5.5. The bicarbonate should be omitted from the Krebs-Ringer-bicarbonate solution (Cubeddu and Vargas, 1977). (e) The sample collection time should be carefully determined, particularly in perfused organs. After a period of stimulation the overflow of DBH lags behind that of catecholamines, both in sympathetically innervated organs and in the adrenal medulla. Therefore, samples for determination of DBH activity should be collected for longer periods. In the perfused cat spleen a significant output of enzyme was present in samples collected even 11 m after the period of nerve stimulation (5 Hz, 300 pulses, 1 m). The duration of the DBH overflow was directly related to the degree of spleen contraction (Cubeddu et al., 1974a, b).

3. Either the NA present in LDCV alone was released by exocytosis or, alternatively, all the NA was released by exocytosis from both large and small vesicles. Thus the lower DBH:NA ratios found in the perfusates would simply have been due to the lack of soluble proteins in the small vesicles.

E. The Vesicle is Capable of
Exocytotic Release in the Absence of Stored NA

One of the functional aspects to be considered is whether the presence of NA or of the *NA-storage complex* within the vesicle is a necessary requirement for exocytosis, or if the components involved in the interaction that brings about the exocytotic release of transmitter are in the vesicle membrane.

We have discussed in one of the preceding sections the fact that phenylethylamine derivatives can be taken up, β-hydroxylated, stored in vesicles, and released upon nerve stimulation (see exocytosis section of this paper and Muscholl, 1972). These experiments suggest that, because of the lack of specificity of the sympathetic neuron in some of its important functions, other transmitters can replace NA in the vesicle. However, the experiments do not indicate whether the reserpine-sensitive uptake or the β-hydroxylation of the amines are previous requirements for the vesicle to become functional for exocytotic release. The answer to this question can be found in the experiment done by Farnebo (1971). He used irises from rats pretreated with reserpine. The irises were then incubated in the presence of metaraminol, a drug which can be taken up into vesicles by a reserpine-resistant uptake process. Under these conditions, metaraminol was released upon stimulation. These experiments indicated that there was release from vesicles when a false transmitter was stored in them and that the storage of NA, the β-hydroxylation, and the amine uptake process were not determinants of the release capability of the vesicle. However, the experiments did not indicate whether the vesicle membrane played a role in exocytosis. Experiments in reserpinized animals have provided this information. Dixon, García, and Kirpekar (1975) showed that when adrenal medullae of reserpinized cats were stimulated, there was a release of DBH, which was not accompanied by a concomitant release of catecholamines. Similarly, the stimulation of the nerves to the vas deferens and spleen of reserpine-pretreated guinea pigs and cats respectively produced release of DBH, which again was not accompanied by a parallel release of NA (Cubeddu et al., 1974a, b; Thoa et al., 1975).

All the above experiments indicate the presence in the vesicle membrane of recognition sites which might be important in the membrane-membrane interaction that brings about exocytosis (see membrane fusion).

F. Conclusions

The proportional release between NA and other soluble vesicle components (chromogranin A and DBH), together with the lack of release of cytosol marker enzymes (lactate dehydrogenase, etc.) during nerve stimulation suggest that exocytosis is the most probable mechanism of transmitter release from sympathetic nerves. In addition, the retention of vesicle membrane components and the absence of release of NA from extragranular compartments during nerve stimulation further support the theory of exocytotic release of transmitter.

The fact that the DBH:NA ratios determined in the perfusate and incubation media of adrenergic tissues during nerve stimulation were smaller than the ratios found in tissue samples causes some doubt about exocytosis as the unique mechanism of transmitter release during nerve stimulation. These observations seem to suggest the possibility of *partial* exocytosis or exocytosis from only *one type* of vesicle. However, it should be taken into consideration that the presence of a heterogeneous store of NA in noradrenergic nerve terminals (large and small vesicles) makes the ratio of DBH to NA an unreliable index of exocytosis. In order to calculate meaningful DBH:NA tissue ratios, it would be necessary to know 1) the exact proportion of each vesicle type in a given terminal, 2) the soluble contents (soluble DBH:NA) of each vesicle type, and 3) the contribution of each type to the total store. For technical reasons, this information is not available at the present time. However, the fact that there is a proportionality between overflow of DBH and transmitter not only at different frequencies (1–20 Hz), but also with different technical procedures and drug treatments, suggests strongly that the release of sympathetic transmitter occurs by the process of exocytosis.

IV. IONIC REQUIREMENTS FOR EXOCYTOSIS

A. Role of Calcium Ions

Early experiments by Houssay and Molinelli (1928) suggested the importance of Ca^{++} in catecholamine secretion. However, it was Douglas and Rubin (1961) who conceived the idea that the role of Ca^{++} in secretion was a general one and who named the events involved in the secretory process stimulus-secretion coupling because of the similarity to the excitation-contraction coupling in muscle (Douglas, 1968). The requirement for Ca^{++} in NA release from sympathetic nerves was demonstrated first by Huković and Muscholl (1962), who stimulated the sympathetic nerves to the heart in the presence or absence of Ca^{++} in the extracellular environment. These observations were extended later to the splenic nerves of the cat (Kirpekar and Misu, 1967) and to the sympathetic nerves to the colon of the cat (Boullin, 1967). Furthermore, and as observed earlier with the adrenal medulla (Douglas and Rubin, 1961, 1963), the inhibitory effect of Mg^{++} on NA release from sympathetic nerves was also shown (Boullin, 1967; Kirpekar and Misu, 1967). In addition, it was demonstrated that both Ba^{++} and Sr^{++} were able to substitute for Ca^{++} in the release process (Boullin, 1967; Kirpekar and Misu, 1967). Not only was the release of NA from stimulated sympathetic nerves Ca^{++} dependent; the secretion of other storage vesicle components, such as dopamine β-hydroxylase and chromogranin A, also required extracellular Ca^{++} (Smith et al., 1970; Cubeddu et al., 1974a; see also exocytosis section of this paper).

The relationship between extracellular Ca^{++} and transmitter release evoked from sympathetic nerves is highly nonlinear, and a sigmoidal relationship exists between the two parameters (Stjärne, 1973d). This is similar to the relationship between extracellular Ca^{++} and acetylcholine release at the neuromuscular junction (Dodge and Rahamimoff, 1967). In the Michaelis-Menten equation, when velocity was replaced with fractional ^3H-NA release per nerve impulse and substrate concentration was replaced with the concentration of Ca^{++} in the medium, it was observed that the dependence of NA release for Ca^{++}, after inhibition of negative feedback control, followed Michaelis-Menten kinetics (Stjärne, 1973d). Under these conditions, the Lineweaver-Burk double reciprocal plot of NA release against Ca^{++} concentration yielded a straight line (Stjärne, 1973d). From this, a K_{Ca} (Km) of 2.96 mM Ca^{++} was calculated for the secretory process, a value which is close to the concentration of Ca^{++} in the extracellular environment.

There is evidence that, in many secretory systems, stimulation brings about an increase in the membrane conductance for Ca^{++} with a concomitant increase in Ca^{++} influx (Rahamimoff et al., 1975). When isolated nerve endings (synaptosomes) are incubated *in vitro*, the addition to the medium of the depolarizing concentrations of either K^+ or veratridine stimulates both Ca^{++} uptake and Ca^{++}-dependent release of NA (Blaustein, Johnson, and Needleman, 1972; Blaustein, 1975). Studies on the movement of Ca^{++} in the squid axon and in the adrenal medulla have shown that the entry of Ca^{++} is biphasic: an *early phase* that uses the Na^+ channel and that is blocked by tetrodotoxin but not by the Ca^{++} antagonist methoxyverapamil (Baker and Reuter, 1975; Aguirre, Pinto, and Trifaró, 1977); and a *late phase*, tetrodotoxin insensitive, which is blocked by methoxyverapamil (Baker and Reuter, 1975; Aguirre et al., 1977). Methoxyverapamil (D600) also blocks catecholamine release from the adrenal medulla in response to K^+ and acetylcholine depolarization (Pinto and Trifaró, 1976). Furthermore, the same cations (Mg^{++}, Mn^{++}, Co^{++}, Ni^{++}, La^{+++}) which blocked the Ca^{++} conductance (the late Ca^{++} channel) in the squid axon (Baker and Reuter, 1975) also blocked NA release from sympathetic nerves (Kirpekar, Dixon, and Prat, 1970; Kirpekar et al., 1972). In addition, it also has been suggested that Ca^{++} influx into the terminals might be regulated by alpha-presynaptic receptors (Stjärne, 1973b; Langer, Dubocovich, and Celuch, 1975; see also section of this paper on presynaptic regulation), prostaglandins, and angiotensin (see presynaptic regulation section).

Therefore, under physiological conditions, an increase in intracellular Ca^{++}, due to an enhanced Ca^{++} entry through a specific channel (the *late Ca^{++} channel*) seems to be a necessary requirement for triggering exocytotic release. Where Ca^{++} is needed still remains to be elucidated. Ca^{++} may play a role in membrane fusion (Trifaró, 1977) or may be involved in some kind of contractile event leading to the exocytotic release of transmitter (Trifaró, 1978; also see below). In addition Ca^{++} may also be involved in the termination of the release reaction (Trifaró, 1977; Aguirre et al., 1977). One or more of the following mechanisms may be responsible for this: (a) Inactivation of the late Ca^{++} channel. Perfusion of spleens with carbachol, protoveratrine, or high K^+ decreases the NA release in response to nerve stimulation (Kirpekar et al., 1972). This observation was interpreted as being due to the inactivation of the Ca^{++} channel by the prolonged depolarization produced by these agents (Kirpekar et al., 1972).

Furthermore, the fact that during the stimulation of sympathetic nerves, the output of transmitter decreases with time might also be due to the inactivation of the late Ca^{++} channel. This has been demonstrated to be the case during the catecholamine release from the adrenal medulla elicited by a high concentration of K^+ (Baker and Rink, 1975). (b) Extrusion of Ca^{++} to the cell exterior. A Na-Ca exchange mechanism has been described in the squid axon, in the adrenal medulla, and in synaptosomes prepared from rat brain tissue (Baker and Reuter, 1975; Blaustein and Ector, 1976; Aguirre et al., 1977). In the resting neuron the cytoplasm is negative with respect to the external medium. Therefore, Ca^{++} must be extruded against a large electrochemical gradient. In many tissues, including peripheral nerves and the adrenal medulla, Ca^{++}efflux seems to depend in part upon the presence of Na^+ in the extracellular environment (Baker and Reuter, 1975; Blaustein and Ector, 1976; Aguirre et al., 1977). Thus, Ca^{++} efflux involves a carrier-mediated counterflow exchange of Na^+ for Ca^{++}, where the movement of Na^+ into the cells, down its electrochemical gradient, may provide energy for the "uphill" Ca^{++} extrusion (Blaustein and Ector, 1976; Aguirre et al., 1977). (c) Cellular binding or sequestration of Ca^{++}. The sequestration of Ca^{++} by a Mg-ATP-dependent mechanism has been demonstrated in mitochondria and microsomes prepared from secretory tissues (Trifaró, 1977). It has also been shown that in cholinergic terminals ruthenium red, an inorganic dye which blocks rather specifically the Ca^{++} uptake by mitochondria (Moore, 1971) produced an increase in the release of transmitter (Rahamimoff and Alnaes, 1973). Therefore it is possible that these organelles, specifically mitochondria, are responsible not only for the termination of the release reaction in the varicosities but also for the low Ca^{++} levels present in the cytosol during resting conditions (Trifaró, 1977).

B. Sodium Ions and NA Release

In addition to the well-known role of sodium ions in action potential generation, low extracellular sodium concentrations are known to accelerate the release of catecholamines from the adrenal medulla (Douglas and Rubin, 1961, 1963; Lastowecka and Trifaró, 1974) and of NA from noradrenergic nerve terminals (Keen and Bogdanski, 1970; Blaszkowsky and Bogdanski, 1971; García and Kirpekar, 1973, 1975; Ritzel and Muscholl, 1976; Nakazato, Onoda, and Onga, 1977). However, some discrepancy was found in the calcium dependency and in the mode of secretion of catecholamines by the sodium-free or low-sodium solutions. Whereas in some studies sodium deprivation induced release of catecholamines even in the absence of extracellular Ca^{++} (García and Kirpekar, 1973; Lastowecka and Trifaró, 1974), in others a Ca^{++} dependency was observed (Blaszkowsky and Bogdanski, 1971; Nakazato et al., 1977). In the latter studies, the Ca^{++} requirement for the release of NA induced by Na^+ deprivation was greater in the presence of choline than in the presence of sucrose when used as substitutes for sodium ions.

Regarding the mode of secretion, it should be pointed out that whereas in the adrenal medulla Na^+ deprivation produced a proportional release of catecholamines, DBH, and ATP (Lastowecka and Trifaró, 1974), this was not the case in the spleen, where only the release of catecholamines was observed (García and Kirpekar, 1973, 1975). Furthermore, increasing the concentration of extracellular Mg^{++} blocked the catecholamine release from the adrenal medulla without modifying NA release from the spleen in response to Na^+ deprivation (Lastowecka and Trifaró, 1974). In addition to organ and species differences, the experimental conditions employed by García and Kirpekar (1973, 1975) did not allow the study of an immediate effect of Na^+ deprivation on the release of NA. These authors evaluated the release of catecholamines produced by the exposure of spleen slices to a Na^+-free solution for a total of 30 or more m, whereas in the adrenal medulla the exocytotic release was observed only in the first minutes (1–3 m) of exposure to the Na^+-free solution (Lastowecka and Trifaró, 1974). A short exocytotic event could have been obscured by the long period of incubation. It is possible that exposure to low sodium could lead to an early increase in exocytotic release of NA from sympathetic nerves followed by an accelerated nonexocytotic efflux of transmitters. With regard to this latter mechanism, low sodium is known to accelerate the efflux of ^3H-NA from tissues pretreated with reserpine and monoamine-oxidase inhibitors by a calcium-independent, carrier-mediated effect (Paton, 1973; Graefe and Fuchs, personal communication, 1978). In addition, prolonged tissue exposure to low-sodium media could induce catecholamine release due to cell damage and could impair the release of amines in response to physiological stimuli (Banks, 1967; Lastowecka and Trifaró, 1974). The possibility of cell damage was also postulated by García and Kirpekar (1973) as a possible mechanism by which prolonged exposure to Na^+-deprived solutions would induce noradrenaline release from sympathetic nerves. However, evaluation of cell damage by the release of cytoplasmic markers was not performed by those authors.

Several mechanisms could be postulated to explain the Na^+-free-evoked exocytotic release of catecholamines from the adrenal medulla: increased calcium influx (Banks et al., 1969; Baker, 1972), reduced calcium efflux (Blaustein and Hodgkin, 1969; Aguirre et al., 1977), or reduced sequestration or greater release of calcium from intracellular binding sites (Carafoli et al., 1975; Aguirre et al., 1977; section of this paper on calcium). An analysis of the immediate effects of Na^+-deprived solutions on the release of NA and DBH would allow one to determine whether Na^+-free medium evokes exocytotic transmitter release from noradrenergic nerve terminals.

C. Sodium-Potassium Adenosine Triphosphatase and NA Release

Recent studies on the release of acetylcholine and catecholamines have focused attention on the possible role of the adenosine triphosphatase (Na^+-K^+-ATPase) in stimulus-secretion coupling and its participation in the alpha-presynaptic regulation of release in noradrenergic neurons (see section on alpha-presynaptic receptors). The interest comes from experimental results which revealed that conditions (K^+-free medium, ouabain) known to lead to inhibition of the Na^+-K^+ATPase activity are able to trigger acetylcholine release from Auerbach's plexus, cortical slices, and motor nerve terminals, even in the absence of extracellular calcium (Paton et al., 1971; Vizi, 1972, 1974, 1975a, b; Baker and Crawford, 1975). Similarly, for the adrenal medulla (Banks, 1967; Banks et al., 1969; Lastowecka and Trifaró, 1974; Gutman and Boonyaviroj, 1977; Horga et al., 1978) and for sympathetic nerves (Vizi, 1975b, 1977), an increase in the release of catecholamines has been induced by K^+-free medium and by ouabain in the absence of extracellular calcium. On the other hand, diphenylhydantoin (a stimulant of Na^+-K^+-ATPase) reduced the release of catecholamines from rat adrenal medulla, an effect abolished by preincubation of the glands in a K^+-free medium (Gutman and Boonyaviroj, 1977). From these observations it seems apparent that inhibition of Na^+-K^+-ATPase induces transmitter release. The physiological relevance of these findings has been stretched: several authors have postulated that the sodium pump per se is directly involved in the stimulus-secretion coupling. Inhibition of the pump would induce release, and ATPase stimulation would inhibit either resting or nerve-stimulation-evoked transmitter release. Because of the inhibitory properties of calcium on ATPase activity, it has been proposed that the influx of calcium that occurs during neuronal depolarization could cause transmitter release by inhibiting the Na^+-K^+-ATPase (Paton et al., 1971; Garciá and Kirpekar, 1975; Vizi, 1977). According to this view, inhibition of this enzyme would be a necessary event in stimulus-secretion coupling. However, on the basis of additional experimental evidence these results could be interpreted differently. It is known that conditions which increase the $[Na^+]_i$:$[Na^+]_o$ ratio—as, for example, inhibition of the sodium pump—favor the accumulation of intracellular calcium (Trifaró, 1977). In fact, the accumulation of calcium by the mitochondria is dependent on intracellular Na^+ (Carafoli et al., 1975; Baker and Schlaepfer, 1975). It is then possible that a greater intracellular Na^+ concentration due to pump inhibition could raise the cytoplasmic Ca^{++} levels as a result of either reduced sequestration or a greater calcium release from intracellular binding sites. In addition, the reversal of the sodium gradient has been reported to produce an outward movement of Na^+ coupled with an inward transport of calcium (Baker, 1972, in squid giant axon); and Banks et al. (1969) suggested that under physiological conditions the intracellular levels of Na^+ could probably regulate the influx of calcium. Thus, the increase in free-cytoplasmic Ca^{++} levels by either of the mechanisms mentioned could be directly responsible for the exocytotic release observed when the Na^+-K^+-ATPase is inhibited. If this were to be the case, ATPase inhibition would not be a necessary event in stimulus-secretion coupling. Although at present the possible physiological participation of the Na^+-K^+-ATPase in the mechanism of release of noradrenaline from sympathetic nerves is not clear, drugs that modify this enzyme's activity can markedly affect transmitter release.

V. MECHANISMS OF RELEASE

The sequence of the molecular events taking place during the exocytotic release of transmitters and hormones has not yet been elucidated. A large amount of circumstantial and indirect evidence has been accumulated about the possible molecular mechanisms involved in exocytosis. In general terms, the large majority of the studies have been focused on two aspects: (a) the mechanisms involved in the fusion of both the vesicle and plasma membranes and (b) the possible role of contractile elements (microtubules and microfilaments) as triggers of exocytosis. Some of these observations are discussed in this section.

A. Membrane Fusion

Release by exocytosis involves the interaction of both the vesicle and the plasma membrane, and a process of membrane fusion seems to be an early event during exocytosis. The experiments in membrane fusion have been carried out in different secretory systems (including the adrenal medulla), and there are practically no data available on membrane fusion in noradrenergic neurons. However, because of the implications that membrane fusion may have in exocytotic release in sympathetic neurons, some of these observations will be discussed here.

It is possible that some kind of rearrangement of the lipids of the vesicle and plasma membranes takes place during exocytosis. It has been suggested that the configuration of the lipid molecules of the membranes is of primary importance in the process of membrane fusion and that fusion will occur only if the lipid molecules are appropriately oriented (Lucy, 1970). Membrane fusion may not occur if the lipids of one or both membranes are in the bimolecular leaflet configuration. For membrane fusion to occur, the two membranes in question should have a high proportion of their phospholipid in the miscellar configuration (Lucy, 1970). Therefore, any situation that would produce a transition from bilayer to miscellar configuration would facilitate membrane fusion. This type of transition (lamellar → miscellar) may be the result of the incorporation of perturbing molecules into the lipids of the membranes. One of the molecules capable of producing such a transition is lysolecithin. Interestingly enough, chromaffin granules have a large content (13%–17%) of lysolecithin (Douglas et al., 1966; Blaschko et al., 1967; Trifaró, 1973), and that led to the suggestion that, during stimulation, this lipid is involved in the process of membrane fusion (Blaschko et al., 1967). However, lysolecithin is not formed during stimulation, and it is present in the same concentration in granule membranes during resting conditions (Trifaró, 1969a, b). Moreover, no fusion among chromaffin granules is observed in the resting cell. The content of lysolecithin in LDCV is only between 0% and 3% of the total phospholipids. Therefore, the role of lysolecithin, if any, in the secretory process remains to be elucidated.

As discussed above, Ca^{++} may be another important factor in membrane fusion. An electrostatic function for Ca^{++} in exocytosis has been proposed recently (Dean, 1975; Dean and Matthews, 1975). According to this proposal, one possible function of Ca^{++} ions in exocytosis is to reduce the potential at the surface of both the vesicle and cell membranes, thus decreasing the potential energy barrier for granule-membrane interaction (Dean, 1975; Dean and Matthews, 1975). This would enable contact or coalition to occur between the two membranes (Dean, 1975; Dean and Matthews, 1975). It has been also shown that in some secretory systems, like intact leukocytes, Ca^{++} causes the attachment of the granules to the plasma membrane (Woodin, French, and Marchesi, 1963). Furthermore, in an *in vitro* system formed by vasopressin-containing vesicles and neurohypophyseal plasma membranes, the addition of Ca^{++} induces fusion, and the degree of fusion is proportional to the *in vitro* release of vasopressin (Gratzl et al., 1977). It seems, therefore, that by combining with anionic groups, Ca^{++} would neutralize the negative charges of the granules and of the interior of the plasma membrane. In fact, it has been shown that, at physiological pH, chromaffin granules have surface negative charges and that Ca^{++} can cause aggregation of chromaffin granules (Banks, 1966). This effect of Ca^{++} could be due to an interaction with membrane lipids (Poisner and Trifaró, 1967). In connection with this, it has been demonstrated that ATP induces the synthesis of diphosphatidyl inositol (DPI) in chromaffin granule membranes (Trifaró, 1973; Trifaró and Dworkind, 1975). The formation of diphosphatidyl inositol in chromaffin granule membranes is catalyzed by a granule membrane phosphatidyl inositol kinase (Trifaró, 1973). An increased synthesis of DPI has been demonstrated in chromaffin granules during catecholamine release from the adrenal medulla in response to acetylcholine stimulation (Trifaró and Dworkind, 1975). Diphosphatidyl inositol has great affinity for Ca^{++}; and in some membranes, there is a direct correlation between Ca^{++} binding and

DPI content (Buckley and Hawthorne, 1972). At the present time it is not known whether LDCV and other secretory vesicles contain PIKinase, and no information is available about the presence or synthesis of DPI in these storage vesicles. Therefore, the functional implications of the DPI metabolism and content in secretory vesicles should be determined in future experiments.

Freeze-fracturing EM studies on chromaffin granules have shown that the granules exhibit a smooth surface with a random distribution of membrane-associated particles (Schober et al., 1977). These freeze-etching studies revealed that the addition of Ca^{++} (10 mM) to chromaffin granules induced their aggregation. The contact areas of the granules were always free of particles on both faces of the membrane. At the margin of the contact area, the particles aggregated around the circumference, forming a rosette-like structure (Schober et al., 1977). This rosette-like structure was, in this case, induced by a large and perhaps unphysiological concentration of Ca^{++}. However, similar rosette-like structures have been observed in the plasma membrane of the nerve terminals of the neurohypophysis during electrical or K^+-induced stimulation (Dreifuss et al., 1976). Furthermore, a similar pattern of particle aggregates has been described in mammalian central synapses (Pfenninger et al., 1972) and in the plasma membrane of the Tetrahymena (Satir, Schooley, and Satir, 1973). In this protozoan, it has been convincingly demonstrated that the rosette identifies the membrane site where fusion between the secretory vesicle (mucocist) and the plasma membrane takes place prior to secretion. It is, therefore, tempting to speculate that in the other secretory systems the rosettes also mark membrane sites pre-determined for vesicle fusion and exocytosis. Further experiments should determine if these rosette-like structures are also present in adrenergic varicosities and other secretory systems.

A paper has recently been published on the isolation of a protein (synexin) from the adrenal medulla that causes a Ca-dependent aggregation of isolated chromaffin granules. This protein is activated in a positively cooperative manner by a small concentration of Ca^{++} (6 μM) causing aggregation. On the other hand, Mg^{++}, Sr^{++}, and Ba^{++} were ineffective in this regard. The authors suggested that synexin may be the intracellular receptor for Ca^{++} in the process of exocytosis (Creutz, Pazoles, and Pollard, 1978). However, it remains to be determined if this protein is the cytosol factor described earlier by Oka, Izumi, and Kashimoto (1972).

As discussed above, charge neutralization may play a major role in exocytotic release. A new hypothesis has been advanced in this regard; it involves the carboxymethylation of chromaffin granule proteins (Diliberto, Viveros, and Axelrod, 1976). In the adrenal medulla, 97% of the protein carboxymethylase was free in the cytosol and, among all subcellular organelles, the chromaffin granules had the highest concentration of substrates for protein carboxymethylase. After methylation, a large proportion of carboxymethylated proteins was detached from the granule membranes. Therefore, carboxymethylation of chromaffin granule membrane proteins could participate in the two major steps necessary for membrane fusion; (a) the neutralization of the charges, allowing membrane contact; and (b) the removal of surface proteins, thus exposing the lipid layers.

In summary, the above observations seem to indicate that there are at least two requirements for membrane fusion: (a) neutralization of the membrane surface negative charges and (b) rearrangement of components (lipids and proteins) of the vesicle and plasma membrane. However, further experiments are necessary to elucidate the molecular mechanisms involved in membrane fusion.

B. Microtubules

It has been proposed that microtubules are involved in the mechanisms of hormone and transmitter release in a variety of tissues (Lacy et al., 1968; Poisner and Bernstein, 1971; Labrie et al., 1973; Thoa et al., 1972, 1975). This hypothesis is based on indirect observations that agents which disrupt microtubules, such as colchicine and vinblastine, inhibit the release process. The first observation on the effects of these agents was made by Lacy et al. (1968), who showed that colchicine inhibits glucose-induced release of insulin from the pancreas. Lacy suggested that the storage granules that are attached to microtubules, and not those that are free in the cytosol of the β cell, are available for immediate release; and that Ca^{++} may trigger contraction or change in the phsyiological conformation in the microtubule system, which results in granule extrusion (Lacy and Greider, 1972). A similar interpretation was made of the blocking effects of colchicine and vinblastine on catecholamine release from the adrenal medulla (Poisner and Bernstein, 1971) and sympathetic nerves (Thoa et al., 1972, 1975). This hypothesis is subject to criticism for reasons provided by the following observations:

1. The glucose-induced release of insulin is a biphasic event (Grodsky et al., 1969; Hoshi and Shreeve, 1973): an immediate and acute release response (phase I, which is due to exocytosis) is followed by a late and long-lasting release response (phase II, which depends on the rate of insulin synthesis, the rate of conversion of proinsulin to insulin, and the intracellular transport of secretory granules). These two phases of secretion are observed when the pancreas is perfused (Trifaró, 1977). Colchicine blocks phase II of glucose-induced insulin release without affecting phase I (Lacy, Walker, and Fink, 1972). It is well known that colchicine and vinblastine block the intracellular transport and the axonal transport of hormones (Trifaró, 1977) and neurotransmitter substances (Livett, 1976) respectively. This differential

effect of colchicine was not observed in the early experiments where β cell pancreatic islets were incubated for 90 m (Lacy et al., 1968). Similarly, in the experiments with sympathetic nerve preparations, the collection periods of the hypogastric nerve vas deferens preparations incubated *in vitro* were 30 m (Thoa et al., 1975) and 60 m (Thoa et al., 1972). Therefore, an important condition for the study of the effect of these agents on the secretory process seems to be an adequate preparation of perfused tissue, in which exocytosis per se can be temporarily separated from the exocytotic process which follows the intracellular transport of secretory vesicles (Trifaró, 1977). This prerequisite has not always been complied with, and many of the studies on hormone and transmitter release have been carried out in pieces, slices, or organs incubated *in vitro* and exposed to these agents for long periods of time. In the presence of these agents, a decrease in the amount of hormone and transmitter collected during the stimulation was observed in some cases (Lacy et al., 1968; Labrie et al., 1973; Kraicer and Milligan, 1971; Douglas and Sorimachi, 1972a, b; Sundberg et al., 1973; Temple et al., 1972; Thoa et al., 1972, 1975); and no change (Kraicer and Milligan, 1971; Temple et al., 1972) or even the potentiation of release (Sundberg et al., 1973) was observed in others.

2. Results obtained with agents that disrupt microtubules are also difficult to interpret because of other effects of these drugs on biological systems (Trifaró, 1977). Some of these effects are an inhibition by colchicine and its analogues of nucleoside uptake (Mizel and Wilson, 1972), a reduction by colchicine and vincristine of ATP production (Jamieson, 1972), the binding of colchicine to cell membranes (Stadler and Franke, 1974), the tubocurarine effects of colchicine and vinblastine (Spoor and Ferguson, 1965), and the anticholinergic effects of colchicine and vinblastine (Trifaró et al., 1972). This latter effect was observed in experiments with perfused adrenal glands and sympathetic ganglia (Trifaró et al., 1972). The exocytotic release of catecholamines from the adrenal medulla in response to either nicotine (Poisner and Bernstein, 1971) or acetylcholine (Poisner and Bernstein, 1971; Trifaró et al., 1972; Douglas and Sorimachi, 1972a, b) was blocked by colchicine and vinblastine. However, catecholamine release induced by either depolarizing concentrations of K^+ (Trifaró et al., 1972; Douglas and Sorimachi, 1972a) or angiotensin (Trifaró et al., 1972) was unaffected. This suggested an anticholinergic effect of these agents, which was confirmed in experiments with perfused superior cervical ganglia. Colchicine and vinblastine were able to block ganglionic transmission during either preganglionic nerve stimulation or acetylcholine administration without affecting the release of acetylcholine from the preganglionic nerve terminals (Trifaró et al., 1972).

3. Lacy's suggestions that Ca^{++} triggers contraction of microtubules also seems unlikely, since Ca^{++} blocks microtubule polymerization

(Weisenberg, 1972). It has been demonstrated in experiments carried out *in vitro* that Ca^{++} seems to be as effective in blocking microtubule polymerization as low temperatures and colchicine (Weisenberg, 1972). Furthermore, the intracellular levels of free Ca^{++} may control microtubule polymerization (Shelanski, 1973). If this is the case, the polymerization of microtubules should decrease during the exocytotic release reaction, a condition in which an increase in free intracellular Ca^{++} has been assumed (Trifaró, 1977; see this paper, section on Ca^{++}). The above results suggest that, although microtubules might be involved in the intracellular transport of secretory vesicles, they are not involved in the exocytotic process itself. Therefore, the true role of microtubules in the secretory process still remains to be elucidated.

C. Contractile Proteins

The events involved in the secretory process of nerve terminals, the adrenal medulla, and other secretory tissues have many features in common with the process of muscle contraction (Smith and Winkler, 1972; Douglas, 1974, 1975; Trifaró, 1977). The common physiological features between two apparently different processes, contraction and secretion, have been reviewed and discussed in detail elsewhere (Douglas, 1974, 1975; Trifaró, 1977). However, it is worthwhile noting that on the basis of their own work, Poisner and Trifaró (1967) suggested that the molecular mechanism involved in the exocytosis of chromaffin cells was a true contractile event. Under certain experimental conditions, ATP, in the presence of Mg^{++}, induced the release from chromaffin granules of catecholamines and other soluble components (Poisner and Trifaró, 1967; Trifaró and Poisner, 1967; Poisner and Trifaró, 1968, 1969). It was concluded from these experiments that ATP was hydrolyzed by the chromaffin granule ATPase and that this hydrolysis was followed by the production of some conformational change (contractile event?) in the granule membrane leading to the release of the granule components (Poisner and Trifaró, 1967; Trifaró and Dworkind, 1971). ATP-induced release of substances from cholinergic and other secretory vesicles has also been reported (Trifaró, 1977; 1978).

The idea that exocytosis is a true contractile event raises questions about the presence and the possible role of contractile proteins in neurons and other related cells. In this connection, the following observations have been made: (1) myosin and actin have been isolated from brain tissue (Berl, Puszkin, and Nicklas, 1973); (2) actin has been identified in sympathetic neurons (Fine and Bray, 1971); (3) actin has been isolated from the adrenal medulla (Phillips and Slater, 1975; Trifaró and Lee, 1979); (4) myosin has been isolated from the adrenal medulla (Trifaró and Ulpian, 1976; Creutz, 1977); (5) *in vitro* interaction between muscle myosin, muscle actin, and chromaffin granules has been described (Burridge and Phillips, 1975); (6)

the regulatory proteins, tropomyosin and troponin, have been isolated from brain and adrenal medulla (Fine et al., 1973; Fine and Blitz, 1976; Kuo and Coffee, 1976a, b); (7) the binding to chromaffin granules of antibodies against actinin has been observed (Jockusch et al., 1977); and (8) part of the neuronal actin has been observed to form a tridimensional meshwork of microfilaments at the level of the terminals, and this meshwork has been observed to attach not only to the synaptic membranes but also to intracellular organelles, including synaptic vesicles (Le Beux and Willemot, 1975a, b).

On the basis of their own work on actin and myosin of brain tissue, Berl et al. (1973) proposed that exocytosis was indeed, as suggested earlier by Poisner and Trifaró (1967), a contractile event. According to Berl et al. (1973), exocytosis and the expulsion of the vesicular content into the extracellular space was the result of the interaction between vesicular myosin and synaptic membrane actin. This attractive hypothesis has not yet been confirmed. There is little doubt that chromaffin granules and adrenergic and cholinergic vesicles contain an *intrinsic ATPase* (Banks, 1965; Hosie, 1965; Trifaró and Warner, 1972; Lagercrantz, 1976). However, the identification of the vesicle ATPase as myosin has not yet been made (Trifaró, 1978). Electron microscopy negative staining studies have shown that adrenal and brain myosin molecules are of shapes and dimensions (1600 Å) similar to those of muscle myosin (Burridge and Bray, 1975; Trifaró and Ulpian, 1976). It would therefore be unlikely for a myosin molecule to be contained in large adrenergic (700 Å), small adrenergic (400 Å), or cholinergic (400 Å) vesicles, since the length of the myosin molecule is several times the diameter of a vesicle (Trifaró, 1978). Moreover, the similarity in shape between muscle, adrenal, and brain myosins suggests that the interaction of myosin with actin might be similar to that which takes place in muscle and that the sliding mechanism of contraction may also operate in nervous tissues (Trifaró, 1978). Therefore it is unlikely that a large myosin molecule could be accommodated within a storage vesicle in a coiled manner. However, this argument does not negate the possibility of the interaction of myosin and actin with vesicle membranes. In fact, it has been demonstrated that chromaffin granules have the ability to bind muscle actin and myosin (Burridge and Phillips, 1975). Furthermore, actin and regulatory proteins can interact with synaptic vesicles *in vitro* and, after the activation of the *intrinsic* vesicle ATPase, induce the release of transmitter (Puszkin and Kochwa, 1974). In addition, it is not known at the present time whether the microfilament meshwork, which seems to be attached to storage vesicles, plays a role in either the release reaction or in the retrieval process which follows exocytosis (Trifaró, 1978). However, the use of cytochalasin B, a drug known to interact with microfilaments (Wessels et al., 1971), has provided some circumstantial evidence. It has been shown that cytochalasin B blocks catecholamine release from the adrenal medulla (Douglas and Sorimachi, 1972b), sympathetic nerves (Thoa et al., 1972), and synaptosomal preparations (Nicklas and Berl, 1974). Although the blocking effect of this drug may be due to its other metabolic inhibitor properties (Mizel and Wilson, 1972; Nakazato and Douglas, 1973; Trifaró, 1977), it is worthwhile noting that cytochalasin B blocks the polymerization of G actin into F actin (Himes et al., 1976) and the ATPase activity of actin-myosin complexes (Nicklas and Berl, 1974; Spudich and Lin, 1972).

In conclusion, it should be pointed out that although the presence of actin, myosin, and regulatory proteins in neurons and chromaffin cells may be related to cell functions other than exocytosis (Trifaró, 1978), the possible role of these contractile proteins in secretion deserves further investigation.

VI. REGULATION OF EXOCYTOTIC RELEASE OF NORADRENALINE

In the last decade great attention has been focused on the mechanisms by which the amount of noradrenaline release per pulse could be modified, both under physiological conditions and by administration of drugs. Investigations on the mechanisms by which drugs, particularly alpha receptor antagonists, affected the overflow of noradrenaline evoked by nerve stimulation progressively led to the discovery of receptors in noradrenergic nerve terminals. These presynaptic receptors, contrary to those present in the effector organ (postsynaptic) may, when activated, modulate the exocytotic release of the transmitter. Thus exogenous or endogenous compounds acting on presynaptic sites could modify the amount of transmitter released during neuronal activation.

In this section, special attention will be devoted to the effect of frequency of stimulation on noradrenaline release, to how the trends in alpha presynaptic modulation of noradrenaline release emerged, and to the possible physiological relevance of this process. When required, reference to relevant findings in other secretory tissues will be provided.

A. Frequency of Stimulation and NA Release

Changes in the duration and in the rate of sympathetic nerve stimulation are known to modify effector organ responses and NA overflow. In general, frequency-response or frequency-overflow curves are performed by varying the frequency and the duration of the stimulation period in such a way that a constant number of pulses is applied to the nerves. When such a procedure is employed, the average overflow of NA per pulse in many tissues increases with increasing frequencies of stimulation—e.g., cat and dog spleen (Brown and Gillespie, 1957; Kirpekar and Cervoni, 1963; Haefely, Hürlimann and

Thoenen, 1965; Davies, Robinson and Withrington, 1969; De Potter et al., 1971; Cubeddu and Weiner, 1975a); guinea pig uterine artery (Bell and Vogt, 1971); myenteric-longitudinal muscle preparation (Henderson, Hughes and Thompson, 1972; Henderson, Hughes and Kosterlitz, 1975) and vas deferens (Stjärne, 1973a); rabbit portal vein and vas deferens (Hughes, 1972); and human omental arteries and veins (Stjárne and Brundin, 1977).

In other tissues (cat nictitating membrane and mouse vas deferens), the average NA overflow per pulse either is rather constant over a wide range of frequencies (Farnebo and Malmfors, 1971; Henderson and Hughes, 1974; Henderson et al., 1975) or decreases with increasing frequencies of stimulation (rat cerebral cortex and rabbit superior cervical ganglion) (Montel, Starke, and Weber, 1974; Noon and Roth, 1975). Initial studies by Brown and Gillespie (1957), Kirpekar and Cervoni (1963), and Haefely et al. (1965) in the perfused cat spleen were interpreted by these authors as demonstrating that inhibition of neuronal uptake of NA occurred during higher frequencies of stimulation. Therefore it was presumed that a constant amount of NA was released by nerve impulse and that the observed increase in transmitter overflow with higher frequencies of stimulation simply represented a decrease in the inactivation of the NA released from the nerve endings.

Although changes in neuronal uptake have been suggested to occur during depolarization of nerve terminals (Gillis, 1963; Chang and Chiueh, 1969; Häggendal and Malmfors, 1969b; Yamamoto and Kirpekar, 1972; Cubeddu and Weiner, 1975a; Dubocovich and Langer, 1977), they do not seem to account for the marked increase in NA overflow elicited by high frequencies of stimulation. In fact, the enhancement in the stimulation-evoked transmitter overflow produced by drugs that block neuronal uptake is rather small. In addition, a greater output of DBH was observed with increasing frequencies of nerve stimulation (De Potter et al., 1972; Cubeddu and Weiner, 1975a). Stimulating the cat and dog splenic nerves from 5 to 20 Hz, these authors observed a proportional increase in the overflow of NA and DBH; in fact, the ratios for the overflow of both substances were rather similar at the different frequencies of stimulation employed. These results suggested that the greater overflow of NA observed with higher frequencies of stimulation (at least in the perfused spleen) is due mainly to an increase in exocytotic release of transmitter per nerve impulse, although the possibility cannot be ruled out that part of the increasing NA overflow is due to inhibition of the amine pump during neuronal depolarization. Concerning the mechanism by which changes in frequency of stimulation modify transmitter release, an increase in the calcium influx with higher frequencies has been postulated. In fact, Baker, Hodgkin, and Ridgway (1971) demonstrated a greater entry of calcium into the squid giant axon with higher frequencies of stimulation.

Whether an enhancement in exocytotic release of NA occurs in other organs or tissues with positive frequency-overflow relationships has not been investigated. In addition, measurements of the release of DBH have not been performed in tissues with negative frequency-overflow relationships (Montel et al., 1974; Noon and Roth, 1975) nor in those in which there is not such a relationship (Farnebo and Malmfors, 1971; Henderson and Hughes, 1974; Henderson et al., 1975). Therefore, whether all frequency-induced changes in NA overflow are related to changes in exocytotic transmitter release remains to be elucidated.

The effects of most drugs on transmitter release are dependent on the frequency of stimulation employed. In fact, most compounds that inhibit the release of NA elicited by nerve stimulation are more potent and effective at low frequencies of stimulation. In addition, agents acting on presynaptic receptors to modify NA release are less effective at high frequencies of stimulation (see the following section). Studies concerning the effects of drugs on the release of NA should be performed at several frequencies of stimulation before it can be concluded that a certain compound has no effect on evoked transmitter release.

B.

    1. Presynaptic receptors and NA release Studies on peripheral and central noradrenergic neurons have demonstrated that the amount of NA released per pulse could be modulated through presynaptic receptors. This regulatory mechanism has been described not only for noradrenergic neurons but also for dopaminergic, GABAergic, cholinergic, and possibly serotoninergic neurons. In fact, these neurons appear to secrete less transmitter the higher the concentration of the respective transmitter in the biophase, suggesting that nerve terminals have presynaptic receptors for release regulation that are sensitive to the transmitter of the nerve terminal. However, neurons appear to possess a variety of presynaptic receptor sites that when activated may affect transmitter release. For noradrenergic neurons, basically two facilitatory modulators have been described: angiotensin (Ackerly, Blumberg and Peach, 1976; Starke, 1977) and beta agonists (Langer, 1976; Dixon, Mosimann, and Weiner, 1978). The latter probably act through cyclic AMP, whereas alpha agonists (Langer, 1976; Starke, 1977), prostaglandins of the E series (Starke, 1977; Malik, 1978), oxogenous and endogenous opioids (Starke, 1977; Subramanian et al., 1977), adenosine and adenosine nucleotides (Su, 1978; Fredholm and Hedqvist, 1978), dopamine agonists (Langer, 1973; Dixon et al., 1978), and cholinergic-muscarinic agonists (Löffelholz and Muscholl, 1970; Sharma and Banerjee, 1978) act on specific presynaptic receptors to inhibit transmitter release.

With the exception of the alpha presynaptic receptors, large species and tissue differences have been observed for the other prejunctional modulators. Therefore, the variable distribution patterns of presynaptic receptor systems in noradrenergic neurons indicate that these neurons, though basically similar, can undergo different degrees of specialization.

The presence of presynaptic receptors does not imply their participation in the normal physiological regulation of transmitter release. In fact, with the exception of presynaptic muscarinic receptors in noradrenergic neurons of the heart (Löffelholz and Muscholl, 1970; Sharma and Banerjee, 1978), only alpha presynaptic receptors appear to play an important physiological role in the regulation of NA release from noradrenergic neurons.

2. Role of presynaptic alpha receptors and NA release Brown and coworkers were the first to observe that phenoxybenzamine and other alpha-adrenergic blocking agents greatly enhanced the amount of NA appearing in the venous circulation after stimulation of the sympathetic nerves to the spleen, colon, and small intestine (Brown and Gillespie, 1957; Brown, Davies and Gillespie, 1958; Brown, 1965; Gillespie and Kirpekar, 1966; Kirpekar and Wakade, 1970). To account for these results, these investigators proposed that a fraction of the NA released was ordinarily bound to alpha receptors and, when the receptors were blocked, more NA could escape receptor binding and could therefore exit from the organ. Boullin, Costa, and Brodie (1967) elaborated a somewhat more sophisticated hypothesis, in which the NA released would ordinarily form a complex with the alpha receptor sites. This complex would act as a brake to diffusion of the amine from the site of release into the circulation. The NA would then be available for a longer time for recapture into the nerve terminals.

On the basis of similar observations, Thoenen, Hürlimann, and Haefely (1963; 1964a, b) postulated that the enhancement in the nerve-stimulation-mediated overflow of NA produced by alpha-adrenergic blocking agents was related to prevention of the recapture into the nerve endings of the NA released by nerve stimulation. These authors observed that the alpha receptor antagonists had inhibitory properties on neuronal uptake of NA (as shown by Iversen, 1967) and that there was a dissociation between the concentrations of phenoxybenzamine that blocked alpha receptors and those that inhibited neuronal uptake. The inhibition of the amine uptake pump by these agents correlates better with the enhanced overflow of transmitter. However, Thoenen and coworkers' view had several important drawbacks. In fact, when potent and more specific inhibitors of the neuronal uptake of NA, which lack alpha blocking properties, were examined, only a small increase or no change in the nerve-stimulation-mediated overflow of NA was observed (Blakeley, Brown, and Ferry, 1963; Geffen, 1965; Boullin et al., 1967; Kirpekar and Wakade, 1970; Farnebo and Hamberger, 1970a; Starke, Montel, and Schümann, 1971a). In addition, evidence was presented that alpha blockers increased transmitter overflow either at concentrations that failed to inhibit neuronal uptake (Starke, 1971; Starke et al., 1971a; Enero et al., 1972) or in the presence of potent inhibitors of the neuronal amine pump (Starke et al., 1971a; Starke, 1977).

Blockers of alpha receptors can also inhibit the extraneuronal uptake and metabolism of NA (Eisenfeld, Axelrod, and Krakoff, 1967; Avakian and Gillespie, 1968; Iversen and Langer, 1969; Gillespie, Hamilton and Hosie, 1970; Draskocsy and Trendelenburg, 1970); this finding was offered as an explanation for the increased transmitter overflow observed with these compounds (Iversen and Langer, 1969; Langer, 1970). However, no increase in NA overflow was obtained with concentrations of normetanephrine at which the extraneuronal accumulation of NA was markedly inhibited (Farnebo and Hamberger, 1971a, b). More recently, it was demonstrated that the concentrations of alpha antagonists required to inhibit extraneuronal uptake and metabolism of NA were much greater than those required to enhance NA overflow (see Cubeddu et al., 1974a; Cubeddu, Langer, and Weiner, 1974c; Starke, 1977) and that their effects on transmitter overflow were observable in the presence of agents that blocked the extraneuronal disposition of NA (Starke, 1977).

These observations made independent laboratories suggest that an increase in the amount of NA released by nerve impulse could occur in the presence of alpha receptor antagonists (Häggendal, 1970; Langer, 1970; Farnebo and Hamberger, 1971a, b; Starke, 1971; Starke et al., 1971a; Starke, Montel, and Wagner, 1971b; Kirpekar and Puig, 1971; Kirpekar et al., 1972; McCulloch, Rand, and Story, 1972). In support of this are the observations that DBH is also released in greater amounts in the presence of phenoxybenzamine (De Potter et al., 1971; Johnson et al., 1971; Cubeddu et al., 1974a; Cubeddu and Weiner, 1975a) and phentolamine (De Potter et al., 1971; Cubeddu et al., 1974a; Dixon, Mosimann and Weiner, 1977; Langley and Weiner, 1978). These results suggest that alpha receptor antagonists markedly increase the exocytotic release of NA induced by nerve stimulation. They also indicate that the increase in NA overflow observed with these agents is probably due to a combination of factors, i.e., enhancement of exocytotic release, inhibition of neuronal and extraneuronal uptake and metabolism, and possibly prevention of the binding of NA to alpha receptors.

On the basis of the enhanced exocytotic release of NA observed with alpha-adrenergic blocking agents, the presence of presynaptic alpha receptors involved in the regulation of NA release was postulated (Langer et al., 1971; Farnebo and Hamberger, 1971a, b; Starke, 1971, 1972b; Kirpekar and Puig, 1971; Enero et al., 1972). Activation of these alpha receptors presumably inhibits NA release, and it has been suggested that they form part of a negative feedback control mechanism by which the transmitter may regulate its own release (for review see Langer, 1974, 1976; Starke, 1977). *The following pieces of evidence support this hypothesis:*

1. Alpha receptor blocking agents increase and alpha agonists reduce the stimulation-evoked exocytotic release of NA independently of the predominant postsynaptic receptor (α or β). The inhibitory effect of alpha agonists is prevented by alpha antagonists (Adler-Graschinsky, Rubio, and Langer, 1970; Starke et al., 1971a, b).

2. The effects of alpha receptor agonists and antagonists on NA release are dependent on the concentration of the transmitter in the synaptic space. Partial or total depletion of tissue NA with either alpha-methyl-p-tyrosine or reserpine markedly reduced or abolished, respectively, the effects of phenoxybenzamine and phentolamine in increasing the overflow of NA and/or DBH induced by nerve stimulation (Enero and Langer, 1973; Cubeddu and Weiner, 1975a; Dixon et al., 1977). The higher the synaptic cleft concentration of NA, the smaller the effects of alpha agonists in inhibiting NA release. A negative relationship between the percentage of inhibition of NA release induced by oxymethazoline and the amount (in nanograms) of NA overflow induced by nerve stimulation has been reported. In addition, at higher frequencies of stimulation (higher NA output), the alpha agonists are less effective in inhibiting NA release (Starke, 1972a; Starke and Altmann, 1973; Starke, 1977).

3. A certain threshold concentration of NA should be reached in the synaptic space for activation of alpha presynaptic receptors. In fact, a greater fractional release of adrenergic transmitter (fraction of tissue NA released per pulse) is observed after tissue depletion of NA by alpha-methyl-p-tyrosine or reserpine. The reduced quantity of NA released by nerve stimulation (because of the diminished NA tissue content) determines a smaller activation of alpha presynaptic receptors, which in turn leads to a greater release of NA and DBH (Enero and Langer, 1973; Cubeddu and Weiner, 1975a; Dixon et al., 1977).

4. Although pre- and postsynaptic alpha receptors are stimulated by adequate concentrations of alpha agonists and blocked by alpha antagonists, there seem to be differences in these receptors. In fact, on the basis of agonist and antagonist specificity, a classification for alpha receptors has been proposed: $alpha_1$ and $alpha_2$ receptors. Tramazoline, xylazine, alpha-methyl-noradrenaline, clonidine, and oxymetazoline are potent $alpha_2$ receptor agonists, whereas phenylephrine and methoxamine characterize $alpha_1$ receptors. For NA, adrenaline, and naphazoline an almost similar potency has been reported for $alpha_1$ and $alpha_2$ receptors. Regarding the antagonist specificity, phenoxybenzamine, prazosin, and WB-4101 appear to be more potent antagonists of $alpha_1$ receptors, whereas piperoxane,

yohimbine, and mianserine are more selective alpha$_2$ receptor blocking agents. An almost equal affinity for alpha$_1$ and alpha$_2$ receptors has been observed for phentolamine. In most cases, alpha presynaptic receptors behave pharmacologically as alpha$_2$ receptors, and the postsynaptic alpha receptors are generally identified as alpha$_1$ receptors (Dubocovich and Langer, 1974; Cubeddu et al., 1974a; Starke, Borowski, and Endo, 1975a; Starke, Endo, and Taube, 1975b; Borowsky, Ehrl, and Starke, 1976; Starke, 1977). However, differences in agonist and antagonist specificity have been observed, depending on the tissue and species studied (see above references). Binding studies have also provided evidence about the existence of two classes of alpha receptors. The displacement of specific binding of ^{3}H-dihydroergocryptine to rat brain plasma membranes by wide ranges of concentrations of prazocin and yohimbine (peripheral *post* (α_1) and presynaptic (α_2) antagonists, respectively) gave biphasic displacement curves. Blockade of yohimbine sites (*presynaptic*) permitted ^{3}H-dihydroergocryptine to bind to prazocine sites. Clonidine did not produce any additional displacement with yohimbine, but it did after prazosin (Miach, Dausse and Meyer, 1978).

5. The following pieces of evidence favor the presynaptic location of alpha receptors: a) alpha agonists and antagonists modify NA release in organs in which the postsynaptic receptors are of the beta type; b) alpha blocking agents increase NA overflow in the absence of postsynaptic structures, i.e., from neurons in tissue culture (Vogel et al., 1972) and in salivary glands whose secretory cells have been atrophied after duct ligation (Langer, 1976); and c) binding studies reveal a loss of alpha sites after chemical sympathectomy. In fact, a 55%–70% reduction in the binding of ^{3}H-dihydroergocryptine and WB-4101 to membrane fragments prepared from rat cardiac ventricle was observed after pretreatment with 6-hydroxydopamine (Story, Briley, and Langer, 1978). These results suggest the existence of alpha receptor sites in noradrenergic nerve terminals.

Postulated mechanisms by which alpha presynaptic receptor activation reduces transmitter release: Although the studies mentioned support the alpha presynaptic theory for the regulation of NA release, the mechanism by which the activation of alpha presynaptic receptors reduced transmitter release is not known. It is clear from previous studies that the release process regulated by alpha receptors is exocytotic and thus Ca^{++} dependent. Studies by Stjärne (1973b, c) on the guinea pig vas deferens revealed that the alpha receptor blocking agents straighten out the curved shape of the relationship between NA and extracellular calcium concentration (see section on the role of Ca^{++} ions). This author suggested that alpha receptor activation leads to calcium restriction during depolarization, which is disinhibited in the presence of alpha receptor blockade. In addition, Langer et al. (1975) found that the inhibition of transmitter release obtained by exposure to exogenous NA is more pronounced when the calcium concentration in the medium is reduced from 2.6 to 0.26 mmol/L. The potentiation of the inhibitory effects of alpha receptor agonists on neurotransmission by a decreased calcium concentration was interpreted by these authors as an indication that activation of alpha receptors may reduce the availability of calcium for the secretory process. Although this possibility cannot be excluded, both studies could be interpreted differently. Since the effects of alpha antagonists and agonists on NA release depend on the concentration of the amine in the synaptic space, it is possible that the effects observed by Stjärne and Langer and coworkers would not be directly related to calcium, but to the degree of activation of alpha presynaptic receptors existent when the alpha agonists and antagonists were tested. A reduction in extracellular calcium diminishes the amount of exocytotic transmitter released by nerve stimulation and thus the degree of activation of alpha presynaptic receptors. Under these conditions, a greater effectiveness of alpha agonists in inhibiting NA release would be expected, as found by Langer et al. (1975); and within a range, a greater potentiation of NA release would be observed with alpha antagonists (Stjärne, 1973c, d).

The possible role of the Na^+-K^+-ATPase in the alpha regulation of release comes from experiments performed in the rat adrenal medulla incubated *in vitro* (Gutman and Boonyaviroj, 1977; Gutman, 1978). In such preparations, alpha receptor agonists (phenylephrine and naphazoline) reduced acetylcholine-induced release of catecholamines but had no effect on the release evoked by conditions that inhibited the Na^+-K^+-ATPase activity (K^+-free medium, ouabain). In addition, phenoxybenzamine and phentolamine enhanced acetylcholine-induced catecholamine release, but not that induced by K^+-free medium and ouabain. These results were interpreted as showing that activation of alpha presynaptic receptors could lead to depression of release by stimulating the Na^+-K^+-ATPase activity. In favor of this view are the results from *in vitro* studies indicating that an activation of this enzyme could be produced by NA and other alpha agonists. In fact, NA increased the Na^+-K^+-ATPase activity of synaptosomes, an effect prevented by alpha blockade (Gilbert, Wylie, and Davison, 1975). In addition, NA activated the Na^+ pump in frog skeletal muscle, and both naphazoline and phenylephrine stimulated the microsomal ATPase (Na^+-K^+) obtained from rat adrenals and had no effect on the Mg^{++}-ATPase activity of this subcellular fraction (Gutman and Boonyaviroj, 1977).

More recently, in membrane preparations from atrophied submaxillary glands produced by duct ligation, clonidine induced a 50% increase in the Na^+-K^+-ATPase activity, and denervation of the ligated gland abolished this effect (Gutman, 1978). However, as discussed in the section on ATPase, the catecholamine release induced by ATPase inhibition (K^+-free, ouabain) occurs rather slowly when compared with that evoked by acetylcholine, nerve stimulation, and/or K^+; and there is much controversy about the role of ATPase inhibition in the enhancement of exocytotic release of NA from sympathetic nerve terminals. Therefore, much has to be learned about the role of the Na^+-K^+-ATPase in the normal release process before it can be considered responsible for the alpha presynaptic regulation of NA release.

Recently, in rat pineal glands, Pelayo, Dubocovich, and Langer (1978) postulated that the inhibition of NA release by alpha presynaptic receptor activation could be mediated by an increase in the intraneuronal level of cyclic GMP.

Although the mechanism by which alpha presynaptic receptor activation decreases transmitter release is not known, this negative feedback control mechanism for regulating exocytotic release of NA has been shown to be present in all peripheral and central noradrenergic tissue studies. In addition, the magnitude of the increase in transmitter release observed with alpha receptor antagonists is much greater than that obtained with any of the other antagonists of presynaptic modulators (Starke, 1977), an indication of its important physiological role in the modulation of noradrenergic transmission.

C. Changes in NA Release Induced by
Drugs Apparently Non-Acting on Presynaptic Receptors

Drug-induced changes in the size and duration of action potentials are known to affect the amount of transmitter released per nerve impulse. Local anesthetics, tetrodotoxin, bretylium, guanethidine, and other neuron blocking agents are believed to reduce transmitter release by interfering with the development and propagation of action potentials in the nerve terminals (Jaanus, Miele, and Rubin, 1967; Haeusler, Haefely, and Huerlimann, 1969; Shand, Morgan, and Oates, 1973; Nickerson and Collier, 1975; Thoa et al., 1975). On the other hand, tetraethylammonium, 4-aminopyridine, and possibly scorpion toxins, which reduce potassium conductance and hence prolong the duration of the action potential, markedly enhance the release of noradrenaline evoked by nerve stimulation. The prolonged duration of the action potential would allow the calcium channels to remain open longer, leading to a greater entry of calcium and thus increasing the amount of transmitter released by an action potential (Thoenen, Haefely, and Staehelin, 1967; Kirpekar et al., 1972; Moss, Thoa, and Kopin, 1974; Kirpekar, Wakade, and Prat, 1976; Kirpekar, Kirpekar, and Prat, 1977). In addition to these agents, there is a group of structurally different compounds (papaverine, dypiridamole, RO-4-1284) which share as common characteristics an effect on storage granules (Brodie, 1960; Leitz and Stefano, 1971; Langer, 1973; Cubeddu et al., 1974b; Cubeddu and Weiner, 1975b) and a marked facilitation of noradrenaline overflow evoked by nerve stimulation (Langer, 1973; Cubeddu et al., 1974b; Cubeddu and Weiner,

1975b). Their effect on storage vesicles is demonstrated by the fact that these drugs markedly accelerate the efflux of ^{3}H-catechol-deaminated metabolites (^{3}H-3,4-dihydroxyphenylglycol, ^{3}H-DOPEG) from tissues prelabeled with ^{3}H-NA (Langer, 1974). The enhanced efflux of ^{3}H-DOPEG is dose related and calcium independent. On the other hand, the facilitatory effect of the above compounds on the stimulation-evoked transmitter release is calcium dependent and, at least for papaverine and RO-4-1284 (a benzoquinolizine), is accompanied by a greater output of DBH, indicating greater exocytotic transmitter release.

Dypiridamole and papaverine, but not RO-4-1284, are potent inhibitors of cyclic nucleotide phosphodiesterase (Weinryb et al., 1972). However, their effects on storage vesicles and on stimulation-elicited transmitter release do not seem to be mediated by cyclic nucleotide accumulation. In fact, treatment with cyclic nucleotide analogs and phosphodiesterase inhibitors not only had no effect on storage and only minimal effects on transmitter release but also failed to modify the effects of papaverine on basal and stimulation-induced transmitter release (Cubeddu et al., 1974b, 1975). Although the mechanism by which these agents increase exocytotic release is not clear, a relationship between an effect on storage vesicles and enhanced neurotransmitter secretion has been proposed (Cubeddu et al., 1974b; Cubeddu and Weiner, 1975a, b). However, no correlation was observed for one concentration of papaverine between its effects on storage (basal efflux of ^{3}H-DOPEG) and on stimulation-evoked release. In addition, propranolol reduced papaverine effects on transmitter release, even though its granular effect was enhanced (Celuch et al., 1976). Therefore, further studies are required to determine whether an effect on storage vesicles could modify exocytotic transmitter release and to determine the intrinsic mechanism by which stimulus-secretion coupling is facilitated. It should be emphasized that this group of drugs, together with alpha receptor antagonists and with agents that prolong the duration of the action potentials, are the compounds which produce the greater increase in transmitter release elicited by nerve stimulation.

VII. REFERENCES

Ackerly, J.; Blumberg, A.; Peach, M.: Angiotensin Interactions with Myocardial Sympathetic Neurons. Enhanced Release of Dopamine-β-Hydroxylase during Nerve Stimulation. Proc Soc Exp Biol (NY) 151(1976)650–653

Adler-Graschinsky, E.; Rubio, M.C.; Langer, E.Z.: Caminos metabólicos selectivos de la noradrenalina tritiada liberada por estímulos nerviosos y por agentes farmacológicos en aurículas aisladas de cobayo. Resúmenes de Comunicaciones de la Tercera Reuníon de la Sociedad Argentina de Farmacología Experimental (1970)10–11

Aguirre, J.; Pinto, J.E.B.; Trifaró, J.M.: Calcium Movements during the Release of Catecholamines from the Adrenal Medulla: Effects of Methoxyverapamil and External Cations. J Physiol (Lond) 269(1977)371–394

Akert, K.; Pfenniger, K.; Sandri, C.; Moor, H.: Freeze Etching and Cytochemistry of Vesicles and Membrane Complexes in Synapses in the Central Nervous System. In: Structure and Function of Synapses, pp 67–86, ed. by G.D. Pappas, D.P. Purpura. Raven, New York, 1972

Avakian, O.V.; Gillespie, J.S.: Uptake of Noradrenaline by Adrenergic Nerves, Smooth Muscle and Connective Tissue in Isolated Perfused Arteries and its Correlation with the Vasoconstrictor Response. Br J Pharmacol 32(1968)168–184

Bacq, Z.M.: Recherches sur la physiologie du système nerveux autonome. III: Les propriétés biologiques et physicochimiques de la sympathine comparées à celles de l'adrénaline. Arch Int Physiol 36(1933)167–246

Baker, P.F.: Transport and Metabolism of Calcium Ions in Nerve. In: Prog Biophys Mol Biol, Vol. XXII, pp. 177–223, ed. by J.A.V. Butler, D. Noble. Pergamon, Oxford-New York, 1972

Baker, P.F.; Crawford, A.C.: A Note on the Mechanism by Which Inhibitors of the Sodium Pump Accelerate Spontaneous Release of Transmitter from Motor Nerve Terminals. J Physiol 247(1975)209–226

Baker, P.F.; Hodgkin, A.L.; Ridgway, E.B.: Depolarization and Calcium Entry in Squid Giant Axons. J Physiol 218(1971)709–755

Baker, P.F.; Reuter, H.: Calcium Movement in Excitable Cells. Pergamon, New York, 1975

Baker, P.F.; Rink, T.J.: Catecholamine Release from Bovine Adrenal Medulla in Response to Maintained Depolarization. J Physiol 253(1975)593–620

Baker, P.F.; Schlaepfer, W.: Calcium Uptake by Axoplasm Extruded from Giant Axons of Loligo. J Physiol (Lond) 241(1975)37P-38P

Banks, P.: The Adenosine-Triphosphatase Activity of Adrenal Chromaffin Granules. Biochem J 95(1965)490–496

Banks, P.: An Interaction Between Chromaffin Granules and Calcium Ions. Biochem J 101(1966)18C-20C

Banks, P: The Effect of Ouabain on the Secretion of Catecholamines and on the Intracellular Concentration of Potassium. J Physiol 193(1967)631–637

Banks, P.; Biggins, R.; Bishop, R.; Christian, B.; Currie, N.: Sodium Ions and the Secretion of Catecholamines. J Physiol 200(1969)797–805

Banks, P.; Helle, K.: The Release of Protein from the Stimulated Adrenal Medulla. Biochem J 97(1965)40C-41C

Barbella, Y.R.; Marrero, A.; Israel, A.; Trifaró, J.M.; Cubeddu X., L.: Circulating Dopamine Beta-Hydroxylase and Catecholamines in Dog, Rat and Guinea-Pig During Hemorrhagic and Hypoglycemia Stress. VII Int Cong Pharmacol, Paris, July 16–21, 1978, 2401A

Barger, G.; Dale, H.H.: Chemical Structure and Sympathomimetic Action of Amines. J Physiol (Lond) 41(1910)19–59

Bartlett, S.F.; Lagercrantz, H.; Smith, A.D.: Gel Electrophoresis of Soluble and Insoluble Proteins of Noradrenergic Vesicles from Ox Splenic Nerve: A Comparison With Proteins of Adrenal Chromaffin Granules. Neuroscience 1(1976)339–344

Bell, C.; Vogt, M.: Release of Endogenous Noradrenaline from an Isolated Muscular Artery. J Physiol (Lond) 215(1971)509–520

Bennett, M.R.: An Electrophysiological Analysis of Storage and Release of Noradrenaline at Sympathetic Nerve Terminals. J Physiol (Lond) 229(1973a)515–531

Bennett, M.R.: An Electrophysiological Analysis of the Uptake of Noradrenaline at Sympathetic Nerve Terminals. J Physiol (Lond) 229(1973b)533–546

Berl, S.; Puszkin, S.; Nicklas, W.J.: Actomyosin-Like Protein in Brain. Actomyosin-Like Protein May Function in the Release of Transmitter Material at Synaptic Endings. Science (NY) 179(1973)441–446

Berneis, K.H.; Pletscher, A.; Da Prada, M.: Interaction of Proteins with Aggregates of Catecholamines: Possible Biological Implications. Agents and Actions 2(1971)65–68

Bisby, M.A.; Fillenz, M.: The Storage of Endogenous Noradrenaline in Sympathetic Nerve Terminals. J Physiol (Lond) 215(1971)163–179

Bisby, M.A.; Fillenz, M.; Smith, A.D.: Evidence for the Presence of Dopamine β-Hydroxylase in Both Populations of Noradrenaline Storage Vesicles in Sympathetic Nerve Terminals of the Rat Vas Deferens. J Neurochem 20(1973)245–248

236 / José M. Trifaró and Luigi Cubeddu X.

Blakeley, A.G.H.; Brown, L.; Ferry, C.B.: Pharmacological Experiments on the Release of the Sympathetic Transmitter. J Physiol (Lond) 167(1963)505–514
Blaschko, H.; Firemark, H.; Smith, A.D.; Winkler, H.: Lipids of the Adrenal Medulla: Lysolecithin, a Characteristic Constituent of Chromaffin Granules. Biochem J 104(1967)545–549
Blaschko, H.; Welch, A.D.: Localization of Adrenaline in Cytoplasmic Particles of the Bovine Adrenal Medulla. Naunyn-Schmiedebergs Arch Pharmacol 219(1953)17–22
Blaszkowski, T.P.; Bogdanski, D.F.: Possible Role of Sodium and Calcium Ions in Retention and Physiological Release of Norepinephrine by Adrenergic Nerve Endings. Biochem Pharmacol 20(1971)3281–3294
Blaustein, M.P.: Effects of Potassium, Veratridine and Scorpion Venom on Calcium Accumulation and Transmitter Release by Nerve Terminals In Vitro. J Physiol (Lond) 247(1975)617–655
Blaustein, M.P.; Ector, A.C.: Carrier-Mediated Sodium-Dependent and Calcium-Dependent Calcium Efflux from Pinched-Off Presynaptic Nerve Terminals (Synaptosomes) In Vitro. Biochim Biophys Acta 419(1976)295–308
Blaustein, M.P.; Hodgkin, A.L.: The Effect of Cyanamide on the Efflux of Calcium from Squid Giant Axons. J Physiol (Lond) 200(1969)497–527
Blaustein, M.P.; Johnson, E.M.; Needleman, P.: Calcium-Dependent Norepinephrine Release from Presynaptic Nerve Endings In Vitro. Proc Natl Acad Sci USA 69(1972)2237–2240
Bloom, F.E.: Electron Microscopy of Catecholamine-Containing Structures. In: Handbook of Experimental Pharmacology, Vol. XXXIII, Catecholamines, pp 46–78, ed. by H. Blaschko, E. Muscholl. Springer, Berlin-New York, 1972
Borowsky, E.; Ehrl, H.; Starke, K.: Relative Pre- and Postsynaptic Potencies of Adrenolytic Drugs. Naunyn Schmiedebergs Arch Pharmacol 293(1976)R2
Boullin, D.J.: The Action of Extracellular Cations on the Release of the Sympathetic Transmitter From Peripheral Nerves. J Physiol (Lond) 189(1967)85–99
Boullin, D.J.; Costa, E.; Brodie, B.B.: Evidence That Blockade of Adrenergic Receptors Causes Overflow of Norepinephrine in Cat's Colon after Nerve Stimulation. J Pharmacol Exp Ther 157(1967)125–134
Brodie, B.B.: Selective Release of Norepinephrine and Serotonin by Reserpinelike Compounds. Dis Nerv Sys 21(1960)107–109
Brown, G.L.: The Release and Fate of the Transmitter Liberated by Adrenergic Nerves. Proc R Soc Lond (Biol) 162(1965)1–19
Brown, G.L.; Davies, B.N.; Gillespie, J.S.: The Release of Chemical Transmitter From the Sympathetic Nerves of the Intestine of the Cat. J Physiol (Lond) 143(1958)41–54
Brown, G.L.; Gillespie, J.S.: The Output of Sympathetic Transmitter from the Spleen of the Cat. J Physiol (Lond) 138(1957)81–102
Buckley, J.T.; Hawthorne, J.N.: Erythrocyte Membrane Polyphosphoinositide Metabolism and the Regulation of Calcium Binding. J Biol Chem 247(1972)7218–7223
Burnstock, G.; Costa, M.: Adrenergic Neurons. Wiley, New York, 1975
Burridge, K.; Bray, D.: Purification and Structural Analysis of Myosins from Brain and Other Non-Muscle Tissues. J Mol Biol 99(1975)1–14
Burridge, K.; Phillips, J.M.: Association of Actin and Myosin with Secretory Granule Membranes. Nature 254(1975)526–529
Carafoli, E.; Malström, K.; Capana, M.; Sigel, E.; Crompton, M.: Mitochondria and the Regulation of Cell Calcium. In: Calcium Transport in Contraction and Secretion, pp. 53–64, ed. by E. Carafoli, F. Clementi, W. Drabikowski, A. Margreth. North-Holland, Amsterdam-Oxford, 1975
Celuch, S.M.; Dubocovich, M.L.; Langer, S.Z.; Redondo, J.: Influencia de la temperatura sobre los mecanismos que regulan la liberación de noradrenalina inducida por la estimulación nerviosa, a traves de receptores alfa y beta presinápticos, en el bazo perfundido del gato. Proc VI Latin Amer Cong of Pharmacology, Buenos Aires, 1976, 22A
Chang, C.C.; Chiueh, C.C.: Modulation of Noradrenaline Incorporation by Nerve Activities in the Rat Submaxillary Gland. J Physiol (Lond) 203(1969)145–157
Chubb, I.W.; De Potter, W.P.; De Schaepdryver, A.F.: Two Populations of Noradrenaline-Containing Particles in the Spleen. Nature 228(1970)1203–1204
Cramer, W.: Further Observations on the Thyroid-Adrenal Apparatus. A Histochemical

Method for the Demonstration of the Adrenalin Granules in the Suprarenal Gland. J Physiol (Lond) 52(1918)viii-x

Creutz, C.E.: Isolation, Characterization and Localization of Bovine Adrenal Medullary Myosin. Cell Tissue Res 178(1977)17–38

Creutz, C.E.; Pazoles, C.J.; Pollard, H.B.: Identification and Purification of an Adrenal Medullary Protein (Synexin) That Causes Calcium Dependent Aggregation of Isolated Chromaffin Granules. J Biol Chem 253(1978)2858–2866

Cubeddu X., L.; Barnes, E.M.; Langer, S.Z.; Weiner, N.: Release of Norepinephrine and Dopamine-Beta-Hydroxylase by Nerve Stimulation. I. Role of Neuronal and Extraneuronal Uptake and of Alpha Presynaptic Receptors. J Pharmacol Exp Ther 190(1974a)431–450

Cubeddu X., L.; Barnes, E.M.; Weiner, N.: Release of Norepinephrine and Dopamine-β-Hydroxylase by Nerve Stimulation. II. Effects of Papaverine. J Pharmacol Exp Ther 191(1974b)444–457

Cubeddu X., L.; Barnes, E.; Weiner, N.: Release of Norepinephrine and Dopamine-β-Hydroxylase by Nerve Stimulation. IV. An Evaluation of a Role for Cyclic Adenosine Monophosphate. J Pharmacol Exp Ther 193(1975)105–127

Cubeddu X., L.; Langer, S.Z.; Weiner, N.: The Relationships between Alpha Receptor Block, Inhibition of Norepinephrine and the Release and Metabolism of ^{3}H-Norepinephrine. J Pharmacol Exp Ther 188(1974c)368–385

Cubeddu X., L.; Talmaciu, R.; Pinardi, G.; Santiago, E.: Arterial, Venous and Lymph Dopamine Beta-Hydroxylase and Catecholamines During Hemorrhagic Hypotension, in Dogs. VII Int Cong Pharmacol, Paris, July 16–21, 1978, 2400 A

Cubeddu X., L.; Vargas, A.M.: Effects of Sodium Chloride on Phenylethanolamine N-Methyltransferase Activity. Molec Pharmacol 13(1977)172–180

Cubeddu X., L.; Weiner, N.: Nerve Stimulation-Mediated Overflow of Norepinephrine and Dopamine-β-hydroxylase. III. Effects of Norepinephrine Depletion on the Alpha Presynaptic Regulation of Release. J Pharmacol Exp Ther 192(1975a)1–14

Cubeddu X., L.; Weiner, N.: Release of Norepinephrine and Dopamine-β-hydroxylase by Nerve Stimulation. V. Enhanced Release Associated With a Granular Effect of a Benzoquinolizine Derivative with Reserpine-Like Properties. J Pharmacol Exp Ther 193(1975b)757–774

Davies, B.N.; Robinson, B.H.; Withrington, P.G.: The Effects of Graded Doses of Phenoxybenzamine on the Vascular and Capsular Responses of the Isolated Blood Perfused Dogs Spleen to Sympathetic Nerve Stimulation and Catecholamines. Arch Int Pharmacodyn Ther 180(1969)143–154

Dean, P.M.: Exocytosis Modelling: An Electrostatic Function for Calcium in Stimulus-Secretion Coupling. J Theor Biol 54(1975)289–308

Dean, P.M.; Matthews, E.K.: The London-Van der Walls Attraction Constant of Secretory Granules and its Significance. J Theor Biol 54(1975)309–321

De Potter, W.P.; Chubb, I.W.: Biochemical Observations on the Formation of Small Noradrenergic Vesicles in the Splenic Nerve of the Dog. Neuroscience 2(1977)167–174

De Potter, W.P.; Chubb, I.W.; De Schaepdryver, A.F.: Pharmacological Aspects of Peripheral Noradrenergic Transmission. Arch Int Pharmacodyn 196(1972)258–287

De Potter, W.P.; Chubb, I.W.; Put, A.; De Schaepdryver, A.F.: Facilitation of the Release of Noradrenaline and Dopamine β-Hydroxylase at Low Stimulation Frequencies by α-Blocking Agents. Arch Int Pharmacodyn 193(1971)191–197

De Potter, W.P.; De Schaepdryver, A.F.; Moerman, E.J.; Smith, A.D.: Evidence for the Release of Vesicle-Proteins Together with Noradrenaline upon Stimulation of the Splenic Nerve. J Physiol (Lond) 204(1969a)102P–104P

De Potter, W.P.; Moerman, E.J.; De Schaepdryver, A.F.; Smith, A.D.: Release of Noradrenaline and Dopamine β-Hydroxylase Upon Splenic Nerve Stimulation. IV Int Cong Pharmacol, p 146, 1969b

De Potter, W.P.; Smith, A.D.; De Schaepdryver, A.F.: Subcellular Fractionations of Splenic Nerve: ATP, Chromogranin A and Dopamine β-Hydroxylase in Noradrenergic Vesicles. Tissue & Cell 2(1970)529–546

De Robertis, E.; Vaz Ferreira, A.: Electron Microscope Study of the Secretion of Catechol-Containing Droplets in the Adrenal Medulla. Exp Cell Res 12(1957)568–574

Diliberto, E.J.; Viveros, O.H.; Axelrod, J.: Subcellular Distribution of Protein Carboxy-methylase and Its Endogenous Substrates in the Adrenal Medulla: Possible Role in Excitation-Secretion Coupling. Proc Natl Acad Sci USA 73(1976)4050–4054

Diner, O: L'Expulsion des granules de la médullosurrénale chez le hamster. CR Acad Sci (Paris) 265(1967)616–619

Dixon, W.R.; García, A.G.; Kirpekar, S.M.: Release of Catecholamines and Dopamine β-Hydroxylase from the Perfused Adrenal Gland of the Cat. J Physiol (Lond) 244 (1975)805–824

Dixon, W.R.; Mosimann, W.F.; Weiner, N.: The Role of Presynaptic Feedback Mechanisms Regulation of Norepinephrine Release by Nerve Stimulation. Pharmacologist 19(1977)239

Dixon, W.R.; Mosimann, W.F.; Weiner, N.: Effect of Dopamine on the Nerve Stimulation Mediated Release of Norepinephrine (NE) and Dopamine-β-Hydroxylase (DBH) from the Isolated Perfused Cat Spleen, 4th Int Catecholamine Symp (1978) Abst 393

Dodge, F.A.; Rahamimoff, R.: Co-operative Action of Calcium Ions in Transmitter Release at the Neuromuscular Junction. J Physiol (Lond) 193(1967)419–432

Douglas, W.W.: Stimulus-Secretion Coupling: The Concept and Clues from Chromaffin and Other Cells. Br J Pharmacol 34(1968)451–474

Douglas, W.W.: Mechanism of Release of Neurohypophysial Hormones. Stimulus-Secretion Coupling. In: Handbook of Physiology, Endocrinology, Vol. IV, pp. 191–224, ed. by E. Knobil, W.H. Sawyer. American Physiological Society, Washington, 1974

Douglas, W.W.: Secremotor Control of Adrenal Medullary Secretion: Synaptic, Membrane and Ionic Events in Stimulus-Secretion Coupling. In: Handbook of Physiology, Endocrinology, Vol. VI, pp. 367–388, ed. by H. Blaschko, G. Sayers, A.D. Smith. American Physiological Society, Washington, 1975

Douglas, W.W.; Poisner, A.M.; Rubin, R.P.: Efflux of Adenine Nucleotides from Perfused Adrenal Glands Exposed to Nicotine and Other Chromaffin Cell Stimulants. J Physiol (Lond) 179(1965)130–137

Douglas, W.W.; Poisner, A.M.; Trifaró, J.M.: Lysolecithin and Other Phospholipids in The Adrenal Medulla of Various Species. Life Sci 5(1966)809–815

Douglas, W.W.; Rubin, R.P.: The Role of Calcium in the Secretory Response of the Adrenal Medulla to Acetylcholine. J Physiol (Lond) 159(1961)40–47

Douglas, W.W.; Rubin R.P.: The Mechanism of Catecholamine Release from the Adrenal Medulla and the Role of Calcium in Stimulus-Secretion Coupling. J Physiol (Lond) 167(1963)288–310

Douglas, W.W.; Sorimachi, M.: Cholchicine Inhibits Adrenal Medullary Secretion Evoked by Acetylcholine Without Affecting That Evoked by Potassium. Br J Pharmacol 45 (1972a)129–132

Douglas, W.W.; Sorimachi, M.: Effects of Cytochalasin B and Colchicine on Secretion of Posterior Pituitary and Adrenal Medullary Hormones. Br J Pharmacol Chemother 45(1972b)143–144

Draskocsy, P.R.; Trendelenburg, U.: Intraneuronal and Extraneuronal Accumulation of Sympathomimetic Amines in the Isolated Nictitating Membrane of the Cat. J Pharmacol Exp Ther 174(1970)290–306

Dreifuss, J.J.: Akert, K.; Sandri, C.; Moor, H.: Specific Arrangements of Membrane Particles at Sites of Exo-Endocytosis in the Freeze-Etched Neurohypophysis. Cell Tissue Res 165(1976)317–325

Droz, B.; Rambourg, A.; Koenig, H.: The Smooth Endoplasmic Reticulum: Structure and Role in the Renewal of Axonal Membrane and Synaptic Vesicles by Fast Axonal Transport. Brain Res 93(1975)1–13

Dubocovich, M.L.; Langer, S.Z.: Negative Feed-back Regulation of Noradrenaline Release by Nerve Stimulation in the Perfused Cat's Spleen: Differences in Potency of Phenoxy-benzamine in Blocking the Pre- and Post-Synaptic Adrenergic Receptors. J Physiol (Lond) 237(1974)505–519

Dubocovich, M.L.; Langer, S.Z.: Influence of the Frequency of Nerve Stimulation on the Metabolism of ^{3}H-Norepinephrine Released from the Perfused Cat Spleen: Differences Observed During and After the Period of Stimulation. J Pharmacol Exp Ther 198(1977)83–101

Eisenfeld, A.J.; Axelrod, J.; Krakoff, L.: Inhibition of the Extraneuronal Accumulation and Metabolism of Norepinephrine by Adrenergic Blocking Agents. J Pharmacol Exp Ther 156(1967)107–113

Elliott, T.R.: The Action of Adrenalin. J Physiol (Lond) 32(1905)401–467

Enero, M.A.; Langer, S.Z.: Influence of Reserpine-Induced Depletion of Noradrenaline on the Negative Feed-Back Mechanism for Transmitter Release During Nerve Stimulation. Br J Pharmacol 49(1973)214–225

Enero, M.A.; Langer, S.Z.; Rothlin, R.P.; Stefano, F.J.E.: Role of the α-Adrenoceptor in Regulating Noradrenaline Overflow by Nerve Stimulation. Br J Pharmacol 44(1972)672–688

Farnebo, L.-O.: Effect of Reserpine on Release of (^{3}H)Noradrenaline, (^{3}H)Dopamine and (^{3}H)Metaraminol From Field Stimulated Rat Iris. Biochem Pharmacol 20(1971)2715–2726

Farnebo, L.O.; Hamberger, B.: Effects of Desipramine, Phentolamine and Phenoxybenzamine on the Release of Noradrenaline from Isolated Tissues. J Pharm Pharmacol 22 (1970a)855–857

Farnebo, L.-O.; Hamberger, B.: Release of Norepinephrine From Isolated Rat Iris by Field Stimulation. J Pharmacol Exp Ther 172(1970b)332–341

Farnebo, L.O.; Hamberger, B.: Drug-Induced Changes in the Release of ^{3}H-Monoamines from Field Stimulated Rat Brain Slices. Acta Physiol Scand Suppl 371(1971a)35–44

Farnebo, L.O.; Hamberger, B.: Drug-Induced Changes in the Release of (^{3}H)-Noradrenaline from Field Stimulated Rat Iris. Br J Pharmacol 43(1971b)97–106

Farnebo, L.O.; Malmfors, T.: ^{3}H-Noradrenaline Release and Mechanical Response in the Field Stimulated Mouse Vas Deferens. Acta Physiol Scand Suppl 371(1971)1–18

Fillenz, M.: Fine Structure of Noradrenaline Storage Vesicles in Nerve Terminals of the Rat Vas Deferens. Philos Trans R Soc Lond (Biol) 261(1971)319–323

Fillenz, M; Gagnon, C.; Stoeckel, R.; Thoenen, H.: Selective Uptake and Retrograde Axonal Transport of Dopamine β-Hydroxylase Antibodies in Peripheral Adrenergic Neurons. Brain Res 114(1976)293–303

Fillenz, M.; West, D.P.: Changes in Vesicular Dopamine β-Hydroxylase Resulting from Transmitter Release. J Neurochem 23(1974)411–416

Fine, R.E.; Blitz, A.L.: Chemical and Functional Studies of Tropomyosin and Troponin C from Brain and Other Tissues. In: Cell Motility, pp. 785–795, ed. by R. Goldman, T. Pollard, J. Rosenbaum. Cold Spring Harbor, 1976

Fine, R.E.; Blitz, A.L.; Hitchcock, S.E.; Kaminer, B.: Tropomyosin in Brain and Growing Neurones. Nature (New Biol) 245(1973)182–186

Fine, R.E.; Bray, D.: Actin in Growing Nerve Cells. Nature (New Biol) 234(1971)115–118

Fisher, J.E.; Horst, W.D.; Kopin, J.J.: β-hydroxylated Sympathomimetic Amines As False Neurotransmitters. Br J Pharmacol 24(1965)477–484

Fredholm, B.B.; Hedqvist, P.: Presynaptic Inhibition of Transmitter Release by Adenosine and Its Antagonism by Theophylline. Presynaptic Receptors. VII Int Cong Pharmacol, Paris, July 16–21 (1978) 43

García, A.G.; Kirpekar, S.M.: Release of Noradrenaline from Cat Spleen by Sodium Deprivation. Br J Pharmacol 47(1973)720–747

García, A.G.; Kirpekar, S.M.: Inhibition of Na-K-activated ATPase and Release of Neurotransmitters. Nature 257(1975)722

Geffen, L.B.: The Effect of Desmethylimipramine upon the Overflow of Sympathetic Transmitter From the Cat's Spleen. J Physiol (Lond) 181(1965)69–70P

Geffen, L.B.; Livett, B.G.: Axoplasmic Transport of ¹⁴C-Noradrenaline and Protein and Their Release by Nerve Impulses. Proc Int Union Physiol Sci 7(1968)152

Geffen, L.B.; Livett, B.G.: Origin, Functions and Fate of Synaptic Vesicles in Sympathetic Neurones. Physiol Rev 51(1971)98–157

Geffen, L.B.; Livett, B.G.; Rush, R.A.: Immunological Localization of Chromogranins in Sheep Sympathetic Neurones, and Their Release by Nerve Impulses. J Physiol (Lond) 204(1969)58–59P

Geffen, L.B.; Livett, B.G.; Rush, R.A.: Immunohistochemical Localization of Chromogranins in Sheep Sympathetic Neurones and Their Release by Nerve Impulses. In: New Aspects of Storage and Release Mechanism of Catecholamines (Bayer Symposium II), pp. 58–72, ed. by H.J. Schümann, G. Kroneberg, Springer, Berlin, 1970

Gewirtz, G.P.; Kopin, I.J.: Release of Dopamine β-Hydroxylase with Norepinephrine during Cat Splenic Nerve Stimulation. Nature (Lond) 227(1970)406–407

Gilbert, J.C.; Wylie, M.G.; Davison, D.V.: Nerve Terminal ATPase As Possible Trigger for Neurotransmitter Release. Nature 255(1975)237–238

Gillespie, J.S.; Hamilton, D.N.H.; Hosie, R.J.A.: The Extraneuronal Uptake and Localization of Noradrenaline in the Cat Spleen and the Effects on This of Some Drugs, of Cold and of Denervation. J Physiol (Lond) 206(1970)563–590

Gillespie, J.S.; Kirpekar, S.M.: The Uptake and Release of Radioactive Noradrenaline by the Splenic Nerves of Cats. J Physiol (Lond) 187(1966)51–58

Gillis, C.N.: Increased Retention of Exogenous Norepinephrine by Cat Atrica After Electrical Stimulation of the Cardioaccelerator Nerves. Biochem Pharmacol 12(1963)593–595

Glassman, P.M.; Angelakos, E.T.; McNary, W.F.: Catecholamine-Containing Fractions of Dog Heart Homogenates. Life Sci 4(1965)1727–1734

Goldstein, D.J.; Cubeddu X., L.: Dopamine-Beta-Hydroxylase Activity in Human Cerebrospinal Fluid. J Neurochem 261(1976)193–195

Goldstein, M.; Freedman, L.S.; Bonnay, M.: An Assay for Dopamine-Beta-Hydroxylase Activity in Tissues and Serum. Experientia 27(1971)632–633

Gratzl, M.; Dahl, G.; Russell, J.T.; Thorn, N.A.: Fusion of Neurohypophyseal Membranes in Vitro. Biochim Biophys Acta 470(1977)45–57

Grillo, M.A.: Electron Microscopy of Sympathetic Tissues. Pharmacol Rev 18(1966)387–399

Grodsky, G.M.; Landahl, H.; Curry, D.; Bennett, L.: In Vitro Studies Suggesting a Two-Compartmental Model for Insulin Secretion. In: Structure and Metabolism of the Pancreatic Islets, pp. 409–420, ed. by S. Falkmer, B. Hellman, I.B. Täljedal. Pergamon, Oxford, 1969

Gutman, Y.: Molecular Mechanism in the Modulation of Catecholamine Release from the Adrenal Medulla. VII Int Cong Pharmacol (1978) 222O A

Gutman, Y.; Boonyaviroj, P.: Inhibition of Catecholamine Release by Alpha-Adrenergic Activation: Interaction with Na,K-ATPase. J Neural Transm 40(1977)245–252

Haefely, W.; Hürlimann, A.; Thoenen, H.: Relation between the Rate of Stimulation and the Quantity of Noradrenaline Liberated from Sympathetic Nerve Endings in the Isolated Perfused Spleen of the Cat. J Physiol (Lond) 181(1965)48–58

Haeusler, G.; Haefely, W.; Huerlimann. A.: On the Mechanism of the Adrenergic Nerve Blocking Action of Bretylium. Naunyn Schmiedebergs Arch Pharmacol 265(1969)260–277

Häggendal, J.: Some Further Aspects on the Release of the Adrenergic Transmitter. In: New Aspects of Storage and Release Mechanism of Catecholamines (Bayer Symposium II), pp. 100–109, ed by H.J. Schümann, G. Kroneberg. Springer, Berlin, 1970

Häggendal, J.; Malmfors, T.: The Effect of Nerve Stimulation on Catecholamines Taken Up in Adrenergic Nerves After Reserpine Pretreatment. Acta Physiol Scand 75(1969a)33–38

Häggendal, J.; Malmfors, T.: The Effect of Nerve Stimulation on the Uptake of Noradrenaline into the Adrenergic Nerve Terminals. Acta Physiol Scand 75(1969b)28–32

Helle, K.B.; Lagercrantz, H.; Stjärne, L.: Biochemistry of Catecholamine Storage: Some Similarities between Whole Sympathetic Nerve Trunk Vesicles and the Membranes of Adrenomedullary Vesicles. Acta Physiol Scand 81(1971)565–567

Henderson, G.; Hughes, J.: Modulation of Frequency-Dependent Noradrenaline Release by Calcium, Angiotensin and Morphine. Br J Pharmacol 52(1974)455–465P

Henderson, G.; Hughes, J.; Kosterlitz, H.W.: The Effects of Morphine on the Release of Noradrenaline from the Cat Isolated Nictitating Membrane and the Guinea-Pig Ileum Myenteric Plexus. Longitudinal Muscle Preparation. Br J Pharmacol 53(1975)505–512

Henderson, G.; Hughes, J.; Thompson, J.W.: The Variation of Noradrenaline Output with Frequency of Nerve Stimulation and the Effect of Morphine on the Cat Nictitating Membrane and on the Guinea-Pig Myenteric Plexus. Br J Pharmacol 46(1972)524–525P

Hillarp, N.Å.: Different Pools of Catecholamines Stored in the Adrenal Medulla. Acta Physiol Scand 50(1960)8–22

Hillarp, N.Å.; Lagerstedt, S., Nilson, B.: The Isolation of a Granular Fraction from the Suprarenal Medulla, Containing the Sympathomimetic Catecholamines. Acta Physiol Scand 29(1953)251–263

Himes, R.H.; Kersey, R.N.; Ruscha, M.; Houston, L.L.: Cytochalasin A Inhibits the in Vitro

Polymerization of Brain Tubulin and Muscle Actin. Biochem Biophys Res Commun 68(1976)1362-1370

Hökfelt, T.: Distribution of Noradrenaline Storing Particles in Peripheral Adrenergic Neurons as Revealed by Electron Microscopy. Acta Physiol Scand 76(1969)427-440

Hökfelt, T.: Neuronal Catecholamine Storage Vesicles. In: Frontiers in Catecholamine Research, pp. 439-446, ed by E. Usdin, S. Snyder. Pergamon, New York-Oxford, 1973

Holman, M.E.: Junction Potentials in Smooth Muscle. In: Smooth Muscle, pp. 244-288, ed. by E. Bülbring, A.F. Brading, A.W. Jones, T. Tomita. Edward Arnold, London, 1970

Horga, J.F.; Hernandez, M.; García, A.G.; Esquerro, E.; Sánchez-García, P: Ouabain Induces Release of Catecholamines and Dopamine-Beta-Hydroxylase from the Perfused Cat Adrenal Gland. VII. Int Cong Pharmacol, Paris, July 16-21 (1978)2407 A

Hörtnagl, H.; Hörtnagl, H.; Winkler, H.: Bovine Splenic Nerve: Characterization of Nora-drenaline-Containing Vesicles and Other Cell Organelles by Density Gradient Centrifugation. J Physiol (Lond) 205(1969)103-114

Hoshi, M.; Shreeve, W.W.: Release and Production of Insulin by Isolated, Perifused Rat Pancreatic Islets. Diabetes 22(1973)16-24

Hosie, R.J.A.: The Localization of Adenosine Triphosphatases in Morphologically Characterized Fractions of Guinea-Pig Brain. Biochem J 96(1965)404-412

Houssay, B.A.; Molinelli, E.A.: Excitabilité des fibres adrénalino-sécrétoires du nerf grand splanchnique. Fréquences, seuil et optimum des stimulus. Rôle de l'ion calcium. C R Soc Biol 99(1928)172-174

Hughes, J.: Evaluation of Mechanism Controlling the Release and Inactivation of the Adrenergic Transmitter in the Rabbit Portal Vein and Vas Deferens. Br J Pharmacol 44(1972)472-491

Huković, S.; Muscholl, E.: Die Noradrenalin-Abgabe aus dem isolierten Kaninchenherzen bei sympatischer Nervenreizung und ihre pharmakologische Beeinflussung. Naunyn-Schmiedebergs Arch Pharmacol 244(1962)81-96

Iijima, K.; Awazi, N.: Histochemical Studies on the Morphology of the Golgi Apparatus and Its Relationship to Catecholamine Biosynthesis in the Locus Coeruleus of the Rat. Z Zellforsch Mikrosk Anat 136(1973)329-348

Iversen, L.L.: The Uptake and Storage of Noradrenaline in Sympathetic Nerves. The University Press, Cambridge, 1967

Iversen, L.L.; Glowinski, J.; Axelrod, J.: The Uptake and Storage of [^{3}H] Norepinephrine in the Reserpine-Pretreated Rat Heart. J Pharmacol Exp Ther 150(1965)173-183

Iversen, L.L.; Langer, S.Z.: Effects of Phenoxybenzamine on the Uptake and Metabolism of Noradrenaline in the Rat Heart and Vas Deferens. Br J Pharmacol 37(1969)627-637

Jaanus, S.D.; Miele, E.; Rubin, R.P.: The Analysis of the Inhibitory Effect of Local Anesthetics and Propranolol on Adrenomedullary Secretion Evoked by Calcium or Acetylcholine. Br J Pharmacol Chemother 31(1967)319-330

Jacobowitz, D.M.; Ziegler, M.G.; Thomas, J.A.: In Vivo Uptake of Antibody to Dopamine β-Hydroxylase into Sympathetic Elements. Brain Res 91(1975)165-170

Jamieson, J.D.: Transport and Discharge of Exportable Proteins in Pancreatic Exocrine Cells: In Vitro Studies. Curr Top Membr Transp 3(1972)273-338

Jockusch, B.M.; Burger, M.M.; Da Prada, M.; Richards, J.G.; Chaponnier, C.; Gabbiani, G.: α-Actinin Attached to Membranes of Secretory Vesicles. Nature 270(1977)628-629

Johnson, D.G.; Thoa, N.B.; Weinshilboum, B.; Axelrod, J.; Kopin, I.J.: Enhanced Release of Dopamine-β-Hydroxylase from Sympathetic Nerves by Calcium and Phenoxybenzamine and its Reversal by Prostaglandins. Proc Natl Acad Sci (USA) 68(1971)2227-2230

Kanno, Y.; Loewenstein, W.R.: Cell-to-Cell Passage of Large Molecules. Nature 212(1966)629-630

Kapeller, K.; Mayor, D.: The Accumulation of Noradrenaline in Constricted Sympathetic Nerves as Studied by Fluorescence and Electron Microscopy. Proc R Soc Lond (Biol) 167(1967)282-292

Kaufman, S.; Friedman, S.: Dopamine-β-Hydroxylase. Pharmacol Rev 17(1965)71-100

Keen, P.M.; Bogdanski, D.F.: Sodium and Calcium Ions in Uptake and Release of Norepinephrine by Nerve Endings. Am J Physiol 219(1970)677-682

Kirpekar, S.M.; Cervoni, P.: Effect of Cocaine, Phenoxybenzamine and Phentolamine on the Catecholamine Output from Spleen and Adrenal Medulla. J Pharmacol Exp Ther 142(1963)59–70

Kirpekar, S.M.; Dixon, W.; Prat, J.C.: Inhibitory Effect of Manganese on Norepinephrine Release from the Splenic Nerves of Cats. J Pharmacol Exp Ther 174(1970)72–76

Kirpekar, M.; Kirpekar, S.M.; Prat, J.C.: Effect of 4-Aminopyridine on Release of Noradrenaline from the Perfused Cat Spleen by Nerve Stimulation. J Physiol 272(1977)517–528

Kirpekar, S.M.; Misu, Y.: Release of Noradrenaline by Splenic Nerve Stimulation and its Dependence Upon Calcium. J Physiol (Lond) 188(1967)219–234

Kirpekar, S.M.; Prat, J.D.; Puig, M.; Wakade, A.R.: Modification of the Evoked Release of Noradrenaline from the Perfused Cat Spleen by Various Ions and Agents. J Physiol (Lond) 221(1972)601–615

Kirpekar, S.M.; Puig, M.: Effect of Flow-Stop on Noradrenaline Release from Normal Spleens Treated with Cocaine, Phentolamine or Phenoxybenzamine. Br J Pharmacol 43(1971)359–369

Kirpekar, S.M.; Wakade, A.R.: Effects of Phenoxybenzamine on the Uptake and Metabolism of Noradrenaline in the Cat Heart and Vas Deferens. Br J Pharmacol 39(1970)533–541

Kirpekar, S.M.; Wakade, A.R.; Prat, J.C.: Effect of Tetraethylammonium and Barium on the Release of Noradrenaline from the Perfused Cat Spleen by Nerve Stimulation and Potassium. Naunyn-Schmiedebergs Arch Pharmacol 294(1976)23–29

Kirpekar, S.M.; Wakade, A.R.; Steinsland, O.S.; Prat, J.C.; Furchgott, R.F.: Inhibition of the Evoked Release of Norepinephrine (NE) by Sympathomimetic Amines. Fed Proc 31(1972)566A

Kirshner, N.; Sage, H.J.; Smith, W.J.; Kirshner, A.G.: Release of Catecholamines and Specific Protein from Adrenal Glands. Science 154(1966)529–531

Klein, R.L.: A Large Second Pool of Norepinephrine in the Highly Purified Vesicle Fraction from Bovine Splenic Nerve. In: Frontiers in Catecholamine research, pp. 423–425, ed. by E. Usdin, S. Snyder. Pergamon, New York, 1973

Klein, R.L.; Harden, T.K.: Accumulation of Newly Synthesized Norepinephrine in the Fast Release Pool of Purified Adrenergic Vesicle Fraction. Life Sci 16(1975)315–322

Kraicer, J.; Milligan, J.W.: Effect of Colchicine on in Vitro ACTH Release Induced by High K+ and by Hypothalamus-Stalk-Median Eminence Extract. Endocrinology 89(1971)408–412

Kristensson, K.; Olsson, Y.; Sjöstrand, J.: Axonal Uptake and Retrograde Transport of Exogenous Proteins in the Hypoglosal Nerve. Brain Res 32(1971)399–406

Kuo, I.C.Y.; Coffee, C.J.: Bovine Adrenal Medulla Troponin-C. Demonstration of a Calcium-Dependent Conformation Change. J Biol Chem 251(1976a)6315–6319

Kuo, I.C.Y.; Coffee, C.J.: Purification and Characterization of a Troponin-C-Like Protein from Bovine Adrenal Medulla. J Biol Chem 251(1976b)1603–1609

Labrie, F.; Gauthier, M.; Pelletier, G.; Borgeat, P.; Lemay, A.; Gouge, J.J.: Role of Microtubules in Basal and Stimulated Release of Growth Hormone and Prolactin in Rat Adenohypophysis in Vitro. Endocrinology 93(1973)903–914

Lacy, P.E.; Greider, M.H.: Ultrastructural Organization of Mammalian Pancreatic Islets. In: Handbook of Physiology, Endocrinology 1, pp. 77–89, ed. by D.F. Steiner, N. Freinkel. American Physiological Society, Washington, DC, 1972

Lacy, P.E.; Howell, S.L.; Young, D.A.; Fink, C.J.: New Hypothesis of Insulin Secretion. Nature 219(1968)1177–1179

Lacy, P.E.; Walker, M.M.; Fink, C.J.: Perifusion of Isolated Rat Islets in Vitro. Participation of the Microtubular System in the Biphasic Release of Insulin. Diabetes 21(1972)987–998

Lagercrantz, H.: Lipids of the Sympathetic Nerve Trunk Vesicles. Comparison with Adrenomedullary Vesicles. Acta Physiol Scand 82(1971)567–570

Lagercrantz, H.: On the Composition and Function of Large Dense Cored Vesicles in Sympathetic Nerves. Neuroscience 1(1976)81–92

Lagercrantz, H.; Kirksey, D.F.; Klein, R.L.: On the Development of Sympathetic Nerve Vesicles during Axonal Transport. J Neurochem 23(1974)769–773

Lagercrantz, H.; Stjärne, L.: Evidence That a Major Proportion of the Noradrenaline is

Stored with ATP in Sympathetic Large Dense Core Nerve Vesicles. Nature 249 (1974)843–845

Lagercrantz, H.; Thureson-Klein, Å.: On the Soluble Phase of Adrenergic Nerve Vesicles. Correlations of Matrix Density and Biochemical Composition. Histochemistry 43(1975)173–183

Langer, S.Z.: The Metabolism of (³H-)-Noradrenaline Released by Electrical Stimulation from the Isolated Nictitating Membrane of the Cat and from the Vas Deferens of the Rat. J Physiol (Lond) 208(1970)515–546

Langer, S.Z.: The Regulation of Transmitter Release Elicited by Nerve Stimulation Through a Presynaptic Feed-Back Mechanism. In: Frontiers in Catecholamine Research, pp. 543–549, ed. by E. Usdin, S.H. Snyder. Pergamon, New York, 1973

Langer, S.Z.: Selective Metabolic Pathways for Noradrenaline in the Peripheral and Central Nervous System. Med Biol 52(1974)372–383

Langer, S.Z.: The role of α and β-Presynaptic Receptors in the Regulation of Noradrenaline Release Elicited by Nerve Stimulation. Clin Sci Mol Med 51(1976)423–426

Langer, S.Z.; Adler, E.; Enero, M.A.; Stefano, F.J.E.: The Role of Alpha-Receptors in Regulating Noradrenaline Overflow by Nerve Stimulation. Proc Int Union Physiol Sci 9(1971)9

Langer, S.Z.; Dubocovich, M.L.; Celuch, S.M.: Prejunctional Regulatory Mechanism for Noradrenaline Release Elicited by Nerve Stimulatin. In: Chemical Tools in Catecholamine Research, Vol. II, pp. 183–191, ed. by O. Almgren, A. Carlsson, J. Engel. North-Holland, Amsterdam-Oxford, 1975

Langley, J.N.: Observations of the Physiological Actions of Extracts of the Supra-Renal Bodies. J Physiol (Lond) 27(1901)237–256

Langley, A.E.; Weiner, N.: Enhanced Exocytotic Release of Norepinephrine Consequent to Nerve Stimulation by Low Concentrations of Cyclic Nucleotide in the Presence of Phenoxybenzamine. J Pharmacol Exp Ther 205(1978)426–437

Lastowecka, A.; Trifaró, J.M.: The Effect of Sodium and Calcium Ions on the Release of Catecholamines from the Adrenal Medulla. Sodium Deprivation Induces Release by Exocytosis in the Absence of Extracellular Calcium. J Physiol (Lond) 236(1974)681–705

Leaders, F.E.; Dayrit, C.: The Cholinergic Component in the Sympathetic Innervation to the Spleen. J Pharmacol Exp Ther 147(1965)145–152

Le Beux, Y.J.; Willemot, J.: An Ultrastructural Study of the Microfilaments in Rat Brain by Means of Heavy Meromyosin Labeling. I—The Perikaryon, the Dendrites and the Axon. Cell Tissue Res 160(1975a)1–36

Le Beux, Y.J.; Willemot, J.: An Ultrastructural Study of the Microfilaments in Rat Brain by Means of E-PTA Staining and Heavy Meromyosin Labeling. II—The Synapses. Cell Tissue Res 160(1975b)37–68

Leitz, F.H.; Stefano, F.J.E.: The Effects of Tyramine, Amphetamine and Metaraminol on the Metabolic Disposition of ³H-Norepinephrine Released from the Adrenergic Neuron. J Pharmacol Exp Ther 178(1971)464–473

Lever, J.D.; Findlay, J.A.: Similar Structural Basis for the Storage and Release of Secretory Material in Adrenomedullary and β-Pancreatic Cells. Z Zellforsch Mikrosk Anat 74(1966)317–324

Livett, B.G.: Axonal Transport and Neuronal Dynamics: Contributions to the Study of Neuronal Connectivity. In: International Revue of Physiology, Vol. X, pp. 37–124, ed. by R. Porter. University Park Press, Baltimore, 1976

Livett, B.G.; Geffen, L.B.; Austin, L.: Proximo Distal Transport of [¹⁴C] Noradrenaline and Protein in Sympathetic Nerves. J Neurochem 15(1968)931–939

Loewi, O.: Uber Humorale Ubertragbarkeit der Herznervenwirkung. Pflüg Arch Ges Physiol 189(1921)239–242

Löffelholz, K.; Muscholl, E.: Inhibition by Parasympathetic Nerve Stimulation of the Release of the Adrenergic Transmitter. Naunyn Schmiedebergs Arch Pharmacol 267(1970)181–184

Lucy, J.A.: The Fusion of Biological Membranes. Nature 227(1970)815–817

Lundborg, P.: Studies on the Uptake and Subcellular Distribution of Catecholamines and Their Alpha-Methylated Analogues. Acta Physiol Scand Suppl 302(1967)1–34

McCulloch, M.W.; Rand, M.J.; Story, D.F.: Inhibition of ³H-Noradrenaline Release from Sympathetic Nerves of Guinea-Pig Atria by a Presynaptic α-Adrenoceptor Mechanism. Br J Pharmacol 46(1972)523–524P

Malamed, S.; Poisner, A.M.: Trifaró, J.M.; Douglas, W.W.: The Fate of the Chromaffin Granule During Catecholamine Release from the Adrenal Medulla. III. Recovery of a Purified Fraction of Electron-Translucent Structures. Biochem Pharmacol 17(1968)241–246

Malik, K.U.: Prostaglandins—Modulation of Adrenergic Nervous System. Fed Proc 37(1978)203–207

Malmfors, T.: Studies on Adrenergic Nerves. The Use of Rat and Mouse Iris for Direct Observations on their Physiology and Pharmacology at Cellular and Subcellular Levels. Acta Physiol Scand 64 Suppl 248(1965)1–93

Melville, K.I.: The Antisympathomimetic Action of Dioxame Compounds (F883 and F933) with Special Reference to the Vascular Responses to Dihydroxyphenyl Ethanolamine (Arterenol) and Nerve Stimulation. J Pharmacol Exp Ther 59(1937)317–327

Miach, P.J.; Dausse, J.P.; Meyer, P.: Direct Biochemical Demonstration of Two Types of Alpha Adrenoceptors in Rat Brain. Presynaptic Receptors. VII Int Cong Pharmacol, Paris, July 16–21 (1978) 9A pp. 34

Mizel, S.B.; Wilson, L.: Nucleoside Transport in Mammalian Cells. Inhibition by Colchicine. Biochemistry 11(1972)2573–2578

Molinoff, P.B.; Weinshilboum, R.; Azelrod, J.: A Sensitive Enzymatic Assay for Dopamine-β-Hydroxylase. J Pharmacol Exp Ther 178(1971)425–431

Montel, H.; Starke, K.; Weber, F.: Influence of Morphine and Naloxone on the Release of Noradrenaline from Rat Brain Cortex Slices. Naunyn Schmiedebergs Arch Pharmacol 283(1974)357–369

Moore, C.L.: Specific Inhibition of Mitochondrial Ca^{++} Transport by Ruthenium Red. Biochem Biophys Res Comm 42(1971)298–305

Moss, J.; Thoa, N.B.; Kopin, I.J.: On the Mechanism of Scorpion Toxin-Induced Release of Norepinephrine from Peripheral Adrenergic Neurons. J Pharmacol Exp Ther 190(1974)39–48

Musacchio, J.; Kopin, I.J.; Weise, V.K.: Subcellular Distribution of Some Sympathomimetic Amines and Their β-Hydroxylated Derivatives in the Rat Heart. J Pharmacol Exp Ther 148(1965)22–28

Muscholl, E.: Adrenergic False Transmitters. In: Handbook of Exp Pharmacol, Vol. XXXIII, Catecholamines, pp. 618–652, ed. by H. Blaschko, E. Muscholl. Springer, Berlin, 1972

Muscholl, E.; Maître, L.: Release by Sympathetic Stimulation of α-Methylnoradrenaline Stored in the Heart After Administration of α-Methyldopa. Experientia (Basel) 19(1963)658–659

Nagasawa, J.; Douglas, W.W.; Schulz, R.A.: Ultrastructural Evidence of Secretion by Exocytosis and 'Synaptic Vesicle' Formation in Posterior Pituitary Glands. Nature 227(1970)407–409

Nakazato, Y.; Douglas, W.W.: Cytochalasin Blocks Sympathetic Ganglionic Transmission: A Presynaptic Effect Antagonized by Pyruvate. Proc Natl Acad Sci USA 70(1973)1730–1733

Nakazato, Y.; Onoda, Y.; Onga, A.: Role of Calcium in the Release of Noradrenaline Induced by Sodium Deprivation from the Guinea-Pig Vas Deferens. Pflugers Arch 372(1977)63–67

Nelson, D.L.; Molinoff, P.B.: Distribution and Properties of Adrenergic Storage Vesicles in Nerve Terminals. J Pharmacol Exp Ther 196(1976)346–359

Ngai, S.H.; Dairman, M.; Marchelle, M.; Spector, S.: Dopamine β-Hydroxylase in Dog Lymph—Effect of Sympathetic Activiation. Life Sci 14(1974)2431–2439

Nickerson, M.; Collier, B.: Drugs Inhibiting Adrenergic Nerves and Structures Innervated by Them. In: The Pharmacological Basis of Therapeutics, 5th ed., pp. 533–564, ed. by L.S. Goodman, A. Gilman. Macmillan, New York, 1975

Nicklas, W.J.; Berl, S.: Effects of Cytochalasin B on Uptake and Release of Putative Transmitters by Synaptosomes and on Brain Actomyosin-Like Protein. Nature 247 (1974)471–473

Noon, J.P.; Roth, R.H.: Some Physiological and Pharmacological Characteristics of the Stimulus Induced Release of Norepinephrine from the Rabbit Superior Cervical Ganglion. Naunyn Schmiedebergs Arch Pharmacol 291(1975)163–174

Norberg, K.A.; Hamberger, B.: The Sympathetic Adrenergic Neuron. Acta Physiol Scand Suppl. 238(1964)1–42

Oka, M.; Izumi, F.; Kashimoto, T.: Effects of Cytoplasmic and Microsomal Fractions on

ATP-Mg^{++} Stimulated Catecholamine Release from Isolated Adrenomedullary Granules. Jpn J Pharmacol 22(1972)207–214

Paton, D.M.: Evidence of a Carrier-Mediated Efflux of Noradrenaline from the Axoplasm of Adrenergic Nerves in Rabbit Atria. J Pharm Pharmacol 25(1973)265–267

Paton, W.D.M.; Vizi, E.S.; Zar, M. Aboo: The Mechanism of Acetylcholine Release from Parasympathetic Nerves. J Physiol 215(1971)819–848

Pelayo, F.; Dubocovich, M.L.; Langer, S.Z.: Possible Role of Cyclic Nucleotides in Regulation of Noradrenaline Release From Rat Pineal through Presynaptic Adrenoceptors. Nature 274(1978)76–78

Pfenninger, K.; Akert, K.; Moor, M.; Sandri, C.: The Fine Structure of Freeze-Fractured Presynaptic Membranes. J Neurocytol 1(1972)129–149

Phillips, J.H.; Slater, A.: Actin in the Adrenal Medulla. FEBS Lett 56(1975)327–331

Pinto, J.E.B.; Trifaró, J.M.: The Different Effects of D-600 (Methoxyverapamil) on the Release of Adrenal Catecholamines Induced by Acetylcholine, High Potassium or Sodium Deprivation. Br J Pharmacol 57(1976)127–132

Poisner, A.M.; Bernstein, J.: A Possible Role of Microtubules in Catecholamine Release from the Adrenal Medulla. Effect of Colchicine, Vinca Alkaloids and Deuterium Oxide. J Pharmacol Exp Ther 171(1971)102–108

Poisner, A.M.; Trifaró, J.M.: The Role of ATP and ATPase in the Release of Catecholamines from the Adrenal Medulla—I. ATP-Evoked Release of Catecholamines, ATP, and Protein from Isolated Chromaffin Granules. Mol Pharmacol 3(1967)561–571

Poisner, A.M.; Trifaró, J.M.: Release of Catecholamines from Isolated Adrenal Chromaffin Granules by Endogenous ATP. Mol Pharmacol 4(1968)196–199

Poisner, A.M.; Trifaró, J.M.: The Role of Adenosine Triphosphate and Adenosine Triphosphatase in the Release of Catecholamines from the Adrenal Medulla. III. Similarities between the Effects of Adenosine Triphosphate on Chromaffin Granules and on Mitochondria. Mol Pharmacol 5(1969)294–299

Poisner, A.M.; Trifaró, J.M.; Douglas, W.W.: The Fate of the Chromaffin Granule during Catecholamine Release from the Adrenal Medulla. II. Loss of Protein and Retention of Lipid in Subcellular Fractions. Biochem Pharmacol 16(1967)2101–2108

Potter, L.T.: Storage of Norepinephrine in Sympathetic Nerves. Pharmacol Rev 18(1966)439–451

Potter, L.T.: Role of Intraneuronal Vesicles in the Synthesis, Storage and Release of Noradrenaline. Cir Res 21 Suppl 3(1967)13–24

Puszkin, S.; Kochwa, S.: Regulation of Neurotransmitter Release by a Complex of Actin with Relaxing Protein Isolated from Rat Brain Synaptosomes. J Biol Chem 249(1974)7711–7714

Rahamimoff, R.; Alnaes, E.: Inhibitory Action of Ruthenium Red on Neuromuscular Transmission. Proc Natl Acad Sci (USA) 70(1973)3613–3616

Rahamimoff, R.; Erulkar, S.D.; Alnaes, E.; Meiri, H.; Rotshenker, S.; Rahamimoff, H.: Modulation of Transmitter Release by Calcium Ions and Nerve Impulses. Cold Spring Harbor Symp Quant Biol 40(1975)107–116

Ritzel, H.; Muscholl, E.: Differences in Time Course and Ca^{++} Dependency of Noradrenaline (NA) Release from the Heart Evoked by High K$^+$ and/or Low Na$^+$ Solutions. Naunyn Schmiedeberg's Arch Pharmakol 293(1976)R2

Ross, S.B.; Eriksson, H.E.; Hellström, W.: On the Fate of Dopamine-β-Hydroxylase After Release from the Peripheral Sympathetic Nerves in the Cat. Acta Physiol Scand 92(1974)578–580

Satir, B.; Schooley, C.; Satir, P.: Membrane Fusion in a Model System. Mucocyst Secretion in Tertrahymena. J Cell Biol 56(1973)153–176

Schneider, F.H.; Smith, A.D.; Winkler, H.: Secretion from the Adrenal Medulla: Biomedical Evidence for Exocytosis. Br J Pharmacol 31(1967)94–104

Schober, R.; Nitsch, C.; Rinne, U.; Morris, S.J.: Calcium-Induced Displacement of Membrane-Associated Particles upon Aggregation of Chromaffin Granules. Science 195(1977)495–497

Schwab, M.; Thoenen, H.: Selective Trans-Synaptic Migration of Tetanus Toxin after Retrograde Axonal Transport in Peripheral Sympathetic Nerves: A Comparison with Nerve Growth Factor. Brain Res 122(1977)459–474

Scott, F.H.: On the Metabolism and Action of Nerve Cells. Brain 28(1905)506–526

Shand, D.G.; Morgan, D.H.; Oates, J.A.: The Release of Guanethidine and Bethanidine by Splenic Nerve Stimulation: A Quantitative Evaluation Showing Dissociation from Adrenergic Blockade. J Pharmacol Exp Ther 184(1973)73–80

Sharma, V.K.; Bannerjee, S.P.: Presynaptic Muscarinic Cholinergic Receptors. Nature 272(1978)276–278

Shelanski, M.L.: Chemistry of the Filaments and Tubules of Brain. J Histochem Cytochem 21(1973)529–539

Slotkin, T.: Hypothetical Model of Catecholamine Uptake into Adrenal Medullary Storage Vesicles. Life Sci 13(1973)675–683

Smith, A.D.: Cellular Control of the Uptake, Storage and Release of Noradrenaline in Sympathetic Nerves. Biochem Soc Symp 36(1972)103–131

Smith, A.D.; De Potter, W.P.; Moerman, E.J.; De Schaepdryver, A.F.: Release of Dopamine β-Hydroxylase and Chromogranin A upon Stimulation of the Splenic Nerve. Tissue & Cell 2(1970)547–568

Smith, A.D.; Winkler, H.: Fundamental Mechanisms in the Release of Catecholamines. In: Handbook of Experimental Pharmacology, Vol. XXXIII, pp. 538–617, ed. by H. Blaschko, E. Muscholl. Springer, Berlin, 1972

Smith, U.; Smith, D.S.; Winkler, H.; Ryan, J.W.: Exocytosis in the Adrenal Medulla Demonstrated by Freeze-Etching. Science 179(1973)79–82

Spoor, R.P.; Ferguson, F.C.: Colchicine. IV. Neuromuscular Transmission in Isolated Frog and Rat Tissues. J Pharm Sci 54(1965)779–780

Spudich, J.A.; Lin, S.: Cytochalasin B, Its Interaction with Actin and Actomyosin from Muscle. Proc Natl Acad Sci USA 69(1972)442–446

Stadler, J.; Franke, W.W.: Characterization of the Colchicine Binding of Membrane Fractions from Rat and Mouse Liver. J Cell Biol 60(1974)297–303

Starke, K.: Influence of α-Receptor Stimulants of Noradrenaline Release. Naturwissenschaften 58(1971)420

Starke, K.: Alpha Sympathomimetic Inhibition of Adrenergic and Cholinergic Transmission in the Rabbit Heart. Naunyn Schmiedebergs Arch Pharmacol 274(1972a)18–45

Starke, K.: Influence of Extracellular Noradrenaline on the Stimulation-Evoked Secretion of Noradrenaline from Sympathetic Nerves: Evidence for an α-Receptor-Mediated Feed-Back Inhibition of Noradrenaline Release. Naunyn Schmiedebergs Arch Pharmacol 275 (1972b)11–23

Starke, K.: Regulation of Noradrenaline Release by Presynaptic Receptor Systems. Rev Physiol Biochem Pharmacol 77(1977)1–124

Starke, K.; Altman, K.P.: Inhibition of Adrenergic Neurotransmission by Clonidine: An Action on Prejunctional α-Receptors. Neuropharmacol 12(1973)339–347

Starke, K.; Borowski, E.; Endo, T.: Preferential Blockade of Presynaptic α-Adrenoceptors by Yohimbine. Eur J Pharmacol 34(1975a)385–388

Starke, K.; Endo, T.; Taube, H.D.: Relative Pre- and Postsynaptic Potencies of β-Adrenoceptor Agonists in the Rabbit Pulmonary Artery. Naunyn Schmiedebergs Arch Pharmacol 291(1975b)55–78

Starke, K.; Montel, H.: Schümann, H.J.: Influence of Cocaine and Phenoxybenzamine on Noradrenaline Uptake and Release. Naunyn Schmiedebergs Arch Pharmacol 270 (1971a)210–214

Starke, K.; Montel, H.; Wagner, J.: Effect of Phentolamine on Noradrenaline Uptake and Release. Naunyn Schmiedebergs Arch Pharmacol 271(1971b)181–192

Stelzner, D.J.: The Relationship between Synaptic Vesicles, Golgi Apparatus, and Smooth Endoplasmic Reticulum: A Development Study Using the Zinc Iodide-Osmium Technique. Z Zellforsch Mikrosk Anat 120(1971)332–345

Stjärne, L.: Studies of Catecholamine Uptake, Storage and Release Mechanism. Acta Physiol Scand 62(1964) Suppl 228

Stjärne, L.: Storage Particles in Noradrenergic Tissues. Pharmacol Rev 18(1966)425–432

Stjärne, L.: The Synthesis, Uptake and Storage of Catecholamines in the Adrenal Medulla. The Effect of Drugs. In: Handbook of Experimental Pharmacology, Vol. XXXIII, Catecholamines, pp. 231–261, ed. by H. Blaschko, E. Muscholl. Springer, Berlin 1972

Stjärne, L.: Frequency-Dependence of Dual Negative Feedback Control of Secretion of Sympathetic Neurotransmitter in Guinea-Pig Vas Deferens. Br J Pharmacol 49(1973a)358–360

Stjärne, L.: Kinetics of Secretion of Sympathetic Neurotransmitter As a Function of External Calcium: Mechanism of Inhibitory Effect of Prostaglandin E. Acta Physiol Scand 87(1973b)428–430

Stjärne, L.: Michaelis-Menten Kinetics of Secretion of Sympathetic Neurotransmitter as a Function of External Calcium: Effects of Graded Alpha-Adrenoceptor Blockade. Naunyn Schmiedebergs Arch Pharmacol 278(1973c)323–327

Stjärne, L.: Mechanisms of Catecholamine Secretion. Dual Feedback Control of Sympathetic Neurotransmitter Secretion; Rôle of Calcium: In: Frontiers in Catecholamine Research, pp. 491–496, ed. by E. Usdin, S. Snyder. Pergamon, New York-Oxford, 1973(d)

Stjärne, L.; Brundin, J.: Frequency-Dependence of ^{3}H-Noradrenaline Secretion from Human Vasoconstrictor Nerves. Modification by Factors Interfering with α- or β-Adrenoceptor or Prostaglandin E_2-Mediated Control. Acta Physiol Scand 101(1977)199–210

Stjärne, L.; Roth, R.H.; Lishajko, F.: Noradrenaline Formation from Dopamine in Isolated Subcellular Particles from Bovine Splenic Nerve. Biochem Pharmac 16(1967)1729–1739

Story, D.F.; Briley, M.S.; Langer, S.Z.: The Effects of 6-Hydroxy-Dopamine on the Binding of ^{3}H-Quinuclidinyl Benzilate, ^{3}H-Dihydroergocryptine and ^{3}H-WB 4101 to Rat Heart Ventricular Membranes. Presynaptic Receptors. VII Int Cong Pharmacol 11A(1978)17

Su, C.: Purinergic Inhibition of Adrenergic Transmission in Rabbit Blood Vessels. J Pharmacol Exp Ther 204(1978)351–361

Subramanian, N.; Mitznegg, P.; Sprügel, W.; Domschke, W.; Domschke, S.; Wünsch, E.; Demling, L.: Influence of Enkephalin on K^+-Evoked Efflux of Putative Neurotransmitter and Dopamine Release. Selective Inhibition of Acetylcholine and Dopamine Release. Naunyn Schmiedebergs Arch Pharmacol 299(1977)163–165

Sundberg, D.K.; Krulich, L.; Fawcett, C.P.; Illner, P.; McCann, S.M.: The Effect of Colchicine on the Release of Rat Anterior Pituitary Hormones In Vitro. Proc Soc Exp Biol Med 142(1973)1097–1100

Taugner, G.: The Membrane of Catecholamine Storage Vesicles of Adrenal Medulla. Naunyn Schmiedebergs. Arch Pharmacol 270(1971)392–406

Taugner, G.; Hasselbach, W.: Uber den Mechanismus der CA-Speicherung en den "chromafinen Granula" des Nebennierenmarks. Naunyn Schmiedebergs Arch Pharmacol 255(1966)266–286

Taxi, J.: Morphological and Cytochemical Studies on the Synapses in the Autonomic Nervous Systems. Progr Brain Res 31(1969)5–20

Temple, R.; Williams, J.A.; Wilber, J.F.; Wolff, J.: Colchicine and Hormone Secretion. Biochem Biophys Res Commun 46(1972)1454–1461

Thoa, N.B.; Wooten, G.F.; Axelrod, J.; Kopin, I.J.: Inhibition of Release of Dopamine-β-Hydroxylase and Norepinephrine from Sympathetic Nerves by Colchicine, Vinblastine, or Cytochalasin-B. Proc Natl Acad Sci (USA) 69(1972)520–522

Thoa, N.B.; Wooten, G.F.; Axelrod, J.; Kopin, I.J.: On the Mechanism of Release of Norepinephrine from Sympathetic Nerves Induced by Depolarizing Agents and Sympathomimetic Drugs. Mol Pharmacol 11(1975)10–18

Thoenen, H.; Haefely, W.; Staehelin, H.: Potentiation by Tetraethylammonium of the Response of the Cat Spleen to Postganglionic Sympathetic Nerve Stimulation. J Pharmacol Exp Ther 157(1967)532–540

Thoenen, H.; Hürlimann, A.; Haefely, W.: Removal of Infused Norepinephrine by the Cat's Spleen, Mechanism of Its Inhibition by Phenoxybenzamine. Experientia 19(1963)601–604

Thoenen, H.; Hürlimann, A.; Haefely, W.: Dual Site of Action of Phenoxybenzamine in the Cat's Spleen. Blockade of α-Adrenergic Receptors and Inhibition of Re-Uptake of Neurally Released Norepinephrine. Experientia (Basel) 20(1964a)272–273

Thoenen, H.; Hürlimann, A.; Haefely, W.: Wirkungen von Phenoxybenzamin, Phentolamin und Azapetin auf adrenergische Synapsen der Katzenmils. Helf Physiol Pharmacol Acta 22(1964b)148–161

Tranzer, J.P.: A New Amine Storing Compartment in Adrenergic Axons. Nature (New Biol) 237(1972)57–58

Tranzer, J.P.: New Aspects of the Localization of Catecholamines in Adrenergic Neurons. In:

Frontiers in Catecholamine Research, pp. 453–458, ed. by E. Usdin, S. Snyder. Pergamon, New York-Oxford, 1973

Tranzer, J.P.; Thoenen, H.; Snipes, R.L.; Richards, J.D.: Recent Developments on the Ultrastructural Aspects of Adrenergic Nerve Endings in Various Experimental Conditions. Progr Brain Res 31(1969)33–46

Trifaró, J.M.: The Effect of Ca^{2+} Omission on the Secretion of Catecholamines and the Incorporation of Orthophosphate-^{32}P into Nucleotides and Phospholipids of Bovine Adrenal Medulla During Acetylcholine Stimulation. Mol Pharmacol 5(1969a)420–431

Trifaró, J.M.: Phospholipid Metabolism and Adrenal Medullary Activity. I. The Effect of Acetylcholine on Tissue Uptake and Incorporation of Orthophosphate-^{32}P into Nucleotides and Phospholipids of Bovine Adrenal Medulla. Mol Pharmacol 5(1969b)382–393

Trifaró, J.M.: The Secretory Process of the Adrenal Medulla. Endocrinologia Experimentalis 4(1970)225–251

Trifaró, J.M.: Phospholipids of the Chromaffin Granule Membrane and Catecholamine Release. In: Frontiers in Catecholamine Research, pp. 501–503, ed. by E. Usdin; S. Snyder. Pergamon, New York-Oxford, 1973

Trifaró, J.M.: Common Mechanisms of Hormone Secretion. Ann Rev Pharmacol Toxicol 17(1977)27–47

Trifaró, J.M.: Contractile Proteins in Tissues Originating in the Neural Crest. Neuroscience 3(1978)1–24

Trifaró, J.M.; Collier, B.; Lastowecka, A.; Stern, D.: Inhibition by Colchicine and by Vinblastine of Acetylcholine-Induced Catecholamine Release from the Adrenal Gland: An Anticholinergic Action, Not an Effect upon Microtubules. Mol Pharmacol 8(1972)264–267

Trifaró, J.M.; Duerr, A.C.; Pinto, J.E.B.: Membranes of the Adrenal Medulla: A Comparison between the Membranes of the Golgi Apparatus and Chromaffin Granules. Mol Pharmacol 12(1976)536–545

Trifaró, J.M.; Dworkind, J.: A New and Simple Method for Isolation of Adrenal Chromaffin Granules by Means of an Isotonic Density Gradient. Anal Biochem 34(1970)403–412

Trifaró, J.M.; Dworkind, J.: Phosphorylation of Membrane Components of Adrenal Chromaffin Granules by Adenosine Triphosphate. Mol Pharmacol 7(1971)52–65

Trifaró, J.M.; Dworkind, J.: Phosphorylation of the Membrane Components of Chromaffin Granules: Synthesis of Diphosphatidylinositol and Presence of Phosphatidylinositol Kinase in Granule Membranes. Can J Physiol Pharmacol 53(1975)479–492

Trifaró, J.M.; Lee, R.: Actin and Myosin in Chromaffin Cells: Characterization and Roles in Cell Function. In: Catecholamines: Basic and Clinical Frontiers. Proceedings of the Fourth International Catecholamine Symposium, pp. ed. by E. Usdin. Pergamon Press, N.Y. 1979, 558–560

Trifaró, J.M.; Poisner, A.M.: The Role of ATP and ATPase in the Release of Catecholamines from the Adrenal Medulla. II—ATP-Evoked Fall in Optical Density of Isolated Granules. Mol Pharmacol 3(1967)572–580

Trifaró, J.M.; Poisner, A.M.; Douglas, W.W.: The Fate of the Chromaffin Granule during Catecholamine Release from the Adrenal Medulla. I. Unchanged Efflux of Phospholipid and Cholesterol. Biochem Pharmacol 16(1967)2095–2100

Trifaro, J.M.; Ulpian, C.: Isolation and Characterization of Myosin from the Adrenal Medulla. Neuroscience 1(1976)483–488

Trifaró, J.M.; Warner, M.: Membranes of Adrenal Chromaffin Granules. Solubilization and Partial Characterization of the Mg^{2+} Dependent ATPase. Mol Pharmacol 8(1972)159–169

Van Orden, L.S.; Bensch, K.G.; Giarman, N.J.: Histochemical and Functional Relationships of Catecholamines in Adrenergic Nerve Endings. 2. Extravesicular Noradrenaline. J Pharmacol Exp Ther 155(1967)428–439

Viveros, O.H.; Arqueros, L.; Connett, R.J.; Kirshner, N.: Mechanism of Secretion from the Adrenal Medulla. 3. Studies of Dopamine β-Hydroxylase As a Marker for Catecholamine Storage Vesicle Membrane in Rabbit Adrenal Glands. Mol Pharmacol 5(1969a)60–68

Viveros, O.H.; Arqueros, L.; Connett, R.J.; Kirshner, N.: Mechanism of Secretion from the Adrenal Medulla. 4. The Fate of the Storage Vesicles Following Insulin and Reserpine Administration. Mol Pharmacol 5(1969b)69–82

Viveros, O.H.; Arqueros, L.; Kirshner, N.: Release of Catecholamines and Dopamine β-Oxidase from the Adrenal Medulla. Life Sci 7(1968)609–618

Viveros, O.H.; Arqueros, L.; Kirshner, N.: Quantal Secretion from Adrenal Medulla: All or None Release of Storage Vesicle Content. Science 165(1969c)911–913

Vizi, E.S.: Stimulation, by Inhibition of (Na^+-K^+,Mg^{2+})-activated ATPase, of Acetylcholine Release in Cortical Slices from Rat Brain. J Physiol 226(1972)95–117

Vizi, E.S.: Possible Connection between the Release of Acetylcholine and the Activity of Na^+-K^+-Activated ATPase. In: Neurobiological Basis of Memory Formation, pp. 96–116, ed. by H. Matthies. VEB Volk and Gesundheit, Berlin, 1974

Vizi, E.S.: Release Mechanisms of Acetylcholine and the Role of Na^+-K^+-activated ATPase. In: Cholinergic Mechanisms, pp. 199–211, ed. by P.G. Waser. Raven, New York, 1975a

Vizi, E.S.: The Role of Na^+-K^+-Activated ATPase in Transmitter Release: Acetylcholine Release from Basal Ganglia, Its Inhibition by Dopamine and Noradrenaline. In: Subcortical Mechanism and Sensorimotor Activities, pp. 63–87, ed. by T.L. Frigyesi. Hans Huber, Bern, 1975b

Vizi, E.S.: Termination of Transmitter Release by Stimulation of Sodium-Potassium Activated ATPase. J Physiol 267(1977)261–280

Vogel, S.A.; Silberstein, S.D.; Berr, K.R.; Kopin, I.J.: Stimulation-Induced Release of Norepinephrine from Rat Superior Cervical Ganglia in Vitro. Eur J Pharmacol 20(1972)308–311

von Euler, U.S.: A Specific Sympathomimetic Ergone in Adrenergic Nerve Fibres (Sympathin) and its Relations to Adrenaline and Nor-Adrenaline. Acta Physiol Scandinav 12(1946)73–97

von Euler, U.S.: Twenty Years of Noradrenaline. Pharmacol Rev 18(1966)29–38

von Euler, U.S.: Synthesis, Uptake and Storage of Catecholamines in Adrenergic Nerves, the Effect of Drugs. In: Handbook of Experimental Pharmacology, Vol. 33, Catecholamines, pp. 187–230, ed. by H. Blaschko; E. Muscholl. Springer-Verlag, Heidelberg-New York, 1972

von Euler, U.S.; Hillarp, N.-A.: Evidence for the Presence of Noradrenaline in Submicroscopic Structures of Adrenergic Axons. Nature (Lond) 177(1956)44–45

Weiner, N.: Regulation of Norepinephrine Biosynthesis. Ann Rev Pharmacol 10(1970)273–289

Weinryb, I.; Chasin, M.; Free, C.A.; Harris, D.N.; Goldenberg, H.; Michel, I.M.; Park, V.S.; Phillips, M.; Samaniego, S.; Hess, S.M.: Effect of Therapeutic Agents of Cyclic AMP Metabolism in Vitro. J Pharmacol Sci 61(1972)1556–1567

Weinshilboum, R.M.; Thoa, N.B.; Johnson, D.G.; Kopin, I.J.: Proportional Release of Norepinephrine and Dopamine β-Hydroxylase from Sympathetic Nerves. Science 174(1971)1349–1351

Weisenberg, R.C.: Microtubule Formation in Vitro in Solutions Containing Low Calcium Concentrations. Science 177(1972)1104–1105

Wessells, N.K.; Spooner, B.S.; Ash, J.F.; Bradley, M.O.; Ludueña, M.A.; Taylor, E.L.; Wrenn, J.T.; Yamada, K.M.: Microfilaments in Cellular and Developmental Processes. Contractile Microfilament Machinery of Many Cell Types is Reversibly Inhibited by Cytochalasin B. Science 171(1971)135–143

Winkler, H.: The Composition of Adrenal Chromaffin Granules: An Assessment of Controversial Results. Neuroscience 1(1976)65–80

Woodin, A.M.; French, J.E.; Marchesi, V.T.: Morphological Changes Associated with the Extrusion of Protein Induced in the Polymorphonuclear Leucocyte by Staphylococcal Leucocidin. Biochem J 87(1963)567–571

Yamamoto, H.; Kirpekar, S.M.: Effects of Nerve Stimulation on the Uptake of Norepinephrine by the Perfused Spleen of the Cat. Eur J Pharmacol 17(1972)25–33

Yen, S.S.; Kleen, R.L.; Chen-Yen, S.H.; Thureson-Klein, A.: Norepinephrine:Adenosine-Triphosphate Ratios in Purified Adrenergic Vesicles. J Neurobiol 7(1976)11–22

Ziegler, M.G.; Thomas, J.A.; Jacobowitz, D.M.: Retrograde Axonal Transport of Antibody to Dopamine β-Hydroxylase. Brain Res 104(1976)390–395

Desensitization Phenomena in Smooth Muscle

Leon Hurwitz and Linda J. McGuffee

I. INTRODUCTION

Excessive exposure of a tissue to a high level of an excitatory agent may result in a profound change in the functional activity of the tissue. This change is seen as a partial or complete loss of sensitivity of the tissue to the biological action of the excitatory agent. When this phenomenon occurs, the tissue may be said to have developed some degree of desensitization. The phenomenon of desensitization has been recognized for over seventy years and has been shown to occur in a great many different kinds of cells and tissues. It would appear that the process of desensitization constitutes one of the important means by which homeostasis is maintained in the living organism. Although the underlying molecular changes producing desensitization are not well understood, there is good reason to believe that this phenomenon can occur by a number of different mechanisms. On the basis of the experimental observations that have been made thus far, it is highly likely that a single agent such as isoproterenol may induce different kinds of desensitization reactions in different types of cells or tissues; and further, that two different excitatory agents, such as acetylcholine and serotonin, may each induce a different kind of desensitization reaction in the same tissue. The primary aim in this article is to examine the prominent features and possible mechanisms of desensitization as it occurs in smooth muscle cells.

II. DESENSITIZATION IN CELLS OTHER THAN SMOOTH MUSCLE

The extent to which the desensitization process in smooth muscle mimics or differs from this process in other types of cells may be judged by briefly considering some general aspects of the desensitization phenomenon. As an example of a prominent mechanism by which desensitization develops in a variety of cell types, the experimental findings of Mukherjee, Caron, and Lefkowitz (1975) may be cited. These investigators injected frogs with β-adrenergic agonists for 1- to 24-h periods and thereby produced a profound subsensitivity of the adenylate cyclase enzyme in the erythrocyte membrane. The subsensitization was found to be specific for the catecholamine-stimulated adenylate cyclase activity. Basal and fluoride stimulation of the enzyme was unaffected. Mukherjee and coworkers also carried out binding studies with the competitive β-adrenergic antagonist $(-)$ [^{3}H] alprenolol and found a 60% fall in the number of β-adrenergic receptor binding sites in the erythrocyte membranes from desensitized animals. The binding affinity of these sites was not markedly altered. These data suggested that the underlying mechanism for the desensitization was a reduction in the number of specific receptors with which the desensitizing agent must normally interact to produce its biological effect.

Similar results were obtained in experiments with the insulin receptor. Gavin et al. (1974) exposed cultured human lymphocytes to elevations in the ambient concentration of insulin. They found that cells that were preincubated with 10^{-3}M insulin for 5 h would subsequently bind [^{125}I] insulin up to about 70% of the control level. After a 16-h preincubation period, the level of binding of [^{125}I] insulin was about 45% of control level. Based on the configurations and the positions of the binding curves that were obtained, these workers concluded that the decrease in insulin binding could be accounted for by a decrease in the effective concentration of the insulin receptors and not by a significant alternation in the affinity of the receptors for insulin.

Kobayashi and Olefsky (1978), using rats, studied the effects of high concentrations of insulin *in vivo*. They found that experimental hyperinsulinemia led to a 40% decrease in the number of insulin receptors on isolated adipocytes. When the effect of insulin on glucose transport was plotted against insulin bound per unit plasma membrane surface area, the curves from control and hyperinsulinemic rats were superimposed. These data suggested that the hyperinsulinemia caused a reduction in the number of insulin receptors present on the adipocytes but did not interfere with the mechanism coupling the insulin-receptor interaction to the glucose transport process.

The phenomenon of receptor modulation (change in number of ligand-binding sites) brought about by varying the concentration of a specific binding ligand has also been shown to occur with epinephrine and α adrenergic receptors in the parotid cell (Strittmatter, Davis, and Lefkowitz, 1977) and with growth hormone and its receptors in cultured human lymphocytes (Lesniak and Roth, 1976).

The cellular events that lead to a reduction in the number of receptor binding sites subsequent to the interaction between these binding sites and specific agonists has not been clearly established. Various suggestions have been made to account for this phenomenon. These include such hypothetical possibilities as (a) the reversible inactivation of receptors that occurs as a result of some conformational alteration induced by the agonist (Williams and Lefkowitz, 1978), (b) the induction of an increased degradation or decreased synthesis of receptors (Gavin et al., 1974), (c) the release of receptors into the medium (Gavin et al., 1974), (d) the translocation of receptors into an intracellular site (Gavin et al., 1974), and others. The possibility that receptors may be internalized derives some degree of credibility from the fact that in some types of cells the transport of surface proteins to an intracellular location has been demonstrated (Raff and DePetris, 1973; Unanue, Perkins, and Karnovsky, 1972).

Although the reports cited above support the concept that receptor modulation is an important and widespread mechanism for achieving tissue desensitization, evidence for alternative mechanisms of desensitization also exists. As a case in point, Kebabian et al. (1975), working with the rat pineal gland, found that a mild isoproterenol-induced desensitization was associated with a loss of both hormone-sensitive adenylate cyclase activity and specific $(-)$ [^{3}H] alprenolol binding sites. The binding sites that remained in the desensitized gland did not exhibit any change in affinity for isoproterenol or $(-)$ alprenolol. These findings are similar to those made by Mukherjee et al. (1975) in the erythrocyte membrane of the frog. However, when a more intense desensitization of the gland was induced, both the hormone-sensitive and the basal adenylate cyclase activity were decreased. Furthermore, the desensitized pineals exhibited substantially less fluoride-stimulated adenylate cyclase activity. Thus, in contrast to the observations made on the frog erythrocyte membrane, the pineals of the rat may develop a subsensitivity attributable to both a reduction in the functional β receptor binding sites and a decrease in the activity of the enzyme, adenylate cyclase.

Neither a reduction in receptor binding sites nor a direct inhibition of the cellular processes activated by the drug-receptor interaction are considered to be responsible for the desensitized state produced by a cholinergic agonist in skeletal muscle. In a paper published in 1957, Katz and Thesleff developed a model that pictured desensitization of the nicotinic cholinergic receptor as a consequence of a change in the conformation of the receptor molecule subsequent to a prolonged interaction between it and acetylcholine or some other cholinergic agonist. The altered receptor molecule exhibits a greater affinity for the cholinergic agonist, but its interaction with the agonist does not lead to the opening of monovalent ion channels in the muscle membrane (Katz and Thesleff, 1957). Most, but not all, workers who have studied biological preparations containing the nicotinic cholinergic receptors view the model presented by Katz and Thesleff as an acceptable interpretation of the available data dealing with the desensitization of the nicotinic cholinergic receptors (Nastuk, 1977; Rang and Ritter, 1970).

A somewhat unusual type of desensitization has been found by Cox and Padhya (1977). These investigators studied the inhibition of acetylcholine release by opiate drugs in the myenteric plexus of the guinea pig ileum. The data they obtained showed that higher-than-normal concentrations of morphine were required to produce 50% inhibition of the electrically stimulated contractions of myenteric-plexus–longitudinal-muscle preparations isolated from morphine-pretreated animals. There was also an increase in the slope of linearized dose-response curves in opiate-tolerant preparations. The maximum effect induced by the opiates was not modified in these tolerant preparations, and responses to exogenous acetylcholine were not affected. This opiate-induced tolerance to opiate drugs was not accompanied by a change in the affinity or the number of stereospecific binding sites for [³H] etorphine. In order to explain these results, the assumption was made that in tolerant preparations a certain minimal fraction of the opiate receptor population must be occupied so that a threshold level is exceeded. Below threshold level, the drug effects cannot be elicited. It was suggested that the tissue adapts toward a threshold level the magnitude of which bears some relationship to the mean receptor occupancy attained during the period of opiate drug pretreatment.

In a study (DeVellis and Brooker, 1974) carried out on cultured C6 glioma cells, the development of desensitization to norepinephrine was linked to the possible synthesis of some inhibitory protein. This association was inferred from experimental data indicating that the presence of cyclohexamide, an inhibitor of protein synthesis, caused a striking impairment in the development of the desensitization process. The type of refractoriness that Su, Cubeddu, and Perkins (1976) have uncovered in human astrocytoma cells represents still another type of desensitization. They found that the interaction between norepinephrine and specific catecholamine receptors will, after some period of time, effect a reduction in the capacity of prostaglandin E_1, as well as norepinephrine, to stimulate the production of cyclic AMP. The reverse was also found to occur. Prostaglandin E_1, by interacting with its receptors for a prolonged period, reduced the capacity of both norepinephrine and prostaglandin E_1 to stimulate the production of cyclic AMP. The cross-reaction that Su et al. (1976) observed was termed heterologous desensitization. Their experimental results, in addition to the outcome of the several other studies cited above, leave little doubt that desensitization may be achieved by a variety of dissimilar cellular mechanisms.

III. DESENSITIZATION IN SMOOTH MUSCLE CELLS

The work performed to characterize the desensitization reaction in smooth muscle cells also negates any notion that a single mechanism is involved. Workers have shown that both specific and nonspecific desensitization may occur. Barsoum and Gaddum (1935) reported that the rectal cecum of the fowl could be desensitized to histamine by exposing the tissue preparation to a high concentration of the drug. Conversely, exposure to large doses of histamine only slightly diminished responses to acetylcholine, barium, and other agonists. Cantoni and Eastman (1946) have reported opposite findings. Working with an intestinal strip from the guinea pig, they observed that the mechanical response to a test dose of histamine was impaired after prior administration of a large dose of histamine. However, if the initial high dose of drug administered was pilocarpine, subsequent test doses of histamine were also decreased. By increasing the potassium ion in the medium to twice the usual concentration, they were able to administer large doses of histamine without impairing the contractile responses of the intestinal smooth muscle to subsequent test doses of this drug. Thus, the desensitization phenomenon that these investigators observed was nonspecific and could be abolished by potassium ion.

In a more recent study, Morgenstern and Bluth (1976) have noted that the specificity of the desensitization reaction in smooth muscle could be complete, partial, or essentially nonexistent. Their studies were performed on the guinea pig ileum. The procedure they employed consisted of exposing the smooth muscle preparation to a high concentration of an agonist for a 10-m period. The high desensitizing concentration of the agonist was then washed out, and resensitization of the tissue preparation was periodically tested by introducing smaller test doses of an agonist. The degree to which these smooth muscle cells become desensitized is a function of both the concentration of the desensitizing agent employed and the length of time that the muscle preparation is exposed to the desensitizing agent. Resensitization of the muscle preparation appears to progress as a linear function of time. Morgenstern and Bluth (1976) measured the linear progression of resensitization with time for a variety of desensitizing and test drugs. The intercepts of their regression lines denoted the percentage of the normal contractile response that a test dose of agonist would elicit immediately after washing out the desensitizing agent. It disclosed, in essence, the maximum degree of desensitization that the ileal muscle developed as a result of being exposed to the desensitizing agent. The slopes of their regression lines denoted the rate at which the contractile responses of the smooth muscle returned to a normal magnitude. When acetylcholine was used as the desensitizing agonist, responses to test doses of acetylcholine, carbachol, histamine, and serotonin were clearly diminished. Resensitization to all test agonists showed little difference. The intercepts of all linear regression lines were found to be near zero, and the slopes were found to be quite steep (greater than 1.6). When histamine was used as the desensitizing agonist, responses to test doses of acetylcholine, carbachol, and serotonin were only weakly affected. In contrast to an intercept of 18.7% and a rather steep slope of 2.0 for histamine, the intercepts of the lines for acetylcholine, carbachol, and serotonin were found to be between 72.4% and 85.0%, and the slopes were much more shallow. When serotonin was used as the desensitizing agent, responses to test doses of acetylcholine, carbachol and histamine were not affected significantly. Whereas the regression line for serotonin had an intercept of 25% and a rather steep slope, the lines for acetylcholine, carbachol, and histamine had intercepts that were between 99% and 108% and slopes that were extremely shallow. Thus, acetylcholine appeared to act as a nonspecific desensitizing agent, histamine as a partially specific desensitizing agent, and serotonin as a completely specific desensitizing agent.

Although it may be reasonable to speculate that receptor modification in smooth muscle cells leads to the development of a specific desensitization, some alternative explanation must be sought for the appearance of nonspecific desensitization. Studies carried out on the longitudinal muscle of the guinea pig ileum have raised the possibility that sodium ion may be involved in the nonspecific desensitization produced by acetylcholine (Joiner, 1973; Paton and Rothschild, 1965). It appears that in the presence of acetylcholine the smooth muscle initially gains sodium ions, which are later extruded. The electrogenic extrusion of sodium ions is thought to oppose the depolarizing action of the cholinergic agonist and as a consequence may induce the development of nonspecific desensitization. Experimental findings consistent with this hypothesis are (a) the observation that ouabain, which prevents the extrusion of sodium ions, reduced the decline of the acetylcholine-induced contraction that occurred during the continued presence of the cholinergic agonist (Joiner, 1973) and (b) the observation that calcium deficiency, which reduced the entry of sodium into the cell in the presence of acetylcholine, also reduced the intensity of the desensitization that developed (Paton and Rothschild, 1965).

Electrophysiological studies performed in two different laboratories have shown that desensitization is indeed accompanied by a repolarization of the smooth muscle membrane. This observation was made in the guinea pig tenia coli exposed to 5.5×10^{-5}M carbachol (Magaribuchi, Ito, and Kuriyama, 1973) and in the rat myometrium exposed to $3-6 \times 10^{-4}$M carbachol or $3-6 \times 10^{-6}$M oxytocin (Johnson and Marshall, 1972). In both cases the introduction of the agonist induced an intial depolarization of the membrane and a rise in muscle tension. However, during the continued presence of the agonist, these events were followed by a repolarization of the membrane and a fall in muscle tension. In the guinea pig tenia coli membrane resistance was also monitored. Initially it was reduced, but during the desensitization phase it increased again. In bathing solutions in which sodium ion was reduced or calcium ion was increased, the desensitization reaction in the tenia coli was accelerated. In solutions in which calcium ion or chloride ion was reduced or potassium ion was increased, the desensitization reaction was suppressed. Several speculative suggestions involving ionic mechanisms have been offered to account for some of these findings, but the underlying basis for the development of desensitization is still to be established. The problem is complicated by the fact that the desensitization process in different types of smooth muscle cells does not seem to be influenced by the same external factors. In the vas deferens of the rat (Miranda, 1976), for example, a norepinephrine-induced desensitization was reported to be unaffected by drastic modifications in the sodium and calcium ion concentrations in the bathing solution. The reduction in sensitivity produced by the norepinephrine appeared to be nonspecific because responses to test doses of serotonin and acetylcholine, as well as those of norepinephrine, were attenuated. In the myometrium of the rat (Johnson and Marshall, 1972), the time course of desensitization to carbachol and oxytocin was also unaffected by alterations in the extracellular calcium ion concentration over a range of 1.0–7.5 mM. In this case, however, the agonists carbachol and oxytocin were both deemed to be inducers of a specific desensitization. This latter conclusion was based on the demonstration that a myometrial preparation, after undergoing desensitization to carbachol, would remain fully responsive to a high concentration of oxytocin and vice versa. The responsiveness of the desensitized muscle preparation to submaximal test doses of each of the agonists was never investigated and might have yielded different results.

The factors influencing the desensitization reaction induced by β-adrenergic agonists in smooth muscle also vary from one type of smooth muscle cell to another. In isolated tracheal smooth muscle from the guinea pig (Douglas et al., 1977), desensitization to the relaxant action of isoproterenol was induced by preincubating the muscle preparation in a high concentration of the catecholamine. If the muscle was pretreated with an inhibitor of prostaglandin synthetase, indomethacin, the desensitization to the relaxant effect of isoproterenol was prevented. On the other hand, incubation with dibutyryl cyclic AMP; dibutyryl cyclic GMP; norepinephrine; or the phosphodiesterase inhibitors papaverine, theophylline, and ICI 58301 also desensitized the tracheal muscle to isoproterenol. Attempts to influence the sensitivity of the tracheal preparation to the action of isoproterenol with sodium nitrite, methoxamine, or adenosine were not successful. The investigators (Douglas et al., 1977) who obtained these results concluded that their data were inconsistent with the concept that desensitization produced in the guinea pig tracheal preparation results from a perturbation of the β-adrenergic receptor. They noted, however, that desensitization to β-adrenergic agonists could be produced by agents which appear to enhance the levels of intracellular cyclic AMP, but not by agents which do not affect cyclic AMP content. On this basis, they speculated that prolonged elevations of cyclic AMP in the smooth muscle may possibly result in a feedback inhibition of adenylate cyclase or stimulation of phosphodiesterase or both.

In this regard, Murad and Kimura (1974) have reported that both epinephrine and prostaglandin E_1 cause a transitory increase in cyclic AMP levels in tracheal rings from the rat. The concentration of cyclic AMP reached a peak in 2 to 3 m and then declined. Introducing the β-adrenergic blocking agent, propranolol, served to inhibit the epinephrine-induced increase in cyclic AMP but did not modify the increase in cyclic AMP produced by prostaglandin E_1. The α-adrenergic blocker, phenoxybenzamine, was found to have no effect on either the epinephrine- or the prostaglandin E_1-induced increase in cyclic AMP. This finding suggested that the two agonists increase adenylate cyclase activity and the accumulation of cyclic AMP by different pathways but that desensitization to both these excitatory agents results from a decrease in cyclic AMP synthesis or an increase in cyclic AMP hydrolysis.

The fact that Douglas et al. (1977) could prevent the development of an isoproterenol-induced desensitization in tracheal muscle with indomethacin suggested a possible relationship between the loss of sensitivity to β-adrenergic agonists and prostaglandin biosynthesis. This type of association has also been reported for vascular smooth muscle by Gryglewski and Ocetkiewicz (1974). The latter workers found that the infusion of norepinephrine in the cat produced an immediate increase in blood pressure, which was followed by a slow decline to a normal level of blood pressure over a 30-m period. In addition, they observed that during the early stages of the acute tolerance to norepinephrine, a substance appeared in the venous blood that acted much like prostaglandin when tested by a bioassay procedure. In the presence of indomethacin, the tolerance developed to norepinephrine was relieved and the prostaglandinlike substance did not appear to be present in the bloodstream. On the basis of these findings, the authors postulated that vasoconstriction induced by norepinephrine elicits a release of prostaglandins in vascular beds. The prostaglandins, in turn, exert a vasodilatory action on the vascular beds, thus decreasing peripheral resistance and inducing tolerance.

Shaw, Jessup, and Ramwell (1972) have offered a suggestion that combines the concept of the linkage of desensitization to β agonists and prostaglandin synthesis with the concept that desensitization involves a feedback inhibition of adenylate cyclase or stimulation of phosphodiesterase. They postulate that prostaglandins are formed as a consequence of the production of cyclic AMP and that these prostaglandins act as the negative feedback inhibitors of cyclic AMP accumulation in the smooth muscle cell. A precedent for this suggestion derives from studies that have been performed on rat adipocytes. It has been found that elevations of cyclic AMP levels in the adipocytes will induce the generation of an adenylate cyclase inhibitor (Ho and Sutherland, 1971) that has been identified as a prostaglandin precursor, prostaglandin endoperoxide, PGH_2 (Gorman, Hamberg, and Samuelsson, 1976). Whether a similar type of reaction occurs in smooth muscle cells has yet to be determined.

Using isolated strips of tracheal smooth muscle from the rat, rather than the guinea pig, Lin et al. (1977) demonstrated a completely different type of desensitization process. These workers found that the muscle became considerably less sensitive to the relaxing action of isoproterenol after incubation with $5 \times 10^{-6}M$ isoproterenol for 30 m. Pretreatment with propranolol protected the tracheal muscle against the isoproterenol-induced desensitization. Moreover, an isoproterenol-desensitized muscle exhibited diminished sensitivity to other β agonists, but not to the spasmolytic actions of D600, hydralazine, sodium nitrite, or aminophylline. The authors concluded that these data support the concept that the β-adrenergic receptor is specifically involved in the desensitization produced by isoproterenol. Subsequent experiments did not permit them to reach any definite conclusion with respect to a possible reduction in receptor binding sites in the desensitized tracheal muscle, but the experiments provided ample evidence that the affinity of the β-adrenergic receptor for propranolol was significantly decreased. The dissociation constant for the propranolol-β receptor complex in the desensitized tissue was found to be 180-fold larger than that in normal tissue. This finding was considered to be an indirect indication that at least one of the underlying causes for the development of desensitization of rat tracheal strips to isoproterenol and other β agonists is a diminution in the affinity of the β-adrenergic receptor for both β agonists and antagonists. Whether the reduction in affinity is due to some conformational change in the receptor molecule or to the formation of some competitive inhibitory substance that occupies the β receptor could not be determined from the results obtained in this study.

In order to determine whether a decrease in the affinity of the β receptor of the rat tracheal muscle for propranolol would also occur in vivo, Avner and Noland (1978) injected various concentrations of isoproterenol or terbutaline into rats for a period of 3 to 7 days. The rats were then sacrificed, the tracheal muscle was isolated, and the dissociation constant for the propranolol-β receptor complex was determined. They found a highly significant difference between the dissociation constants determined in tissues from control (saline-treated) rats and those determined in tissues from isoproterenol- or terbutaline-treated rats. The degree to which the magnitude of the dissociation constant was elevated depended both on the concentration of isoproterenol used and on the length of time that the agonist was administered to the animals.

The results of this work stand in sharp contrast to the observations made in other smooth muscle preparations, which suggested a cyclic-AMP–prostaglandin negative feedback mechanism as the underlying cause of the desensitization that was produced by catecholamines. It also differs from the observation made in a number of non-muscle-cell types in which desensitization resulted from a reduction in the number of β-adrenergic receptors.

In the aortic smooth muscle of the rat, the relaxation produced by repeated applications of high concentrations of isoproterenol not only diminished, but usually changed into a contractile effect (Fleisch and Titus, 1972). No evidence of an eventual desensitization to the contractile effect of the isoproterenol was detected. The inference drawn from these observations was that the β receptor action of isoproterenol can undergo desensitization, whereas the α receptor action of the isoproterenol is resistant to desensitization. The presence of phentolamine, bromolysergic acid diethylamide, aminophylline, caffeine, theobromine, tetracaine, papaverine, and nitroglycerin inhibited the isoproterenol-induced desensitization and prevented the conversion of the action of isoproterenol from one that induced relaxation to one that induced contraction. Since none of these agents appear to interact with the β receptor per se, the postulate put forth was that this diverse group of drugs may exert an effect on the smooth muscle membrane. This effect may involve an allosterically mediated stabilization of receptors and thereby permit the β receptors to function without undergoing desensitization. This suggestion is, of course, a highly speculative one, and the extent to which it is valid cannot be assessed at the present time.

A considerable effort has also been made to elucidate the underlying basis for the desensitization produced by angiotensin in smooth muscle cells. The reader is referred to the review by Stewart (1974) for a thorough examination of the work done prior to 1974. More recently, Moore and Khairallah (1976) have examined the effectiveness of a number of analogues of angiotensin in producing desensitization. Although rabbit aorta and rat stomach do not readily exhibit a loss of responsiveness to angiotensin, they do develop a subsensitivity to several specific analogues of this agonist. On the other hand, the rat uterus can develop a subsensitivity to both angiotensin and analogues of the peptide. The desensitization produced in all these tissues, although qualitatively different, was reported to be related to the affinity of the angiotensin analogue for the receptor. The higher the affinity of an angiotensin analogue for the angiotensin receptor, the more readily is the desensitization produced (Moore, Bumpus, and Khairallah, 1977; Moore and Khairallah, 1976).

An alternative hypothesis has been proposed by Freer and Stewart (1972) and Stewart (1974) and by Paiva et al. (1974) and Paiva, Mendes, and Paiva (1977). Working independently, these two groups have suggested that desensitization is produced by an abnormal binding of angiotensin to an anionic site that normally binds calcium. This anionic calcium site is located close to the receptor. By virtue of the binding of angiotensin to the anionic site, an abnormal folding of the angiotensin molecule occurs. Thus the change in receptor conformation that is required for the development of a contractile response does not occur. As long as the angiotensin molecule is in combination with the abnormal binding site, the cell is desensitized to subsequent doses of angiotensin. The difference between the theories of Freer and Stewart (1972) and Stewart (1974) and Paiva et al. (1974, 1977) relates to the specific chemical group of the angiotensin molecule that is involved in the interaction with the desensitization-inducing tissue binding site. According to Freer and Stewart (1972), the interaction is between the protonated imidazole on the histidine residue of the angiotensin molecule and the binding site. However, Paiva et al. (1974) contend that the interaction is between the protonated amino group of angiotensin and the binding site. It has subsequently been suggested that both protonated imidazole and amino groups may be involved in the production of desensitization (Stewart et al., 1976). Data confirming that the anionic site is indeed a calcium site can be found by examining the effect of calcium ion concentration and pH on the induction of desensitization. At a physiological calcium ion concentration, desensitization does not occur in rat uterus even at low pH. However, at normal pH and low calcium ion concentration, desensitization does occur. At low pH and low calcium-ion concentration, desensitization is induced and can be reversed by increasing either the pH or the calcium ion concentration (Freer and Stewart, 1972; Stewart, 1974). These findings suggest that the anionic site responsible for desensitization may be saturated with calcium under normal conditions. Along these same lines of investigation, Paiva et al. (1977) showed that recovery from the desensitized state requires the displacement of angiotensin from the binding site by calcium ions and that this displacement is an active process. However, the investigators warn that the proposed interaction between the angiotensin molecule and the calcium binding site may not be simply a competitive phenomenon, since they could not inhibit desensitization in the guinea pig ileum simply by raising the calcium ion concentration.

In an effort to understand why a tissue such as the rat uterus undergoes a reduction in responsiveness to angiotensin, whereas under the same experimental conditions the rabbit aorta does not, Freer (1975) examined the sources of calcium for contraction in these two tissues. He found that a tissue such as the uterus, which requires for the most part external calcium for an angiotensin-induced contraction, can become desensitized; whereas a tissue such as the aorta, which requires primarily internal calcium for contraction, does not undergo desensitization. This hypothesis provides an alternative to that of Khairallah et al. (1966), in which it is suggested that the rabbit aorta is resistant to the development of desensitization because it contains a larger concentration of angiotensinase, which can eliminate the presence of an effective concentration of the desensitizing agent.

At the present time, neither the anionic theories as proposed by Paiva and coworkers (Paiva et al., 1974, 1977) and Freer and Stewart (1972) nor the affinity theory of Moore and coworkers (Moore and Khairallah, 1976; 1977; Moore et al., 1977) can be excluded from consideration as possible mechanisms of angiotensin-induced desensitization. It is very possible, as suggested by Stewart (1974), that there may be different mechanisms for the induction of desensitization to angiotensin in different smooth muscles.

IV. GENERAL CONCLUSIONS

From a consideration of the currently available data on desensitization two general conclusions may be drawn. First, the diminution or loss of responsiveness of cells to excitatory stimuli appears to be a highly important adaptive process that can occur in many different kinds of tissue, including smooth muscle. This adaptive process serves to counteract the potentially detrimental effects of very high levels of excitatory agents that remain in the vicinity of the reactive cells for excessively long periods of time. Second, it is incorrect to view the development of desensitization as the final outcome of some single specific series of biochemical and/or physiological reactions. Current evidence would indicate that the desensitization that develops in different types of cells or the desensitization induced by different agonists in the same cell type may be achieved by a variety of dissimilar molecular mechanisms. Consequently, one must use extreme caution when attempting to explain the basis for desensitization in one type of cell from evidence obtained in another type of cell.

V. REFERENCES

Avner, B.P.; Noland, B.: *In Vivo* Desensitization to Beta Receptor Mediated Bronchodilator Drugs in the Rat: Decreased beta receptor affinity. J Pharmacol Exp Ther 207(1978)23

Barsoum, G.S.; Gaddum, J.H.: The Pharmacological Estimation of Adenosine and Histamine in Blood. J Physiol (Lond) 85(1935)1

Cantoni, G.L.; Eastman, G.: On the Response of the Intestine to Smooth Muscle Stimulants. J Pharmacol Exp Ther 87(1946)392

Cox, B.M.; Padhya, R.: Opiate Binding and Effect in Ileum Preparations from Normal and Morphine Pretreated Guinea-Pigs. Br J Pharmacol 61(1977)271

DeVellis, J.; Brooker, G.: Reversal of Catecholamine Refractoriness by Inhibitors of RNA and Protein Synthesis. Science 186(1974)1221

Douglas, J.S.; Lewis, A.J.; Ridgway, P.; Brink, C.; Bouhuys, A.: Tachyphylaxis to β-Adrenoceptor Agonists in Guinea Pig Airway Smooth Muscle *in Vivo* and *in Vitro*. Eur J Pharmacol 42(1977)195

Fleisch, J.H.; Titus, E.: The Prevention of Isoproterenol Desensitization and Isoproterenol Reversal. J Pharmacol Exp Ther 181(1972)425

Freer, R.J.: Calcium and Angiotensin Tachyphylaxis in Rat Uterine Smooth Muscle. Am J Physiol 228(1975)1423

Freer, R.J.; Stewart, J.M.: Some Characteristics of Uterine Angiotensin Receptors. In: Structure-Activity Relationships of Protein and Polypeptide Hormones, pp. 490–495, ed. by M. Margoulies, F.C. Greenwood, Excerpta Medica, Amsterdam, 1972

Gavin, J.R., III; Roth, J.; Neville, D.M.; DeMeyte, P.; Buell, D.N.: Insulin-Dependent Regulation of Insulin Receptor Concentrations: A Direct Demonstration in Cell Culture. Proc Nat Acad Sci USA 71(1974)84

Gorman, R.R.; Hamberg, M.; Samuelsson, B.: Inhibition of Adenylate Cyclase in Adipocyte Ghosts by the Prostaglandin Endoperoxide PGH_2. In: Advances in Prostaglandin and Thromboxane Research, Vol. I, pp. 325–330, ed. by B. Samuelsson, R. Paoletti. Raven, New York, 1976

Gryglewski, R.J.; Ocetkiewicz, A.: A release of Prostaglandins May Be Responsible for Acute Tolerance to Norepinephrine Infusions. Prostaglandins 8(1974)31

Ho, R.-J; Sutherland, E.W.: Formation and Release of a Hormone Antagonist by Rat Adipocytes. J Biol Chem 246(1971)6822

Johnson, P.N.; Marshall, J.M.: Desensitization in the Rat Myometrium. Am J Physiol 223(1972)249

Joiner, P.D.: Studies on the Loss of Acetylcholine Sensitivity in Ileal Muscle. J Pharmacol Exp Ther 186(1973)552

Katz, B.; Thesleff, S.: A Study of the Desensitization Produced by Acetylcholine at the Motor Endplate. J Physiol (Lond) 138(1957)63

Kebabian, J.W.; Zatz, M.; Romero, J.A.; Axelrod, J.: Rapid Changes in Rat Pineal β-Adrenergic Receptor: Alterations in 1-[³H]Alprenolol Binding and Adenylate Cyclase. Proc Nat Acad Sci USA 72(1975)3735

Khairallah, P.A.; Page, I.H.; Bumpus, F.M.; Türker, R.K.: Angiotensin Tachyphylaxis and Its Reversal. Circ Res 19(1966)274

Kobayashi, M.; Olefsky, J.M.: Effect of Experimental Hyperinsulinemia on Insulin Binding and Glucose Transport in Isolated Rat Adipocytes. Am J Physiol 235(1978)E53

Lesniak, M.A.; Roth, J.: Regulation of Receptor Concentration by Homologous Hormone. J Biol Chem 251(1976)3720

Lin, C.-S.; Hurwitz, L.: Jenne, J.; Avner, B.P.: Mechanism of Isoproterenol-Induced Desensitization of Tracheal Smooth Muscle. J Pharmacol Exp Ther 202(1977)12

Magaribuchi, T.; Ito, Y.; Kuriyama, H.: Desensitization of Smooth Muscle Cells in the Guinea Pig Taenia Coli to Prolonged Application of Carbachol. Jpn J Physiol 23(1973)447

Miranda, H.: Vas Deferens Desensitization by Noradrenaline and Other Drugs. Arch Int Pharmacodyn Ther 221(1976)223

Moore, A.; Khairallah, P.A.: Further Studies on Angiotensin Tachyphylaxis. J Pharmacol Exp Ther 197(1976)575

Moore, A.F.; Bumpus, F.M.; Khairallah, P.A.: New Approaches to the Study of Angiotensin Tachyphylaxis. Mayo Clin Proc 52(1977)446

Morgenstern, R.; Bluth R.: Studies on the Loss of Sensitivity in Smooth Muscle. Acta Biol Med Ger 35(1976)K69

Mukherjee, C.; Caron, M.G.; Lefkowitz, R.J.: Catecholamine-Induced Subsensitivity of Adenylate Cyclase Associated with Loss of β-Adrenergic Receptor Binding Sites. Proc Nat Acad Sci USA 72(1975)1945

Murad, F.; Kimura, H.: Cyclic Nucleotide Levels in Incubations of Guinea Pig Trachea. Biochim Biophys Acta 343(1974)275

Nastuk, W.L.: Cholinergic Receptor Desensitization. In: Synapses, pp. 177–201, ed. by G.A. Cottrell, P.N.R. Usherwood. Academic, New York, 1977

Paiva, T.B.; Juliano, L.; Nouailhetas, V.L.A.; Paiva, A.C.M.: The Effect of pH on Tachyphylaxis to Angiotensin Peptides in the Isolated Guinea Pig Ileum and Rat Uterus. Eur J Pharmacol 25(1974)191

Paiva, T.B.; Mendes, G.B.; Paiva, A.C.M.: Specific Desensitization (tachyphylaxis) of the Guinea Pig Ileum to Angiotensin II. Am J Physiol 232(1977)H223

Paton, W.D.M.; Rothschild, A.M.: The Changes in Response and in Ionic Content of Smooth Muscle Produced by Acetylcholine Action and by Calcium Deficiency. Br J Pharmacol 24(1965)437

Raff, M.C.; DePetris, S.: Movement of Lymphocyte Surface Antigens and Receptors: The Fluid Nature of the Lymphocyte Plasma Membrane and Its Immunological Significance. Fed Proc Fed Am Soc Exp Biol 32(1973)48

Rang, H.P., and Ritter, J.M.: On the Mechanism of Desensitization at Cholinergic Receptors. Mol Pharmacol 6(1970)357

Shaw, J.E.; Jessup, S.J.: Ramwell, P.W.: Prostaglandin–Adenyl Cyclase Relationships. In: Advances in Cyclic Nucleotide Research, Vol. I, pp. 479–491, ed. by P. Greengard, R. Paoletti, G.A. Robison. Raven, New York, 1972

Stewart, J.M.: Tachyphylaxis to Angiotensin. In: Angiotensin, pp. 170–184, ed. by I.H. Page, F.M. Bumpus. Springer, New York, 1974

Stewart, J.M.; Freer, R.J.; Rezende, L.; Peña, C.; Matsueda, G.R.: A Pharmacological Study of the Angiotensin Receptor and Tachyphylaxis in Smooth Muscle. Gen Pharmacol 7(1976)177

Strittmatter, W.J.; Davis, J.N.; Lefkowitz, R.J.: Alpha-Adrenergic Receptors in Rat Parotid Cells. II. Desensitization of Receptor Binding Sites and Potassium Release. J Biol Chem 252(1977)5478

Su, Y.-F.; Cubeddu, L.Y.; Perkins, J.P.: Regulation of Adenosine 3':5'-Monophosphate Content of Human Astrocytoma Cells: Desensitization to Catecholamines and Prostaglandins. J Cyclic Nucleotide Res 2(1976)257

Unanue, E.R.; Perkins, W.D.; Karnovsky, M.J.: Ligand-Induced Movement of Lymphocyte Membrane Macromolecules. J Exp Med 136(1972)885

Williams, L.T.; Lefkowitz, R.J.: Regulation of Adrenergic Receptors. In: Receptor Binding Studies in Adrenergic Pharmacology. pp. 127–149. Raven, New York, 1978

Termination of Agonist Action on Autonomic Receptors

Stanley Kalsner

I. INTRODUCTION

The interaction of neurotransmitter substances and their analogues with responsive tissues has traditionally been assessed in terms of the magnitude of the characteristic response of the organ system under study—for example, tension development in muscle, frequency or rate of response in cardiac or nervous tissue, and the quantitative volume of secretion in exocrine glands. Except for work concerned specifically with the dynamics of agonist-receptor interactions, the dissipation of agonist-induced responses with time has, until recent years, received little attention.

In some early studies, note was made of the duration of the effects produced by sympathomimetic or cholinomimetic agents, and occasionally even the rate of decline of the effect was recorded. For example, Elliot (1905) showed that contractions of a smooth muscle *in vivo* to an agonist such as adrenaline are increased in both duration and magnitude after nerve section, and Cannon and Rosenblueth (1949) observed that cocaine prolongs as well as enhances the contraction of the nictitating membrane and the rise in blood pressure induced by noradrenaline or adrenaline. However, the fact is still not commonly appreciated that many alterations in the physiological state of innervated systems are reflected not only in the magnitude but also in the duration of the induced response.

A number of contemporary theories in autonomic pharmacology, particularly adrenergic mechanisms, rest heavily on postulates that could be investigated by studying the rate of decay of the effects of agonists on responsive tissues; and this undoubtably accounts for the encouraging current trend toward evaluating the response as a holistic event involving its development, maintenance, and decline, rather than monocularly in terms of peak response magnitude alone.

Termination of action is a homeostatic process. The cells of an effector, in a state of heightened or diminished activity due to receptor activation, are released from external control as the number of inciting agonist molecules diminishes. For our purposes here, response termination is "concerned strictly with the reduction in the number of active agonist molecules at the locus of action, the processes which enforce this dilution and its consequences on magnitude and duration of response" (Kalsner, 1977, p. 315). This article will survey briefly the variety of agonist removal processes likely to be operative in typical autonomic effector systems and their relationships to each other and to termination of action. In the article it will also emerge that although terminating mechanisms are operative throughout the temporal contours of the response, the consequences of their inhibition on response magnitude are not always easily predictable.

II. ACCESS BARRIERS VERSUS TERMINATION OF ACTION

Perhaps the most debated sensitization in adrenergic pharmacology is that induced by cocaine on responses to catecholamines. In preparations as diverse in structure and function as rabbit ear artery and cat nictitating membrane, profound magnification of responses to exogenous noradrenaline and adrenaline is elicited by this agent. It is now appreciated that some (but not all) of the effect of cocaine is attributable to the inhibition of an active neuronal uptake process for catecholamines located at sympathetic nerve terminals. However, rather than resolving the long-standing dispute regarding the mechanisms terminating the action of the sympathetic transmitter, as is widely assumed, it illuminates the consequences of confounding access barriers with terminating mechanisms.

This can be understood easily by an analysis of the rabbit ear preparation of De La Lande et al. (1967), where the nerve plexus is discretely wrapped about the outer face of the media, an arrangement not uncommon in vascular tissue. Thus, if a section of vessel is cannulated at both ends for intraluminal perfusion, and also mounted in a muscle chamber so that Krebs solution separately bathes the outer surface, the noradrenaline can be selectively applied through one surface of the preparation only. This allows a fairly precise assessment of the influence of the nerve plexus on response magnitude. Extraluminally applied noradrenaline passes through the nerve plexus to reach responsive muscle cells, whereas access to the muscle layer is unrestricted by the intraluminal route. Since it was found that the potentiation of responses to extraluminally applied noradrenaline by cocaine is considerably greater than to intraluminally applied noradrenaline, it was widely assumed to represent a definitive demonstration of uptake acting as a potent terminating mechanism in one but not the other case. However, whereas access barriers metabolize, impede, bind, or in other ways limit the number of free agonist molecules en route to the receptors, they do not decide the rate of removal from the receptors and thus the duration of the response (Kalsner, 1976a). For once at the sites of action, the agonist molecules are subject to a host of additional processes, such as extraneuronal uptake, diffusive dilution, enzymatic degradation and passive binding; and it is the relative activity of these processes, along with neuronal uptake, all drawing on a common pool of active agonist molecules, that determines agonist duration.

It is imperative to note, however, that when magnitude of response alone is considered, inhibition of an access barrier may have impressive consequences. As shown in Figure 1, a functional access barrier can reduce the passage of 100 molecules per unit time to 50, 10, 1, or even less, whereas a terminating mechanism is confined to the number of molecules already available for and participating in action at the receptors.

The action of cocaine to enhance responses to exogenous catecholamines in numerous preparations is, at least partially, a measure of the effectiveness of a dense and active nerve plexus, in some cases interwoven throughout the tissue, acting as an absorption barrier to free passage of amine to its receptors rather than in a terminating capacity. For example, a 100-fold increase in responses to noradrenaline (dose ratio) in the nictitating membrane, due solely to block of a terminating mechanism, would be feasible only if the gradient for noradrenaline toward the nerve terminals from the receptors is the only pathway involved in reducing the agonist concentration at the biophase (which it is not) and—an important point—if, after its inhibition by cocaine, the nerve plexus acts as a virtual physical barrier to free diffusion. If amine, which would otherwise be extracted by the nerves, could diffuse, even only fractionally, through and past the nerve plexus or be transported extraneuronally, then termination of action would not be drastically reduced. That diffusion past an inhibited nerve uptake process can rapidly dilute noradrenaline released by nerve activity is abundantly clear (Brown, 1965; Su and Bevan, 1970; Bevan and Osher, 1970), as is the widespread presence of an extraneuronal uptake process (Avakian and Gillespie, 1968; Kalsner and Nickerson, 1968a; Kalsner and Nickerson, 1969b; Trendelenburg and Henseling, 1976).

The problem of distinguishing between access barriers and terminating mechanisms is not confined to adrenergic mechanisms, but holds for other transmitter substances and their actions as well. Even the intense amplification of acetylcholine-induced responses by inhibition of cholinesterase

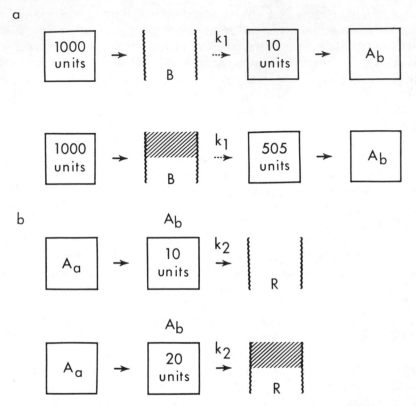

Figure 1. A schema depicting the effects on agonist concentration in the biophase of a disposition mechanism functioning either as access barrier or as terminating mechanism. a:*Top*, the functional access barrier B (e.g., nerve uptake, enzymatic pathway) reduces the passage of 1,000 units to 10 units; *bottom*, a 50% inhibition of the activity of the disposition mechanism leads to an increase of over 50-fold in the number of penetrating agonist molecules en route to receptors. b: *Top*, 50% inhibition of the termination process R (e.g., extraneuronal uptake, enzymatic pathway) leads maximally to a doubling of agonist at receptors under steady-state conditions (*bottom*) and to a twofold prolongation of response duration after decline of A_a. A_a and A_b represent agonist in the external (aqueous) phase and biophase (receptor region), respectively; k_1 and k_2 are rate constants for approach of agonist to and removal from receptor region (A_b). B represents access barriers and R the terminating processes. (Reproduced by permission of the National Research Council of Canada from Can J Physiol Pharmacol 54[1976]177–187.)

appears to involve blockade of enzyme operating to cleave acetylcholine en route to its receptors (Zupančič, 1953; Eccles and Jaegar, 1958).

Since the functions of access barriers and terminating mechanisms differ, it is not surprising that the consequences of their inhibition also differ, not only on response magnitude and duration, but also on other parameters of response performance. These include the slopes of concentration-response curves, the influence of routes of agonist administration on response, and interactions with other inactivation processes. The reader is referred to a recent review for an in-depth analysis of these often critical differences (Kalsner, 1976a).

III. THE MAGNITUDE OF SENSITIZATIONS

There are many forms of sensitization, only some of which are linked to deficits in agonist inactivation. The complex postsynaptic origin of several sensitizations are just now under scrutiny; the enhanced maximal responses observed in certain sensitizations, the nonspecificity of decentralization and reserpine supersensitivities, and direct evidence for a postsynaptic action of reserpine and even for cocaine have been significant factors in this trend. Continued study of these processes is essential if durable models of sensitization are to be formulated. For example, responses to noradrenaline and other sympathomimetic amines can be enhanced by drug-induced modulation of effector cell physiology, to a magnitude sometimes comparable or even materially greater than that elicited by interruption with termination of action. Thus, in vascular tissue, responses to noradrenaline are increased two- to threefold by agents that interfere with the rebinding of calcium released into the environment of the contractile elements or by those that promote the use of extracellular and/or loosely bound calcium for contraction (Kalsner, 1970; 1973). Chronic reserpine treatment enhances contractions of some vascular smooth muscle to catecholamines much more than does total inhibition of all its endogenous inactivation pathways, and it does this without material interruption in tissue rates of agonist inactivation (Kalsner and Nickerson, 1969a).

The well-established procedure for assessing sensitization of responses of an autonomic effector to an agonist, regardless of the origin of the sensitization, has been to determine the horizontal distance between dose-response curves, analogous to the use of the dose ratio in the study of drug antagonism (Trendelenburg, 1963). However, this procedure is inadequate in separating sensitizations related to interruption of agonist disposition pathways from those involving changes in the physiology of the responding tissue itself (Kalsner, 1974a). Sensitizations need to be placed in two main categories: type I, those attributable to increases in the effective concentration of agonist at the receptors; and type II, those due to changes in the effector, presumably demonstrable at some point between drug-receptor combination and ultimate tissue response. This is illustrated in Figure 2.

If a sensitization is linked to an increase in the effective concentration of agonist at the receptors, it is correctly expressed by determining the reduction in the administered concentration necessary to produce the same response as in the control condition (e.g., at the ED_{50}). This is the procedure of assessing the horizontal shift of the dose-response curve, and it is obvious that the determined value will vary from agonist to agonist, depending on the relative importance of the inhibited process (e.g., access barrier, terminating mechanism) in reducing its concentration at the receptors. If the sensitization is linked to an alteration in the responding tissue itself, however, then it must be assessed in the direction of response magnitude. Thus it can be seen, for example, that a magnification in the strength of the signal moving through a to c, or e to f, or f to g (in fig. 2) would result in a uniform magnification of a given quantity of response (g) for all agonists acting on receptor systems R_1–R_3 in the first instance or R_1–R_7 in the second and third instances, regardless of the shapes of the agonist-induced concentration-response curves. This is so because the intensity of the signal moving along any common path in the schema must be the same for all elicited responses of equivalent magnitude, regardless of agonist employed or receptor system activated to initiate it.

Horizontal assessment of such data could lead to gross misrepresentations of the degree of sensitization and even to the erroneous conclusion that responses are depressed when in fact they are enhanced (Kalsner, 1974a). Thus, when reserpine-induced sensitization in aortic strips is measured by the dose ratio procedure, an unpredictable variation in sensitization is obtained, depending on agonist and response level selected for comparison. However, when type II procedures are applied, it is found that the mm

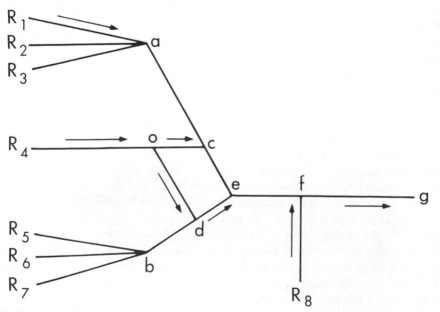

Figure 2. A schema depicting the sequence of steps between agonist receptor systems (R_1–R_7) and response (g) in an effector. (Reprinted courtesy of Br J Pharmacol 51[1974]427–434.)

increment in final recorded contraction amplitude approaches a constant value for the entire group of sympathomimetics analyzed. Responses to potassium, which by horizontal procedures were assessed among the least increased, were enhanced the most when a vertical evaluation was made.

In calculating sensitizations linked to depressed agonist inactivation routes, it is the type I approach that should be used. However, another concern arises. The assumption must be avoided that there is a parallel shift of the concentration-response curve such that comparisons at the ED_{50} are made representative of the entire curve. This is unlikely often to be the case. Type I sensitizations involve modifications of dynamic, saturable, and competing processes; and the role of a given pathway in the metabolism of an agonist is unlikely to remain constant over the broad concentration range generally required for a concentration-response curve. The lack of parallelism in the concentration-response curve after inhibition of individual inactivation pathways has been demonstrated (Kalsner, 1974a), and it is clear that a single value such as the ED_{50} is probably inadequate and potentially misleading when used alone to describe a sensitization involving altered agonist disposition.

IV. SENSITIZATION AND TERMINATION OF ACTION

The processes terminating action are operative not only during the dissipation of the response but during its development and maintenance as well. The response plateau is an expression of equilibrium between agonist accumulation and removal at the pertinent tissue receptors. Interference with termination of action will produce the same proportionate increase in response magnitude in the presence of agonist (type I sensitization) and in duration of response, once the concentration of drug in the external phase wanes or nerve excitation abates, since they are kinetically linked. Accordingly, response potentiation under steady-state conditions can be a valid monitor of terminating events, but only under certain specified terms: (a) if inhibition of access barriers is eliminated as a contributing factor to the sensitization and (b) if all incidental effects of the inhibitor that might account for the sensitization are rigorously excluded from participation. This latter point deserves some commentary.

Sensitization agents rarely have a simple profile of action. For example, potentiation by cocaine was at one time attributed to its weak activity as a monoamine oxidase inhibitor, and that induced by Catron to its high potency as an inhibitor of the same enzyme. Neither assignment was correct. Similarly, a number of cholinesterase inhibitors enhance responses to agonists that are not substrates for the enzyme. Other examples are available in a recent review (Kalsner, 1976a) and elsewhere. It is obviously critical that the specificity of the induced sensitization in the particular tissue under study be examined with a range of agonists, some of which are not substrates for the pathway under consideration, to determine whether potentiation develops or fails to develop when expected. It is preferable and far more secure to study termination of action directly; this is discussed below.

V. TERMINATION OF ACTION

A. Limitations of Measurements of Tissue Metabolites

Termination of action is a physiological event describing a process of recovery from agonist-induced excitation in an effector tissue; yet it has most often been explored remotely, by biochemical measurements of the amount of agonist and its metabolites present in particular tissues under incubation conditions. Although we no longer are subjected to analyses of terminating pathways based on the incubation of disrupted tissue homogenates or minces with the agonist under study, similar analyses done with intact tissues are also, by themselves, of limited worth in describing terminating events in functioning autonomic effectors.

For example, the presence of active cholinesterase in intact rabbit aorta, capable of rapidly hydrolyzing added acetylcholine, gives little insight into termination of action when it is observed separately that even complete inhibition of the enzyme does not enhance contractile responses to the choline ester (Ehrenpreis, Bigo-Gullimo, and Anery, 1965). In addition, the enthusiasm for presynaptic uptake of catecholamines as the only important terminating process in sympathetically innervated tissues derives from the identification of a neuronal transport process for noradrenaline so effective that it "is capable of clearing the entire extracellular space of the heart in approximately 10 seconds" (Iversen, 1971, p. 573). However, such a feat presumes that all the free and active noradrenaline in a tissue be presented directly to the nerve transport sites within that time interval and additionally that no other competing processes—perhaps less rapid, but strategically placed with respect to the receptors—also function. This is an unlikely assumption.

For example, guinea pig ileum shows a catecholamine content, a Km of amine uptake, and an ED_{50} for drug inhibiting uptake in the nerves of Auerbachs' plexus comparable to the values reported for heart; yet blockade of neuronal uptake with either cocaine or desipramine does not sensitize inhibitory responses to noradrenaline (Govier, Sugrue, and Shore, 1969). As Govier states, "There must exist a finite distance over which this uptake mechanism is operative . . . if the distance between nerve terminals and effector organ receptor is greater . . . then the amine uptake mechanism will not alter significantly the amine concentration at the receptor" (Govier, 1968, p. 76). A similar explanation appears to hold for myocardial alpha receptors, since the positive inotropic effect attributable to their activation is not enhanced by cocaine (Govier, 1968), and other recent work indicates that a number of beta-receptor-mediated responses in smooth muscle are generally terminated by extraneuronal processes, as are some responses mediated by α receptors (Kalsner, 1978).

As our understanding of the intricacies of cellular microanatomy increases, it becomes clearer that pathways of agonist metabolism most relevant to the response are those situated strategically with respect to the pertinent receptors, and these can be appropriately defined only when attention is paid to the tissue response itself. The generalized assumption that the inactivation process accounting for the largest amount of agonist in the tissue or having the greatest turnover capacity is the most influential in terminating action is clearly unwarranted. The reader is also referred to the above discussion on access barriers for another such illustration.

A further essential limitation of simple assessment of the quantity of agonist and its metabolites present in the tissue at a particular point in time is that no differentiation can be made between primary events terminating action and secondary processes acting on already inactivated molecules—or, for that matter, between free and active agonist and loosely sequestered agonist unavailable for action. The sequential character of inactivation processes appears to be fairly common when established or putative transmitter substances are considered. Free extracellular catecholamine may be withdrawn into neuronal cytoplasm, a possible terminating event, and subsequently deaminated or contained in granules. Extraneuronal uptake may reduce the active agonist concentration at its effector sites of action, but definitive disposal rests with O-methylating and deaminating enzymes. Histamine may be N-methylated and also deaminated, but only one of the two structural modifications is needed to disrupt agonist efficacy. Again, agonist dilution by diffusion is certainly a contributor to termination of action in a number of systems, particularly when release is from a point source such as nerve terminals close to the receptor sites (Kalsner, 1977); but it is by necessity ignored when only biochemical assessments are made. Evidence for this is particularly clear in the case of 5-hydroxytryptamine release from mollusk ganglia (Gershenfeld and Stefani, 1968), where diffusive dilution appears to terminate action. It is important, that analyses of metabolites could only show the inadequacy of deamination at the ganglia, and physiologically oriented studies were necessary to demonstrate the primacy of diffusion in ending agonist action. The role of diffusion is also usually neglected in preparations where the transmitter outflow from innervated organs after nerve stimulation is collected (see below).

B. Techniques for Assessing Duration of Action

Termination of action is applicable only to that fraction of administered agonist or nerve-released mediator that reaches the immediate environment of and acts upon appropriate tissue receptors, and the responding tissue itself appears to provide the only reliable measure of this moiety now available. However, early workers with smooth muscle preparations, in particular, often assumed that whereas recovery from the response is initiated by removal of agonist from the biophase, the latter phases of the process were attributable to mechanical properties of the responding tissue unrelated to the rate of agonist removal. This assumption has been shown not to be the case. Kalsner and Nickerson (1968b) demonstrated that the relaxation of aortic strips in Krebs solution from agonist-induced contractions after washout of the agonist from the muscle baths is directly attributable, almost throughout its entire course, to the declining agonist concentration in the vicinity of the receptors. This has been amply confirmed not only for vascular tissue but for some other smooth muscles as well. The relaxation of contracted tissues after washout of agonist in Krebs solution is now routinely employed for the direct study of termination of action (Brandão, 1976, Trendelenburg and Henseling, 1976; Guimarães and Paiva, 1977), especially when diffusion of agonist out from the tissue is of prime concern.

It is obvious that when smooth muscles are mounted in a muscle chamber, diffusion of agonist from the responding tissue into the aqueous medium is maximized. The bath concentration drops to negligible levels at washout, and the usual repeated changes of bath fluid assure that a maximal concentration gradient is maintained. This maximization of diffusion out of the tissue as a mechanism terminating action can easily obscure tissue mechanisms of physiological importance, particularly with low concentrations of agonist, where relaxation is usually rapid. For that reason, the technique of oil immersion was developed (Kalsner and Nickerson, 1968a, b). After the response to the agonist under study has reached a plateau value in aqueous solution, the chamber is drained and refilled with warmed and oxygenated light mineral oil or silicone oil. The external source of drug is thus removed, trapping a fixed amount in the tissue; and the rate of relaxation becomes a direct measure of the capacity of intrinsic processes to terminate action. The use of this technique is illustrated in figures 3 and 4.

It has been shown that the oil itself has no detectable pharmacological action and that a reduction of the extracellular space from an essentially infinite volume to one only slightly greater than that of the interstitial compartment of the test tissue does not alter any parameter of the environment to an extent detectable by the performance of the tissue (Kalsner and Nickerson, 1968a, b). Although the statement cannot be made categorically

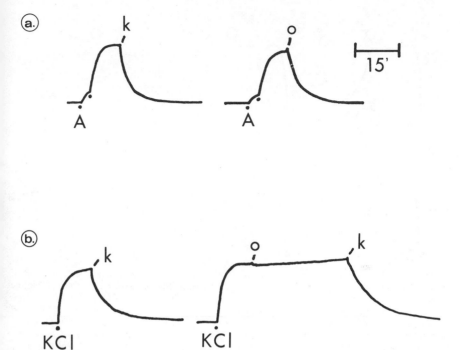

Figure 3. Behavior of aortic strips contracted by angiotensin and by KCl in Krebs solution and after oil immersion. a: Records of a strip contracted by angiotensin (A) (1 and 3 × 10⁻⁸ g/ml) and washed in Krebs solution (k) (left) or immersed in oil (o) (right). b: Records of a strip contracted by KCl (0.1 M) and washed in Krebs solution (left) or immersed in oil for about 30 m. (Reproduced by permission of the National Research Council of Canada from Can J Physiol Pharmacol 46[1968]719-730.)

for all drugs, there appears to be little or no escape of drug from the tissue during oil immersion, and the technique has now been extended to a variety of vascular and nonvascular preparations (Garg et al., 1971; Osswald, Guimarães, and Coimbra, 1971; Rudinger, Pliska, and Krejci, 1972; Guimarães and Brandão, 1973; Regoli et al., 1974; Wyse, 1976; Guimarães and Paiva, 1977). It has also proved valuable in studies with nerve-released transmitter (e.g., Brandão, 1976).

C. Limitations and Advantages of Oil Immersion

The results of studies with the oil immersion technique must be interpreted with a full appreciation of the differences between it and other test systems. Termination of agonist action in oil cannot be equated directly with termination of action *in vivo* or in an isolated tissue in an aqueous medium. The oil immersion procedure intentionally minimizes efflux of agonist into the

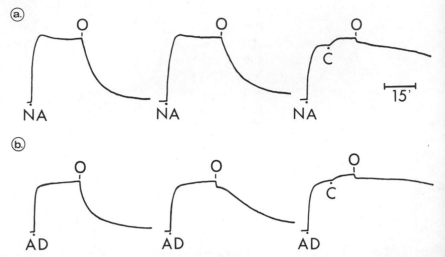

Figure 4. Effects of cocaine and of enzyme inhibitors on the termination of action in oil of aortic strips contracted by noradrenaline or adrenaline. a: Strips contracted by noradrenaline (NA) (1 × 10⁻⁸ g/ml); left, control strip; center, strip treated with the COMT inhibitor tropolone; right, strip treated with the MAO inhibitor iproniazid, tropolone, and cocaine (C), all added prior to oil immersion (O). b: The same as a, except that strips were contracted by adrenaline (AD) (1 × 10⁻⁸ g/ml) instead of noradrenaline. (Reproduced by permission of the American Society for Pharmacology and Experimental Therapeutics from J Pharm Exp Ther 165[1969]152–165)

environment of the tissue to focus on intrinsic mechanisms of drug disposition, their identification, and their relative contributions to termination of action.

The detailed analysis of mechanisms of agonist disposition requires a combination of the oil immersion technique with the use of drugs to inhibit individual pathways of uptake, metabolism, and binding; and the specificity of these inhibitors must be carefully established. From a study of several chemical candidates, concentration ranges, and periods of exposure, an attempt should be made to establish conditions that 1) produce a maximal reduction in the rate of relaxation in oil after contractions produced by an agonist known to be handled by the system in question; 2) do not alter either the contractile response to or the rate of relaxation following contraction by an agonist that is known to act on the same tissue receptors, but that is known to be resistant to the inactivation pathway under scrutiny; and 3) do not themselves alter the basal tone of the preparation in either Krebs solution or oil. Ideally, these conditions should be fulfilled over an inhibitor concentration range of at least 10-fold, to allow for variations in the sensitivity of different preparations with oil immersion. The utility of the technique and certain recently noted complications regarding its use, particularly with adrenergic mechanisms, will be described in a later section.

When dealing with tissue inactivation processes for agonists, it has been most difficult to exclude the participation of still unidentified processes of agonist binding or degradation. With the oil immersion technique, however, the absence of relaxation over a considerable period of time after the inactivation of known pathways of disposition, or with certain agonists even without such intervention, appears to provide sound evidence that the tissue has no unidentified mechanism for terminating the action of the agonist in question. Thus, aortic strips contracted by the sympathomimetic methoxamine do not relax even after 60 m immersion in oil; and this compound is known to be resistant to neuronal uptake or metabolism by monoamine oxidase (MAO) and catechol-O-methyltransferase (COMT). After inhibition of COMT, MAO, and neuronal uptake, aortic strips do not relax in oil after contractions by noradrenaline; but Wyse (1976) has observed a residual relaxation in rat tail artery and has suggested an additional route of amine inactivation still to be determined. However, incomplete inhibition of one of the established enzymatic pathways is a more likely explanation of his data.

Oil immersion was also used to demonstrate that aortic tissue of the rabbit, although responsive to the prostaglandins, has no intrinsic mechanism, presently defined or undefined, capable of terminating their action when they are presented to intact functional strips (Kalsner, 1974b). Contractions mediated by moderate concentrations of PGE_1, E_2, and $F_{2\alpha}$ were sustained during 60 m of oil immersion, although relaxation in Krebs solution was abrupt. Thus, although prostaglandins may act as local hormones in vascular tissue, it appears that any such action *in vivo* would be terminated by diffusion out of the tissue and subsequent metabolism at distant loci, such as the lungs and liver.

D. Complicating Factors

Trendelenburg and colleagues have raised some concerns regarding the view that the rate of relaxation after oil immersion is a valid index of the rate of amine inactivation in the region of the receptors (Trendelenburg and Henseling, 1976; Henseling, Rechtsteiner, and Trendelenburg, 1978). These workers comment that measurements of the half time for relaxation are dependent on the height of the initial response to noradrenaline and that sensitization of the response by an inhibitor may consequently modify the subsequent relaxation rate. This is, of course, a possibility, as was pointed out in an early publication by Kalsner and Nickerson (1969c) in dealing with reserpine-induced sensitization. It was shown in that paper, however, that correction for differences in response magnitudes resulting from potentiation in aortic strips (i.e., any given percentage of relaxation corresponded to different residual concentrations in the reserpine-treated and untreated preparations) did not appreciably alter interpretation of the results. Trendelenburg and Henseling (1976) reached a similar conclusion for aortic strips. However, in other tissues where the magnification of responses by inhibitors may be greater than in vascular tissue, it is appropriate to correct for changes in response magnitude.

A more serious factor, which complicates the direct study of termination of action with sympathomimetics, is the possibility that under certain circumstances the recovery of preparations involves not only the removal of agonist from the biophase (receptor region) but also the efflux of unchanged catecholamine from tissue sites past the receptors (Trendelenburg, 1974; Kalsner, 1975b). Trendelenburg and Henseling (1976) maintain that such efflux will prolong the decline of the response and lead to erroneous estimates of the contribution of individual processes. It has been shown, however, that during oil immersion no evidence for reflux of agonist could be obtained; and the data on termination of action formulated by use of this procedure, at least when the 50% recovery time is used, are not compromised by neuronal or extraneuronal efflux (Kalsner, 1977). Perhaps if late stages of relaxation were analyzed, some perturbation would be apparent; but terminal relaxation is unsuitable for the study of agonist inactivation for other reasons as well (Kalsner & Nickerson, 1968b). It has also been shown that relaxation of untreated aortic strips in Krebs solution is a direct measure of termination of action and that inhibitors of neuronal or extraneuronal uptake appear to induce a slowing of relaxation proportional to their role in termination of action (Kalsner 1975b). These agents block not only termination of action but also any cellular accumulation of amine that could subsequently distort the relaxation process. However, if MAO and COMT are directly inhibited, allowing tissue accumulation of intact noradrenaline, the subsequent relaxation will reflect the outward movement of intact agonist past the receptors rather than solely the rate of elimination of agonist from its sites of action. Recent efflux experiments of Henseling et al. (1978) to determine precisely the sources and magnitudes of ^{3}H-noradrenaline and its metabolites leaving the tissue cannot transfer directly to the kinetics of response termination unless the assumption is made that total tissue and receptor specific events do not differ materially from each other in space or in time. There is at present no basis for such a simplifying assumption; in fact, there is evidence to the contrary (see below), and such data should be interpreted with this in mind.

E. Alternate and Multiple Pathways of Agonist Inactivation

Unfortunately, the lack of any sensitization or prolongation of the response after inhibition of a suspected pathway of agonist inactivation does not establish the irrelevance of that route to termination of action. Inhibition of a mechanism that inactivates agonist in the region of the receptors to the same extent in two different systems may initiate a considerable sensitization and response prolongation in one but not the other. This seeming discrepancy is due to the function of alternate or backup mechanisms of agonist disposition so that an important terminating mechanism may be inhibited but termination of action not delayed. Alternate pathways of disposition take over the role of the inhibited pathway by an apparent increase in their rate constants for agonist removal from the biophase.

For example, blockade of monoamine oxidase or catechol-O-methyltransferase alone has little effect on response magnitude or termination of action for noradrenaline in rabbit aortic strips, but simultaneous blockade of both yields considerable effects on both parameters (Kalsner & Nickerson, 1969a; Levin and Furchgott, 1970). Evidence indicates a topographical arrangement of extraneuronal COMT and MAO in some tissues such that presentation of intact noradrenaline to the one enzyme is favored over that to the other (e.g., Kalsner & Nickerson, 1969a; Brandão, 1977; Garrett and Branco, 1977). Extraneuronal MAO may be routinely presented with the O-methylated metabolite in rabbit aorta (Kalsner and Nickerson, 1969a). However, after inhibition of O-methylation the deaminating enzyme inactivates the intact agonist molecule, rendering it an alternate mechanism of inactivation and preventing any material delay in termination of action. In general, there is abundant support for the extraneuronal location of functional MAO and COMT in smooth muscle (e.g., Burnstock and Costa, 1975; Brandão, 1977; O'Donnell and Saar, 1978). A recent report also suggests that centrally released noradrenaline, by stimulation of the locus ceruleus, is rapidly metabolized after release by the sequential operation of COMT and MAO (Van Wijk and Korf, 1976). Further, granular storage and deamination after neuronal uptake of catecholamine appear in certain circumstances to function as alternate pathways of inactivation (e.g., Langer and Enero, 1974).

In contrast, multiple mechanisms compete for a common pool of intact agonist in the biophase, in a way similar to that in which diffusion out of the tissue and extraneuronal and neuronal uptake might operate in sympathetically innervated systems (Kalsner, 1977). In such a case, inhibition of one of the routes produces a magnification of the response and a delay in termination of action at a given biophase concentration of agonist that is proportional to the reduction in the total sum of the rate constants for inactivation. In this connection it should be emphasized again that diffusion of agonist away from the site of action often functions both as an alternate and as a multiple pathway of agonist dissipation in many systems, and this often confounds analyses of termination of action when endogenous mechanisms are involved.

It is most difficult to establish if the effect of inhibition of a given pathway on termination of action reflects its real role or is an underestimate due to the presence of alternate mechanisms of inactivation. The commonly encountered relationships between multiple and alternate mechanisms, the complexity of the problem, and some solutions have been discussed at length elsewhere (Kalsner, 1977).

VI. TERMINATION OF NORADRENALINE ACTION

What ends the action of noradrenaline by reducing its effective concentration at its sites of action in autonomic effectors? There is no shortage, but rather an abundance, of terminating candidates. Since the initial enzymatic explanation of deamination by monoamine oxidase (Blaschko, Richter, and Schlossman, 1937; Burn and Robinson, 1952), we have seen the advocacy of O-methylation (Axelrod, 1960) yield to a persistent enthusiasm for neuronal uptake, with the concept of inactivation by effector cell uptake (Kalsner, 1966; Eisenfeld et al., 1967; Avakian and Gillespie, 1968; Kalsner and Nickerson, 1968a, 1969a, b) now being increasingly considered as important in a number of systems (Burnstock and Costa, 1975; Kalsner, 1975a; Gillespie, 1976).

It is only recently that the direct participation of neuronal uptake in termination of action has been closely studied. It seemed sufficient in early studies merely to emphasize the rapidity and efficiency of the uptake process in accumulating intraneuronally intact ^{3}H-noradrenaline, far in excess of that accounted for proportionately by any other available inactivation process (Iversen, 1965). This, coupled with the well-known sensitization induced by cocaine, a potent blocker of neuronal uptake, and the lack of uptake of noradrenaline in sympathetically denervated systems, along with a denervation sensitization comparable to that induced by cocaine and nonadditive with it, provided all that appeared needed for the acceptance of presynaptic inactivation in its most encompassing form.

However, the evidence for neuronal uptake as the only significant terminating mechanism in sympathetically innervated systems is not consistently impressive. Sympathetic nerve activation of perfused or bathed organs yields an outflow of intact noradrenaline that is often only negligibly or modestly increased by cocaine (Kirpekar and Cervoni, 1963; Geffen, 1965; Bouillin, Costa, and Brodie, 1967; Blakeley, Brown, and Ferry, 1963; Kirpekar and Puig, 1971) or by the similarly acting desipramine (e.g., Geffen, 1965), although responses may be demonstrably enhanced. Others have noted that although the total outflow of radioactivity in previously primed tissues may not be reliably increased in the presence of neuronal uptake blockade (e.g., Farnebo and Hamberger, 1971), less of it appears as a deaminated metabolite during and after cessation of stimulation (Langer and Enero, 1974; Dubocovich and Langer, 1976). To explain this, Dubocovich and Langer considered that amine transported intraneuronally during the response is promptly released as a deaminated metabolite, rather than stored for subsequent reuse. However, if this occurs to a measurable extent proximal to the excited receptors, then inhibitors of monoamine oxidase would be expected to materially enhance response magnitude and duration, since, in their presence, intact rather than deaminated molecules would be released at the synaptic gap; however, they do not. These workers also concluded on the basis of an analysis of deaminated metabolites that neuronal uptake operates with decreasing effectiveness as the frequency of stimulation is increased from 0.5 to 5.0 Hz. But if the failure of neuronal uptake at moderate frequencies does occur, then one is left with an unrelated explanation for the often substantial sensitization of nerve-induced responses seen in some tissues with cocaine at these frequencies—the backbone of the neuronal uptake hypothesis. More probably what is again illustrated is the improbability that examination of effluent metabolites can accurately define conditions at the synaptic gulf. Further, much early work interpreting the enhanced outflow of transmitter after treatment with phenoxybenzamine (e.g., Su and Bevan, 1970) as key support for the dominance of neuronal uptake is now reinterpretable, according to many, as an action on presynaptic receptors controlling transmitter release rather than an expression of a reduction of a presynaptic inactivation process.

Experiments of a similar design with blockers of extraneuronal uptake reveal that inhibitors such as normetanephrine increased somewhat the efflux of transmitter from cat spleen (Cripps and Dearnaley, 1971), rabbit heart (Junstad, Stjärne, and Wennmalme, 1973), and rabbit vas deferens (Hughes, 1972); but some others report negligible effects (e.g., Bell and Vogt, 1971; Story and McCulloch, 1972). Numerous experiments demonstrate a decreased formation of normetanephrine or of deaminated-O-methylated metabolites after block of extraneuronal uptake (e.g., Luchelli-Fortis and Langer, 1975; Brandão, 1977), confirming the involvement of the effector cell in inactivation.

That both extraneuronal and neuronal metabolism of noradrenaline occurs in most sympathetically innervated systems is no longer in doubt (e.g., Burnstock and Costa, 1975; Gillespie, 1976; Kalsner, 1977); but the contributions of these processes to termination of action cannot be delineated by measurements of the outflow of noradrenaline and its metabolites, any more than whole tissue estimates of retained material are valid monitors of a physiological event (as was described at some length in an earlier section of this article). There is no substantial evidence and no a priori reason to assume that noradrenaline and its products leaving a perfused or bathed organ during and after stimulation reconstruct accurately the spatial and temporal dynamics of agonist accumulation and decay at specific receptor sites proximal to the source of release. This is immediately obvious, for instance, when the possibility of local action of the released transmitter coupled with myogenic propagation of the response is considered (Burnstock and Costa, 1975; Bevan, 1978). The resultant out-flow, instead, is probably a distorted summary of relevant and irrelevant inactivation, primary and secondary processes, intimate and remote from the sites of action. In addition, the mobility of the mediator in all its various conditions (e.g. intact, metabolite, loosely-bound, receptor-exciting and from varying intra- and extra-cellular loci) is sure to be unequal (Chidsey et al., 1963; Andén, Carlsson, and Waldick, 1963; Levin, 1974) and not a relia-ble measure of events during the course of the response. Further, there is little solid evidence that the outflow of radioactivity in a tissue previously primed with ^{3}H-noradrenaline is a completely acceptable index of the endogenous transmitter released with nerve stimulation. See, for example, Schrold and Nedergaard (1977) for evidence of the extraneuronal origin of some of the ^{3}H-noradrenaline released by field stimulation. Diffusion away from the site of action is consistently ignored as a terminating process in outflow studies, yet intact transmitter routinely appears and may account for over 50% of the total released radioactivity (e.g., Dubocovich and Langer, 1976).

The essential and unavoidable criterion to define terminating mechanisms, to which all other estimates must yield, is that their interrup-tion gives a prolongation of response duration coincident upon prolonged concentrations of agonist at the pertinent receptors, taking into account the compensatory function of alternate pathways. Many new data bear on this, since studies with the oil immersion technique first emphasized the importance of direct examination of the decay of the response (Kalsner, 1966; Kalsner and Nickerson, 1968a, c). This work done initially with rabbit aortic strips showed that termination to exogenous noradrenaline is mainly through extraneuronal uptake followed by definitive inactivation through the sequential operation of catechol-O-methyl-transferase and monoamine oxidase (Kalsner and Nickerson, 1969a, b). This technique was employed to provide the first evidence, subsequently confirmed, that extraneuronal metabolism of noradrenaline is a terminating event and that it was inhibited by haloalkylamines and by a number of steroids (Kalsner, 1969a, b; Kalsner & Nickerson, 1969b).

The essential observations made with the oil immersion technique in rabbit aorta have been confirmed, and the procedure has been extended to other vascular and nonvascular preparations to study termination of action of noradrenaline and adrenaline (Osswald et al., 1971; Guimarães et al., 1971; Guimaraes and Brandão, 1973; Wyse, 1976; Brandão, 1977; Guimarães and Paiva, 1977). An analysis of these reports reveals varying degrees of involvement of neuronal and extraneuronal processes in termina-tion of action when assessed directly by measurements of recovery times. Recent extension of the technique to neurally released transmitter nora-drenaline (Brandão, 1977) supports the previously defined role for extraneuronal processes in rabbit aorta (Kalsner & Nickerson, 1969a, b); but these may be somewhat less important in saphenous vein, where the terminal innervation spreads throughout the media rather than being limited to the adventitial-medial junction.

Other studies of termination of action done in Krebs medium (to allow diffusion to participate maximally in agonist dissipation) again revealed a prominent role for extraneuronal inactivation. For example, Bell and Grabsch (1976) found that after blockade of either neuronal or extraneuronal uptake in rat isolated atrium the time for recovery of heart rate following a brief period of nerve stimulation is substantially delayed. Numerous studies have, of course, shown sensitization of response magnitudes induced by exogenous and nerve-released noradrenaline by neuronal and extraneuronal uptake inhibitors (e.g., Langer and Enero, 1974; Kalsner, Frew, and Smith, 1975; Head et al., 1975; Belfrage, Fredholm, and Rosell, 1977; Kalsner, 1978); the magnitudes varied from preparation to preparation and with the experimental system used, but access barriers were not considered when evaluating them and possible direct postsynaptic sensitization by cocaine (Kalsner and Nickerson, 1969d), not often ruled out.

An initial report—not easily reconciled with the body of available evidence on termination of action—that responses of perfused noradrenaline are increased in magnitude by oxytetracycline, presumably by blockade of catecholamine binding to collagen and elastin in the vascular wall (Powis, 1973), has not been substantiated. It was found that the compound, an inhibitor of amine binding to connective tissue, neither sensitized the central ear artery of the rabbit to sympathetic nerve activation or noradrenaline nor prolonged the duration of the responses (Kalsner, 1976b). Similarly, aortic strips of the rabbit, rich in connective tissue, did not show heightened contractions to noradrenaline in the presence of oxytetracycline. Thus, although binding of catecholamine to connective tissue may occur, it is unlikely that it is an additional independent factor of any significance in termination of action, especially with moderate concentrations of amine.

VII. CONCLUSIONS

Termination of action is a complex event describing the restoration of a responsive system to its resting state as agonist is eliminated from the sites of action. The rate of removal of agonist from the receptor region, along with the rate of its supply, also determines the magnitude and plateau during the response. This process, long neglected, is now under scrutiny in many laboratories. Rather than indirect measurements of tissue and effluent levels of intact agonist and its metabolic products, the response decay itself is being examined. Recovery of a smooth muscle to basal tone or of a heart, gland, or nerve cell to its resting parameters, either in aqueous medium or in oil, provides a direct assessment of termination of action. Although the use of inhibitors to block pathways of inactivation is fraught with complications, and interpretation correspondingly complex, only direct analyses of response contours can yield definitive answers. The presence of alternate and multiple pathways of inactivation in many systems further compounds analysis, but these must not be neglected. With regard to smooth muscle and adrenergic mechanisms, study of relaxation rates permits us to conclude with some confidence that the long-sought terminating mechanisms can be identified; extraneuronal and neuronal pathways each are involved in most systems, as is the process of simple diffusion. Their relative importance varies from system to system and according to whether endogenous neurotransmitter or exogenous amine is used to provoke the response.

When the techniques described here for study of termination of action are applied to other systems and with other neurotransmitters, they should yield correspondingly fruitful results.

VIII. REFERENCES

Andén, N-E.; Carlsson, A.; Waldick, B.: Reserpine-Resistant Uptake Mechanisms of Noradrenaline in Tissues. Life Sci 2 (1963) 889–894

Avakian, O.V.; Gillespie, J.S.: Uptake of Noradrenaline by Adrenergic Nerves, Smooth Muscle and Connective Tissue in Isolated Perfused Arteries and Its Correlation with the Vasoconstrictor Response. Br J Pharmacol 32(1968)168–184

Axelrod, J.: The Fate of Adrenaline and Noradrenaline. In: Ciba Symposium on Adrenergic Mechanisms, pp 28–39, ed. by J.R. Vane, G.E.W. Wolstenholme, M. O'Connor. J. & A. Churchill, London, 1960

Belfrage, E.; Fredholm, B.B.; Rosell, S.: Effect of Catechol-O-Methyltransferase (COMT) Inhibition on the Vascular and Metabolic Responses to Noradrenaline, Isoprenaline and Sympathetic Nerve Stimulation in Canine Subcutaneous Adipose Tissue. Arch Pharmacol 300(1977)11–17

Bell, C.; Grabsch, B.: Involvement of Uptake$_2$ in the Termination of Activity of Neurogenic Noradrenaline in the Rat Isolated Atrium. J Physiol 254(1976)203–212

Bell, C.; Vogt, M.: Release of Endogenous Noradrenaline from an Isolated Muscular Artery. J Physiol 215(1971)509–520

Bevan, J.A.: Response of Blood Vessels to Sympathetic Nerve Stimulation. Blood Vess 15(1978)17–25

Bevan, J.A.; Osher, J.V.: Distribution of Norepinephrine Released from Adrenergic Motor Terminals in Arterial Wall. Eur J Pharmacol 13(1970)55–58

Blakeley, A.G.H.; Brown, G.L.; Ferry, C.B.: Pharmacological Experiments on the Release of the Sympathetic Transmitter. J Physiol 167(1963)505–514

Blaschko, H.; Richter, D.; Schlossmann, H.: The Oxidation of Adrenaline and Other Amines. Biochem J 31(1937)2187–2196

Bouillin, D.J.; Costa, E.; Brodie, B.B.: Evidence that Blockade of Adrenergic Receptors Causes Overflow of Norepinephrine in Cats' Colon after Nerve Stimulation. J Pharmacol Exp Ther 157(1967)125–134

Brandão, F.: A Comparative Study of the Role Played by Some Inactivation Pathways in the Disposition of the Transmitter in the Rabbit Aorta and the Saphenous Vein of the Dog. Blood Vess 13(1976)309–318

Brandão, F.: Inactivation of Norepinephrine in an Isolated Vein. J Pharmacol Exp Ther 202(1977)23–29

Brown, G.L.: The Release and Fate of the Transmitter Liberated by Adrenergic Nerves. Proc. R Soc Lond Ser B 162(1965)1–19

Burn, J.H.; Robinson, J.: Effect of Denervation on Amine Oxidase in Structures Innervated by the Sympathetic. Br J Pharmacol 7(1952)304–318

Burnstock, G.; Costa, M.: Adrenergic Neurons. Chapman & Hall, London, 1975

Cannon, W.B.; Rosenblueth, A.: The Supersensitivity of Denervated Structures. Macmillan, New York, 1949

Chidsey, C.A.; Kahler, R.L.; Kleminson, L.L.; Braunwald, E.: Uptake and Metabolism of Tritiated Norepinephrine in the Isolated Canine Heart. Circ Res 12(1963)220–227

Cripps, H.; Dearnaley, D.P.: Evidence Suggesting Uptake of Noradrenaline at Adrenergic Receptors in the Isolated Blood-Perfused Cat Spleen. J Physiol 216(1971)55P–56P

De La Lande, I.S.; Frewin, D.; Waterson, J.G.; Cannell, V.: Factors Influencing Supersensitivity to Noradrenaline in the Isolated Perfused Artery; Comparative Effects of Cocaine, Denervation, and Serotonin. Circ Res Suppl 3(1967)177–181

Dubocovich, M.; Langer, S.Z.: Influence of the Frequency of Nerve Stimulation on the Metabolism of ^{3}H-Norepinephrine Released from the Perfused Cat Spleen: Differences Observed during and after the Period of Stimulation. J Pharmacol Exp Ther 198 (1976)83–101

Eccles, J.C.; Jaegar, J.C.: The Relationship between the Mode of Operation and the Dimensions of the Junctional Regions at Synapses and Motor End-Organs. Proc R Soc Lond Ser B 148(1958)38–56

Ehrenpreis, S.; Bigo-Gullimo, M.; Anery, M.A.: The Effect of Cholinesterase Inhibitors and Lipid Soluble Quaternary Ammonium Compounds on Contractions of Rabbit Aortic Strip. Arch Int Pharmacodyn 156(1965)1–21

Eisenfeld, A.J.; Krakoff, L.; Iversen, L.L.; Axelrod, J.: Inhibition of the Extraneuronal Metabolism of Noradrenaline in the Isolated Heart by Adrenergic Blocking Agents. Nature 213(1967)297–298

Elliot, T.R.: The Action of Adrenalin, J Physiol 32(1905)401–467

Farnebo, L-O.; Hamberger, B.: Drug-Induced Changes in the Release of [^{3}H]-Noradrenaline from Field Stimulated Rat Iris. Br J Pharmacol 43(1971)97–106

Garg, B.; Buckner, C.; Sethi, O.; Sokoloski, T.; Patil, P.N.: Steric Aspects of Adrenergic Drugs. XVII. Influence of Tropolone on the Magnitude and Duration of Action of Catecholamine Isomers. Arch Int Pharmacodyn Ther 189(1971)281–294

Garrett, J.; Branco, D.: Uptake and Metabolism of Noradrenaline by the Mesenteric Arteries of the Dog. Blood Vess 14(1977)43–54

Geffen, L.: The Effect of Desmethylimipramine upon the Overflow of Sympathetic Transmitter from the Cat's Spleen. J Physiol 181(1965)69P–70P

Gershenfeld, H.M.; Stefani, E.: Evidence for an Excitatory Transmitter Role of Serotonin in Molluscan Central Synapses. Adv Pharmacol 6A(1968)369–392

Gillespie, J.S.: Extraneuronal Uptake of Catecholamines in Smooth Muscle and Connective Tissues. In: The Mechanism of Neuronal and Extraneuronal Transport of Catecholamines, pp. 325–354, ed. by D.M. Paton. Raven, New York, 1976

Govier, W.C.: Myocardial Alpha Adrenergic Receptors and Their Role in the Production of a Positive Ionotropic Effect by Sympathomimetic Agents. J Pharmacol Exp Ther 159(1968)82–90

Govier, W.C.; Sugrue, M.F.; Shore, P.A.: On the Inability to Produce Supersensitivity to Catecholamines in Intestinal Smooth Muscle. J Pharmacol Exp Ther 165(1969)71–77

Guimarães, S.; Brandão, F.: Comparison between the Effects Produced by Chronic Denervation and by Cocaine on the Sensitivity to, and on the Disposition of, Noradrenaline in Isolated Spleen Strips. Arch Pharmacol 277(1973)163–174

Guimarães, S.; Osswald, W.; Cardoso, W.; Bronco, D.: The Effects of Cocaine and Denervation on the Sensitivity to Noradrenaline, Its Uptake and the Termination of Its Action in Isolated Venous Tissue. Arch Pharmacol 271(1971)262–273

Guimarães, S.; Paiva, M.Q.: The Role Played by the Extraneuronal System in the Disposition of Noradrenaline and Adrenaline in Vessels. Arch Pharmacol 296(1977)279–287

Head, R.J.; Johnson, S.M.; Berry, D.; De La Lande, I.S.: Denervation and O-Methylation of Noradrenaline in the Rabbit Ear Artery. Clin Exp Pharmacol Phys Suppl 2(1975)39–42

Henseling, M.; Rechtsteiner, D.; Trendelenburg, U.: The Influence of Monoamine Oxidase and Catechol-O-Methyltransferase on the Distribution of ^{3}H-($\pm$)-Noradrenaline in Rabbit Aortic Strips. Arch Pharmacol 302(1978)181-194

Hughes, J.: Evaluation of Mechanisms Controlling the Release and Inactivation of the Adrenergic Transmitter in the Rabbit Portal Vein and Vas Deferens. Br J Pharmacol 44(1972)472-491

Iversen, L.L.: The Inhibition of Noradrenaline Uptake by Drugs. In: Advances in Drug Research, Vol. II, pp. 1-46, ed. by N.J. Harper, A.B. Simmonds. Academic, London-New York, 1965

Iversen, L.L.: Role of Transmitter Uptake Mechanisms in Synaptic Neurotransmission. Br J Pharmacol 41(1971)571-591

Junstad, M.; Stjärne, L.; Wennmalme, A.: On the Relative Importance of Extraneuronal Uptake of Noradrenaline Released by Nerve Stimulation in the Rabbit Heart. Acta Physiol Scand 88(1973)67-70

Kalsner, S.: Studies on the Mechanisms Terminating the Action of the Sympathetic Nerve Mediator (Noradrenaline). Ph.D. thesis, 1966, University of Manitoba

Kalsner, S.: Mechanism of Hydrocortisone Potentiation of Responses to Epinephrine and Norepinephrine in Rabbit Aorta. Circ Res 24(1969a)383-396

Kalsner, S.: Steroid Potentiation of Responses to Sympathomimetic Amines in Aortic Strips. Br J Pharmacol 36(1969b)582-593

Kalsner, S.: The Potentiating Effects of Ethanol on Responses of Aortic Strips to Stimulant Drugs. J Pharm Pharmacol 22(1970)877-879

Kalsner, S.: Mechanism of Potentiation of Vascular Responses by Tetraethyl-Ammonium: A Novel Form of Sensitization. Can J Physiol Pharmacol 51(1973)451-457

Kalsner, S.: A New Approach to the Measurement and Classification of Forms of Supersensitivity of Autonomic Effector Responses. Br J Pharmacol 51(1974a)427-434

Kalsner, S.: Responses to and Termination of Action of Prostaglandins in Vascular Tissue of the Rabbit. Can J Physiol Pharmacol 52(1974b)1020-1025

Kalsner, S.: The Importance of Adrenergic Neuronal Uptake in Termination of Action; Another view—Response to I.S. de la Lande. Blood Vess 12(1975a)316-322

Kalsner, S.: Role of Extraneuronal Mechanisms in the Termination of Contractile Responses to Amines in Vascular Tissue. Br J Pharmacol 53(1975b)267-277

Kalsner, S.: Sensitization of Effector Responses by Modification of Agonist Disposition Mechanisms. Can J Physiol Pharmacol 54(1976a)177-187

Kalsner, S.: The Lack of Effect of Oxytetracycline on Responses to Sympathetic Nerve Stimulation and Catecholamines in Vascular Tissue. Br J Pharmacol 58(1976b)261-266

Kalsner, S.: Termination of Effector Responses to Agonists: An Analysis of Agonist Disposition Mechanisms. Can J Physiol Pharmacol 55(1977)315-331

Kalsner, S.: Mechanisms of Inactivation of Noradrenaline in this Iris Sphincter, Tracheal Muscle and Facial Artery of Cattle: Implications for Beta-Adrenoceptor Mediated Responses. Br J Pharmacol, 64(1978)545-552

Kalsner, S.; Frew, R.D.; Smith, G.: Mechanism of Methylxanthine Sensitization of Norepinephrine Responses in a Coronary Artery. Am J Physiol 228(1975)1702-1707

Kalsner, S.; Nickerson, M.: Disposition of Phenylephrine in Vascular Tissue, Determined by the Oil Immersion Technique. J Pharmacol Exp Ther 163(1968a)1-10

Kalsner, S.; Nickerson, M.: A Method for the Study of Mechanisms of Drug Disposition in Smooth Muscle. Can J Physiol Pharmacol 46(1968b)719-730

Kalsner, S.; Nickerson, M.: Disposition of Norepinephrine and Epinephrine in Vascular Tissue, Determined by the Technique of Oil Immersion. J Pharmacol Exp Ther 165(1969a)152-165

Kalsner, S.; Nickerson, M.: Effects of a Haloalkylamine on Responses to and Disposition of Sympathomimetic Amines. Br J Pharmacol 35(1969b)440-455

Kalsner, S.; Nickerson, M.: Effects of Reserpine on the Disposition of Sympathomimetic Amines in Vascular Tissue. Br J Pharmacol 35(1969c)394-405

Kalsner, S.; Nickerson, M.: Mechanism of Cocaine Potentiation of Responses to Amines. Br J Pharmacol 35(1969d)428-439

Kirpekar, S.M.; Cervoni, P.: Effect of Cocaine, Phenoxybenzamine and Phentolamine on the

Catecholamine Output from Spleen and Adrenal Medulla. J Pharmacol Exp Ther 142(1963)59–70

Kirpekar, S.M.; Puig, M.: Effect of Flow-Stop on Noradrenaline Release from Normal Spleens and Spleens Treated with Cocaine, Phentolamine or Phenoxybenzamine. Br J Pharmacol 43(1971)359–369

Langer, S.Z.; Enero, M.A.: The Potentiation of Responses to Adrenergic Nerve Stimulation in the Presence of Cocaine: Its Relationship to the Metabolic Fate of Released Norepinephrine. J Pharmacol Exp Ther 191(1974)431–443

Levin, J.A.: The Uptake and Metabolism of ^{3}H-l and ^{3}H-dl Norepinephrine by Intact Rabbit Aorta and by Isolated Adventitia and Media. J Pharmacol Exp Ther 190(1974)219–226

Levin, J.A.; Furchgott, R.F.: Interactions between Potentiating Agents of Adrenergic Amines in Rabbit Aortic Strips. J Pharmacol Exp Ther 172(1970)320–331

Luchelli-Fortis, M.A.; Langer, S.Z.: Selective Inhibition by Hydrocortisone of ^{3}H-Normetanephrine Formation during ^{3}H-Transmitter Release Elicited by Nerve Stimulation in the Isolated Nerve-Muscle Preparation of the Cat Nictating Membrane. Arch Pharmacol 287(1975)261–275

O'Donnell, S.R.; Saar, N.: The Uptake Kinetics and Metabolism of Extraneuronal Noradrenaline in Guinea-Pig Trachea As Studied with Quantitative Fluorescence Microphotometry. Br J Pharmacol 62(1978)235–239

Osswald, W.; Guimarães, S.; Coimbra, A.: The Termination of Action of Catecholamines in the Isolated Venous Tissue of the Dog. Arch Pharmacol 269(1971)15–31

Powis, G.: Binding of Catecholamines to Connective Tissue and the Effect upon the Responses of Blood Vessels to Noradrenaline and to Nerve Stimulation. J Physiol Lond 234(1973)145–162

Regoli, D.; Rioux, F.; Park, W.K.; Choi, C.: Role of the N-Terminal Amino Acid for the Biological Activities of Angiotensin and Inhibitory Analogues. Can J Physiol Pharmacol 52(1974)39–49

Rudinger, J.; Pliska, V.; Krejci, I.: Oxytocin Analog in the Analysis of Some Phases of Hormone Action. In: Recent Progress in Hormone Research, Vol. XXVIII, pp. 131–172, ed. by E.B. Eastwood. Academic, New York, 1972

Schrold, J.; Nedergaard, O.A.: Neuronal and Extraneuronal Outflow of ^{3}H-Noradrenaline Induced by Electrical-Field Stimulation of an Isolated Blood Vessel. Acta Physiol Scand 101(1977)129–143

Story, D.F.; McCulloch, M.W.: Effect of Phenoxybenzamine on the Release of ^{3}H-Noradrenaline from Isolated Guinea-Pig Atria. Proc Aust Physiol Soc 3(1972)84–85

Su, C.; Bevan, J.A.: The Release of H^3-Norepinephrine in Arterial Strips Studied by the Technique of Superfusion and Transmural Stimulation. J Pharmacol Exp Ther 172(1970)62–68

Trendelenburg, U.: Supersensitivity and Subsensitivity to Sympathomimetic Amines. Pharmacol Rev 15(1963)225–276

Trendelenburg, U.: The Relaxation of Rabbit Aortic Strips after a Preceding Exposure to Sympathomimetic Amines. Arch Pharmacol 281(1974)13–46

Trendelenburg, U.; Henseling, M.: Factors Determining the Rate of Relaxation of Rabbit Aortic Strips after an Exposure to Noradrenaline. Arch Pharmacol 293(1976)235–244

Van Wijk, M.; Korf, J.: Metabolism of Centrally Released Noradrenaline by Extraneuronal Monoamine Oxidase and Catechol-O-Methyltransferase. Brain Res 106(1976)403–406

Wyse, D.G.: Inactivation of Neural and Exogenous Norepinephrine in Rat Tail Artery Studied by the Oil Immersion Technique. J Pharmacol Exp Ther 198(1976)102–111

Zupančič, A.O.: The Mode of Action of Acetylcholine. A Theory Extended to a Hypothesis on the Mode of Action of Other Biologically Active Substances. Acta Physiol Scand 29(1953)63–71

The Interconversion of Adrenoceptors

Bruno G. Benfey

I. INTRODUCTION

Adrenoceptors are commonly classified into two types, α or β, according to their sensitivity to agonists and antagonists. A response is said to be mediated by α-adrenoceptors when measurement of the potency of a series of agonists shows that adrenaline or noradrenaline is highest, phenylephrine is somewhat lower, and isoprenaline is very low, and when the response is inhibited by a relatively low concentration of an α-adrenoceptor blocking drug. A response is considered to be mediated by β-adrenoceptors when the relative potency of a series of agonists indicates that isoprenaline is highest and phenylephrine lowest, and when the response is inhibited by a relatively low concentration of a β-adrenoceptor blocking drug (Furchgott, 1972).

In the past few years radioligand binding methods have been developed for the study of adrenoceptors (Lefkowitz, 1978). Radioligand binding methods usually use homogenates or membrane fractions of tissues rather than intact tissues. Both the radioligand binding methods and the pharmacological procedures can estimate affinities (reciprocals of dissociation constants) of a receptor for agonists and competitive antagonists. However, only radioligand binding methods can give an estimate of the concentration of receptors, and only pharmacological procedures can

Acknowledgments. The author's studies were supported by grants from the Medical Research Council of Canada.

evaluate the efficacies of agonists acting on the receptor for producing a stimulus that leads to a response (Furchgott, 1978).

Dale (1906) first suggested that there are two kinds of receptors for adrenaline. He observed that ergot converted the vasoconstrictor effect of the drug to a vasodilator effect and proposed that one kind of receptor causes vasoconstriction and a second vasodilatation. Normally the action of the receptors for vasoconstriction masks that of the receptors for dilatation, but in the presence of ergot the receptors for constriction are blocked and those for dilatation are unmasked.

Burn and Robinson (1951) and Burn (1956) speculated that there is only one adrenoceptor. They proposed that a drug that reverses the effect of adrenaline from constriction to dilatation causes adrenaline to combine with the receptor in an abnormal manner. As a result the receptor is inactivated and the contractile mechanism of the blood vessel wall relaxes. Belleau (1963) speculated that the adrenoceptor contains α and β sites and that the response depends on the site attacked by the agonist.

The adrenoceptor interconversion hypothesis was proposed by Kunos and Szentivanyi (1968), whose paper begins as follows:

> The fact that adrenaline can act differently in various organs has often been explained by assuming that there are different kinds of receptors. A simpler explanation of these differences in adrenaline action is that a single adrenoceptor, influenced in different ways by the different metabolic milieu in various organs, is sufficient to interpret all kinds of adrenaline effects. If this assumption is correct, the well-defined receptor quality of the adrenaline effect, as tested by the effectiveness of different types of receptor blocking agents, can be transformed into another receptor quality in one organ, by changing its metabolic milieu. (p. 1077)

Nickerson and Kunos (1977) "consider adrenoceptor interconversion to be one of the mechanisms that adapts the response of an organ or tissue to its metabolic state" (p. 2583). This paper examines critically the evidence marshaled to support the interconversion of α- and β-adrenoceptors.

II. THE EVIDENCE FOR ADRENOCEPTOR INTERCONVERSION

A. Effect of Low Temperature on Amphibian Heart

1. The first experiment Using the isolated cardiac ventricle, Kunos and Szentivanyi (1968) found in the summer frog that lowering the bath temperature from 22–24°C to 5–10°C reduced the potency of the β-adrenoceptor blocking drug propranolol as an antagonist of the inotropic effect of adrenaline, and in the winter frog that raising the bath temperature from 22–24°C to 32–34°C reduced the potency of the α-adrenoceptor blocking drug phentolamine as an adrenaline antagonist. They concluded that "the prerequisites for the existence of a metabolically influenced single adreno-ceptor—as far as myocardium is concerned—have been fulfilled" (p. 1078). Objections must be raised. This and the following studies supporting the notion of adrenoceptor interconversion have not been done under "optimal conditions in experiments for the pharmacological characterization of adrenoceptors in isolated tissues" (Furchgott, 1972, p. 293). Thus in tissues containing both receptors the potency of a β-adrenoceptor blocking drug should have been determined after blockade of α-adrenoceptors and vice versa. The catecholamine uptake processes (both neuronal and extraneuronal) that affect drug potencies should have been blocked. Furthermore, Kunos and Szentivanyi (1968) used the Straub technique, in which a cannula is put through the aorta and the fluid passes up and down from the cannula into the ventricle. There is a considerable volume of tidal fluid, and the dead space in the aortic cannula greatly reduces the oxygen supply to the heart. Clark et al. (1938) find the Straub technique "not very suitable for measuring quantitatively the effect of drugs on the mechanical response." (p. 275).

2. The use of irreversible α-adrenoceptor blocking drugs Buckley and Jordan (1970) were the first to test the adrenoceptor interconversion hypothesis. Using the technique of Symes (1918), they perfused the frog heart at 7°C with 15 μM phenoxybenzamine (an irreversible α-adrenoceptor blocking drug) for 90 m and found that the inotropic and chronotropic effects of adrenaline were inhibited at 7°C but that the blockade disappeared when the drug was withdrawn and the temperature raised to 24°C. The authors concluded that the adrenoceptors are not interconvertible but that the frog heart possesses two pools of adrenoceptors, the availability of which is governed by temperature.

Buckley and Jordan's (1970) observation agrees with earlier results of Nickerson and Nomaguchi (1950). A low concentration of dibenamine (3.4 μM), a β-haloalkylamine related to but 20 times less potent than phenoxybenzamine, inhibited the chronotropic effect of adrenaline on the winter frog heart, but the blockade disappeared when dibenamine was withdrawn. (The inotropic effect of adrenaline was not inhibited, unless high concentrations of dibenamine were used that depressed the heart.) Nickerson and Nomaguchi (1950) modified the Straub technique by introducing Ringer's solution through a fine needle that extended to the tip of the cannula, provided a continuous flow of perfusate, and "largely eliminated the 'dead space' of the single cannula."

Kunos, Yong, and Nickerson (1973) and Kunos and Nickerson (1976) then incubated the frog ventricle for four 10-m periods with 7.3 μM phenoxybenzamine. Treatment at 14°C inhibited the inotropic effect of adrenaline at 14°C, and the blockade remained when the temperature was raised to 24°C. The authors concluded that at the low temperature phenoxybenzamine irreversibly blocked the adrenoceptor in "α-conformation" so that temperature elevation did not convert it to the "β-conformation." Kunos et al. (1973) and Kunos and Nickerson (1976) used the unmodified Straub technique, as Kunos and Szentivanyi (1968) had done before.

The results were not confirmed with the new irreversible α-adrenoceptor blocking drug BHC (N,N'-bis[6-(o.methoxybenzylamino)-n-hexyl]cystamine[Melchiorre et al., 1978]). Perfusion of the heart of the pithed frog with BHC at 14°C and test at 22°C revealed no inhibition of the inotropic effect of adrenaline, phenylephrine, or isoprenaline (Benfey, 1978).

3. **Tissue retention of radiolabeled α- and β-adrenoceptor blocking drugs** Kunos and Nickerson (1976) found that the isolated frog ventricle infused with the Straub cannula retained more [^{14}C]propranolol at 24°C than at 14°C and more [^{3}H]phenoxybenzamine at 14°C than at 24°C and took this as additional evidence that low temperature converts β-adrenoceptors to α-adrenoceptors. It is a doubtful claim.

The frog ventricle was exposed to propranolol for only 10 m; and that is not long enough to obtain a full blockade, particularly at low temperature. At 37°C it took 90 m to achieve a 98% equilibration with propranolol in guinea pig atria (Potter, 1967) and 75 m to obtain an 80%–90% equilibration in guinea pig trachea (Furchgott, Jurkiewicz, and Jurkiewicz, 1973). The specific activity of the [^{14}C]propranolol—6.15 mCi/mmole—was very low, which required the use of high concentrations. Even with low concentrations of preparations with high specific activity, nonspecific binding has been a problem in the use of radiolabeled propranolol for β-adrenoceptor assay (Potter, 1967; Vatner and Lefkowitz, 1974; Lefkowitz, 1975; Wolfe, Harden, and Molinoff, 1977).

The concentration of phenoxybenzamine used by Kunos and Nickerson (1976)—four 10-m incubations with 7.3 μM—was very high; and the specific activity of the tritiated compound—33.13 mCi/mmole—was low. At 24°C phenoxybenzamine "binding" was about 50% lower than at 14°C (Kunos and Nickerson, 1976), but at 24°C phenoxybenzamine is active and exerts a variety of irreversible effects. Thus it potentiated the inotropic effect of adrenaline (Kunos and Nickerson, 1976) and inhibited the intropic effect of acetylcholine on the frog ventricle (Benfey, 1975).

Phenoxybenzamine exhibits irreversible antagonism toward a great variety of receptors, which indicates that it is not to be regarded as a specific α-adrenoceptor blocking drug (Triggle and Triggle, 1976; Triggle, 1978). Furthermore, tissues have a high binding capacity for the highly lipid soluble unchanged phenoxybenzamine. Phenoxybenzamine alkylates nucleophilic centers, including those in α-adrenoceptors, muscarinic and nicotinic receptors, receptors for histamine, 5-hydroxytryptamine and opiate, and neuronal and extraneuronal uptake sites for noradrenaline, after forming an aziridinium ion on neutralization. Low temperature stabilizes the intermediate aziridinium ring and reduces its reactivity (Rosen and Ehrenpreis, 1972). Phenoxybenzamine also forms a nonalkylating alcohol upon reaction of the aziridinium ion with water. Tissues retain the alcohol (Berry and Miller, 1975).

4. Potency of sympathomimetic and adrenergic blocking drugs Kunos and Nickerson (1976) reported that in frog ventricle low temperature reduces both the inotropic potency of adrenaline and the potency of propranolol as an adrenaline antagonist. This is at variance with other observations. Thus in the pithed toad lowering the temperature from 25° to 12°C increased both the chronotropic potency of adrenaline and the potency of propranolol as an adrenaline antagonist (Harri, 1973). In the pithed frog lowering the temperature from 25° to 12°C increased the chronotropic potency of adrenaline (Tirri et al., 1974). Benfey (1975, 1976) began to question the validity of the adrenoceptor interconversion hypothesis when he found in the frog ventricle that lowering the bath temperature from 24° to 14°C did not reduce the inotropic potency of isoprenaline or the potency of propranolol as an isoprenaline antagonist. Vernikov (1975) observed in the frog ventricle that low temperature did not increase the inotropic potency of phenylephrine.

Harri (1973) reported that in the pithed toad phenoxybenzamine inhibited the chronotropic effect of phenylephrine at 12°C but not at 25°C, and this has been taken as evidence that low temperature converts β-adreno-ceptors to α-adrenoceptors. It is an example of the nonspecific effect of a high concentration of an α-adrenoceptor blocking drug, because the dose of phenoxybenzamine used to inhibit the phenylephrine effect at low tempera-ture (not at high temperature) inhibited the chronotropic effect of adrenaline at both the low and the high temperature (Harri, 1973). At 15°C phentolamine did not inhibit the inotropic effect of phenylephrine on frog ventricle (Keenan, 1978). Positive inotropic and chronotropic actions of adrenaline on the perfused heart of winter frogs were blocked by β-adreno-ceptor blocking drugs and not by α-adrenoceptor blocking drugs (Singh et al., 1978).

The concentrations of phenoxybenzamine used by Buckley and Jordan (1970)—15 μM—and by Kunos et al. (1973) and Kunos and Nickerson (1976)—four 10-m incubations with 7.3 μM—to block the adrenaline effect on the frog heart at low temperature are very high. A lower concentration of phenoxybenzamine-2.9 μM-inhibited the inotropic effect of acetylcholine on the frog ventricle (Benfey, 1975). The concentration of phentolamine employed by Kunos and Nickerson (1976) to inhibit the inotropic effect of adrenaline, 26.5 μM, is also exceedingly high. The conclusion that the high concentrations of the α-adrenoceptor blocking drugs did not inhibit the adrenaline effect by receptor blockade is consistent with the observation that at low temperature phenoxybenzamine inhibited the inotropic effect of isoprenaline (Benfey, 1975; Kunos and Nickerson, 1976), although there is evidence that isoprenaline did not act on α-adrenoceptors (Benfey, 1975). Low temperature greatly increases the contractility of the amphibian heart, and as a consequence the inotropic drug effect is small (Nayler and Wright, 1963; Benfey, 1977a). It should be easier to inhibit nonspecifically the small effect at low temperature than the much larger effect at higher temperature.

Low temperature did not change adenylate-cyclase-coupled β-adrenoceptors in frog ventricle (Benfey, Kunos and Nickerson, 1974) or in frog erythrocytes (Caron and Lefkowitz, 1974).

5. Conclusion There is no good evidence that the frog heart contains α-adrenoceptors, at both low and higher temperatures. A critical review of the experimental data lends no support to the notion of adrenoceptor interconversion.

B. Effect of Low Temperature on Mammalian Heart

1. α-Adrenoceptors in mammalian heart In contrast to the amphibian heart, the mammalian heart possesses inotropic α-adrenoceptors, and these have been demonstrated at normal temperature (Wenzel and Su, 1966; Benfey and Varma, 1967; Govier, 1967, 1968; Leong and Benfey, 1968; Wagner and Brodde, 1978). Alpha- and β-adrenoceptor-mediated mechanisms differ. Thus, unlike β-adrenoceptor stimulation, α-adrenoceptor stimulation is not associated with activation of myocardial adenylate cyclase (Benfey, 1971; Osnes and Øye, 1975).

The concentrations of α-adrenoceptor blocking drugs that antagonize the inotropic effect of phenylephrine on mammalian heart are similar to those that block α-adrenoceptors in smooth muscle. Thus the K_B for phentolamine was 28 nM in rabbit atrium (Benfey, 1973) and 23 nM in rabbit aorta (Besse and Furchgott, 1976). The pA_2 of phentolamine in rabbit papillary muscle was 7.35 (Schümann et al., 1974). Presynaptic α-adrenoceptors in guinea pig atrium were blocked by 0.31 μM phentolamine (Langer, Adler-Graschinsky, and Giorgi, 1977). Higher concentrations of phentolamine have unspecific effects. Thus 3.1 μM phentolamine inhibited the chronotropic effect of sympathetic nerve stimulation on guinea pig atrium (Langer et al., 1977).

Phenoxybenzamine is a highly potent α-adrenoceptor blocking drug. One nanomolar phenoxybenzamine inhibited the inotropic effect of phenylephrine on rabbit atrium (Benfey, 1973), and a 5-m incubation with 0.3 nM phenoxybenzamine inhibited the noradrenaline-induced contraction of isolated cat spleen (Davidson and Innes, 1972). A 5-m exposure of the isolated rabbit aorta to phenoxybenzamine in a concentration of 29 nM or less caused a significant adrenaline blockade (Nickerson and Chan, 1961). Dibenamine, which is about 20 times less potent than phenoxybenzamine (Graham, 1962), had a pA_2 of 8.3 on 20-m incubation in guinea pig vas deferens (Graham and Al Katib, 1966).

The high potency is deceptive; phenoxybenzamine is not selective. Beta-halo alkylamines have inhibitory effects on mammalian heart that are unrelated to α-adrenoceptor blockade. Thus 0.1 μM phenoxybenzamine inhibited the inotropic and chronotropic effects of acetylcholine on guinea pig atrium (Benfey and Grillo, 1963), 0.78 μM phenoxybenzamine caused a 50% inhibition of neuronal noradrenaline uptake, and 2.8 μM phenoxybenzamine caused a 50% inhibition of extraneuronal noradrenaline uptake in rat heart (Iversen, 1973); 10 μM dibenamine inhibited the chronotropic effect of isoprenaline (Krell and Patil, 1969), and 29 μM phenoxybenzamine inhibited the chronotropic effect of noradrenaline on guinea pig atrium (Adler-Graschinsky, Langer, and Rubio, 1972).

2. Studies relating to adrenoceptor interconversion Kunos and Nickerson (1977) found "increases in α-adrenoceptor properties" (p. 603) in rat atria at low temperature. Their data are complex. In spontaneously beating atria, lowering the temperature reduced the inotropic and chronotropic potency of isoprenaline; but in driven left atria, lowering the temperature from 31° to 17°C increased the inotropic potency of isoprenaline, noradrenaline, and phenylephrine and reduced the potency of propranolol as a noradrenaline antagonist. Following 6-hydroxydopamine treatment, lowering the temperature increased the potency of propranolol in driven atria. Phenoxybenzamine (four 10-m incubations with 7.3 μM) inhibited the inotropic effect of noradrenaline at 17°C but not at 24° or 31°C. Phentolamine (2.6 μM) inhibited the inotropic effect of phenylephrine more at 17°C than at 31°C. It was not explained why the phentolamine antagonism was noncompetitive at 17°C; phentolamine is known to act competitively on α-adrenoceptors.

It has been difficult to repeat these experiments. Benfey (1977a) found that at 17°C the rat atrium often did not respond to sympathomimetic drugs. At 17°C the positive inotropic effect of sympathomimetic drugs was absent or greatly reduced; only noradrenaline produced a significant effect, and it was not possible to evaluate the potency of phenylephrine or isoprenaline (Martinez and McNeill, 1977).

Martinez and McNeill (1977) tested the adrenoceptor interconversion hypothesis in rat left atria directly. Exposure to 1 μM phenoxybenzamine for 45 m at 17°C led to no inhibition of the contractile response or the cyclic AMP response to noradrenaline at 37°C, and the authors concluded that "there is no interconversion of α- and β-adrenoceptors mediated by temperature" (p. 457). Wagner and Brodde (1978) determined the effect of 1 μM phenoxybenzamine on the positive inotropic response to phenylephrine in strips of rat right ventricle at 37 and 24°C. The $-\log EC_{50}$ for phenylephrine was lower at 37°C than at 24°C. When the strips were incubated with phenoxybenzamine at 24°C and when after removal of phenoxybenzamine the bath temperature was raised to 37°C, the $-\log EC_{50}$ did not differ from that determined after incubation with phenoxybenzamine at 37°C. The same held true when the procedure was reversed—i.e., when the strips were incubated with phenoxybenzamine at 37°C and the dose-response curve of phenylephrine was determined at 24°C. The result was the same in driven rat atria. The authors concluded that the rat heart contains two distinct and not interconvertible adrenoceptor types.

Other studies also do not agree with the results of Kunos and Nickerson (1977). Bennett and Kemp (1978) measured inotropic and chronotropic responses of rat atria to phenylephrine at 37° and 21°C. Reduction in temperature produced no change in the potency of phenylephrine nor any greater susceptibility of the responses to blockade by phentolamine rather than propranolol. In rat atria lowering the temperature from 37° to 22°C did not alter the chronotropic potency of isoprenaline, adrenaline, noradrenaline, or phenylephrine (Sadavongvivad et al., 1977). In the anesthetized dog, lowering the temperature to 22°C did not change or only moderately reduced the effects of adrenaline and phenylephrine on contractile force and heart rate; the effect of phenylephrine on contractile force was slight at 37° and 22°C (Cotten and Brown, 1957). In mouse atria, lowering the temperature from 37° to 26°C increased the chronotropic potency of isoprenaline and the potency of propranolol as an isoprenaline antagonist (Munoz-Ramirez, Haavik, and Ryan, 1973; Munoz-Ramirez, Ryan, and Buckner, 1975). In guinea pig atria, lowering the temperature from 37° or 30°C to 27°, 26°, or 25°C increased the chronotropic potency of isoprenaline (Oppermann, Ryan, and Haavik, 1972; Wöppel and Trendelenburg, 1973; Duncan and Broadley, 1977). In spontaneously beating guinea pig atria, lowering the temperature from 42° or 30°C to 27° or 25°C increased the inotropic potency of isoprenaline (Duncan and Broadley, 1977, 1978b; Reinhardt et al., 1978). In driven guinea pig atria, lowering the temperature from 33° to 25°C increased the potency of practolol as an antagonist of the inotropic effect of isoprenaline (Reinhardt, Wagner, and Schümann, 1972).

From studies in rat atria Amer and Byrne (1975) concluded that the β-adrenoceptors that trigger the synthesis of cyclic AMP at 37°C promote the synthesis of cyclic GMP at 24°C. The authors speculate that this may be due to changes in substrate specificity of the catalytic subunit of adenylate cyclase from ATP to GTP with no change in the receptor unit or the coupling of the β-adrenoceptor subunit at 24°C with the catalytic subunit of guanylate cyclase. No further work has been reported on this topic. In guinea pig atria, lowering the temperature from 38° to 22.5°C led to parallel changes in mechanical and cyclic AMP responses to the β-adrenoceptor stimulant orciprenaline, and there was "no evidence of α-adrenoceptor activation at any temperature" (Duncan and Broadley, 1978a). Adenylate-cyclase-coupled β-adrenoceptors in rat ventricle slices (Benfey et al., 1974) and rat heart membranes (Caron and Lefkowitz, 1974) did not change when the temperature was reduced from 37°C to 17° or 15°C.

3. **Conclusion** The mammalian heart contains both inotropic α- and β-adrenoceptors, and there is no good evidence that low temperature converts inotropic or chronotropic β-adrenoceptors to α-adrenoceptors.

C. Effect of Low Temperature on Tissues Other Than the Heart

1. **Physiological studies** In the isolated rabbit ear artery, cooling from 37° to 11°C did not cause a decrease in the dilator activity of isoprenaline nor a change in the β-adrenoceptor quality (Glover, 1972). In the isolated rabbit aorta, lowering the temperature from 42° to 25°C increased the dilator potency of isoprenaline and decreased the constrictor potency of phenylephrine (Wagner, Reinhardt, and Huppertz, 1975). In the isolated dog saphenous vein, cooling from 43° or 37°C to 29°, 25°, or 24°C increased the dilator potency of isoprenaline and noradrenaline; the constrictor potency of acetylcholine, 5-hydroxytryptamine, and noradrenaline; and the potency of phentolamine (Vanhoutte and Shepherd, 1970a, b; Janssens and Vanhoutte, 1978).

In the isolated rabbit iris dilator muscle, noradrenaline increases and isoprenaline and terbutaline decrease tension. Lowering the bath temperature from 37° to 25°C increased the potency of noradrenaline and decreased the potency of isoprenaline and terbutaline (Matheny and Ahlquist, 1976). Ahlquist (1977) took this as evidence of adrenoceptor interconversion.

In the isolated rabbit ileum both α- and β-adrenoceptors mediate relaxation. Lowering the temperature from 42° or 37°C to 25°C increased the potency of isoprenaline and phenylephrine as β-adrenoceptor stimulants, increased the potency of practolol as an isoprenaline antagonist, and decreased the potency of phenylephrine as an α-adrenoceptor stimulant (Wagner, Reinhardt, and Schümann, 1972, 1973).

The α- and β-adrenoceptor activities of the isolated rat uterus during the estrous cycle are influenced by temperature changes (Butterworth and Jarman, 1974). During diestrus, lowering the bath temperature from 40° to 25°C increased the β-adrenoceptor-mediated inhibition by isoprenaline, adrenaline, noradrenaline, and phenylephrine, During estrus, adrenaline, noradrenaline, and phenylephrine produced biphasic responses of contraction followed by inhibition at 40°C; and isoprenaline produced only inhibition. At 25°C the contractile α-responses were either abolished (phenylephrine) or greatly reduced (adrenaline and noradrenaline), whereas the inhibitory β effects of all four amines were increased.

Beta-adrenoceptor stimulation relaxes the isolated guinea pig trachea. Lowering the temperature from 37° to 25°C increased the potency of isoprenaline and of practolol as an isoprenaline antagonist (Wagner et al., 1972). Lowering the temperature from 37.5° to 17.5°C increased the potency of isoprenaline more than 10-fold (Foster, 1967).

Incubation of rat erythrocytes and mouse thymus cells with propranolol at 5°C led to inhibition of the action of isoprenaline on cyclic AMP production that persisted after the temperature had been raised to 24°C and the cells washed, an effect which "most likely results from specific and tight binding of the antagonist to the beta receptor" (Sheppard and Burghardt, 1978, p. 223).

2. Radioligand-binding studies Beta-adrenoceptors in turkey erythrocyte membranes were identified by [³H]dihydroalprenolol binding (Pike and Lefkowitz, 1978). Lowering the temperature from 37° to 4°C increased the affinity of agonists but not of antagonists. The dissociation constants of [¹²⁵I]iodohydroxybenzylpindolol in turkey erythrocytes were similar at 37° and at 20°C (Brown et al., 1976). The same amount of steady-state binding of [³H]dihydroalprenolol to frog erythrocytes was attained at 4°C as was attained at 25° and 37°C (Limbird and Lefkowitz, 1976). In membrane preparations of rat and monkey brain, similar dissociation constants were obtained for [³H]dihydroalprenolol at 37°, 23°, and 0°C (Bylund and Snyder, 1976).

The binding of [³H]adrenaline and [³H]noradrenaline to calf cortical membranes had properties indicating an association with α-adrenoceptors (U'Prichard and Snyder, 1977). At 25° and 4°C the [³H]catecholamines and agonist competitors had 2–4 times greater affinity for the binding sites than at 37°C, partial agonists had approximately the same affinity, and antagonists were 2–10 times weaker.

3. Conclusion Studies in isolated mammalian tissues have provided no good evidence that low temperature converts β-adrenoceptors to α-adrenoceptors.

D. Effect of Thyroid Hormone Deficiency on Rat Heart

1. Rate and contractility Kunos, Vermes-Kunos, and Nickerson (1974) and Kunos (1977) obtained results in rat atria "indicating thyroid hormone-dependent interconversion of myocardial α- and β-adrenoceptors" (Kunos, 1977, p. 177) and "suggested that this interconversion is similar to that observed earlier in frog hearts at different temperatures and that both effects may reflect an allosteric transition between two forms of a single basic structure" (Kunos, 1977, p. 177). It was observed that thyroidectomy reduced the chronotropic and inotropic potency of isoprenaline and noradrenaline and increased that of phenylephrine, reduced the potency of propranolol as a noradrenaline antagonist, and caused α-adrenoceptor blocking drugs to inhibit the inotropic and chronotropic effects of noradrenaline. Conversely, thyroid treatment increased the potency of propranolol as a noradrenaline antagonist in the driven atrium (not in the spontaneously beating atrium) and did not change the potency of isoprenaline or noradrenaline.

Studies by Wagner and Brodde (1978) do not support the concept of adrenoceptor interconversion. Propylthiouracil treatment of rats did not cause a change in the pA_2 value for phentolamine as an antagonist of the inotropic effect of phenylephrine on the left atrium.

Nakashima et al. (1971); Nakashima and Hagino (1972); and Nakashima, Tsura, and Shigei (1973); had earlier reported that propylthiouracil treatment increased the inotropic and chronotropic potency of phenylephrine on rat atria and decreased that of isoprenaline. Hashimoto and Nakashima (1978) reported that thyroid treatment reduced the potency of phenylephrine and phentolamine and increased the potency of isoprenaline and propranolol on contractility of guinea pig atrium and rabbit papillary muscle. Since reduction of the phenylephrine response occurred after 2 days of thyroxine treatment and potentiation of the isoprenaline effect required longer treatment, the authors concluded that the changes in the effects mediated by α- and β-adrenoceptors induced by thyroxine are independent of each other.

2. Cyclic AMP Kunos et al. (1976) found in working but not in resting rat atria that following thyroidectomy the adrenoceptor-mediated rise in cyclic AMP was inhibited by phenoxybenzamine (7.3 μM), whereas in normal animals it was inhibited by a β-adrenoceptor blocking drug. The authors concluded that "the results indicate that adrenoceptors mediating the rise in cyclic AMP and contractility are similarly interconvertible" (p. 781).

These results have not been confirmed. Thus in the perfused heart of hypothyroid rats, the positive inotropic effect following α-adrenoceptor stimulation was not associated with a rise in myocardial cyclic AMP (Osnes, 1976). In propylthiouracil-treated working rat atria and ventricles, α-adrenoceptor stimulation did not elevate cyclic AMP (Wagner and Brodde, 1978).

3. Radioligand-binding studies The data are not clear. Thyroid hormone pretreatment of normal rats increased [³H]dihydroalprenolol binding capacity in purified heart membranes (Williams et al., 1977; Ciaraldi and Marinetti, 1977, 1978) but not in crude heart membrane preparations (Banerjee and Kung, 1977) and reduced [³H]dihydroergocryptine binding capacity in frozen hearts (Ciaraldi and Marinetti, 1977) but not in fresh hearts (Ciaraldi and Marinetti, 1978).

Thyroidectomy (Banerjee and Kung, 1977) or propylthiouracil treatment (Ciaraldi and Marinetti, 1977, 1978) reduced the binding capacity for the β-adrenoceptor blocking drug; and in addition, propylthiouracil treatment reduced the binding capacity for the α-adrenoceptor blocking drug (Ciaraldi and Marinetti, 1977, 1978).

Thyroid hormone treatment of thyroidectomized rats increased the [³H]dihydroalprenolol binding capacity (Banerjee and Kung, 1977) and decreased the [³H]dihydroergocryptine binding capacity—changes that might be independent of one another (Sharma and Banerjee, 1978).

4. Conclusion There is no firm evidence that thyroid hormone deficiency converts β-adrenoceptors in rat heart to α-adrenoceptors.

E. α-Adrenoceptor Subsensitivity in Rat Heart

Isolated atria of rats subjected to cold acclimation (Harri, Melender, and Tirri, 1974), to daily injections of phenylephrine or isoprenaline (Tirri, Siltuvuori, and Harri, 1976), or to physical training by swimming or repeated injections of ACTH (Siltovuori, Tirri, and Harri, 1977) were subsensitive to the chronotropic and inotropic effects of phenylephrine; but the sensitivity to isoprenaline did not change, which "indicated that there was no interconversion of these receptors" (Siltovuori et al., 1977, p. 459).

F. Effect of Driving Rate on Isolated Hearts

In rabbit papillary muscle, the positive inotropic effect of methoxamine was greater at 0.5 and 1 Hz than at 1.5 Hz (Endoh and Schümann, 1975). In guinea pig ventricle strips, the inotropic effect of phenylephrine was greater at 1 Hz than at 2.5 Hz (Ledda, Marchetti, and Mugelli, 1975). The inotropic effect of low concentrations of adrenaline on guinea pig ventricle strips was inhibited by phentolamine at 1 Hz but not at 2.5 Hz and by practolol at 2.5 Hz but not at 1 Hz (Mugelli, Ledda, and Mantelli, 1976).

Nickerson and Kunos (1977) and Kunos (1978) take these observations as further evidence of adrenoceptor interconversion. A simpler explanation is that only at the low driving rate could the α-adrenoceptor-mediated inotropic effect develop fully. The α-adrenoceptor-mediated inotropic effect differs from that mediated by β-adrenoceptors in that time to peak tension and time of relaxation are not shortened and may be prolonged (Ledda et al., 1975; Benfey, 1977b).

G. Effect of Muscle Activity on Skeletal Muscle Blood Flow

Szentivanyi et al. (1970) measured the vasoconstrictor effect of noradrenaline in the dog hindlimb at rest and during electrical stimulation of the sciatic nerve. Stimulation of the sciatic nerve inhibited the constrictor response to noradrenaline and propranolol reestablished the constrictor effect of noradrenaline, although it had no effect on noradrenaline constriction in resting muscle.

Hence, adrenergic reaction lost its alpha character in the active muscle by giving place to a beta-sensitive inhibition of the alpha constrictor response. These changes in the receptor quality could be ascribed to a factor which was released when metabolic rate was elevated and which modified the quality of the receptor. Accordingly, perfusing the resting hindlimb with blood obtained from the heart which displays 'beta' qualities and thus contains this factor in a greater amount, resulted in the same changes in the adrenergic response as it was the case during locally increased metabolic level. The disappearance of adrenergic vasoconstriction in the vessels of the active muscle may be due to a transformation of the activity of alpha receptors into beta, evoked by a modulator substance.

Further work on the "modulator substance" has not been reported.

H. Effect of Alloxan Treatment on Rabbit Aorta

Czeuz et al. (1973) found in rabbits pretreated with alloxan that the constrictor effect of noradrenaline on the isolated aorta was inhibited not only by phentolamine but also by propranolol and suggested that "the phenomenon may reflect the formation of new receptor sites or conformational changes in structures with previously different reactivity" (p. 755). Further work on this topic has not been published.

I. Isoprenaline Resistance in Bronchial Asthma

Szentivanyi (1968) suggested that an inherent defect of the β-adrenoceptor is a major factor in bronchial asthma, and Kunos (1978) quotes this suggestion as an example of adrenoceptor interconversion: changes in adrenoceptor characteristics of airways and leukocytes in patients with bronchial asthma are compatible with a "shift in receptor balance from β to α" (p. 304). A simpler explanation is desensitization of β-adrenoceptors by exposure to isoprenaline (Lefkowitz, 1978). Prolonged exposure to isoprenaline produced isoprenaline resistance in man and dog (Conolly et al., 1971). Isolated rat tracheal muscle became considerably less sensitive to the relaxing effect of isoprenaline after being incubated with a high concentration of the drug for 30 m (Lin et al., 1977). Beta-adrenoceptor function was tested in lymphocytes of normal subjects, asthmatic patients taking large doses of β-adrenergic bronchodilators, and comparable asthmatics treated exclusively with nonadrenergic medication (Conolly and Greenacre, 1976). Maximal increase in cyclic AMP in lymphocytes from normal subjects and in asthmatics on nonadrenergic medication was much greater than in asthmatics taking large doses of sympathomimetics. Withdrawal of β-adrenergic drugs was followed by a reversion of the cyclic AMP response to normal values, which suggests that the depression was drug-induced rather than an inherent feature of the disease.

J. Additional Radioligand-Binding Studies Relating to Adrenoceptor Interconversion

Roberts et al. (1977) tested the adrenoceptor interconversion hypothesis in subcellular preparations of rabbit uterus. Contraction, mediated by α-adrenoceptors, occurs in uteri from estrogen-treated rabbits, whereas relaxation, mediated by β-adrenoceptors, predominates with progesterone treatment or during pregnancy. Progesterone treatment reduced the binding capacity for [³H]dihydroergocryptine but did not change the binding capacity for [³H]iodohydroxypindolol. There was no change in the affinity of the adrenoceptor blocking drugs. The authors concluded that this direct estimate of α- and β-adrenoceptors did not support the hypothesis that the receptors are simply alternate configurations of one structure.

Guellaen et al. (1978) tested the adrenoceptor interconversion hypothesis in rat liver membranes. Adrenalectomy shifts the response of rat liver, in terms of glucose production, from a pure α to a mixed α-β type. Catecholamine-stimulated cyclic AMP production is increased by adrenalectomy. Since adrenalectomy enhanced [³H]dihydroalprenolol binding capacity and did not change [³H]dihydroergocryptine binding capacity or the affinity for either ligand, the authors wrote that "it thus appears that α- and β-adrenergic receptors in rat liver plasma membranes may be under independent physiological control" (p. 1114).

In rabbits, denervation by removal of the superior cervical ganglion led to an increased density of β-adrenoceptors (as measured by [³H]dihydroalprenolol binding) in membranes prepared from iris with no increase in the density of α-adrenoceptors (as measured by [³H]dihydroergocryptine binding) (Page and Neufeld, 1978).

III. CONCLUSION

Both the analysis of the experimental data and the review of the literature have shown that the adrenoceptor interconversion hypothesis is not based on sound evidence. The pharmacological experiments supporting the notion that α- and β-adrenoceptors are interconvertible have not been done under properly controlled conditions, and their results have not been critically evaluated. Radioligand-binding methods have demonstrated that the concentrations of α- and β-adrenoceptors can be altered (Kahn, 1976), but they have not shown that adrenoceptors are interconvertible.

IV. REFERENCES

Adler-Graschinsky, E.; Langer, S.Z.; Rubio, M.C.: Metabolism of Norepinephrine Released by Phenoxybenzamine in Isolated Guinea-Pig Atria. J Pharmacol Exp Ther 180(1972) 286–301

Ahlquist, R.P.: Adrenoceptor Sensitivity in Disease As Assessed through Response to Temperature Alteration. Fed Proc 36(1977)2572–2574

Amer, M.S.: Byrne, J.E.: Interchange of Adenyl and Guanyl Cyclases as an Explanation for Transformation of β- to α-Adrenergic Responses in the Rat Atrium. Nature 256(1975) 421–424

Banerjee, S.P.; Kung, L.S.: β-Adrenergic Receptors in Rat Heart: Effects of Thyroidectomy. Eur J Pharmacol 43(1977)207–208

Belleau, B.: An Analysis of Drug-Receptor Interactions. In: Proceedings of the First International Pharmacological Meeting, Vol. VII, pp. 75–95, ed. by K.J. Brunings, P. Lindgren. Pergamon, Oxford, 1963

Benfey, B.G.: Lack of Relationship between Myocardial Cyclic AMP Concentrations and Inotropic Effects of Sympathomimetic Amines. Br J Pharmacol 43(1971)757–763

Benfey, B.G.: Characterization of α-Adrenoceptors in the Myocardium. Br J Pharmacol 48(1973)132–138

Benfey, B.G.: Temperature Dependence of Phenoxybenzamine Effects and the Adrenoceptors Transformation Hypothesis. Nature 256(1975)745–747

Benfey, B.G.: Temperature, Phenoxybenzamine and Adrenoceptor Transformation. Nature 259(1976)252

Benfey, B.G.: Cardiac Adrenoceptors at Low Temperature: What Is the Experimental Evidence for the Adrenoceptor Interconversion Hypothesis? Fed Proc 36(1977a)2575–2579

Benfey, B.G.: Theophylline and Phenylephrine Effects on Cardiac Relaxation. Br J Pharmacol 59(1977b)75–81

Benfey, B.G.: Discussion of Evidence Regarding Adrenoceptor Interconversion. Fed Proc 37(1978)686

Benfey, B.G.; Grillo, S.A.: Antagonism of Acetylcholine by Adrenaline Antagonists. Br J Pharmacol Chemother 20(1963)528–533

Benfey, B.G.; Kunos, G.; Nickerson, M.: Dissociation of Cardiac Inotropic and Adenylate Cyclase Activating Adrenoceptors. Br J Pharmacol 51(1974)253–257

Benfey, B.G.; Varma, D.R.: Interactions of Sympathomimetic Drugs, Propranolol and Phentolamine on Atrial Refractory Period and Contractility. Br J Pharmacol Chemother 30(1967)603–611

Bennett, T.; Kemp, P.A.: Lack of Evidence for a Temperature-Mediated Change of Adrenoceptor Type in the Rat Heart. Naunyn Schmiedebergs Arch Pharmacol 301(1978)217–222

Berry, D.G.; Miller, J.W.: Binding of Phenoxybenzamine to Rat Platelets and Platelet Fractions. J Pharmacol 31(1975)176–184

Besse, J.C.; Furchgott, R.F.: Dissociation Constants and Relative Efficacies of Agonists on Alpha Adrenergic Receptors in Rabbit Aorta. J Pharmacol Exp Ther 197(1976)66–78

Brown, E.M.; Aurbach, G.D.; Hauser, D.; Troxler, F.: β-Adrenergic Receptor Interactions. Characterization of Iodohydroxybenzylpindolol As a Specific Ligand. J Biol Chem 251(1976)1232–1238

Buckley,G.A.; Jordan, C.C.: Temperature Modulation of α- and β-Adrenoceptors in the Isolated Frog Heart. Br J Pharmacol 38(1970)394–398

Burn, J.H.: Functions of Autonomic Transmitters, pp. 143–146. Williams & Wilkins, Baltimore, 1956

Burn, J.H.; Robinson, J.: Reversal of the Vascular Response to Acetylcholine and Adrenaline. Br J Pharmacol Chemother 6(1951)110–119

Butterworth, K.R.; Jarman, D.A.: Effect of Temperature on Changes, Induced by Oestrus, in α- and β-Adrenoceptor Activities of the Rat Uterus. Br J Pharmacol 51(1974)462–464

Bylund, D.B.; Snyder, S.H.: Beta Adrenergic Receptor Binding in Membrane Preparations from Mammalian Brain. Mol Pharmacol 12(1976)568–580

Caron, M.G.; Lefkowitz, R.J.: Temperature Immutability of Adenyl Cyclase-Coupled β Adrenergic Receptors. Nature 249(1974)258–260

Ciaraldi, T.; Marinetti, G.V.: Thyroxine and Propylthiouracil Effects in Vivo on Alpha and Beta Adrenergic Receptors in Rat Heart. Biochem Biophys Res Commun 74(1977)984–991

Ciaraldi, T.P.; Marinetti, G.V.: Hormone Action at the Membrane Level. VIII. Adrenergic Receptors in Rat Heart and Adipocytes and Their Modulation by Thyroxine. Biochim Biophys Acta 541(1978)334–346

Clark, A.J.; Eggleton, M.C.; Eggleton, P.; Gaddie, R.; Stewart, C.P.: The Metabolism of the Frog's Heart. Oliver & Boyd, Edinburgh and London, 1938

Conolly, M.E.; Davies, D.S.; Dollery, C.T.; George, C.F.: Resistance to β-Adrenoceptor Stimulants (a Possible Explanation for the Rise in Asthma Deaths). Br J Pharmacol 43(1971)389–402

Conolly, M.E.; Greenacre, J.K.: The Lymphocyte β-Adrenoceptor in Normal Subjects and Patients with Bronchial Asthma. J Clin Invest 58(1976)1307–1316

Cotten, M. DeV.; Brown, Jr., T.G.: Effects of Pressor Amines and Ouabain on the Heart and Blood Pressure During Hypothermia. J Pharmacol Exp Ther 121(1957)319–329

Czeuz, R.; Wenger, T.L.; Kunos, G.; Szentivanyi, M.: Changes of Adrenergic Reaction Patterns in Experimental Diabetes Mellitus. Endocrinol 93(1973)752–755

Dale, H.H.: On Some Physiological Actions of Ergot. J Physiol 34(1906)163–206

Davidson, W.J.; Innes, I.R.: Lack of Spare α-Adrenoceptors in the Cat Spleen. Can J Physiol Pharmacol 50(1972)1210–1213

Duncan, C.; Broadley, K.J.: The Influence of Temperature upon Reserpine-Induced Supersensitivity of Guinea-Pig Isolated Atria to Isoprenaline and Salbutamol. Naunyn Schmiedebergs Arch Pharmacol 297(1977)163–170

Duncan, C.; Broadley, K.J.: Correlation Between cAMP Production in Guinea-Pig Left and Right Atria and their Inotropic and Chronotropic Responses to Orciprenaline at Different Temperatures. Mol Pharmacol 14(1978a)1063–1072

Duncan, C.; Broadley, K.J.: Possible Sites of Temperature-Dependent Changes in Sensitivity of the Positive Inotropic and Chronotropic Responses to Sympathomimetic Amines by Comparisons of the Temperature Optima for a Range of Agonists. Arch Int Pharmacodyn 231(1978b)196–211

Endoh, M.; Schümann, H.J.: Frequency Dependence of the Positive Inotropic Effect of Methoxamine and Naphazoline Mediated by α-Adrenoceptors in the Isolated Rabbit Papillary Muscle. Naunyn Schmiedebergs Arch Pharmacol 287(1975)377–389

Foster, R.W.: The Potentiation of the Responses to Noradrenaline and Isoprenaline of the Guinea-Pig Isolated Tracheal Chain Preparation by Desipramine, Cocaine, Phentolamine, Phenoxybenzamine, Guanethidine, Metanephrine and Cooling. Br J Pharmacol Chemother 31(1967)466–482

Furchgott, R.F.: The Classification of Adrenoceptors (Adrenergic Receptors). An Evaluation from the Standpoint of Receptor Theory. In: Catecholamines, pp. 283–335, ed. by H. Blaschko, E. Muscholl. Springer, Berlin, 1972

Furchgott, R.F.: Pharmacological Characterization of Receptors: Its Relation to Radioligand-Binding Studies. Fed Proc 37(1978)115–120

Furchgott, R.F.; Jurkiewicz, A.; Jurkiewicz, N.H.: Antagonism of Propranolol to Isoproterenol in Guinea-Pig Trachea: Some Cautionary Findings. In: Frontiers in Catecholamine Research, pp. 295–299, ed. by E. Usdin, S.H. Snyder. Pergamon, New York, 1973

Glover, W.E.: Effect of Cooling on Beta-Adrenergic Responses in the Rabbit Ear Artery. J Physiol 224(1972)91P–92P

Govier, W.C.: A Positive Inotropic Effect of Phenylephrine Mediated through α Adrenergic Receptors. Life Sci 6(1967)1361–1365

Govier, W.C.: Myocardial Alpha Adrenergic Receptors and Their Role in the Production of a Positive Inotropic Effect by Sympathomimetic Agents. J Pharmacol Exp Ther 159 (1968)82–90

Graham, J.D.P.: 2-Haloalkylamines. In: Progress in Medicinal Chemistry, Vol. II, pp. 132–175, ed. by G.P. Ellis, G.B. West. Butterworths, London, 1962

Graham, J.D.P.; Al Katib, H.: The Action of Trypsin on Blockade by 2-Halogenoalkylamines: Speculation on the Nature of the Alpha Receptor for Catecholamine. Br J Pharmacol Chemother 28(1966)1–14

Guellaen, G.; Yates-Aggerbeck, M.; Vauquelin, G.; Strosberg, D.; Hanoune, J.: Characterization with [³H]Dihydroergocryptine of the α-Adrenergic Receptor of the Hepatic Plasma Membrane. J Biol Chem 253(1978)1114–1120

Harri, M.N.E.: Temperature-Dependent Sensitivity of Adrenoceptors in the Toad's Heart. Acta Pharmacol Tox 33(1973)273–279

Harri, M.N.E.; Melender, L.; Tirri, R.: Changed Chronotropic Sensitivity to Sympathomimetic Amines in Isolated Atria from Rats Following Cold Acclimation. Experientia 30(1974)1041–1043

Hashimoto, H.; Nakashima, M.: Influences of Thyroid Hormone on the Positive Inotropic Effects Mediated by α- and β-Adrenergic Receptors in Isolated Guinea Pig Atria and Rabbit Papillary Muscles. Eur J Pharmacol 50(1978)337–347

Iversen, L.L.: Catecholamine Uptake Processes. Br Med Bull 29(1973)130–135

Janssens, W.J.; Vanhoutte, P.M.: Instantaneous Changes of Alpha-Adrenoceptor Affinity Caused by Moderate Cooling in Canine Cutaneous Veins. Am J Physiol 234(1978) H330–H337

Kahn, C.R.: Membrane Receptors for Hormones and Neurotransmitters. J Cell Biol 70(1976)261–286

Keenan, A.K.: The Temperature-Dependent Action of Phenylephrine in Frog Cardiac Muscle. Abstracts, 7th Int Congr Pharmacol (1978)240

Krell, R.D.; Patil, P.N.: Combinations of Alpha and Beta Adrenergic Blockers in Isolated Guinea Pig Atria. J Pharmacol Exp Ther 170(1969)262–271

Kunos, G.: Thyroid Hormone-Dependent Interconversion of Myocardial α- and β-Adrenoceptors in the Rat. Br J Pharmacol 59(1977)177–189

Kunos, G.: Adrenoceptors. Ann Rev Pharmacol Tox 18(1978)291–311

Kunos, G.; Mucci, L.; Jaeger, V.: Interconversion of Myocardial Adrenoceptors: Its Relationship to Adenylate Cyclase Activation. Life Sci 19(1976)1597–1602

Kunos, G.; Nickerson, M.: Temperature-Induced Interconversion of α- and β-Adrenoceptors in the Frog Heart. J Physiol 256(1976)23–40

Kunos, G.; Nickerson, M.: Effects of Sympathetic Innervation and Temperature on the Properties of Rat Adrenoceptors. Br J Pharmacol 59(1977)603–614

Kunos, G.; Szentivanyi, M.: Evidence Favouring the Existence of a Single Adrenergic Receptor. Nature 217(1968)1077–1078

Kunos, G.; Vermes-Kunos, I.; Nickerson, M.: Effects of Thyroid State on Adrenoceptor Properties. Nature 250(1974)779–781

Kunos, G.; Yong, M.S.; Nickerson, M.: Transformation of Adrenergic Receptors in the Myocardium. Nature New Biol 241(1973)119–120

Langer, S.Z.; Adler-Graschinsky, E.; Giorgi, O.: Physiological Significance of α-Adrenoceptor Mediated Negative Feedback Mechanism Regulating Noradrenaline Release during Nerve Stimulation. Nature 265(1977)648–650

Ledda, F.; Marchetti, P.; Mugelli, A.: Studies on the Positive Inotropic Effect of Phenylephrine: A Comparison with Isoprenaline. Br J Pharmacol 54(1975)83–90

Lefkowitz, R.J.: Identification of Adenylate Cyclase-Coupled Beta-Adrenergic Receptors with Radiolabeled Beta-Adrenergic Antagonists. Biochem Pharmacol 24(1975)1651–1658

Lefkowitz, R.J.: Identification and Regulation of Alpha- and Beta-Adrenergic Receptors. Fed Proc 37(1978)123–129

Leong, L.S.K.; Benfey, B.G.: The Alpha-Receptors in the Driven Rabbit Heart and Their Absence in the Spontaneously Beating Rabbit Heart and Driven Frog Heart. Proc Can Fed Biol Soc 11(1968)129

Limbird, L.E.; Lefkowitz, R.J.: Negative Cooperativity Among β-Adrenergic Receptors in Frog Erythrocyte Membranes. J Biol Chem 215(1976)5007–5014

Lin, C.S.; Hurwitz, L.; Jenne, J.; Avner, B.P.: Mechanism of Isoproterenol-Induced Desensitization of Tracheal Smooth Muscle. J Pharmacol Exp Ther 203(1977)12–22

Martinez, T.T.; McNeill, J.H.: The Effect of Temperature on Cardiac Adrenoceptors. J Pharmacol Exp Ther 203(1977)457–466

Matheny, J.L.; Ahlquist, R.P.: Role of Neuronal and Extraneuronal Factors in Temperature Mediated Responsiveness of Adrenoceptors. Arch Int Pharmacodyn 224(1976)180–189

Melchiorre, C.; Yong, M.S.; Benfey, B.G.; Belleau, B.: Molecular Properties of the Adrenergic α-Receptor II. Optimum Covalent Inhibition by Two Different Prototypes of Polyamine Disulfides. J Med Chem 21(1978)1126–1132

Mugelli, A.; Ledda, F.; Mantelli, L.: Frequency Dependence of the α-Adrenoceptor-Mediated Inotropic Effect in Guinea Pig Heart. Eur J Pharmacol 36(1976)215–220

Munoz-Ramirez, H.; Haavik, C.O.; Ryan, C.F.: Temperature-Dependent Supersensitivity to Isoprenaline in Mouse Atria. Eur J Pharmacol 22(1973)43–46

Munoz-Ramirez, H.; Ryan, C.F.; Buckner, C.K.: Studies on the Temperature-Dependent Sensitivity of Mouse Atria to Adrenergic Drugs. Eur J Pharmacol 30(1975)73–78

Nakashima, M.; Hagino, Y.: Evidence for the Existence of Alpha Adrenergic Receptors in Isolated Rat Atria. Jpn J Pharmacol 22(1972)227–233

Nakashima, M.; Maeda, K.; Sekiya, A.; Hagino, Y.: Effect of Hypothyroid Status on Myocardial Responses to Sympathomimetic Drugs. Jpn J Pharmacol 21(1971)819–825

Nakashima, M.; Tsuru, H.; Shigei, T.: Stimulant Action of Methoxamine in the Isolated Atria of Normal and 6-Propyl-2-Thiouracil-Fed Rats. Jpn J Pharmacol 23(1973)307–312

Nayler, W.G.; Wright, J.E.: Effect of Epinephrine on the Mechanical and Phosphorylase Activity of Normo- and Hypothermic Hearts. Circ Res 13(1963)199–206

Nickerson, M.; Chan, G.C.: Blockade of Responses of Isolated Myocardium to Epinephrine. J Pharmacol Exp Ther 133(1961)186–191

Nickerson, M.; Kunos, G.: Discussion of Evidence Regarding Induced Changes in Adrenoceptors. Fed Proc 36(1977)2580–2583

Nickerson, M.; Nomaguchi, G.M.: Blockade of the Epinephrine-Induced Cardioacceleration in the Frog. Am J Physiol 163(1950)484–504

Oppermann, J.A.; Ryan, C.F.; Haavik, C.O.: The Role of Metabolism in Temperature-Dependent Supersensitivity of Guinea-Pig Atria to Sympathomimetic Amines. Eur J Pharmacol 18(1972)266–270

Osnes, J.B.: Positive Inotropic Effect without Cyclic AMP Elevation After α-Adrenergic Stimulation of Perfused Hearts from Hypothyroid Rats. Acta Pharmacol Toxic 39(1976)232–240

Osnes, J.B.; Øye, I.: Relationship between Cyclic AMP Metabolism and Inotropic Response of Perfused Rat Hearts to Phenylephrine and Other Adrenergic Amines. In: Advances in Cyclic Nucleotide Research. Vol. V, pp. 415–433, ed. by G.I. Drummond, P. Greengard, G.A. Robison. Raven, New York, 1975

Page, E.D.; Neufeld, A.H.: Characterization of α- and β-Adrenergic Receptors in Membranes Prepared from the Rabbit Iris before and after Development of Supersensitivity. Biochem Pharmacol 27(1978)953–958

Pike, L.J.; Lefkowitz, R.J.: Agonist-Specific Alterations in Receptor Binding Affinity Associated with Solubilization of Turkey Erythrocyte Membrane Beta Adrenergic Receptors. Mol Pharmacol 14(1978)370–375

Potter, L.T.: Uptake of Propranolol by Isolated Guinea-Pig Atria. J Pharmacol Exp Ther 155(1967)91–100

Reinhardt, D.; Butzheinen, R.; Brodde, O.E.; Schümann, H.J.: The Role of Cyclic AMP in Temperature-Dependent Changes in Contractile Force and Sensitivity to Isoprenaline and Papaverine in Guinea Pig Atria. Eur J Pharmacol 48(1978)107–116

Reinhardt, D.; Wagner, J.; Schümann, H.J.: Influence of Temperature on the Sensitivity of the β-Receptors and the Contractility of Guinea-Pig Atrium. Naunyn Schmiedebergs Arch Pharmacol 275(1972)95–104

Roberts, J.M.; Insel, P.A.; Goldfien, R.D.; Goldfien, A.: α-Adrenoceptors but Not β-Adrenoceptors Increase in Rabbit Uterus with Oestrogen. Nature 270(1977)624–625

Rosen, G.M.; Ehrenpreis, S.: Physical and Pharmacological Properties of a Series of Ultra-Long Acting Local Anesthetics and Neuromuscular Blocking Agents. Trans NY Acad Sci II 34(1972)255–285

Sadavongvivad, C.; Srayavivad, J.; Prachayasittikul, V.; Mo-Suwun, L.: Modification of Relative Potencies of Beta-Adrenoceptor Agonists by Negative Chronotropic Agents in Rat Atrium. Gen Pharmacol 8(1977)263–267

Schümann, H.J.; Endoh, M.; Wagner, J.: Positive Inotropic Effects of Phenylephrine in the Isolated Rabbit Papillary Muscle Mediated by Both Alpha- and Beta-Adrenoceptors. Naunyn Schmiedebergs Arch Pharmacol 284(1974)133–148

Sharma, V.K.; Banerjee, S.P.: α-Adrenergic Receptors in Rat Heart. Effects of Thyroidectomy. J Biol Chem 253(1978)5277–5279

Sheppard, H.; Burghardt, C.R.: Retained Inhibition of the Beta Receptor by Propranolol after Preincubation and Washout. Res Commun Chem Pathol Pharmacol 21(1978)223–235

Siltovuori, A.; Tirri, R.; Harri, M.N.E.: Alpha-Receptor Subsensitivity of Isolated Atria from Rats Following Physical Training or Repeated ACTH-Injections. Acta Physiol Scand 99(1977)457–461

Singh, G.S.; Prabm, S.; Singh, A.G.: Adrenergic Receptors of the Heart of the Frog. J Mol Cell Cardiol 10 suppl 1(1978)108

Symes, W.L.: A Student's Apparatus for the Perfusion of the Suspended Frog's Heart. J Physiol 52(1918)XLVI–XLVII

Szentivanyi, A.: The Beta Adrenergic Theory of the Atopic Abnormality in Bronchial Asthma. J Allergy 42(1968)203–232

Szentivanyi, M.; Kunos, G.; Juasz-Nagy, A.: Modulator Theory of Adrenergic Receptor Mechanism: Vessels of the Dog Hind Limb. Am J Physiol 218(1970)869–875

Tirri, R.; Harri, M.N.E.; Laitinen, L.: Lowered Chronotropic Sensitivity of Rat and Frog Hearts to Sympathomimetic Amines Following Cold Acclimation. Acta Physiol Scand 90(1974)260–266

Tirri, R.; Siltovuori, A.; Harri, M.: Alpha-Receptor Subsensitivity of Isolated Atria from Rats Following Repeated Injections of Phenylephrine or Isoprenaline. Experientia 32(1976) 1283–1284

Triggle, D.J.: Receptor Theory. In: Receptors in Pharmacology, pp. 1–65, ed. by J.R. Smythies, R.J. Bradley. Dekker, New York and Basel, 1978

Triggle, D.J.; Triggle, C.R.: Chemical Pharmacology of the Synapse. Academic, London, New York, San Franciso, 1976

U'Prichard, D.C.; Snyder, S.H.: Binding of ³H-Catecholamines to α-Noradrenergic Receptor Sites in Calf Brain. J Biol Chem 252(1977)6450–6463

Vanhoutte, P.M.; Shepherd, J.T.: Effect of Cooling on Beta-Receptor Mechanisms in Isolated Cutaneous Veins of the Dog. Microvasc Res 2(1970a)454–461

Vanhoutte, P.M.; Shepherd, J.T.: Effect of Temperature on Reactivity of Isolated Cutaneous Veins of the Dog. Am J Physiol 218(1970b)187–190

Vatner, D.E.; Lefkowitz, R.J.: [³H]Propranolol Binding Sites in Myocardial Membranes: Nonidentity with Beta Adrenergic Receptors. Mol Pharmacol 10(1974)450–456

Vernikov, Y.P.: Some Data Contradicting the Transformation of Adrenoceptors in the Myocardium. Russ Pharmacol Toxic 38(1975)41–42

Wagner, J.; Brodde, O.E.: On the Presence and Distribution of α-Adrenoceptors in the Heart of Various Mammalian Species. Naunyn Schmiedebergs Arch Pharmacol 302(1978)239–254

Wagner, J.; Reinhardt, D.; Huppertz, W.: The Influence of Temperature Increase, Elevation of Extracellular H⁺-Concentration, and of Triiodothyronine on the Actions of Phenylephrine, Histamine, and β-Sympathomimetic Drugs on Rabbit Aortic Strips. Arch Int Pharmacodyn 218(1975)40–53

Wagner, J.; Reinhardt, D.; Schümann, H.J.: Sensitivity Changes in Adrenergic β-Receptors of Isolated Ileum and Trachea Preparations Induced by Alteration of Temperature. Arch Int. Pharmacodyn 197(1972)290–300

Wagner, J.; Reinhardt, D.; Schümann, H.J.: Influence of the Metabolic State on the Action of Phenylephrine on Rabbit Ileum, Guinea-Pig Vas Deferens and Atrium. Naunyn Schmiedeberg's Arch Pharmacol 276(1973)63–70

Wenzel, D.G.; Su, J.L.: Interactions between Sympathomimetic Amines and Blocking Agents on the Rat Ventricle Strip. Arch Int Pharmacodyn 160(1966)379–389

Williams, L.T.; Lefkowitz, R.J.; Watanabe, A.M.; Hathaway, D.R.; Besch, Jr., H.R.: Thyroid Hormone Regulation of β-Adrenergic Receptor Number. J Biol Chem 252(1977)2787–2789

Wolfe, B.B.; Harden, T.K.; Molinoff, P.B.: In Vitro Study of β-Adrenergic Receptors. Ann Rev Pharmacol Toxic 17(1977)575–604

Wöppel, W.; Trendelenburg, U.: Temperature-Dependent Supersensitivity of Isolated Atria to Catecholamines. Eur J Pharmacol 23(1973)302–305

The Identification of the Metabolic Receptors For Catecholamines

Dennis G. Haylett

I. INTRODUCTION

The classification of the receptors concerned in the effects of sympathomimetic amines on carbohydrate and fat metabolism and on associated ion movements (particularly calcium and potassium) has engaged the interest of many investigators. Because the resulting literature is now so immense, it has been necessary to restrict the topics considered in this article.

The possible role of dopamine receptors in metabolic responses can be quickly dealt with. An important role for this catecholamine has not been established; and although dopamine has been reported to have both a hyperglycemic action (Neuvonen, Vapaatalo, and Westermann, 1971) and to raise plasma free fatty acids (Pilkington et al., 1966), its known activity at both α- and β-adrenoceptors may account for this.

I am grateful to Dr. D.H. Jenkinson and Dr. K. Koller for helpful comments on the manuscript.

A. General Classification of Adrenoceptors

An important objective in this chapter is to assess the attempts that have been made to accommodate the metabolic responses to catecholamines within Ahlquist's α and β categories (Ahlquist, 1948). Ahlquist's classification, although slow to gain general acceptance, has not been seriously challenged; and with minor modifications, it is now accepted as being both useful and theoretically sound. Attempts to depart from Ahlquist's scheme have included the early rival proposal of Lands (1952) and the later suggestion to extend the classification to include δ and γ receptors (for intestinal inhibition and metabolic responses respectively [Furchgott, 1959]). Although both of these challenges were inadequate, is is important to appreciate that new hypotheses should not be accepted without question. Questions should also be asked, of course, about the more recent subclassification of adrenoceptors. There is good evidence that the receptors labeled β by Ahlquist do not form a homogeneous group (see chapter by Levy in this volume). The proposal made by Lands et al. (1967), which has gained a wide measure of a acceptance, was that two subtypes be recognized and that these be called β_1 (for cardiac mechanical effects and lipolysis) and β_2 (for bronchodilatation and vasodilatation). The suggestion was thus to subclassify rather than to reclassify. In this instance the decision has probably worked out well: the differences in agonist and antagonist potencies are not extreme (though clinically important), and a common mechanism is apparently involved (adenylate cyclase activation). It is important, however, that alternative explanations be explored. For example, it has been pointed out that tissue selectivity (which is readily interpreted as evidence for receptor subtypes) may also, under some circumstances, arise from differences in the events that follow receptor activation (Jenkinson, 1973). Although the β_1/β_2 subclassification is now generally accepted, the reader may care to speculate on what Ahlquist might have concluded if instead of isoprenaline he had used a selective B_2 agonist (such as salbutamol).

That there are also subtypes of α-adrenoceptors has more recently been recognized. The main evidence is the selectivity of certain agonists and antagonists for particular receptors found on sympathetic nerve endings. These receptors are believed to respond physiologically to noradrenaline released by the nerves (they are thus adrenoceptors) and act to reduce further transmitter release. They are considered to be α because of (a) their activation by noradrenaline and adrenaline but low sensitivity to isoprenaline (which may indeed exert the opposite effect by activating presynaptic β receptors) and (b) their blockade by phentolamine, a classical α blocker. The difference from previously defined α receptors lies in their rather selective activation by certain other agonists, in particular clonidine and α-methylnoradrenaline, and also in the fact that some blockers act preferentially at the presynaptic receptor (yohimbine), whereas others (e.g., prazosin) show postsynaptic selectivity. These receptors have been labeled α_1 (postsynaptic) and α_2 (presynaptic) by Langer (1974). (For reviews of the α receptor subclassification, see Langer, 1977; Starke, 1977; and Berthelsen and Pettinger, 1977). In contrast to the situation with β receptors, however, little is known about the mechanisms immediately underlying α_1 and α_2 receptor activation; therefore the arguments in favor of subclassification are not so complete.

B. The Metabolic Responses to Catecholamines

The term *metabolic* is so general that it can encompass actions on almost every kind of cell. It is best, certainly in terms of examining the attempts made to classify the receptors concerned in such effects, to restrict attention to the responses where most work has been done and where the position is becoming reasonably clear. Accordingly, consideration will be given to glycogenolysis in liver, skeletal muscle, and heart; gluconeogenesis in the liver; lipolysis in adipose tissue; and ion changes in liver. This last response is included because its relationhip to effects on carbohydrate metabolism has recently been the subject of intense interest.

The detailed mechanisms of these effects will not be described; for these descriptions, reference should be made to the excellent reviews by Himms-Hagen (1972) and Fain (1973, 1977). Some knowledge of the general mechanisms is nevertheless important in considering the responses measured. Thus hepatic glycogenolysis could be assessed by any of the following: (a) adenylate cyclase activation (or cAMP production), (b) phosphorylase activation, (c) glucose release (or hyperglycemia), or (d) glycogen breakdown. The use of cyclase activation and the even more recent development of ligand binding methods deserves particular comment. In these instances a receptor event has been divorced from its normal physiological manifestation. For example, β receptors in heart mediate chronotropic and inotropic effects as well as glycogenolysis, and cyclase activation cannot be specifically associated with any one of these separately. Quite different problems are presented by responses at the other end of the chain of events—hyperglycemia, lacticacidemia, and hyperkalemia. These *in vivo* responses are complicated by the possible involvement of several organs and the operation of homeostatic mechanisms. Thus hyperglycemia will result from hepatic glycogenolysis and gluconeogenesis (including that from lactate produced by muscle glycogenolysis, if it is activated at the same time). It will also be modified by the effects of catecholamines on insulin secretion. Interpretation of *in vivo* responses must therefore be most careful; indeed, some authors (e.g., Hornbrook, 1970; Himms-Hagen, 1972) have been inclined to dismiss all results obtained in whole animals for the purpose of receptor classification.

C. Approaches to Receptor Classification

Before looking in detail at the attempts made to classify metabolic responses, it is worthwhile to recall the principles employed in receptor classification and to note any special problems likely to arise in the application of these principles to such responses.

Classification of receptors has since the early days of receptor pharmacology depended mainly on the relative potencies of agonists and selectivity of antagonists. Ligand binding methods may well assume an equally important role in the near future. Analysis of potency ratios and antagonism is often based on the assumption that the drug concentration at the receptor (in the "biophase") is the same as that in the bathing medium. In many cases this will not apply. Furchgott (1972) has clearly outlined the general problems of classification, stressing among other things the need to take account of inactivation processes that would lower drug concentrations in the biophase. The rate of inactivation could be very different for different drugs. In the case of the metabolic responses to catecholamines it is not then surprising that the liver should have proven particularly troublesome, since it is unequaled in its capacity to metabolise a wide variety of compounds. Two important examples can be mentioned. First, noradrenaline given intraperitoneally to mice may be almost completely metabolised (mainly by catechol-O-methyl transferase) during its initial absorption and passage into the general circulation via the hepatic portal system (Carlsson and Waldeck, 1963). This indicates an extremely efficient removal process, which would be expected to markedly reduce noradrenaline concentrations outside the liver cells. A second example of rapid inactivation by the liver concerns propranolol. This has a very high "first pass" hepatic clearance in human beings and other mammals (Shand, Rangno, and Evans, 1972), which again suggests that the concentration of this antagonist at the liver cell membrane might be substantially below that in the bloodstream (or in the solution bathing an isolated preparation).

Another factor modifying the effective drug concentration is protein binding. This would be important *in vivo* and also in *in vitro* systems employing protein-containing solutions. This is a problem which is generally ignored, though such binding may reduce the free, effective concentration of drugs to a small fraction of the total present. This will be discussed in the later consideration of lipolytic responses, where albumin is commonly employed as an acceptor of free fatty acids released from adipose tissue. There is often little information on the extent of protein binding. The situation is improving for β-adrenoceptor antagonists (Zaagsma, Meems, and Boorsma, 1977) where the fractional binding is seen to vary considerably within the class (propranolol being strongly bound). It is unlikely that noradrenaline and adrenaline are highly bound, but there appears to be remarkably little information on this point. Mirkin, Brown, and Ulstrom

(1966) reported the apparent presence of a specific carrier protein for catecholamines in the blood; and earlier work by Antoniades et al. (1958) suggested binding of adrenaline to albumin.

These considerations taken by themselves would indicate that experimental conditions that enable concentrations in the biophase to approach closely the concentration applied in the bulk phase might produce the least ambiguous results. Thus experiments on isolated cell suspensions and membrane preparations have an intrinsic attraction.

Finally, the task of classification is made easier if agents with high affinity for the receptor and also high selectivity are available. High affinity enables low concentrations to be employed, thus reducing nonspecific effects. Thus isoprenaline has proved to be a most useful drug in classification studies. It has a high selectivity for β as compared with α receptors and is active at very low concentrations.

II. METABOLIC RECEPTOR CLASSIFICATION: LIVER

A. Glycogenolysis

Ahlquist in his original classification (1948) did not examine metabolic responses, but it is nevertheless of interest to consider his early views. Thus, in 1954, he was inclined to the opinion that glycogenolysis resulting from the action of adrenaline on the liver was an α response (Ahlquist, 1954). He was mainly influenced by reports of blockade of the increase in blood glucose in rabbits and cats by the α blockers then available, but he also cited the relative ineffectiveness of isoprenaline as a hyperglycemic agent in rabbits. This conclusion is mainly of historical interest, based as it is on relatively few *in vivo* studies. It serves, however, to establish a starting point and also indicates the tools then available, namely a variety of agonists—including, of course, isoprenaline and α blockers. It had indeed been known for many years that first the ergot alkaloids and later the synthetic α blockers would antagonize adrenaline hyperglycemia. Ahlquist did not consider the possibility of species variation, which, as we shall see, is of particular importance in this field. Nearly all the early work was reviewed by Ellis (1956), who, it may be noted, at this time made no reference at all to α and β receptors.

Two major advances in the late 1950s were important for the development of adrenoceptor classification. These were the introduction of β-adrenoceptor antagonists and the discovery of cyclic 3′,5′-adenosine monophosphate (cAMP) and the elucidation of its role as a "second messenger" in the response of many tissues to a variety of hormones.

Slater and Powell first described the antagonist properties of dichloroisoprenaline (DCI) in 1957. Its importance was immediately recognized, and it was soon employed in receptor studies, one of the early outcomes being the consolidation and wider acceptance of Ahlquist's classification. Many other selective β antagonists followed, propranolol (Black et al., 1964) becoming the β blocker to which others were compared.

Cyclic $3',5'$-adenosine monophosphate was described in 1958 by Sutherland and Rall; a comprehensive review of its actions is provided in the monograph by Robison, Butcher, and Sutherland (1971). The main importance of this discovery for the classification of adrenoceptors relates to the close association of adenylate cyclase with the β receptor, since by reverse "logic" it might be concluded that where adrenoceptors elicit a particular response, accompanied by an elevation of cAMP, β receptors are necessarily involved. Two important questions about the relationship of adenylate cyclase to adrenoceptors still remain only partly answered. First, do all β-mediated responses involve the activation of adenylate cyclase? Venter and his colleagues (e.g., Hu and Venter, 1978) are among the main advocates of a dissociation, particularly in the heart. Although there is obviously some uncertainty, most workers currently attribute all β effects to cyclase activation. The second question concerns the involvement of adenylate cyclase in α responses. It has been reported that α receptors stimulate the enzyme (e.g., Chasin et al., 1973) and that they inhibit it (Turtle and Kipnis, 1967; Hittelman, Wu, and Butcher, 1973). The first of these studies, which concerned the measurement of cyclase activity in specified areas of guinea pig brain, requires careful analysis to rule out indirect effects (for example, the release of neurotransmitters). There is more support at the moment for the idea that α receptors do not have a direct influence on cyclase (though they may modify its action indirectly—for example, by changing $[Ca^{++}]i$).

We can now examine progress in classifying metabolic responses to catecholamines following these developments. By the early 1960s, despite the availability of many experimental observations, the overall picture was relatively complicated. One of the clearest images was perhaps that rat liver glycogenolysis was α mediated. Thus VanRoy and Schulhof (1961) found isoprenaline to be quite inactive in rat liver slices; and in intact rats, subcutaneous isoprenaline, unlike adrenaline or noradrenaline, failed to activate hepatic phosphorylase (Hornbrook and Brody, 1963). The very low potency of isoprenaline is suggestive of an action on α receptors. Hornbrook and Brody, however, declined to draw this conclusion, because only ergotamine could produce complete inhibition of the response, phenoxybenzamine as well as DCI and pronethalol causing partial block. An illuminating study was made by Fleming and Kenny (1963), who found in anesthetised rats that hyperglycemia was apparently β mediated in fasted rats but α mediated in fed ones. This finding was based on the relative potencies of agonists, in particular the ineffectiveness of isoprenaline in fed rats. They suggested that in fed animals, with substantial stores of liver glycogen, α-mediated hepatic glycogenolysis was dominant, whereas in starved animals β-mediated muscle glycogenolysis predominated. Similar experiments have been conducted more recently by Potter and Ellis (1975), who made comparable observations but were able to attribute the very low activity of isoprenaline in fed rats to an effect on insulin release; insulin release from pancreatic islets is stimulated by isoprenaline but inhibited by adrenaline and noradrenaline (Porte, 1967). Thus the action of isoprenaline, raising blood glucose, might be masked by the concomitant effect of increased levels of insulin, a decrease in blood glucose. Strong support for this explanation came from Potter and Ellis's studies with alloxan-diabetic rats, which responded to isoprenaline with hyperglycemia (even when fed). Still more recent work (Potter, Barnett, and Woodson, 1978) indicates a role also for α-mediated release of glucagon in the hyperglycemia produced by adrenaline. These *in vivo* studies highlight the problems encountered in whole animals, illustrating the effects of diet and the involvement of several tissues and endogenous regulators.

Cats and dogs had also been well studied, and in these species it appeared that hepatic glycogenolysis was β mediated. Thus Mayer, Moran, and Fain (1961) showed that in dogs DCI would block adrenaline hyperglycemia, which was also induced readily by isoprenaline but rather weakly by noradrenaline. Murad et al. (1962) found that cAMP formation by particulate fractions of dog liver was stimulated by catecholamines with a potency order isoprenaline > adrenaline > noradrenaline, the stimulation being antagonized by DCI. In intact cats Ellis and Eusebi (1965) were able to show that the β blockers sotalol and isopropylmethoxamine (IMA) could block the increase in blood glucose caused by adrenaline (specificity being demonstrated by the lack of blockade of hepatic K loss, and subsequent hyperkalemia, attributable to α receptors). The α antagonist dibozane failed to antagonize the glucose response but did block hyperkalemia. This study provided further evidence for the independence of hyperglycemia and hyperkalemia, already suggested by Ellis and Beckett (1963). This earlier study, in addition to showing a lack of effect of classical α antagonists against hyperglycemia in the cat, had also clearly indicated a blocking action of dihydroergotamine (DHE). Various derivatives of ergot do, however, exhibit a wide variety of actions both at the level of the receptor and at stages beyond receptor activation. For example, Murad et al. (1962) found that ergotamine would inhibit catecholamine-induced cAMP forma- tion in a dog heart preparation—β receptors, of course, being primarily involved. In perfused rat liver, Northrop (1968) found the glycogenolytic effect of cAMP to be abolished by DHE; and Chan, Ellis, and Mühlbachová (1978), following up earlier results with rabbit liver slices, found DHE to inhibit responses to catecholamines, perhaps by an action on β receptors, while leaving glycogenolysis due to glucagon and cAMP relatively unchanged.

Work with β antagonists continued, and the conference on these agents organized by the New York Academy of Science in 1966 contained several papers that provide a convenient summary of the views then prevalent. The dominant role of adenylate cyclase in β-mediated responses was strongly advocated; Robison, Butcher, and Sutherland (1967) proposed "that in most and perhaps all tissues the beta receptor and adenyl cyclase are the same" (p. 720). They introduced the notion of regulatory and catalytic subunits, which is generally accepted today, though they considered the subunits to be part of a single molecular complex and it is currently widely held that discrete molecules are present. Ellis et al. (1967) dealt specifically with metabolic responses, stressing the need to take account of species differences and to avoid high concentrations of blocking agents. Relying mainly on the actions of antagonists, they concluded that the bulk of the evidence indicated that in cats and dogs hepatic glycogenolysis (as well as muscle glycogenolysis and lipolysis) was β mediated. The difficulties encountered with rat liver were approached in an interesting way. Since it was held that hepatic glycogenolysis was mediated by cAMP, Ellis et al. were inclined to classify the receptor as β. They felt obliged, however, to qualify this conclusion by attributing to the receptor a "different" (low) affinity for N-isopropyl groups, such as in isoprenaline. They were thus more strongly influenced by the underlying mechanism than by the binding properties of the receptor. This was a significant departure from the traditional principles of receptor classification based on recognition features rather than mechanism. On the basis of rather less evidence, Ellis et al. thought that liver glycogen breakdown in human beings and rabbits involved receptors similar to those found in rats.

Three other papers at the 1966 conference—those by Moran (1967); Furchgott (1967); and Burns, Salvador, and Lemberger (1967)—were important in raising the question of β receptor subtypes. Analogues of methoxamine, particularly butoxamine, were shown to be more effective in blocking some β responses, including metabolic effects (hyperglycemia, hyperlacticacidemia, and the elevation of plasma FFA), than cardiac effects. (Butoxamine had in fact been referred to as "a specific antagonist of the metabolic actions of epinephrine" by Burns and Lemberger [1965, p. 298].) Furchgott's evidence for at least three β receptor subtypes, based on affinity constants of different tissues for pronethalol, has been overshadowed by the β_1/β_2 subclassification. The main importance of Furchgott's article, however, was to emphasize the importance of quantitative measurement in pharmacological classification. Many of the principles to be dealt with more fully in his 1972 publication were introduced here. It is clear, however, that most other workers then were not aware of the advantages to be gained by constructing complete dose-response curves and by assessing drug antagonism through the changes produced in these curves.

Progress in classifying hepatic adrenoceptors continued, and the views of Hornbrook (1970) are of interest. Like Ellis and coworkers, he was apparently strongly influenced by the association of cAMP with the β receptor and dismissed the evidence suggesting α-mediated hepatic glycogenolysis in the rat. He felt that species differences were more likely to be quantitative than qualitative and concluded that there was little justification in classifying the rat liver receptor as α.

Up to this time most workers had assumed that a single receptor type was involved in particular metabolic effects, if not in all the metabolic effects, of catecholamines—e.g., the receptor for metabolic effects (Furchgott [1959]) or "a specific antagonist of the metabolic actions" (Burns and Lemberger, 1965, p. 298). This was probably, at least partly, because in most instances α and β receptors exert opposite effects in any one tissue, the only exception known at that time being relaxation of certain intestinal smooth muscle that may be both α and β mediated (though by different mechanisms). Substantial evidence for the involvement of both α and β receptors in hepatic glycogenolysis was provided by Haylett and Jenkinson (1968, 1972b). These results will be considered in some detail because the author is well acquainted with them and only too aware of their inadequacies. Guinea pig liver slices were chosen for the study rather than the more widely used rat liver preparations because the former but not the latter exhibited certain responses to catecholamines, related to an effect on cell membrane potassium permeability, which were also of interest (Haylett and Jenkinson, 1972a). Slices were employed because they were particularly suited to the experiments envisaged to investigate ion movements, and also because they would not be subjected to anoxia, secondary to vasoconstriction, which can be troublesome in the perfused liver when α agonists are tested. It has to be kept in mind, however, that liver slices suffer much physical damage during preparation; this leads to alterations in the tissue's biochemical composition, and these are only partially restored during incubation. Glucose release rather than phosphorylase activity was measured as an indicator of glycogenolysis; this indicator must be considered less satisfactory, since glucose release will depend on glycogen content and perhaps also reflect (though probably to only a small extent) effects on gluconeogenesis. A further point deserving comment in this study concerns the use of amidephrine as an α agonist. Furchgott (1967, 1972) suggested the use of phenylephrine as a selective α agonist, and today it is widely accepted as the preferred agonist; it does, however, retain some β-agonist activity at high concentrations. Amidephrine, a close analogue of adrenaline, is more selective for α receptors than phenylephrine, exhibiting only a very weak partial agonist activity at β receptors (Buchthal and

Jenkinson, 1970). It is interesting that earlier studies had not routinely sought to employ the most specific agents available, though it may be noted that two imidazolines, naphazoline and tetrahydrozoline, which are now recognized as selective α stimulants, were shown at an early stage to be hyperglycemic in mice (Hutcheon et al., 1955).

Haylett and Jenkinson found that both isoprenaline and amidephrine could increase glucose release from guinea pig liver slices to a comparable extent (though the parallelism of the log dose-response curves and equivalence of maximum responses was not rigorously tested). This was taken as suggestive of α and β receptor involvement, a conclusion supported by the antagonism of the amidephrine response by phentolamine and the isoprenaline response by propranolol, but not vice versa. Typical results are shown in Figure 1, which is included as an example of standard classification methods. Two receptors are clearly indicated; but how well do they

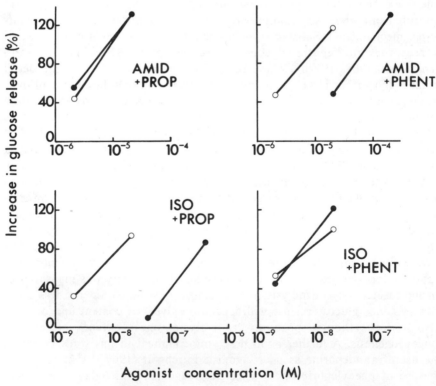

Agonist concentration (M)

Figure 1. Selective antagonism by phentolamine (PHENT, 10^{-5}M) and (±)-propranolol (PROP, 10^{-6}M) of glycogenolysis in guinea pig liver slices mediated by the β agonist (−)-isoprenaline (ISO, lower two graphs) and the α agonist (±)-amidephrine (AMID, upper two graphs). Open circles indicate responses to agonists alone; closed circles indicate those in the presence of the antagonist indicated. (Redrawn from Haylett and Jenkinson, 1972b.)

equate with Ahlquist's α and β types? First, the β receptor: Propranolol, 1 μM, produced a parallel shift of the log dose-response curve to the right with a dose ratio of approximately 40. Since other concentrations of propranolol were not tried, it is not possible to confirm simple competitive antagonism. However, if this is assumed, the equilibrium dissociation constant, K_D, may be estimated to be 25 nM. In other tissues the K_D for propranolol at β receptors varies between 1 nM in rabbit aorta to 1,000 nM in bovine iris sphincter, but for many tissues a value of 2 nM could be considered characteristic of β receptor binding (see Furchgott [1972] for a compilation of values). The value obtained by Haylett and Jenkinson is accordingly on the high side but still within the range compatible with β receptor involvement. Of course, β receptors are also indicated by the activity of low concentrations of isoprenaline (2 nM proving effective). Indeed, this sensitivity might well be an underestimate if drug inactivation is an important factor. Haylett and Jenkinson (1972b) were more cautious in classifying the other receptor involved, preferring, in view of its apparent resistance to blockade by phentolamine, to call it α-like. In guinea pig liver slices 10 μM phentolamine gave a dose ratio against amidephrine of only 6, which—again assuming simple competitive interaction—corresponds to a K_D of 2 μM. In smooth muscle much lower K_D values—5–300 nM—have been reported (Furchgott, 1972). Further work in this laboratory has shown that the apparent insensitivity of the guinea pig liver α receptor extends to other selective α antagonists: thymoxamine, WB 4101, and DHE (Burgess, Koller, Haylett, and Jenkinson, unpublished observations). A possible explanation is that the concentration of the blockers at the receptors is less than that added, as discussed earlier. Studies of antagonist binding to hepatic cell membranes promise to provide decisive information in this respect (see below). The findings with agonists—including phenylephrine, methoxamine, and amidephrine, all of which cause glucose release—are consistent with conventional α receptors (see also subclassification section).

Haylett and Jenkinson thus concluded that two receptor types were involved in the stimulation of glycogenolysis, β receptors giving a response that was likely to involve cAMP and an α response occurring by some other mechanism, perhaps related to ion fluxes (K^+ and Na^+).

Quite independently, Sherline, Lynch, and Glinsmann (1972) also came to the conclusion that in perfused rat liver both α and β mechanisms were involved in glycogen breakdown. In addition to the established cAMP cascade, they identified a cAMP-independent α response, which at that time they believed might be due to anoxia following vasoconstriction. Their result gave greater prominence to the α mechanism, isoprenaline being effective only at high concentrations, when at least a part of its glycogenolytic effect was probably due to α receptor activation (being blocked by phentolamine).

In further experiments with rabbit liver slices at this time, Mühlbachová, Chan, and Ellis (1972) could demonstrate only β-mediated glycogenolysis, since no evidence was obtained for an addition α component. It is important to note, however, that the slices were not incubated in a balanced physiological medium; in particular, the solution lacked calcium. In the light of present-day knowledge, which indicates an important role for Ca in α-mediated glycogenolysis (see below), it can be seen that these circumstances might have selectively impaired any contribution by α receptors.

The reports suggesting both α and β receptor involvement have been amply supported by later work. Exton and his coworkers (Exton and Harper, 1975; Hutson et al., 1976; Cherrington et al., 1976; Assimacopoulos-Jeannet, Blackmore, and Exton, 1977) have provided further evidence for an α-mediated, cAMP-independent glycogenolytic response to catecholamines in rats; and Osborn has provided the same evidence in guinea pigs (1975, 1978). Exton and Harper showed that in perfused rat liver isoprenaline was much more effective in raising cAMP levels than phenylephrine, whereas phenylephrine was at least as effective in causing glucose release. Furthermore, phentolamine, but not propranolol, would inhibit the glucose release caused by adrenaline without reducing cAMP efflux.

Much of the more recent work of Exton and his colleagues has used isolated hepatocytes in suspension. These cells can be prepared in large quantities, relatively free of other cell types, and will remain in a satisfactory condition for some hours. There should be no problem in providing the cells with an adequate oxygen supply, and drug access should be good. A possible drawback with isolated liver cells is that some modification of receptor binding properties may be induced by the isolation procedure, which routinely involves the application of proteolytic enzymes (collagenase) and a period of exposure to calcium-free solution. However, any such effect appears to be relatively unimportant, since isolated cells respond well to a variety of hormones in the expected manner.

The current drive is to elucidate the mechanism underlying α-mediated glycogenolysis. Since α receptors will cause changes in calcium disposition in liver cells (Haylett, 1976; Assimacopoulos-Jeannet et al., 1977; Keppens, Vandenheede, and De Wulf, 1977), and since there is evidence that calcium can activate phosphorylase b kinase in rat liver (e.g., Shimazu and Amakawa, 1975), a central role for calcium appears likely. Support for this hypothesis comes from the action of the Ca-ionophore A 23187, which can also stimulate phosphorylase in isolated rat liver cells (Assimacopoulos-Jeannet et al., 1977).

Two other control points in hepatic glycogen metabolism deserve consideration. First, the results of Shimazu and Amakawa (1975) suggest that phosphorylase phosphatase (the enzyme deactivating phosphorylase) may be an important regulatory step. In their experiments they obtained clear evidence that stimulation of sympathetic nerves to rabbit liver caused enhanced glycogenolysis directly attributable to inhibition of this enzyme and independent of cyclase activation. They suggested that an unknown neurotransmitter might be responsible for the phosphatase inhibition, but the evidence was not sufficiently strong to exclude the possibility that this was a consequence of noradrenaline acting on α receptors (as suggested by Osborn [1978]). The other control point in overall glycogen metabolism is at the level of glycogen synthetase. Although the activity of this enzyme is very sensitive to the increase in cAMP caused by glucagon, the importance of β-mediated rises in cAMP in inhibiting it in rat liver is in doubt. Hutson et al. (1977) obtained results suggesting that synthetase inhibition in rats is mainly an α-mediated event of uncertain mechanism. Currently, then, the relative roles of α and β receptors in the control of glycogen synthetase and phosphorylase phosphatase are not fully evaluated.

To summarize, in rat and guinea pig there is good evidence that hepatic glycogen breakdown in response to catecholamines can be mediated through two distinct receptors using different mechanisms. It seems likely that the adenylate cyclase route will be found in all species, undoubtedly linked to β receptors. There seem to be no grounds for supposing that the β receptor will prove appreciably different from that found in other tissues. (The question of subtypes will be considered shortly.) The alternative route for phophorylase activation may well operate to different extents in different species. In rat liver it appears to dominate—as, indeed, suggested by the early results in favour of α receptor mediation (though diet and hormonal influences may be pronounced—e.g., Preiksaitis and Kunos, 1979). In guinea pig liver slices glycogenolysis seems to be activated to a similar extent by either route. Thus glucose release due to noradrenaline can be inhibited by both phentolamine and propranolol, neither blocker proving as effective against noradrenaline as against selective α or β agonists (Haylett and Jenkinson, 1972b). Both α and β routes appear to operate in rabbit liver (Haylett, 1976). Further work is needed to assess the importance of the α mechanism in cats and dogs, where most evidence favors β predominance. (Kuo, Kamaka, and Lum [1978] have, however, suggested on the basis of *in vivo* experiments with selective agonists and antagonists that the cat has both α- and β-adrenoceptors subserving hepatic glycogenolysis.)

B. Gluconeogenesis

Gluconeogenesis has been less extensively studied than glycogenolysis, and only now is the hormonal control of the enzymes involved becoming at all clear. Studies of catecholamine effects on this process have not, therefore, used the activation of particular enzymes; rather, glucose production from substrates such as lactate has been measured in intact cells.

Early studies of catecholamine action on gluconeogenesis (e.g., Exton and Park, 1966) were not concerned with the receptor types involved; therefore in their reviews Ellis (1967) and Himms-Hagen (1972) could not attempt a classification. However, the observations of increased gluconeogenesis with glucagon and exogenous cAMP (Exton and Park, 1966; Friedmann, 1972) would have suggested that β-mediated increases in cAMP might be important.

Tolbert, Butcher, and Fain (1973) were among the first to attempt a classification of the adrenoceptors concerned in isolated rat liver cells. They obtained evidence that was generally in favor of an α mechanism, independent of cAMP. Thus adrenaline and noradrenaline, as well as phenylephrine, would stimulate glucose formation from lactate, whereas the specific β agonists, isoprenaline and salbutamol, were ineffective. The authors declined, however, to describe the receptors as α because of the poor antagonism with phentolamine and phenoxybenzamine. (The response was, on the other hand, 'remarkably' sensitive to DHE, blockade being evident at 50 nM.) These findings were confirmed by Kneer et al. (1974) also in isolated rat hepatocytes. These workers considered the evidence for α receptors satisfactory, since blockade by phenoxybenzamine (1–5 μM) but not propranolol (10 μM) and the ineffectiveness of isoprenaline were regarded as diagnostic. Exton and Harper (1975) provided further evidence for a cAMP-independent α mechanism but also found a significant β component to gluconeogenesis in isolated rat hepatocytes; there was a prominent response to isoprenaline. The low activity of phentolamine against the α-mediated gluconeogenesis recorded by both Tolbert et al. (1973) and Exton and Harper (1975) is reminiscent of the findings of Haylett and Jenkinson (1972b) for glucose release from guinea pig liver slices and is perhaps similarly attributable to drug metabolism or uptake.

The current view is thus that two mechanisms are probably concerned in the stimulation of hepatic gluconeogenesis by catecholamines. Activation of β receptors (and glucagon receptors) would lead to an increase in cAMP, which perhaps by phosphorylation and thereby inhibition of pyruvate kinase would lead to glucose formation (Felíu, Hue, and Hers, 1976; Kemp and Clark, 1978). Further work is required to explain why the response to isoprenaline appears to be so variable. A cAMP-independent pathway is also indicated (further support coming from Cherrington et al., 1977), results with agonists and antagonists indicating that α receptors are involved. The mechanism in this case is very uncertain.

All the recent work has employed rat liver, and there is no indication whether both α and β systems operate in other species. It is quite conceivable that the relative importance of the two mechanisms will vary between species, as is the case for hepatic glycogenolysis.

C. Hyperkalemia

The physiological significance of the changes in plasma potassium brought about by catecholamines is not clear. However, the possible association of these changes with effects on carbohydrate metabolism has been the subject of considerable study, and the receptors involved are reasonably well established.

D'Silva (1934) provided an early demonstration of the hyperkalemic effect of adrenaline in cats, and his later studies showed that the increase in plama potassium was due to release from the liver. In most species the increase is transient and followed by a more sustained hypokalemia. The rat is an exception; in this animal the initial response of the liver is not to release potassium, but rather to take it up (e.g., Northrop, 1968).

In his early experiments. D'Silva had shown that ergotoxine blocked the hyperkalemic response to adrenaline, but it was Ellis and Beckett (1963) who began the systematic classification of the receptors involved. As already indicated, it was this work that established that potassium efflux and glycogenolysis could be independent; and the further studies of Ellis and Eusebi (1965) firmly categorized hepatic potassium release in the cat as an α response. Their results with α and β antagonists were further supported by the finding that methoxamine, a selective α agonist, would also elevate plasma potassium (Ellis et al., 1967).

Similar observations were made by Todd and Vick (1971) for the dog, in which they found phenylephrine but not isoprenaline to cause hyperkalemia. There was, however, some evidence to suggest a β component to the potassium loss. This was not entirely surprising, since Ellis and Beckett (1963) had previously shown in the cat that glucagon (presumably acting via cAMP) could also elevate plasma potassium. In the rat also, both glucagon and cAMP cause a loss of potassium from the liver (after the initial uptake) (Friedmann, 1972). In guinea pig liver slices (Haylett and Jenkinson, 1972b) and in rabbit liver slices (Haylett, 1976) potassium loss in response to adrenoceptor agonists is predominantly α mediated. Isoprenaline is normally much less effective than either noradrenaline or amidephrine in these preparations. Other studies in this laboratory (Haylett and Jenkinson, 1973; and unpublished observations with K. Koller) have shown, however, that under some circumstances both isoprenaline and cAMP become effective in causing potassium loss. These experiments revealed an interesting interaction between α and β mechanisms, which has been further examined by Jenkinson and Koller (1977).

With regard to the mechanism of the α-mediated potassium release, Haylett and Jenkinson (1972a) obtained evidence to suggest that an increase in the potassium permeability of the cell membrane was important. This leads also to hyperpolarization of the liver cells, a response that can be usefully employed for classification purposes. Hyperpolarization of guinea pig liver cells can be induced by a variety of selective α agonists, including amidephrine, phenylephrine, methoxamine, and several imidazolines (Haylett and Jenkinson, 1972b; Jenkinson and Koller, 1977). It seems likely that the α-mediated increase in potassium permeability, like α-mediated glycogenolysis, is due to changes in the internal Ca ion concentration (Haylett, 1976). The mechanism of K loss from rat liver cells may well be different, since work in this laboratory has failed to demonstrate an early effect of noradrenaline on radioactive potassium loss from rat liver slices; nor is there any immediate effect on membrane potential comparable to that observed with guinea pig liver slices. A delayed hyperpolarization of cells in perfused rat liver has, however, been observed with glucagon, cAMP, and isoprenaline (Friedmann, Somlyo, and Somlyo, 1971).

The hypokalemic phase of catecholamine action has been shown to be largely due to the stimulation of potassium uptake by muscle following β receptor activation (Todd and Vick, 1971; Castro-Tavares, 1976). The evidence is convincing and requires no comment.

D. Receptor Binding Studies

As already discussed, Ahlquist's classification was based primarily on agonist *potency ratios* with supporting evidence from the effects of antagonists. Measurement of agonist *affinities*, like antagonist affinities, could also serve as a basis for classification; but until recently it has been possible to determine the affinity constants only for partial agonists (or for full agonists if an irreversible antagonist for the receptor concerned is available—to effectively remove "spare receptors"). Binding studies should now allow both agonist and antagonist affinities for receptors to be measured directly. (It is important to remember that the relative affinities of agonists may well be different to their relative potencies because of different efficacies.) The equilibrium dissociation constant and number of receptors commonly determined for the radioligand itself by Scatchard analysis, and the affinity of other compounds for the receptor is then assessed by their ability to inhibit binding of the radiolabel.

The earliest binding studies to investigate adrenoceptors employed tritiated catecholamines; but—as has been discussed in detail by Cuatrecasas et al. (1974, 1975); Levitzki (1976) and Wolfe, Harden, and Molinoff (1977)—the outcome with labeled adrenaline and noradrenaline was generally unsatisfactory for a number of reasons, an important one being the presence in the tissues of other binding sites more numerous than the adrenoceptors. The main advance in adrenoceptor binding studies followed the switch to radiolabeled antagonists, which have several advantages over catecholamines (Wolfe et al., 1977). [³H]-propranolol, [³H]-dihydro-alprenolol (DHA), and [¹²⁵I]-iodohydroxybenzylpindolol (IHYP) have been the ligands most commonly employed to investigate β receptors, and [³H] dihydroergocryptine (DHEC) has proved a suitable high-affinity ligand for α-adrenoceptors (though with a comparably high affinity for other receptors, e.g., those for dopamine [Caron et al., 1978].

Table 1 collects data for drug binding to rat liver plasma membranes, and, for comparison, similar results for some other tissues. Rat heart may be considered to illustrate binding to β_1 receptors, rat lung to β_2 receptors (predominantly), and dog aorta and rat uterus to α_1 receptors. The main conclusion to be drawn from these results (and others, not presented, indicating stereospecific binding) is that rat liver plasma membranes possess at least two kinds of binding site with properties expected of α and β receptors. The dissociation constants have unfortunately been measured at a variety of temperatures and cannot therefore be expected to agree exactly. This could partly account for the substantially different K_D values of both nora-drenaline and adrenaline reported for the α receptors in rat liver in the two studies cited. It is not, however, obvious why temperature should modify receptor density, as suggested by the two values given by Guellaen et al. (1978) for rat liver α receptors. Binding conditions were otherwise very similar (if not physiological) in the different studies.

It is evident from the results in Table 1 that the binding of nora-drenaline and adrenaline does not on its own provide a basis for distinguishing α from β receptors; the same is true of phenylephrine. Isoprenaline, phentolamine, and propranolol, on the other hand, are highly discriminative (as are some other α and β antagonists). The value of more selective α agonists (e.g., clonidine) is difficult to assess without further information on their affinity for β receptors. (Although they have very little agonist activity at β receptors, their antagonistic action is poorly described.)

Binding studies thus confirm the presence of α and β adrenoceptors in rat liver and so are consistent with the earlier conclusion that both receptors influence hepatic carbohydrate metabolism. There are no grounds for supposing that the α receptors differ from those found elsewhere in the body (cf. results for dog aorta, Table 1). Indeed, binding studies do not show the discrepant results with phentolamine that were observed in experiments using perfused or sliced liver. Thus phentolamine displaced DHEC at low concentrations, lending support to the earlier contention that concentrations of this antagonist at the receptor are access limited in intact hepatic tissue. The β receptors revealed in these studies with rat liver also appear to be

Table 1. Equilibrium dissociation constants for drugs binding to adrenoceptors, as determined by binding studies

Tissue	References*	Temperature (°C.)	Radioligand	Binding Site Density (pmole/mg protein)	K_D values by competition (nM)									
					ADR	NOR	ISO	PE	SAL	CLON	αMN	PROP	PHENT	YOH
Rat liver	(1)	37	IHYP**	0.039	120	270	24					2.7		
Rat liver	(2)	30	DHA	0.06	150	140	12					12		
Rat adipocytes	(3)	37	DHA	0.24	3,800	1,800	220					17		
Rat heart	(4)	23	DHA	—	150	330	7	6,500	1,800	$>10^5$		0.46	40,000	
Rat lung	(4)	23	DHA	—	110	1,050	70	3,300	320	$>10^5$		0.22	33,000	
Rat liver	(2)	30	DHEC	1.4	1,240		74,000		$>10^5$	600				
Rat liver	(5)	37	DHEC	0.9	2,400	2,400	184,000	4,100				14,000	9.5	
Rat uterus	(6)	25	DHEC	1.7	120	120	59,000	2,300			70,000	6,300*	2.3	78
Dog aorta	(7)	25	DHEC	0.15	230	650	43,000	3,500		160		27,000*	15	220
Rat brain	(8)	25	DHEC	0.14	1,000	2,600	330,000	5,300		260		23,000*	53	200
Rat brain	(8)	25	CLON	—	5.9	17	5,600	270		5.7	7.7	5,900*	22	150

*References: (1) Wolfe et al. (1976); (2) Guellaen et al. (1978); (3) Williams et al. (1978); (4) U'Prichard et al. (1978); (5) Clarke et al. (1978), K_D values estimated from given EC_{50} figures; (6) Williams et al. (1976b); (7) Tsai and Lefkowitz (1978); (8) U'Prichard et al. (1977).

**Abbreviations. IHYP, iodohydroxybenzylpindolol; DHA, dihydroalprenolol; DHEC, dihydroergocryptine; ADR, (−) adrenaline; NOR, (−) noradrenaline; ISO, (−) isoprenaline; PE, (−) phenylephrine; SAL, (±) salbutamol; CLON, clonidine; αMN, α-methylnoradrenaline; PROP, (−) propranolol; PHENT, phentolamine; YOH, yohimbine. (* indicates (±) isomer).

conventional. For example, the K_D for propranolol, 2.7–12 nM, compares well with the values obtained in dose-ratio studies in other tissues (see earlier discussion, where a figure of 2 nM was considered characteristic).

In rat liver, where α receptors appear to be most important in the regulation of carbohydrate metabolism, it is interesting to see that they considerably outnumber the β receptors (by a factor of 20 [Table 1]). Results for other species in which β receptors are more important are eagerly awaited.

E. Subclassification of Hepatic Adrenoceptors

As outlined in the introduction, there are reasonable grounds for supposing that Ahlquist's α and β categories are heterogeneous. Several studies have provided data that allow us to assess the similarity of adrenoceptors responsible for metabolic responses to receptors subserving other responses to catecholamines. Table 2 lists some of the agents that either have proved or promise to prove useful for subclassification purposes (see also chapter by Levy in this volume). So far, β subtypes have received more attention than α subtypes; and their analysis has been helped by the realization that tissues may contain both β_1 and β_2 receptors. The relative proportions of the two may vary from animal to animal (Furchgott et al., 1975), between species (Rugg, Barnett, and Nahorski, 1978), and perhaps even from one part of an organ to another (heart: Carlsson et al., 1977).

1. Hepatic β receptors The earliest information bearing on the subclassification of hepatic β receptors came from studies with methoxamine analogues. Thus Burns et al. (1964) showed that isopropylmethoxamine would block the rise in plasma glucose and free fatty acid and lactate produced by catecholamines in dogs while having relatively little effect on cardiac responses. Supporting evidence came from the work of Robison, Butcher, and Sutherland (1967), who found isopropylmethoxamine to be more effective in antagonizing the stimulation of cAMP formation by isoprenaline in dog liver than in dog heart. This early work thus served to show a difference between heaptic and cardiac β receptors. Following the introduction of the β_1/β_2 scheme, Arnold et al. (1968) attempted a subclassification of the receptors mediating hyperglycemia in dogs. The potency order for selected agonists was adrenaline > isoetharine > noradrenaline (noradrenaline having 1/50 of the potency of adrenaline). This was typical of β_2 receptors, according to the original classification. All subsequent work has been in accord with this conclusion. Kelly and Shanks (1975) found the β_2 agonist, salbutamol, to be more effective in raising blood glucose than FFA in dogs. Lefkowitz (1975), measuring adenylate cyclase activation, showed noradrenaline to be much less active than adrenaline in dog liver as compared with heart; furthermore, butoxamine

Table 2. Drugs showing useful selectivity for adrenoceptor subtypes

	α_1	α_2	β_1	β_2
Agonists	Phenylephrine (8)*	Clonidine (8)	Tazolol (ITP) (3)	Salbutamol (4)
	Methoxamine (8)	α-methylnoradrenaline (8)	Noradrenaline (7)	Isoetharine (7)
	Amidephrine (1)	Tramazoline (8)		OPC 2009 (9)
Antagonists	Phenoxybenzamine (8)	Yohimbine (8)	Practolol (2)	Butoxamine (2)
	Prazosin (5)		Metoprolol (2)	H35/25 (2)
	WB 4101 (1)		Atenolol (2)	IPS 339 (6)
			Acebutolol (2)	

*References:
(1) Butler and Jenkinson (1978); (2) Clark (1976); (3) Clark and Poyser (1977); (4) Cullum et al. (1969); (5) Doxey, Smith, and Walker (1977); (6) Imbs et al. (1977); (7) Lands et al. (1967); (8) Starke (1977); (9) Yabuuchi (1977).

was more effective than practolol in blocking cyclase stimulation in the liver (the reverse being true for heart). The studies of Kuo, Kamaka, and Lum (1977) and Loakpradit and Lockwood (1977) showed that H35/25 but not practolol would antagonize isoprenaline hyperglycemia in cats. There have been fewer conclusive studies with rat liver; but we may note the results of Lacombe et al. (1976), who found that noradrenaline in normal rat liver was significantly less active than adrenaline in stimulating adenylate cyclase and in addition that the β_2 selective agonist, protokylol, was very active in this respect. In a hepatoma cell line, on the other hand, the agonist potency ratios were quite different—in fact suggestive of β_1 receptors. The authors proposed that receptor transformation occurred, but the alternative suggestion of a change in the proportion of β_1 to β_2 receptors seems more compatible with observations described above for other tissues.

Ligand binding studies have so far been of little use in the subclassification of hepatic β receptors. Noradrenaline has been found to displace radioligands from the β receptor with an affinity not too different from that of adrenaline. Table 1 indicates that the factor is 1–2, which may be comared with approximately 10 in favor of adrenaline in rat lung. At face value this might suggest that rat liver possessed mainly β_1 receptors—though, as mentioned earlier, relative affinities need not be the same as relative potencies; information is needed on the efficacies of noradrenaline and adrenaline. Binding studies with selective β-adrenoceptor antagonists might well be more discriminating. At present, then, the evidence is on the whole in favor of β_2 receptors in liver. It is not possible, however, to exclude a minor contribution by β_1 receptors.

2. Hepatic α receptors Studies from this laboratory (Haylett and Jenkinson, 1972b) have shown that amidephrine, phenylephrine, and methoxamine will all hyperpolarize guinea pig liver cells and cause glucose release. More recently we have found (a) clonidine to have only a weak hyperpolarizing action and (b) prazosin to be an effective antagonist of α-mediated hyperpolarization of guinea pig liver cells (but as for phentolamine the dose ratio is less than expected). These results are suggestive of α_1 receptors (see Table 2), though it must be remembered that the selectivity of these agents is not absolute. As described earlier, phenylephrine is also a very effective α agonist in rat liver (e.g., Exton and Harper, 1975). On the other hand, some support for α_2 receptors can be derived from the results of Iwata (1969), who showed clonidine to be hyperglycemic in rats; this was attributed to a direct effect on adrenoceptors.

Binding studies are difficult to interpret, mainly because of a lack of suitable data (particularly for binding to α_2 receptors). Displacement of [³H]-clonidine from receptors appears to be the best indicator currently available and has been examined in rat brain membranes (U'Prichard,

Greenberg, and Snyder, 1977). Binding studies show clonidine to have an affinity for α receptors in rat liver (160–600 nM), which is comparable to those of adrenaline and noradrenaline (Table 1). Although this might be considered indicative of α_2 receptors, clonidine also has a similar affinity for α receptors in rat uterus, which are more likely to be α_1. Furthermore, its affinity for binding sites in the brain (presumably α_2) is much higher (K_D = 5.8 nM). On balance, results with clonidine, although not compelling, favour the classification of α receptors in rat liver as α_1. Results with α-methylnoradrenaline lend support to this conclusion. This agent has a much lower affinity for the α receptors in rat liver than for the clonidine binding sites in rat brain. Results with yohimbine and phenylephrine are less satisfactory: they do not show the expected selectivity of binding. Yohimbine has comparable K_D values, not only for the α receptors in rat liver and uterus and dog aorta, but also for clonidine binding sites in rat brain. This casts doubt either on the selectivity of yohimbine or on the α_1/α_2 subdivision itself. Phenylephrine apparently has a greater affinity for clonidine binding sites in rat brain than for the α receptors in rat liver and uterus and dog aorta. Unless a much lower efficacy of phenylephrine at α_2 receptors can be demonstrated, these results are not consistent with the subclassification. Much more work with agents selective for α_1 and α_2 receptors is required, both to put the subclassification itself on a firmer footing and to clarify the nature of the hepatic adrenoceptors.

III. SKELETAL MUSCLE

The main metabolic effects of catecholamines on skeletal muscle are the breakdown of glycogen and of triglycerides. Lipolysis has as yet been little studied in skeletal muscle and will not be dealt with here. The main pathway for stimulation of glycogenolysis by catecholamines is almost certainly adenylate cyclase and activation of phosphorylase. (A further effect is the inhibition of glycogen synthetase.) In skeletal muscle, breakdown of glycogen leads to a release of lactate into the blood. Thus the response to catecholamines may be assessed by changes in 1) cyclase activity or cAMP levels, 2) phosphorylase activity, and 3) muscle glycogen—alternatively, 4) increases in blood lactate (lacticacidemia). Effects of catecholamines on each have been described and the results reviewed (Ellis, 1967; Himms-Hagen, 1967, 1972; Brody and McNeill, 1970). The adrenoceptor concerned is clearly of Ahlquist's β type; agonists show the appropriate order of potencies (isoprenaline being most potent), and antagonists show the expected selectivity (β but not α blockers inhibiting stimulation).

The remaining point of interest is the subclassification of the β receptors in skeletal muscle. On the basis of agonist potencies, particularly the relatively weak action of noradrenaline coupled with a responsiveness to isoetharine, it was concluded that lacticacidemia in dogs (Arnold et al. [1968]) and rats (Arnold and Selberis [1968]) were β_2 responses. Butoxamine blocks the lacticacidemic response and activation of muscle phosphorylase by isoprenaline in rats (but at doses also having a clear effect on isoprenaline tachycardia) (Burns, Salvador, and Lemberger, 1967). Stanton (1972) confirmed butoxamine's action in rats; it was more effective in blocking glycogen loss induced by catecholamines in skeletal muscle than in cardiac muscle, whereas practolol was more effective in cardiac than in skeletal muscle. This confirmed the difference between cardiac (β_1) receptors and those in skeletal muscle. Lefkowitz (1975), studying cyclase activation in membrane preparations, found noradrenaline to be much less effective relative to isoprenaline in dog diaphragm than in dog heart; he furthermore found butoxamine to be a more effective antagonist than practolol in skeletal muscle, with the reverse holding for the heart. In cats also the evidence favors β_2 receptors: Kuo et al. (1977) found that H35/25 produced a much more effective blockade of lacticacidemia than practolol. The classification of skeletal muscle glycogenolysis as a β_2 response thus seems well founded. (The only observation encountered that is not in keeping with this conclusion is the relative inactivity of salbutamol, a β_2 agonist as a lacticacidemic agent in dogs [Kelly and Shanks, 1975]. Lacticacidemia is, however, a complex response and probably the least discriminatory measure of muscle glycogenolysis.)

It is of interest to consider the classification of other β responses in skeletal muscle, since–unless cAMP levels can be raised selectively in different pools–all β responses will occur simultaneously in response to activation of the same pool of receptors (though the relationship between cAMP concentration and response may, of course, differ for different responses). It is reassuring to find that the hypokalemic effect of catecholamines in cats, attributed mainly to stimulation of potassium uptake by skeletal muscle, is apparently mediated by β_2 receptors. Noradrenaline is relatively ineffective; the β_1 agonist, tazolol (ITP, 1-isopropylamino-3-(2-thiazoloxy)-2-propanol) is completely inactive; and the response is blocked by butoxamine and H35/25 but not by practolol (Lockwood and Lum, 1974). The findings of Bowman and Nott (1970) on the actions of sympathomimetic amines on muscle contraction and their antagonism by various blockers are also indicative of β_2 receptors.

IV. HEART MUSCLE

The metabolic actions of catecholamines on cardiac muscle have been reviewed by Himms-Hagen (1972), Mayer (1974), and Williamson (1975). They include effects on glycogen metabolism and on lipolysis. As for skeletal muscle, only the better studied actions on glycogen metabolism will be discussed here; the main effect is phosphorylase activation (synthetase inhibition apparently being of less consequence in heart than in other tissues [Mayer, 1974]).

The major actions of catecholamines on the heart are, of course, those on rate and force of contraction. The adrenoceptors involved have received much attention and are, indeed, important cornerstones of both Ahlquist's original classification (1948) and Lands et al.'s subsequent subclassification (1967). An important development has been the recognition of an α-mediated inotropic effect in several species. First described by Wenzel and Su (1966) for rat heart, it has since been observed in guinea-pigs, rabbits, and cats. In the dog, however, it appears to be absent (Endoh, Shimizu, and Yanagisawa, 1978). The evidence for this α inotropic effect is well founded on studies with selective agonists, including phenylephrine, methoxamine, naphazoline, and clonidine (e.g., Schümann and Endoh, 1976) and with selective antagonists. Indirect support has come from the binding studies of Ciaraldi and Marinetti (1977), who have obtained results with DHEC and DHA that indeed suggest that α receptors may outnumber β receptors in rat heart by a factor of 3 or so.

Whereas the β-mediated chronotropic and inotropic effects almost certainly involve cAMP (e.g., Tsien, 1977; also see earlier discussion) the α inotropic response probably occurs without the intervention of cAMP (e.g., Osnes and Øye, 1975). There is in fact some suggestion that α receptor activation may lower cAMP in heart muscle (Watanabe et al., 1977). Since a relatively large population of cardiac α receptors may exist in many species, it is relevant to consider whether there are α-mediated effects on cardiac glycogen metabolism because (a) the inotropic effect is likely to be accompanied by an elevation of $[Ca^{++}]i$, and (b) as for skeletal muscle, there is evidence that phosphorylase kinase in heart muscle may be activated by raising $[Ca^{++}]i$ (e.g., Friesen, Oliver, and Allen, 1969). However, the changes in Ca accompanying inotropic effects may not normally be sufficient to activate phosphorylase (Dobson, Ross, and Mayer, 1976); and in keeping with this, the results of Verma and McNeill (1976) suggest that under conditions where an α-mediated inotropic effect is demonstrable, phenylephrine increases phosphorylase activity only via β receptors (following increased cAMP levels). It has to be concluded then, that, although a mechanism may exist whereby α receptors could influence phosphorylase activity, the existing evidence suggests that its role would be minor.

The evidence is, of course, overwhelming for a β-mediated rise in cAMP leading to phosphorylase activation in the heart (Ellis, 1967; Himms-Hagen, 1967; Mayer, 1970). It is of interest to consider the extent to which the cAMP pool involved in the inotropic and chronotropic actions is identifiable with that concerned with phosphorylase activation and whether it might be possible to have both β_1 and β_2 receptors in the same tissue exerting different effects by virtue of discrete pools of cAMP (see also earlier discussion of β responses in skeletal muscle). The quest for a single "metabolic" receptor would bring us directly to this question, since once the β receptor for liver and muscle glycogenolysis is declared (β_2 we might, on such a hypothesis, expect to find β_2 receptors for glycogenolysis in heart coexisting with β_1 receptors for mechanical effects. The work of Carlsson et al. (1977) has already been mentioned as indicating the presence of β_2 receptors at least in some parts of the heart; and Kaumann, Birnbaumer, and Wittmann (1978) also describe the presence of different classes of β-adrenoceptors in guinea pig atria. Is there any further evidence along these lines and in particular for β_2-mediated cardiac glycogenolysis? The early work with methoxamine analogues indicated a relatively weak blocking action of these drugs against both the mechanical effects *and* phosphorylase activation (e.g., Quinn, Hornbrook, and Brody, 1965), suggesting that similar (β_1) receptors were involved. Further support for the classification of glycogenolysis as β_1 comes from the work of Stanton (1972), who found practolol to be more effective than butoxamine and H35/25 in inhibiting breakdown of cardiac glycogen. Where cardiac cylcase activation has been used as a response, the receptors involved have been found to be similar to those revealed by studies of inotropic or chronotropic effects (Kaumann, Birnbaumer, and Yang, 1974) and identifiable as β_1 (Burges and Blackburn, 1972; Lefkowitz, 1975).

Binding studies are more difficult to interpret. Thus, Maguire, Ross, and Gilman (1977) felt that ligand binding results for heart membrane preparations, particularly the relative affinities of adrenaline and noradrenaline (Harden, Wolfe, and Molinoff, 1976), were more in keeping with β_2 than with β_1 receptors. Results with β-blockers are also confusing. Thus Chenieux-Guicheney et al. (1978) found the β_1 selective antagonists practolol, acebutolol, and metoprolol to have low affinities for DHA binding sites in rat heart (butoxamine, however, also exhibiting low affinity); their findings contrast with the work of U'Prichard, Bylund, and Snyder (1978), again with rat heart membranes, who found a higher affinity for practolol (K_D = 350 nM) (but also for many other compounds, suggesting that binding conditions might be exerting some effect). At present, then, results from binding studies are not easily reconciled with observations made using tissue responses and do not rule out a β_2 receptor population.

In summary, then, heart may contain both α- and β-adrenoceptors. The α receptors do not seem to have an important influence on glycogen metabolism, though some effect might perhaps have been expected as a consequence either of changes in $[Ca^{++}]i$ or of inhibition of adenylate cyclase. The β-adrenoceptors are of prime importance in cardiac glycogenolysis, and there is little reason to suppose that they are distinct from those mediating chronotropic and inotropic effects. Accordingly, the general classification of these latter actions as β_1 can probably be directly applied to the actions of catecholamines on phosphorylase. The apparent inconsistencies with ligand binding studies in cardiac muscle should be resolved as methods improve.

V. ADIPOSE TISSUE

The most striking action of catecholamines on fat tissue is to cause the breakdown of triglycerides (lipolysis), releasing fatty acids and glycerol into the bloodstream. There are at the same time effects, probably of lesser importance, on glycogen metabolism that are very similar to those seen in liver and muscle (Steinberg et al., 1975). It is, however, the control of lipolysis that has been studied most extensively and that will be examined here.

The mechanism of fat mobilization by a variety of hormones has been thoroughly investigated and a role for cAMP in the activation of triglyceride lipase clearly established (Himms-Hagen, 1972; Fain, 1977). We should note, however, that an alternative pathway for the activation of triglyceride breakdown by catecholamines has recently been suggested (Wise and Jungas, 1978); the mechanism has not been clearly established. Such a pathway could conceivably rely on different adrenoceptors, and this would require separate investigation.

A. Methodology

Most studies to classify the adrenoceptors for lipolysis have been based on measurements of either (a) the release of free fatty acids (FFA) and glycerol into the blood stream or *in vitro* bathing solution, or (b) the activation of fat cell adenylate cyclase. There have been relatively few attempts, as yet, to use radioligand binding for this purpose. *In vivo* responses have been used extensively; but as for the hyperglycemic actions of catecholamines, the elevation of plasma FFA or glycerol will be influenced by effects on other organs; in this instance, important complications may be produced by changes in plasma glucose and insulin. *In vitro* systems (especially the use of isolated adipocytes) avoid these problems and have allowed rapid progress to be made. A significant factor in *in vitro* experiments is the almost universal inclusion of albumin in the bathing medium as an acceptor for the released fatty acids (in its absence FFA accumulate within the cells and may modify the response and have harmful effects on the tissue). Albumin will, however, bind drugs added to the system; and due allowance should be made for this fact. Zaagsma, Meems, and Boorsma (1977) have observed a 12-fold reduction in the potency of propranolol, due to its high fractional binding to albumin (pA_2 in atria reduced from 9.35 to 8.27). The choice of tissue is also important. Most experiments have been performed using white fat, commonly epididymal. Brown fat may well respond differently; and even for white fat there appear to be significant differences between fat taken either from different sites within a given species or from the same site in different species. Guinea pigs, rabbits, pigs (Rudman, Brown, and Malkin, 1963), and chickens (Steinberg et al., 1975) have been reported to respond poorly to catecholamines, though this may depend on experimental conditions.

B. Results of Classification Studies in Adipose Tissue

The earliest attempts to classify lipolytic responses to catecholamines were befuddled by the actions of α blockers, several workers demonstrating antagonism, particularly with high concentrations. Thus the results of Wenke, Mühlbachová, and Hynie (1962) demonstrated the effectiveness of isoprenaline and its inhibition by DCI (indicative of β receptors) yet also indicated blockade by phentolamine (though at 0.4 mM) and a potent action of noradrenaline (which was viewed primarily as an α agonist). The authors felt unable to attribute the response to either α or β receptors and suggested the presence of an alternative receptor, equivalent to the γ receptor proposed by Furchgott shortly before.

These early difficulties were soon left behind, however, as compelling evidence for β receptor involvement accumulated. Today there can be little doubt that β receptors are of prime importance. Isoprenaline is invariably more potent than adrenaline or noradrenaline, and β blockers produce competitive antagonism. Estimates of the pA_2 value for propanolol have been made and are usually within the normal range associated with antagonism at β receptors—e.g., 7.9 (Miller and Allen, 1971), 6.74 (Harms, Zaagsma, and Van der Wal, 1974), and 8.16 (Bertholet et al., 1979). None of the authors, however, corrected for propranolol's binding to albumin, and the values quoted are almost certainly too low. The last-named investigators, on the other hand, described a significant effect of insulin, present in commercial albumin samples, to reduce the measured pA_2 values (the mechanism of this effect was not investigated).

Pairault and Laudat (1975) found propranolol to be an effective displacer of specific [^{3}H]-noradrenaline binding to plasma membranes of rat adipocytes. The concentration of specific noradrenaline binding sites was estimated to be 0.3–0.35 pmole/mg protein, which compared well with the value of 0.24 pmole/mg protein recorded by Williams, Jarett, and Lefkowitz (1976a) for DHA binding sites, again in rat adipocyte membranes. Williams et al. (1976a) also found propranolol to be a potent competitor ($K_D = 17$ nM) and K_Ds for catecholamines to be consistent with β receptors (table 1). Guidicelli and Pecquery (1978) also report high affinity binding of DHA to rat adipocyte membranes (K_D, 15–20 nM).

C. Inhibitory α Receptors

Early experiments showed that adrenaline and noradrenaline often exhibited bell-shaped lipolytic log dose-response curves in certain species. This has now been clearly attributed to the presence of inhibitory α adrenoceptors, which decrease adenylate cyclase activity in adipocytes. A common finding is a reduced maximum response to agonists possessing both α and β actions and a potentiation of the lipolytic or cAMP response to such agents by α blockade (Pilkington et al., 1966; Robison, Langley, and Burns, 1972). The α inhibitory mechanism may vary in effectiveness between species. It is considered to be weak in white adipose tissue of rats (Robison et al., 1972), though its presence has been reported for rat brown fat (Itaya, 1978).

D. Subclassification of Fat Cell β-Adrenoceptors

Lands et al. (1967) originally classified lipolysis as a β_1 response on the basis of agonist potency ratios. The characteristic high potency of noradrenaline relative to adrenaline as a lipolytic agent had in fact been consistently observed (e.g., Barrett, 1965) and has more recently been found for adenylate cyclase activation in adipose tissue (Lefkowitz, 1975) and for DHA displacement from adipocyte membranes (Williams et al., 1976a; table 1). Fain (1973) reviewed the literature and concluded that Lands et al.'s classification (1967) of lipolysis as β_1 was supported by subsequent findings with selective agents (Salbutamol, practolol, butoxamine). The recent study by Frisk-Holmberg and Östman (1977) with segments of human adipose tissue provides further support for a dominant β_1 receptor population. Salbutamol exhibited a low potency for stimulation of lipolysis; and the cardioselective (β_1) antagonists metoprolol, atenolol, and practolol were all effective inhibitors. Although these results certainly suggest a β_1 classification, the study would have been more informative had the displacement of log dose-response curves been investigated with the further use of Schild plots to determine K_D values. This might have thrown light on the differences that were observed in the effectiveness of the blockers against different agonists.

Although a relatively strong case can thus be made for classifying the β receptors in white adipose tissue as β_1, other studies suggest that the receptors in fat cells differ from those in the heart. Thus early experiments demonstrated a marked antagonism of catecholamine-stimulated lipolysis by isopropylmethoxamine both *in vivo* (dogs) and *in vitro* (rat) at concentrations causing little inhibition of cardiac responses (Burns et al., 1964). (This must, however, be contrasted with the results of Fain, Galton, and Kovacev [1966], who observed a very weak and probably nonspecific antagonism with butoxamine). Zaagsma and colleagues (Harms et al., 1974; De Vente et al., 1978) have thoroughly investigated the relative antagonist action of a series of compounds on lipolysis in isolated rat adipocytes and obtained results that do not simply place lipolytic and cardiac β receptors in the same category. The interesting hypothesis was put forward that β receptors in adipose tissue are neither β_1 nor β_2 but have characteristics of both.

The part of the receptor combining with the side chain of β agonists or antagonists was considered similar to the corresponding component in cardiac β receptors, but the part combining with the catechol moiety of catecholamines (or equivalent region for β antagonists) resembled the same part of the β receptor in trachea. Harms et al. (1974) felt that the correlation overall was better with tracheal β receptors. The results of Lefkowitz (1975), though generally supporting a β_1 classification in rat adipose tissue, also revealed that soterenol (considered a β_2 agonist) had a similar potency to noradrenaline and adrenaline for the activation of adenylate cyclase in adipose tissue but was only a weak agonist in heart muscle. His feeling was that this reflected heterogeneity *within* the β_1 subclass. Differences between heart and fat cell β receptors are also suggested by results with practolol, which (relative to propranolol) is much less effective in adipose tissue than in heart muscle (Kather and Simon, 1977). Evidence that favors β_2 rather than β_1 receptors was obtained by Jolly, Lech, and Menahan (1978). In this study salbutamol was a moderately active lipolytic agent in rat and mouse adipocytes, whereas tazolol (β_1 agonist) was either inactive (mouse) or a weak partial agonist (rat). An alternative view of adipose tissue β receptors is that, rather than differing from β_1 and β_2 receptors found elsewhere, they include both types. Åblad et al. (1975) found the β_1 antagonist, metoprolol, to be more effective in antagonizing the elevation of plasma FFA induced by noradrenaline than that induced by adrenaline in dogs. It was proposed that adrenaline but not noradrenaline exerted a significant part of its action via β_2 receptors that were not blocked by metoprolol.

In summary, there appears to be little doubt that catecholamines cause lipolysis in adipose tissue by interacting with β adrenoceptors; α receptors have been less well studied but where present inhibit lipolysis. It would be interesting to determine the relative concentrations of α and β receptors in this tissue, as has been done for rat liver. The subclassification of the fat cell β receptor presents problems that have yet to be resolved; β_1 and β_2 receptors may both be present.

VI. GENERAL DISCUSSION

In this paper an attempt has been made to determine whether it is possible to make a meaningful classification of the receptors involved in the better studied metabolic responses to catecholamines. In general, the evidence does appear to be well accommodated within Ahlquist's original classification, once it is recognized that allowances must be made for the difficulties arising from 1) the presence of *both* α and β receptors in many tissues, 2) the complexities of *in vivo* responses, 3) factors modifying drug concentrations at the receptors, 4) the existence of receptor subtypes, and 5) nonspecific actions of many drugs when used at high concentrations. Many of these problems have been considered by Furchgott (1972) in his treatise on catecholamine receptor classification; and although it is sometimes difficult or impossible to meet all his suggested criteria or procedures, greater success would surely follow if the attempt were made. The need for careful experimental design and a quantitative approach is particularly important when differences between receptors are small; accordingly, we may reasonably expect the subclassification of adrenoceptors to be more demanding than the relatively straightforward distinction between α and β effects. For metabolic responses many of the data are still of a qualitative nature; one virtue of the ligand binding studies has been that they have brought with them a welcome quantitative approach. Ligand binding results will undoubtedly lead to an improved knowledge of receptor densities and characteristics; but, as noted earlier, they cannot indicate the physiological importance of any particular drug receptor interaction. Thus, in rat liver a preponderance of α receptors is apparently linked to dominant α responses (glycogenolysis, gluconeogenesis); whereas in rat heart, where α receptors may also outnumber β receptors (Ciaraldi and Marinetti, 1977), α responses are nevertheless probably of minor importance.

A large part of this paper has been devoted to the effects of catecholamines on the liver. The reasons for this are, first, that hyperglycemia and hepatic glycogenolysis have been the source of most dispute; and second, that because of the interest engendered, the regulation of hepatic carbohydrate metabolism is becoming reasonably well understood. Much of the early confusion is understandable once we appreciate that both α and β receptors participate in these metabolic responses (albeit using different mechanisms) and that the relative importance of the two systems may vary between species.

Concerning subclassification, it has to be recognized that there is still reluctance in some quarters to accept Lands et al.'s proposals (1967) for β receptors and still less agreement about the subdivision of α receptors. Ahlquist's original classification took nearly ten years to gain general acceptance, and it seems that the same may apply to the β_1/β_2 subtyping. The author, however, takes the view that the evidence must now be considered satisfactory and that no consideration of adrenoceptor classification can be considered complete without some attention to the issue.

An important unresolved problem is whether different β responses occurring within the same cell (e.g., myocardial) might be independently controlled, conceivably through different receptor subtypes. There appears, however, to be no evidence for the existence of the discrete pools of cAMP that would permit such a separation. Following from this, it may be misleading to talk of "metabolic receptors"; rather, we should consider receptors as belonging to a given tissue. Thus it would be reasonable to talk of "hepatic β receptors," activation of which would lead to a variety of responses—including, of course, some metabolic ones (e.g., glycogen breakdown). Where both β_1 and β_2 receptors do coexist in a given tissue, their *actions* would be indistinguishable in the absence of discrete cAMP pools. A complete understanding of the sympathetic regulation of metabolic responses will require much further work: the assessment of the relative importance of nerve released and circulating catecholamines will be aided by a knowledge of the relative potencies of noradrenaline and adrenaline. This, in turn, is determined by the relative densities of the different adrenoceptors in the tissues, their affinities for the catecholamines, and the efficacies of the amines at the receptors. Further information is also required about the relationship of receptor activation to the subsequent biochemical changes, including the relative importance of different second messengers (e.g., cAMP and [Ca^{++}]).

VII. REFERENCES

Åblad, B.; Börjesson, I.; Carlsson, E.; Johnsson, G.: Effects of Metoprolol and Propranolol on some Metabolic Responses to Catecholamines in the Anaesthetized Dog. Acta Pharmacol Toxicol (Kbh) 36 Supp V (1975)85–95

Ahlquist, R.P.: A Study of the Adrenotropic Receptors. Am J Physiol 153(1948)586–600

Ahlquist, R.P.: Adrenergic Drugs. In: Pharmacology in Medicine, pp. 26/1–26/31, ed. by V.A. Drill, McGraw-Hill, New York, Toronto, London, 1954

Antoniades, H.N.; Goldfien, A.; Zileli, S.; Elmadjian, F.: Transport of Epinephrine and Norepinephrine in Human Plasma. Proc Soc Exp Biol Med 97(1958)11–12

Arnold, A.; McAuliff, J.P.; Colella, D.F.; O'Connor, W.V.; Brown, Th.G.: The β-2 Receptor Mediated Glycogenolytic Responses to Catecholamines in the Dog. Arch Int Pharmacodyn Ther 176(1968)451–457

Arnold, A.; Selberis, W.H.: Activities of Catecholamines on the Rat Muscle Glycogenolytic (β-2) Receptor. Experientia 24(1968)1010–1011

Assimacopoulos-Jeannet, F.D.; Blackmore, P.F.; Exton, J.H.: Studies on α-Adrenergic Activation of Hepatic Glucose Output. Studies on Role of Calcium in α-Adrenergic Activation of Phosphorylase. J Biol Chem 252(1977)2662–2669

Barrett, A.M.: The Mobilization of Free Fatty Acids in Response to Isoprenaline in the Rat. Br J Pharmacol 25(1965)545–556

Berthelsen, S.; Pettinger, W.A.: A Functional Basis for Classification of α-Adrenergic Receptors. Life Sci 21(1977)595–606

Bertholet, A.; Milavec, M.; Schild, H.O.; Waite, R.: A Study of Beta-Adrenoceptors in the Guinea-Pig. In preparation

Black, J.W.; Crowther, A.F.; Shanks, R.G.; Smith, L.H.; Dornhorst, A.C.: A New Adrenergic Beta-Receptor Antagonist. Lancet 1(1964)1080–1081

Bowman, W.C.; Nott, M.W.: Actions of some Sympathomimetic Bronchodilator and Beta-Adrenoceptor Blocking Drugs on Contractions of the Cat Soleus Muscle. Br J Pharmacol 38(1970)37–49

Brody, T.M.; McNeill, J.H.: Adrenergic Receptors for Metabolic Responses in Skeletal and Smooth Muscle. Fed Proc 29(1970)1375–1378

Buchthal, A.B.; Jenkinson, D.H.: Effects of Isomers of the α-Agonist Amidephrine on Arterial and Tracheal Muscle *in Vitro*. Eur J Pharmacol 10(1970)293–296

Burges, R.A.; Blackburn, K.J.: Adenyl Cyclase and the Differentiation of β-Adrenoceptors. Nature [New Biol] 235(1972)249–250

Burns, J.J.; Colville, K.I.; Lindsay, L.A.; Salvador, R.A.: Blockade of some Metabolic Effects of Catecholamines by N-Isopropylmethoxamine (B.W. 61-43). J Pharmacol Exp Ther 144(1964)163–171

340 / Dennis G. Haylett

Burns, J.J.; Lemberger, L.: N-Tertiary Butyl Methoxamine, a Specific Antagonist of the Metabolic Actions of Epinephrine. Fed Proc 24(1965)298

Burns, J.J.; Salvador, R.A.; Lemberger, L.: Metabolic Blockade by Methoxamine and its Analogs. Ann NY Acad Sci 139(1967)833–840

Butler, M.; Jenkinson, D.H.: Blockade by WB 4101 of α-Adrenoceptors in the Rat Vas Deferens and Guinea-Pig Taenia Caeci. Eur J Pharmacol 52(1978)303–311

Carlsson, A.; Waldeck, B.: On the Role of the Liver Catechol-O-Methyl Transferase in the Metabolism of Circulating Catecholamines. Acta Pharmacol Toxicol (Kbh) 20(1963)47–55

Carlsson, E.; Dahlof, C.-G.; Hedberg, A.; Persson, H.; Tångstrand, B.: Differentiation of Cardiac Chronotropic and Inotropic Effects of β-Adrenoceptor Agonists. Naunyn Schmiedebergs Arch Pharmacol 300(1977)101–105

Caron, M.G.; Beaulieu, M.; Raymond, V.; Gagné, B.; Drouin, J.; Lefkowitz, R.J.; Labrie, F.; Dopaminergic Receptors in the Anterior Pituitary Gland. Correlation of [³H] Dihydroergocryptine Binding with the Dopaminergic Control of Prolactin Release. J Biol Chem 253(1978)2244–2253

Castro-Tavares, J.: A Comparison Between the Influence of Pindolol and Propranolol on the Response of Plasma Potassium to Catecholamines. Arzneim Forsch 26(1976)238–241

Chan, P.S.; Ellis, S.; Mühlbachová, E.: Differences in Dihydroergotamine Antagonism of Glucose Release by Catecholamines, Glucagon and Adenosine 3′,5′-Monophosphate in Rabbit Liver Slices. Br J Pharmacol 63(1978)593–597

Chasin, M.; Mamrak, F.; Samaniego, S.G.; Hess, S.M.: Characteristics of the Catecholamine and Histamine Receptor Sites Mediating Accumulation of Cyclic Adenosine 3′,5′-Monophosphate in Guinea-Pig Brain. J Neurochem. 21(1973)1415–1427

Chenieux-Guicheney, P.; Dausse, J.P.; Meyer, P.; Schmitt, H.: Inhibition of [³H]-Dihydroalprenolol Binding to Rat Cardiac Membranes by Various β-Blocking Agents. Br J Pharmacol 63(1978)177–182

Cherrington, A.D.; Assimacopoulos, F.D.; Harper, S.C.; Corbin, J.D.; Park, C.R.; Exton, J.H.: Studies on the α-Adrenergic Activation of Hepatic Glucose Output. II. Investigation of the Roles of Adenosine 3′:5′-Monophosphate and Adenosine 3′:5′-Monophosphate-Dependent Protein Kinase in the Actions of Phenylephrine in Isolated Hepatocytes. J Biol Chem 251(1976)5209–5218

Ciaraldi, T.; Marinetti, G.V.: Thyroxine and Propylthiouracil Effects in Vivo on Alpha and Beta Adrenergic Receptors in Rat Heart. Biochem Biophys Res Commun 74(1977)984–991

Clark, B.J.: Pharmacology of Beta-Adrenoceptor Blocking Agents. In: Beta-Adrenoceptor Blocking Agents, pp. 45–76, ed. by P.R. Saxena and R.P. Forsyth, North-Holland, Amsterdam, 1976

Clark, S.J.; Poyser, R.H.: Effect of Tazolol on β-Adrenoceptors in Isolated Preparations of the Guinea-Pig and Rat. J. Pharm. Pharmacol. 29(1977)630–632

Clarke, W.R.; Jones, L.R.; Lefkowitz, R.J.: Hepatic α-Adrenergic Receptors. Identification and Subcellular Localization using [³H] Dihydroergocryptine. J Biol Chem 253(1978) 5975–5979

Cautrecasas, P.; Tell, G.P.E.; Sica, V.; Parikh, I.; Chang, K.-J.: Noradrenaline Binding and the Search for Catecholamine Receptors. Nature 247(1974)92–97

Cuatrecases, P.; Hollenberg, M.D.; Chang, K.-J.; Bennett, V.: Hormone Receptor Complexes and their Modulation of Membrane Function. Recent Prog Horm Res 31(1975)37–94

Cullum, V.A.; Farmer, J.B.; Jack, D.; Levy, G.P.: Salbutamol: a New, Selective β-Adrenoceptive Receptor Stimulant. 35(1969)141–151

De Vente, J.; Bast, A.; Van Bree, L.; Zaagsma, J.: Is the β-Adrenoceptor in Rat Adipocytes a β₁ or β₂ Subtype? The Influence of a Non-Biological Parameter on the Classification. In: Recent Advances in the Pharmacology of Adrenoceptors, pp. 365–366, ed. by E. Szabadi, C.M. Bradshaw, P. Bevan. Elsevier/North-Holland. Amsterdam-New York-Oxford, 1978

Dobson, J.G.; Ross, J.; Mayer, S.E.: The Role of Cyclic Adenosine 3′,5′-Monophosphate and Calcium in the Regulation of Contractility and Glycogen Phosphorylase Activity in Guinea-Pig Papillary Muscle. Circ Res 39(1976)388–395

Doxey, J.C.; Smith, C.F.C.; Walker, J.M.: Selectivity of Blocking Agents for Pre- and Postsynaptic α-Adrenoceptors. Br J Pharmacol 60(1977)91–96

D'Silva, J.L.: The Action of Adrenaline on Serum Potassium. J Physiol (Lond) 82(1934)393–398

Ellis, S.: The Metabolic Effects of Epinephrine and Related Amines. Pharmacol Rev 8(1956)485–562

Ellis, S.; Beckett, S.B.: Mechanism of the Potassium Mobilizing Action of Epinephrine and Glucagon. J Pharmacol Exp Ther 142(1963)318–326

Ellis, S.; Eusebi, A.J.: Dissociation of Epinephrine-Induced Hyperkalemia and Hyperglycemia by Adrenergic Blocking Drugs and Theophylline: Role of Cyclic 3'-5'-AMP. Fed Proc 24(1965)151

Ellis, S.: The Effects of Sympathomimetic Amines and Adrenergic Blocking Agents on Metabolism. In: Physiological Pharmacology. Vol. IV, pp. 179–241, ed. by W.S. Root and F.S. Hofmann. Academic, New York 1967

Ellis, S.; Kennedy, B.L.; Eusebi, A.J.; Vincent, N.H.: Autonomic Control of Metabolism. Ann NY Acad Sci 139(1967)826–832

Endoh, M.; Shimizu, T.; Yanagisawa, T.: Characterization of Adrenoceptors Mediating Positive Inotropic Responses in the Ventricular Myocardium of the Dog. Br J Pharmacol 64(1978)53–61

Exton, J.H.; Park, C.R.: The Stimulation of Gluconeogenesis from Lactate by Epinephrine, Glucagon and Cyclic 3',5'-Adenylate in the Perfused Rat Liver. Pharmacol Rev 18(1966)181–188

Exton, J.H.; Harper, S.C.: Role of Cyclic AMP in the Actions of Catecholamines on Hepatic Carbohydrate Metabolism. Adv Cyclic Nucleotide Res 5(1975)519–532

Fain, J.N.; Galton, D.J.; Kovacev, V.P.: Effect of Drugs on the Lipolytic action of Hormones in Isolated Fat Cells. Mol Pharmacol 2(1966)237–247

Fain, J.N.: Biochemical Aspects of Drug and Hormone Action on Adipose Tissue. Pharmacol Rev 25(1973)67–118

Fain, J.N.: Cyclic Nucleotides in Adipose Tissue. In: Cyclic 3',5',Nucleotides: Mechanisms of Action, pp. 207–228, ed. by H. Cramer and J. Schultz. Wiley, London 1977

Felíu, J.E.; Hue, L.; Hers, H.-G.: Hormonal Control of Pyruvate Kinase Activity and of Gluconeogenesis in Isolated Hepatocytes. Proc Natl Acad Sci USA 73(1976)2762–2766

Fleming, W.W.; Kenny, A.D.: The Effect of Fasting on the Hyperglycaemic Responses to Catechol Amines in Rats. Br J Pharmacol 22(1964)267–274

Friedmann, N.; Somlyo, A.V.; Somlyo, A.P.: Cyclic Adenosine and Guanosine Monophosphates and Glucagon: Effect on Liver Membrane Potentials. Science 171(1971)400–402

Friedmann, N.: Effects of Glucagon and Cyclic AMP on Ion Fluxes in the Perfused Liver. Biochim Biophys Acta 274(1972)214–225

Friesen, A.J.D.; Oliver, N.; Allen, G.: Activation of Cardiac Glycogen Phosphorylase by Calcium. Am J Physiol 217(1969)445–450

Frisk-Holmberg, M.; Östman, J.: Differential Inhibition of Lipolysis in Human Adipose Tissue by Adrenergic Beta Receptor Blocking Drugs. J Pharmacol Exp Ther 200(1977)598–605

Furchgott, R.F.: The Receptors for Epinephrine and Norepinephrine (Adrenergic Receptors). Pharmacol Rev 11(1959)429–441

Furchgott, R.F.: The Pharmacological Differentiation of Adrenergic Receptors. Ann NY Acad Sci 139(1967)553–570

Furchgott, R.F.: The Classification of Adrenoceptors (Adrenergic Receptors). An Evaluation from the Standpoint of Receptor Theory. In: Handbook of Experimental Pharmacology Vol. XXXIII: Catecholamines, pp. 283–335, ed. by H. Blaschko and E. Muscholl. Springer, Berlin-Heidelberg-New York, 1972

Furchgott, R.F.; Wakade, T.D.; Sorace, R.A.; Stollak, J.S.: Occurrence of Both β_1 and β_2 Receptors in Guinea-Pig Tracheal Smooth Muscle, and Variation of the $\beta_1:\beta_2$ Ratio in Different Animals. Fed Proc 34(1975)794

Giudicelli, Y.; Pecquery, R.: β-Adrenergic Receptors and Catecholamine-Sensitive Adenylate Cyclase in Rat Fat-Cell Membranes: Influence of Growth, Cell Size and Aging. Eur J Biochem 90(1978)413–419

Guellaen, G.; Yates-Aggerbeck, M.; Vauquelin, G.; Strosberg, D.; Hanoune, J.: Characterization with [³H]-Dihydroergocryptine of the α-Adrenergic Receptor of the Hepatic Plasma

Membrane: Comparison with the β-Adrenergic Receptor in Normal and Adrenalectomized Rats. J Biol Chem 253(1978)1114–1120

Harden, T.K.; Wolfe, B.B.; Molinoff, P.B.: Binding of Iodinated Beta Adrenergic Antagonists to Proteins Derived from Rat Heart. Mol Pharmacol 12(1976)1–15

Harms, H.H.; Zaagsma, J.; Van der Wal, B.: β-Adrenoceptor Studies III. On the β-Adrenoceptors in Rat Adipose Tissue. Eur J Pharmacol 25(1974)87–91

Haylett, D.G.; Jenkinson, D.H.: Receptors Mediating the Effect of Catecholamines on Glucose Release from Guinea-Pig Liver in Vitro. Br J Pharmacol 34(1968)694P

Haylett, D.G.; Jenkinson, D.H.: Effects of Noradrenaline on Potassium Efflux, Membrane Potential and Electrolyte Levels in Tissue Slices Prepared from Guinea-Pig Liver. J Physiol (Lond) 225(1972a)721–750

Haylett, D.G.; Jenkinson, D.H.: The Receptors Concerned in the Actions of Catecholamines on Glucose Release, Membrane Potential and Ion Movements in Guinea-Pig Liver. J Physiol (Lond) 225(1972b)751–772

Haylett, D.G.; Jenkinson, D.H.: Actions of Catecholamines on the Membrane Properties of Liver Cells. In: Drug Receptors, pp. 15–25, ed. by H.P. Rang. Macmillan, London, 1973

Haylett, D.G.: Effects of Sympathomimetic Amines on ^{45}Ca Efflux from Liver Slices. Br J Pharmacol 57(1976)158–160

Himms-Hagen, J.: Sympathetic Regulation of Metabolism. Pharmacol Rev 19(1967)367–461

Himms-Hagen, J.: Effects of Catecholamines on Metabolism. In: Handbook of Experimental Pharmacology. Vol. XXXIII: Catecholamines, pp. 363–462, ed. by H. Blaschko and E. Muscholl. Springer, Berlin-Heidelberg-New York, 1972

Hittelman, K.J.; Wu, C.F.; Butcher, R.W.: Control of Cyclic AMP Levels in Isolated Fat Cells from Hamsters. Biochim Biophys Acta 304(1973)188–196

Hornbrook, K.R.; Brody, T.M.: Phosphorylase Activity in Rat Liver and Skeletal Muscle after Catecholamines. Biochem Pharmacol 12(1963)1407–1415

Hornbrook, K.R.: Adrenergic Receptors for Metabolic Responses in the Liver. Fed Proc 29(1970)1381–1385

Hu, E.H.; Venter, J.C.: Adenosine Cyclic 3',5'-Monophosphate Concentrations During the Positive Inotropic Response of Cat Cardiac Muscle to Polymeric Immobilized Isoproterenol. Mol Pharmacol 14(1978)237–245

Hutcheon, D.E.; P'An, S.Y.; Gardocki, J.F.; Jaeger, D.A.: The Sympathomimetic and Other Pharmacological Properties of dl 2-(1,2,3,4-tetrahydro-1-naphthyl)-Imidazoline (Tetrahydrozoline). J Pharmacol Exp Ther 113(1955)341–352

Hutson, N.J.; Brumley, F.T.; Assimacopoulos, F.D.; Harper, S.C.; Exton, J.H.: Studies on the α-Adrenergic Activation of Hepatic Glucose Output. I. Studies on the α-Adrenergic Activation of Phosphorylase and Gluconeogenesis and Inactivation of Glycogen Synthase in Isolated Rat Liver Parenchymal Cells. J Biol Chem 251(1976)5200–5208

Imbs, J.L.; Miesch, F.; Schwartz, J.; Velly, J.; Leclerc, G.; Mann, A.; Wermuth, C.G.: A Potent New β_2-Adrenoceptor Blocking Agent. Br J Pharmacol 60(1977)357–362

Itaya, K.: Differences in Responsiveness to Adipokinetic Agents Between White Epididymal and Brown Interscapula Adipose Tissue from Rats. J Pharm Pharmacol 30(1978)632–637

Iwata, Y.: Hyperglycemic Action of 2-(2,6-Dichlorophenylamino)-2-Imidazoline Hydrochloride in Relation to its Hypertensive Effect. Jpn J Pharmacol 19(1969)249–259

Jenkinson, D.H.: Classification and Properties of Peripheral Adrenergic Receptors. Br Med Bull 29(1973)142–147

Jenkinson, D.H.; Koller, K.: Interactions Between the Effects of α- and β-Adrenoceptor Agonists and Adenine Nucleotides on the Membrane Potential of Cells in Guinea-Pig Liver Slices. Br J Pharmacol 59(1977)163–175

Jolly, S.R.; Lech, J.J.; Menahan, L.A.: Comparison of Isoproterenol, Salbutamol and Tazolol as Lipolytic Agents with Isolated Rodent Adipocytes. Biochem Pharmacol 27(1978)1885–1887

Kather, H.; Simon, B.: Catecholamine-Sensitive Adenylate Cyclase of Human Fat Cell Ghosts: A Comparative Study Using Different Beta-Adrenergic Agents. Metabolism 26(1977)1179–1184

Kaumann, A.J.; Birnbaumer, L.; Yang, P.-C.: Studies on Receptor Mediated Activation of

Adenylyl Cyclase. IV. Characteristics of the Adrenergic Receptor Coupled to Myocardial Adenylyl Cyclase: Stereospecificity for Ligands and Determination of Apparent Affinity Constants for β-Blockers. J Biol Chem 249(1974)7874-7885

Kaumann, A.J.; Birnbaumer, L.; Wittmann, R.: Heart β-Adrenoceptors. In: Receptors and Hormone Action. Vol. III. pp. 133-177, ed. by L. Birnbaumer and B.W. O'Malley. Academic, New York-San-Francisco-London 1978

Kelly, J.G.; Shanks, R.G.: Metabolic and Cardiovascular Effects of Isoprenaline and Salbutamol in the Dog. Br J Pharmacol 53(1975)157-162

Kemp, B.E.; Clark, M.G.: Adrenergic Control of the Cyclic AMP-Dependent Protein Kinase and Pyruvate Kinase in Isolated Hepatocytes. J Biol Chem 253(1978)5147-5154

Keppens, S.; Vandenheede, J.R.; De Wulf, H.: On the Role of Calcium as Second Messenger in Liver for the Hormonally Induced Activation of Glycogen Phosphorylase. Biochim Biophys Acta 496(1977)448-457

Kneer, N.M.; Bosch, A.L.; Clark, M.G.; Lardy, H.A.: Glucose Inhibition of Epinephrine Stimulation of Hepatic Gluconeogenesis by Blockade of the α-Receptor Function. Proc Natl Acad Sci USA 71(1974)4523-4527

Kuo, S.-H.; Kamaka, J.K.; Lum, B.K.B.: Adrenergic Receptor Mechanisms Involved in the Hyperglycemia and Hyperlacticacidemia Produced by Sympathomimetic Amines in the Cat. J Pharmacol Exp Ther 202(1977)301-309

Lacombe, M.-L.; Rene, E.; Guellaen, G.; Hanoune, J.: Tranformation of the β_2 Adrenoceptor in Normal Rat Liver into a β_1 Type in Zajdela Hepatoma. Nature 262(1976)70-72

Lands, A.M.: Sympathetic Receptor Action. Am J Physiol 169(1952)11-21

Lands, A.M.; Arnold, A.; McAuliff, J. P.; Luduena, F.P.; Brown, T.G.: Differentiation of Receptor Systems Activated by Sympathomimetic Amines. Nature 214(1967)597-598

Langer, S.Z.: Presynaptic Regulation of Catecholamine Release. Biochem Pharmacol 23(1974)1793-1800

Langer, S.Z.: Presynaptic Receptors and their Role in the Regulation of Transmitter Release. Br J Pharmacol 60(1977)481-497

Lefkowitz, R.J.: Heterogeneity of Adenylate Cyclase-Coupled β-Adrenergic Receptors. Biochem Pharmacol 24(1975)583-590

Levitzki, A.: Catecholamine Receptors. In: Receptors and Recognition, Series A, Vol. 2, pp. 199-229, ed. by P. Cuatrecasas and M.F. Greaves. Chapman and Hall, London, 1976

Loakpradit, T.; Lockwood, R.: Differentiation of Metabolic Adrenoceptors. Br J Pharmacol 59(1977)135-140

Lockwood, R.H.; Lum, B.K.B.: Effects of Adrenergic Agonists and Antagonists on Potassium Metabolism. J Pharmacol Exp Ther 189(1974)119-129

Maguire, M.E.; Ross, E.M.; Gilman, A.G.: β-Adrenergic Receptor: Ligand Binding Properties and the Interaction with Adenylyl Cyclase. Adv Cyclic Nucleotide Res 8(1977)1-83

Mayer, S.E.; Moran, N.C.; Fain, J.N.: The Effect of Adrenergic Blocking Agents on some Metabolic Actions of Catecholamines. J Pharmacol Exp Ther 134(1961)18-27

Mayer, S.E.: Adrenergic Receptors for Metabolic Responses in the Heart. Fed Proc 29(1970)1367-1372

Mayer, S.E.: Effect of Catecholamines on Cardiac Metabolism. Circ Res 35 Supp III(1974)129-135

Miller, D.W.; Allen, D.O.: Antilipolytic Activity of 4-(2-Hydroxy-3-Isopropylaminopropoxy) acetanilide (Practolol). Proc Soc Exp Biol Med 136(1971)715-718

Mirkin, B.L.; Brown, D.M.; Ulstrom, R.A.: Catecholamine Binding Protein: Binding of Tritium to a Specific Protein Fraction of Human Plasma following in Vitro Incubation with Tritiated Noradrenaline. Nature 212(1966)1270-1271

Moran, N.C.: The Development of Beta Adrenergic Blocking Drugs: A Retrospective and Prospective Evaluation. Ann NY Acad Sci 139(1967)649-660

Mühlbachová, E.; Chan, P.S.; Ellis, S.: Quantitative Studies of Glucose Release from Rabbit Liver Slices Induced by Catecholamines and their Antagonism by Propranolol and Phentolamine. J Pharmacol Exp Ther 182(1972)370-377

Murad, F.; Chi, Y.-M.; Rall, T.M.; Sutherland, E.W.: Adenyl Cyclase III. The Effect of Catecholamines and Choline Esters on the Formation of Adenosine 3',5'-Phosphate by Preparations from Cardiac Muscle and Liver. J Biol Chem 237(1962)1233-1238

Neuvonen, P.J.; Vapaatalo, H.I.; Westermann, E.: Some Metabolic Effects of DOPA and Dopamine in Rats. Acta Pharmacol Toxicol (Kbh) 29 Supp 4(1971)40

Northrop, G.: Effects of Adrenergic Blocking Agents on Epinephrine- and 3',5'-AMP-Induced Responses in the Perfused Rat Liver. J Pharmacol Exp Ther 159(1968)22–28

Osborn, D.: Comparison of the Effects of Selective α- and β-Receptor Agonists on Intracellular Cyclic AMP Levels and Glycogen Phosphorylase Activity in Guinea-Pig Liver. Br J Pharmacol 55(1975)286–287P

Osborn, D.: The Alpha Adrenergic Receptor Mediated Increase in Guinea-Pig Liver Glycogenolysis. Biochem Pharmacol 27(1978)1315–1320

Osnes, J.-B.; Øye, I.: Relationship Between Cyclic AMP Metabolism and Intropic Response of Perfused Rat Hearts to Phenylephrine and Other Adrenergic Amines. Adv Cyclic Nucleotide Res 5(1975)415–433

Pairault, J.; Laudat, M.-H.: Selective Identification of 'True' β-Adrenergic Receptors in the Plasma Membranes of Rat Adipocytes. FEBS Lett 50(1975)61–65

Pilkington, T.R.E.; Lowe, R.D.; Foster, R.; Robinson, B.F.; Antonis, A.: Effect of Sympathomimetic Compounds with β-Adrenergic Effects on Plasma Free Fatty Acids in Man. J Lipid Res 7(1966)73–76

Porte, D.: A Receptor Mechanism for the Inhibition of Insulin Release by Epinephrine in Man. J Clin Invest 46(1967)86–94

Potter, D.E.; Ellis, S.: Isoproterenol- and Epinephrine-Induced Changes in Blood Glucose and Tissue Glycogen Levels in Normal and Diabetic Rats: the Influence of Alteration in Endogenous Insulin Levels and State of Nourishment. J Pharmacol Exp Ther 193(1975)576–584

Potter, D.E.; Barnett, J.W.; Woodson, L.C.: Catecholamine-Induced Changes in Plasma Glucose, Glucagon and Insulin in Rabbits: Effects of Somatostatin. Horm Metab Res 10(1978)373–377

Preiksaitis, H.G.; Kunos, G.: Adrenoceptor-Mediated Activation of Liver Glycogen Phosphorylase: Effects of Thyroid State. Life Sci 24(1979)35–42

Quinn, P.V.; Hornbrook, K.R.; Brody, T.M.: Blockade of Catecholamine-Induced Phosphorylase Activation by N-Isopropylmethoxamine (B.W. 61-43) in Certain Tissues. Pharmacologist 7(1965)140

Robison, G.A.; Butcher, R.W.; Sutherland, E.W.: Adenyl Cyclase as an Adrenergic Receptor. Ann NY Acad Sci 139(1967)703–723

Robison, G.A.; Butcher, R.W.; Sutherland, E.W.: Cyclic AMP. Academic, New York, 1971

Robison, G.A.; Langley, P.E.; Burns, T.W.: Adrenergic Receptors in Human Adipocytes—Divergent Effects on Adenosine 3'-5'-Monophosphate and Lipolysis. Biochem Pharmacol 21(1972)589–592

Rudman, D.; Brown, S.J.; Malkin, M.F.: Adipokinetic Actions of Adrenocorticotropin, Thyroid-Stimulating Hormone, Vasopressin, α- and β-Melanocyte-Stimulating Hormones, Fraction H, Epinephrine and Norepinephrine in the Rabbit, Guinea-Pig, Hamster, Rat, Pig and Dog. Endocrinology 72(1963)527–543

Rugg, E.L.; Barnett, D.B.; Nahorski, S.R.: Coexistence of Beta$_1$ and Beta$_2$ Adrenoceptors in Mammalian Lung: Evidence from Direct Binding Studies. Mol Pharmacol 14(1978) 996–1005

Schümann, H.J.; Endoh, M.: α-Adrenoceptors in the Ventricular Myocardium: Clonidine, Naphazoline and Methoxamine as Partial α-Agonists Exerting a Competitive Dualism in Action to Phenylephrine. Eur J Pharmacol 36(1976)413–421

Shand, D.G.; Rangno, R.E.; Evans, G.H.: The Disposition of Propranolol. II. Hepatic Elimination in the Rat. Pharmacology 8(1972)344–352

Sherline, P.; Lynch, A.; Glinsmann, W.H.: Cyclic AMP and Adrenergic Receptor Control of Rat Liver Glycogen Metabolism. Endocrinology 91(1972)680–690

Shimazu, T.; Amakawa, A.: Regulation of Glycogen Metabolism in Liver by the Autonomic Nervous System. VI. Possible Mechanism of Phosphorylase Activation by the Splanchnic Nerve. Biochim Biophys Acta 385(1975)242–256

Slater, J.H.; Powell, C.E.: Blockade of Adrenergic Inhibitory Receptor Sites by 1-(3',4'-dichlorophenyl)-2-isopropylaminoethanol Hydrochloride. Fed Proc 16(1957)336

Stanton, H.C.: Selective Metabolic and Cardiovascular Beta Receptor Antagonism in the Rat. Arch Int Pharmacodyn Ther 196(1972)246–258

Starke, K.: Regulation of Noradrenaline Release by Presynaptic Receptor Systems. Rev Physiol Biochem Pharmacol 77(1977)1–124

Steinberg, D.; Mayer, S.E.; Khoo, J.C.; Miller, E.A.; Miller, R.E.; Fredholm, N.; Eichner, R.: Hormonal Regulation of Lipase, Phosphorylase, and Glycogen Synthase in Adipose Tissue. Adv Cyclic Nucleotide Res 5(1975)549–568

Sutherland, E.W.; Rall, T.W.: Fractionation and Characterization of a Cyclic Adenine Ribonucleotide Formed by Tissue Particles. J Biol Chem 232(1958)1077–1091

Todd, E.P.; Vick, R.L.: Kalemotropic Effect of Epinephrine: Analysis with Adrenergic Agonists and Antagonists. Am. J. Physiol. 220(1971)1964–1969.

Tolbert, M.E.M.; Butcher, F.R.; Fain, J.N.: Lack of Correlation Between Catecholamine Effects on Cyclic Adenosine 3′:5′-Monophosphate and Gluconeogenesis in Isolated Rat Liver Cells. J Biol Chem 248(1973)5686–5692

Tsai, B.S.; Lefkowitz, R.J.: [³H] Dihydroergocryptine Binding to Alpha Receptors in Canine Aortic Membranes. J Pharmacol Exp Ther 204(1978)606–614

Tsien, R.W.: Cyclic AMP and Contractile Activity in Heart. Adv Cyclic Nucleotide Res 8(1977)363–420

Turtle, J.R.; Kipnis, D.M.: An Adrenergic Receptor Mechanism for the Control of Cyclic 3′,5′ Adenosine Monophosphate Synthesis in Tissues. Biochem Biophys Res Commun 28(1967)797–802

U'Prichard, D.C.; Greenberg, D.A.; Snyder, S.H.: Binding Characteristics of a Radiolabeled Agonist and Antagonist at Central Nervous System Alpha Noradrenergic Receptors. Mol Pharmacol 13(1977)454–473

U'Prichard, D.C.; Bylund, D.B.; Snyder, S.H.: (±)-[³H]-Epinephrine and (−)-[³H]-Dihydroalprenolol Binding to β_1 and β_2-Noradrenergic Receptors in Brain, Heart, and Lung Membranes. J Biol Chem 253(1978)5090–5102

Van Roy, F.P.; Schulhof, L.W.: The Effect of Sympathomimetics on Glycogenolysis of Rat Liver Slices in Vitro. Arch Int Pharmacodyn Ther 130(1961)368–373

Verma, S.C.; McNeill, J.H.: Biochemical and Mechanical Effects of Phenylephrine on the Heart. Eur J Pharmacol 36(1976)447–450

Watanabe, A.M.; Hathaway, D.R.; Besch, H.R.; Farmer, B.B.; Harris, R.A.: α-Adrenergic Reduction of Cyclic Adenosine Monophosphate Concentrations in Rat Myocardium. Circ Res 40(1977)596–602

Wenke, M.; Mühlbachová, E.; Hynie, S.: Effects of some Sympathicotropic Agents on the Lipid Metabolism. Arch Int Pharmacodyn Ther 136(1962)104–112

Wenzel, D.G.; Su, J.L.: Interactions between Sympathomimetic Amines and Blocking Agents on the Rat Ventricle Strip. Arch Int Pharmacodyn Ther 160(1966)379–389

Williams, L.T.; Jarett, L.; Lefkowitz, R.J.: Adipocyte β-Adrenergic Receptors. Identification and Subcellular Localization by (−)-(³H) Dihydroalprenolol Binding. J Biol Chem 251(1976a)3096–3104

Williams, L.T.; Mullikin, D.; Lefkowitz, R.J.: Identification of α-Adrenergic Receptors in Uterine Smooth Muscle Membranes by [³H] Dihydroergocryptine Binding. J Biol Chem 251(1976b)6915–6923

Williamson, J.R.: Effects of Epinephrine on Glycogenolysis and Myocardial Contractility. In: Handbook of Physiology, Section 7: Endocrinology, Vol. VI, Adrenal Gland, pp. 605–636, ed. by H. Blaschko, G. Sayers, A.D. Smith. American Physiological Society, Washington, 1975

Wise, L.S.; Jungas, R.L.: Evidence for a Dual Mechanism of Lipolysis Activation by Epinephrine in Rat Adipose Tissue. J Biol Chem 253(1978)2624–2627

Wolfe, B.B.; Harden, T.K.; Molinoff, P.B.: β-Adrenergic Receptors in Rat Liver: Effects of Adrenalectomy. Proc Natl Acad Sci USA 73(1976)1343–1347

Wolfe, B.B.; Harden, T.K.; Molinoff, P.B.: In Vitro Study of β-Adrenergic Receptors. Annu Rev Pharmacol Toxicol 17(1977)575–604

Yabuuchi, Y.: The β-Adrenoceptor Stimulant Properties of OPC-2009 on Guinea-Pig Isolated Tracheal, Right Atrial and Left Atrial Preparations. Br J Pharmacol 61(1977)513–521

Zaagsma, J.; Meems, L.; Boorsma, M.: β-Adrenoceptor Studies. 4. Influence of Albumin on in Vitro β-Adrenoceptor Blocking and Antiarrhythmic Properties of Propranolol, Pindolol, Practolol and Metoprolol. Naunyn Schmiedebergs Arch Pharmacol 298(1977)29–36

The Subclassification of β-Adrenoceptors: Evidence in Support of the Dual β-Adrenoceptor Hypothesis

Michael J. Daly and Geoffrey P. Levy

I. INTRODUCTION

The idea that the β-adrenoceptor, as originally defined by Ahlquist (1948), might actually exist as two or more subtypes was first proposed just over a decade ago (Moran, 1966; Furchgott, 1967; Lands et al., 1967a; Lands, Luduena, and Buzzo, 1967b), and it has provided the stimulus for much subsequent work and conjecture. At least three trends appear evident to us in the developments since 1967.

We thank all the people in the Pharmacology Department, Glaxo-Allenburys Research (Ware) Ltd., who have contributed to the work described in this chapter. In particular, we are indebted to Mr. G.H. Apperley for carrying out many of the experiments in anesthetized guinea pigs and cats, and helping with the references. We especially thank Miss K. Bacon for so cheerfully and efficiently typing the manuscript.

First, after the introduction of the dual β-adrenoceptor hypothesis by Lands and coworkers, the β-1:β-2 terminology quickly achieved a wide usage in the pharmacological and medical literature. We think that this occurred because the introduction of the dual β-adrenoceptor hypothesis coincided with the introduction of a new kind of β-adrenoceptor antagonist, practolol (Dunlop and Shanks, 1968), and a new kind of β-adrenoceptor agonist, salbutamol (Brittain et al., 1968; Cullum et al., 1969). Practolol was shown to be more potent in blocking β-adrenoceptors in cardiac muscle than in airways and vascular smooth muscle and so could be conveniently categorized as a β-1 blocker. On the other hand, salbutamol was shown to be more potent in activating β-adrenoceptors in airways and vascular smooth muscle than in cardiac muscle and so could be conveniently categorized as a β-2 agonist. Of course, practolol and salbutamol were only the first of what rapidly became large groups of β-1 blockers and β-2 agonists respectively; and the β-1:β-2 terminology has enjoyed a correspondingly wide usage.

The second trend arose out of investigations undertaken subsequent to those of Lands and coworkers into the question of the subclassification of β-adrenoceptors. The conclusion from most of these studies was that the dual β-adrenoceptor hypothesis was an oversimplification and that it was necessary therefore to postulate the existence of several subtypes of β-adrenoceptor (see Furchgott, 1972 for references). These two conflicting trends have resulted in the paradox of the wide acceptance of the β-1:β-2 terminology for descriptive purposes on the one hand and the wide rejection of its scientific validity on the other.

The third trend relates to the growing awareness of the possibility that the receptors designated β-1 and β-2 can occur together and can mediate the same response in a single tissue or organ. This idea was first suggested in 1972, but its wider implications are only now becoming appreciated.

II. SCOPE OF THIS CHAPTER

This chapter has two main purposes: first, to summarize evidence for the essential validity of the dual β-adrenoceptor hypothesis that has been obtained in a range of experiments carried out in this laboratory over the past eight years; and second, to review the rapidly growing body of evidence concerning the occurrence of both β-1 and β-2 adrenoceptors in a single tissue or organ. We believe that this concept resolves many of the discrepancies that have led to doubts about the validity of the dual β-adrenoceptor hypothesis. We will then go on to consider briefly some of the implications of these ideas.

It is not our intention to review all the literature relating to the question of the subclassification of β-adrenoceptors. In an authoritative article,

Furchgott (1972) reviewed the evidence available up to 1972 on subtypes of β-adrenoceptor and evaluated the pharmacological procedures used for the characterization and classification of adrenoceptors from the standpoint of receptor theory. We have used his article as the starting point for this chapter, and we recommend that the reader do the same.

III. APPRAISAL OF THE DUAL β-ADRENOCEPTOR HYPOTHESIS

A. Experiments in Isolated Tissues

There are two standard pharmacological procedures for receptor classification: the determination of relative potencies in a series of agonists and the determination of the potencies of competitive antagonists. Lands and coworkers (1967a) used the first procedure in the formulation of their dual β-adrenoceptor hypothesis. However, the two procedures were first applied systematically to the question of the subclassification of β-adrenoceptors by Furchgott (1967). He determined the relative potencies of noradrenaline, adrenaline, isoprenaline, and phenylephrine for responses mediated by β-adrenoceptors in selected isolated tissues from rabbit and guinea pig. In some of the tissues the dissociation constant for pronethalol was also determined. In all of these experiments α-adrenoceptors and the adrenergic neuronal uptake process were blocked. It is of interest to note that two different rank orders of agonist potency were observed. On β-receptors in atrial and gastrointestinal smooth muscle (classified by Lands as β-1) the rank order was isoprenaline > noradrenaline ≥ adrenaline > phenylephrine; on β-receptors in aortic and tracheal smooth muscle (classified by Lands as β-2) the rank order was isoprenaline > adrenaline > noradrenaline > phenylephrine. However, Furchgott was not able to relate his results to the dual β-adrenoceptor hypothesis, since his work was published shortly before Lands and coworkers' papers in 1967. In fact, Furchgott concluded, mainly because of differences in the dissociation constant of pronethalol, that there may be at least three subtypes of β-adrenoceptor even within the limited number of tissues investigated, although he emphasized that a final classification of the subtypes would be premature until further adequately controlled and designed experiments had been completed.

Because of the controversy that arose after the introduction of the dual β-adrenoceptor hypothesis, we decided in 1970–71 to undertake a systematic and wide-ranging study in isolated tissues into the question of the subclassification of β-adrenoceptors. Using Furchgott's (1967) study as the prototype, we determined the relative potencies of agonists and the dissociation constants of antagonists on β-adrenoceptors mediating the pharmacological (but not metabolic) responses originally categorized by Lands and coworkers (1967a, b). We used the three catecholamines that were so important in the formulation of both Ahlquist's and Lands' classifications—isoprenaline, adrenaline, and noradrenaline—and the standard β-adrenoceptor antagonist, propranolol. We also included two of the selectively acting drugs that were not available for the previous investigations, salbutamol and practolol. We took steps to minimize the influence of factors that could distort estimates of agonist and antagonist potency at the level of the β-adrenoceptor. To this end, α-adrenoceptors, uptake$_1$, and uptake$_2$ (and thereby access to the catecholamine-metabolizing enzymes monoamine oxidase and catechol O-methyltransferase) were blocked; and allowance was made for any change in sensitivity of tissues by the use of appropriate controls. Whenever possible, complete concentration-response curves were obtained for the agonists. For the antagonists we determined pA$_2$ values against isoprenaline by the method of Arunlakshana and Schild (1959). Sufficient time was allowed for the antagonists to come into equilibrium with the receptors. Antagonism was judged to be competitive and the pA$_2$ value assumed to correspond to the dissociation constant only 1) when the antagonist caused parallel displacement to the right of the agonist concentration-effect curve with no reduction in the maximum response and 2) when the Schild plot gave a linear regression with a slope not significantly different from unity. If any one of these criteria was not fulfilled, then a pA$_2$ value was not quoted.

We argued that if only one pattern of activity was obtained with the agonists and antagonists over the range of tissues examined, this result would suggest that there is only one type of β-adrenoceptor. If two distinct patterns of activity were obtained, this finding would suggest that there are two subtypes of β-adrenoceptor; if, furthermore, the distribution of the two patterns of activity corresponded to the suggested distribution of β-1 and β-2 adrenoceptors, this correspondence would validate the Lands dual β-adrenoceptor hypothesis. Finally, if several distinct patterns of activity were obtained, this finding would suggest that there are several subtypes of β-adrenoceptor.

Our results and some additional results from other laboratories, where appropriate, are summarized in Table 1. Two distinct patterns of activity are apparent. In tissues said by Lands and coworkers to contain β-1 adrenoceptors, the rank order of potency of the catecholamines was isoprenaline $\geq$ noradrenaline $>$ adrenaline; salbutamol was a very weak, and in some cases a partial, agonist; propranolol was a potent antagonist; and practolol was a relatively potent antagonist. In contrast, in tissues said to contain β-2 adrenoceptors, the rank order of potency of the catecholamines was isoprenaline $>$ adrenaline $>$ noradrenaline, salbutamol was a potent and full agonist, and propranolol was again a potent antagonist; but practolol was a very weak antagonist. Results obtained on guinea pig left atrium and chick rectum, representative of the two distinct patterns of activity, are illustrated in Figure 1. The degrees of precision obtained for the estimates of agonistic and antagonistic potency in these two preparations are representative of those obtained over the range of preparations examined. Plainly, these results are consistent with the idea of two distinct β-adrenoceptor subtypes corresponding to the β-1 and β-2 adrenoceptors of Lands and coworkers.

The evidence on which this conclusion is based is in a sense derived from three independent sources: from the catecholamines, from a noncatecholamine β-adrenoceptor agonist (salbutamol), and from a β-adrenoceptor antagonist (practolol). It is important to recognize that there are limitations associated with the evidence obtained from each of these sources; these will now be considered.

The three catecholamines used in this study are excellent substrates for neuronal and/or extraneuronal uptake; in addition, noradrenaline and adrenaline are potent α-adrenoceptor agonists. Consequently, estimates of catecholamine potency at β-adrenoceptors are especially liable to distortion. The influence of these distorting factors was reduced in the present experiments by the use of appropriate blocking drugs, but it is unlikely to have been entirely eliminated. This has to be borne in mind when assessing the results.

Attention has been drawn to a more fundamental problem associated with the use of agonists for receptor classification. Two quantities are required to define the combination of an agonist with the receptor: its affinity and its efficacy (Stephenson, 1956). These quantities are difficult to measure for strong agonists (Jenkinson, 1973); and for this reason, comparison of relative potency is often used instead, as in the present study. However, there is no reason to suppose that the relationship between the stimulus (as defined by Stephenson, 1956) and the final response is the same for all organs (Furchgott, 1972; Schild, 1973; Jenkinson, 1973). If there were significant differences in this respect, comparison of the relative potency of agonists with unequal efficacies would reveal differences, even though the receptors concerned were identical. For example, an agonist with a low efficacy would be relatively less potent than one with a high efficacy in an organ in which a high stimulus was necessary for threshold response than in an organ in which a low stimulus was necessary. This is unlikely to be a complication with the three catecholamines used here, since they appear to have high and essentially equal efficacies at β-adrenoceptors (Furchgott, 1975). In these circumstances the relative potencies will be the same as the relative affinity constants. It could well be a complication, however, with salbutamol, which clearly has a lower efficacy than isoprenaline in tissues in which it is a partial agonist, but which may also have a lower efficacy than isoprenaline in tissues in which it is normally a

Table 1. Potencies of agonists and antagonists at β-adrenoceptors in isolated tissues

Preparation	Experimental Conditions	Response	Agonist Potency [Equipotent Concentration]				Antagonist Potency [pA$_2$(45 Min) vI (Slope)]		Proposed Receptor Type
			I	N	A	S	Propranolol	Practolol	
Cardiac Muscle									
Guinea Pig Left Atrium (2.5 Hz)	Krebs, 38°C. Animals pretreated with reserpine, 0.5 mg/kg i.p. 24 h prior to experiment. Atria incubated with phenoxybenzamine, 5 µg/ml for 20 m	Increase in force of contraction	1	15	22	616P	8.39 (1.01)	6.73 (0.93)	β-1
Guinea Pig Right Atrium		Increase in rate of beating	1	26	31	581P	8.83 (0.86)	6.70 (0.94)	β-1
Rabbit Left Atrium (2.5 Hz)	Krebs, 37°C. Atria incubated with phenoxybenzamine, 5 µg/ml for 20 m	Increase in force of contraction	1^a	7^a	14^a	2500P	8.61^b (1.03)	6.85^b (0.92)	β-1
Chick Left Atrium (2 Hz)	Krebs, 32°C. Atria incubated with phenoxybenzamine, 1 µg/ml for 20 m	Increase in force of contraction	1	7	15	3700P	—		β-1
Frog Ventricle (1 Hz)	Krebs, 26°C. Atria incubated with phenoxybenzamine, 1 µg/ml for 20 m	Increase in force of contraction	1^c	333^c	8^c	26	8.55 (1.06)	4.85 (1.09)	β-2
Vascular Smooth Muscle									
Rabbit Thoracic Aortic Strip	Krebs, 37°C, plus phenoxybenzamine, 1 µg/ml, cocaine, 10 µg/ml and deoxycorticosterone acetate, 10 µg/ml.	Reduction of KCl-induced concentration	1	358	6	9	9.09 (0.94)	5.05 (0.88)	β-2
Rat Aortic Strip	As above	Reduction of BaCl$_2$-induced contraction	1	303	6	26	9.49 (0.90)	c.a. 5.0	β-2
Dog Skeletal Muscle Artery		Reduction of KCl-induced contraction		21^d	1^d	—	8.62^d	<5.0^d	β-2
Dog Coronary Artery		Reduction of KCl-induced contraction	1^d	6^d	36^d	—	8.81^d	6.83^d	β-1
Pig Coronary Artery		Reduction of KCl-induced				632P^e	8.41^e (1.07)	6.59^e (0.99)	β-1

Tissue	Conditions	Response							Type
Tracheal Smooth Muscle									
Guinea Pig Tracheal Strip	Krebs, 38°C. Tracheal strip incubated with phenoxybenzamine, 5 μg/ml for 20 m	Reduction of methacholine-induced contraction	1	24	9	28	8.33 (0.82)	4.77 (1.07)	β-2
Gastro-Intestinal Smooth Muscle									
Guinea Pig Esophageal Longitudinal Muscle	Krebs, 32°C, plus phentolamine, 1 μg/ml; and cocaine, 10 μg/ml	Reduction of acetylcholine-induced contraction	1	40	74	>1000	8.25 (0.99)	6.68 (0.83)	β-1
Guinea Pig Ileum	Krebs, 32°C, plus phentolamine, 0.1 μg/ml; cocaine, 10 μg/ml; and metanephrine, 10 μg/ml	Reduction of histamine-induced contraction	1	5	23	804	—	—	β-1
Rabbit Duodenum	Krebs, 37°C, plus atropine, 0.1 μg/ml; phentolamine, 1 μg/ml; cocaine 10 μg/ml, and metanephrine, 10 μg/ml	Reduction of spontaneous motility	1	4	27	990	—	—	β-1
Rat Colon	Krebs, 32°C, plus phentolamine, 1 μg/ml; cocaine, 10 μg/ml; and metanephrine, 10 μg/ml	Reduction of methacholine-induced contraction	1	6	13	1215	—	—	β-1
Rat Fundus	Krebs (Mg^{++} excluded, low Ca^{++}), 32°C, plus additions listed above	Reduction of acetylcholine-induced tone	1	7	14	794	—	—	β-1
Mouse Caecum	Krebs (Mg^{++} excluded, low Ca^{++}), 32°C, plus additions listed above	Reduction of spontaneous motility	1	15	17	>1000P	—	—	β-1
Chick Rectum	Krebs, 32°C, plus additions listed above	Reduction of K$^+$ and methacholine-induced tone	1	123	3	32	8.38 (1.14)	4.67 (1.15)	β-2

continued

Table 1—continued

Preparation	Experimental Conditions	Response	Agonist Potency [Equipotent Concentration]				Antagonist Potency [pA$_2$(45 Min) vI (Slope)]		Proposed Receptor Type
			I	N	A	S	Propranolol	Practolol	
Uterine Smooth Muscle									
Rat Uterus	de Jalons, 30°C, plus phentolamine, 1 µg/ml; cocaine, 10 µg/ml; and deoxycorticosterone acetate, 10 µg/ml	Reduction of carbachol-induced contraction	1	370	8	24	8.56 (0.99)	5.12 (0.87)	β-2
Guinea Pig Uterus	Krebs (Mg^{++} excluded, low Ca^{++}) plus phentolamine, 1 µg/ml; cocaine, 1 µg/ml; and deoxycorticosterone acetate, 10 µg/ml	Reduction of BaCl$_2$-induced contraction	1	404	31	3	—	—	β-2
Rat Mesovarium		Reduction of KCl-induced contraction	1^f	344^f	5^f	30^f	8.8^f	5.2^f	β-2

Each value is the mean of at least 6 experiments. (−)-Isoprenaline was included as the reference agonist in each experiment in which agonist potency was determined.

I, (−)-isoprenaline; N, (−)-noradrenaline; A, (−)-adrenaline; S, (±)-salbutamol; P, partial agonist compared to (−)-isoprenaline.

[a] Results from Furchgott (1967).
[b] Results from Bristow, Sherrod, and Green (1970).
[c] Results from Lands et al. (1967b).
[d] Results from Baron et al. (1972).
[e] Results from Drew and Levy (1972).
[f] Results from Apperley et al. (1978).

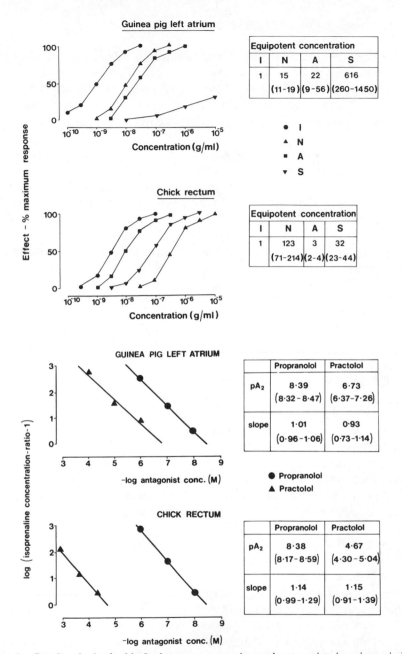

Guinea pig left atrium

Equipotent concentration

I	N	A	S
1	15	22	616
	(11-19)	(9-56)	(260-1450)

- ● I
- ▲ N
- ■ A
- ▼ S

Chick rectum

Equipotent concentration

I	N	A	S
1	123	3	32
	(71-214)	(2-4)	(23-44)

GUINEA PIG LEFT ATRIUM

	Propranolol	Practolol
pA_2	8·39 (8·32-8·47)	6·73 (6·37-7·26)
slope	1·01 (0·96-1·06)	0·93 (0·73-1·14)

- ● Propranolol
- ▲ Practolol

CHICK RECTUM

	Propranolol	Practolol
pA_2	8·38 (8·17-8·59)	4·67 (4·30-5·04)
slope	1·14 (0·99-1·29)	1·15 (0·91-1·39)

Figure 1. Results obtained with β-adrenoceptor agonists and antagonists in guinea pig left atrium (a tissue displaying the typical β-1 adrenoceptor pattern of activity) and chick rectum (a tissue displaying the typical β-2 adrenoceptor pattern of activity). The results of typical experiments are illustrated. Values in the tables are means of at least six experiments, with 95% confidence limits in brackets. Equipotent concentrations were calculated by comparison of EC_{50} values, where the EC_{50} is defined as the concentration of agonist required to produce 50% of the maximum response to that agonist. I, ($-$)-isoprenaline; N, ($-$)-noradrenaline; A, ($-$)-adrenaline; S, ($\pm$)-salbutamol.

355

full agonist. For example, salbutamol is normally a full agonist compared to isoprenaline in guinea-pig tracheal strip, but it becomes a partial agonist when the preparation is strongly contracted by concentrations of carbachol (O'Donnell and Wanstall, 1978). Therefore, the evidence obtained with salbutamol in support of the dual β-adrenoceptor hypothesis cannot by itself be considered definitive.

Evidence obtained with antagonists does not suffer from this drawback because only one quantity, the affinity constant for the combination between the receptor and the antagonist, need be established and the experimental procedure for its determination is relatively simple. Nevertheless, the experimentally determined value may be in considerable error—first, if the preparation used possesses an active saturable removal process for the agonist being used; and second, if the antagonist prevents the removal or inactivation of the agonist (Furchgott, 1972). A particularly pertinent example of the latter has been described recently by Kenakin and Black (1978), who showed that practolol inhibited catechol O-methyltransferase in rat atria, and thereby sensitized the preparation to isoprenaline, at slightly lower concentrations than those at which it inhibited β-adrenoceptors. This additional action resulted in nonlinearity of the Schild plot and in an underestimate of the affinity constant for practolol. We think that such factors are unlikely to have greatly affected the estimates of the affinity constant for practolol in our experiments, however, because of the precautions that were taken. For example, block of uptake$_2$ must have restricted access to catechol O-methyltransferase. Another property of practolol that could complicate estimates of its affinity constant is its intrinsic activity, since prolonged application of agonists, partial or otherwise, may cause receptor desensitization (Jenkinson, 1973). Although the intrinsic activity of practolol is not pronounced (Barrett and Carter, 1970; Kenakin and Black, 1978), there is as yet no means of knowing whether it influenced the affinity-constant values obtained.

We think, therefore, that it would be unwise to conclude that there are two subtypes of β-adrenoceptor on the basis of the data obtained from any one of these three sources of evidence *alone*. But when the data are *combined*, and when the magnitude of the differences between the two patterns of activity is considered, then in our submission there is a strong case in favor of the idea of two subtypes of β-adrenoceptor.

There are several specific points arising out of the results in Table 1 that require comment. First, we were unable to obtain pA_2 estimates for propranolol and practolol in guinea-pig ileum, rabbit duodenum, rat colon, rat fundus, and mouse caecum. Both antagonists caused parallel displacement to the right of the isoprenaline dose-response curves in these preparations; but for reasons that are not yet understood, the displacement could not be extended beyond 10- to 30-fold and was often not dose-dependent even over this range. The only useful information to be derived from these experiments is that the β-adrenoceptor blocking action of propranolol was evident at concentrations as low as 10^{-8} M and that of practolol at concentrations as low as 10^{-6} M, which is at least consistent with the agonist data indicating that the receptor is of the β-1 subtype. Second, although salbutamol is a partial agonist in many preparations that exhibit the typical β-1 adrenoceptor pattern of activity and is a full agonist in many preparations that exhibit the typical β-2 adrenoceptor pattern of activity, this distinction is not invariable. For example, salbutamol is a full agonist compared to isoprenaline on several mammalian gastrointestinal preparations (see Table 1) and was shown to be a full agonist, although 1,000 times less potent than isoprenaline, on the practolol-sensitive β-adrenoceptors in kitten papillary muscle (Kaumann, Birnbaumer, and Wittmann, 1978); conversely, salbutamol can behave as a partial agonist in guinea-pig tracheal strip under certain conditions as noted above. Third, the fact that the racemic form of salbutamol was used in our experiments raises the possibility that its selectivity is due to an interaction between the (−) and (+) isomers in the racemate (Patil, Lapidus, and Tye, 1970). This possibility can be discounted, however, because the (−) isomer has been shown to resemble the racemic compound in being much more active in tracheal muscle than in cardiac muscle (Brittain, Farmer, and Marshall, 1973). Finally, attention should be drawn to two anomalous results in table 1. The potencies of noradrenaline and adrenaline relative to isoprenaline in guinea pig esophageal longitudinal muscle were unusually low; the reason for this is not apparent. The potency of noradrenaline relative to isoprenaline in guinea pig tracheal strip was unusually high; the likely reason for this is presented in section IV A.

B. Experiments in Anesthetized Guinea pigs and Cats

The early clinical trials with salbutamol demonstrated that the most common side effect associated with its systemic administration is an enhancement of physiological tremor. This is now known to be true for all β-stimulant bronchodilator drugs when administered systemically (see Apperley, Daly, and Levy, 1976, for references). The enhancement of physiological tremor is thought to be mediated directly through β-adrenoceptors located on skeletal muscle (Marsden and Meadows, 1968); thus, β-adrenoceptor agonists decrease the degree of fusion and tension developed during submaximal tetanic contractions of the slow-contracting motor units in human muscle (Marsden and Meadows, 1970). The same effects are produced in slow-contracting skeletal muscle from animals—for example, cat and guinea pig soleus muscles (Bowman and Zaimis, 1958; Apperley and Levy, 1975)—and these preparations have been used to predict the tremor-enhancing potential of β-adrenoceptor agonists in man. Two related questions arise: empirically, can the bronchodilator and tremor-enhancing effects of β-adrenoceptor agonists be dissociated; and, more fundamentally, can the β-adrenoceptors mediating these two effects be differentiated? We carried out experiments in anesthetized guinea pigs and cats, the results of which go some way toward answering these two questions and also provide further evidence on the more general question of the subclassification of β-adrenoceptors.

    1. Guinea pig The effects of β-adrenoceptor agonists were compared on the lung, measured as changes in tracheal segment pressure, soleus muscle, and heart rate (Apperley and Levy, 1975) (Table 2 and Figure 2). Blood pressure was also monitored, but the β-adrenoceptor agonists produced either small vasodepressor responses that often were not dose-related, or even, on occasion, vasopressor responses. This is because the

ANAESTHETIZED GUINEA PIG

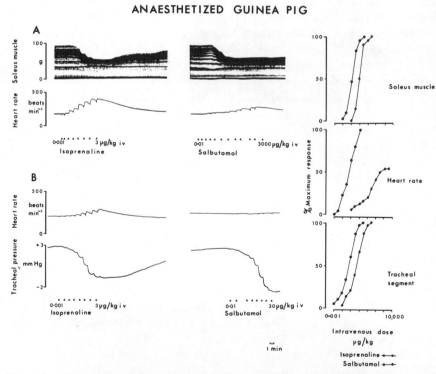

Figure 2. Comparison of the actions of ($-$)-isoprenaline and ($\pm$)-salbutamol in the pentobarbitone-anesthetized guinea pig. Guinea pig (A)—soleus muscle tension and heart rate; guinea pig (B)—tracheal segment pressure and heart rate. Paired experiments were carried out because the time course of the soleus muscle responses was slower than that of the tracheal segment responses. Note that salbutamol was clearly less potent relative to isoprenaline on heart rate than on soleus muscle or tracheal segment and that it was a partial agonist compared to isoprenaline on heart rate, but a full agonist on soleus muscle and tracheal segment.

Table 2.   Activities of β-adrenoceptor agonists in the anesthetized guinea pig

Agonist	Equipotent Dose for		
	Decrease in Tracheal Pressure	Decrease in Soleus Muscle Tension	Increase in Heart Rate
(−)-Isoprenaline	1	1	1
	[ED_{50} = 0.03 μg/kg]	[ED_{50} = 0.03 μg/kg]	[ED_{50} = 0.07 μg/kg]
AH 4553	6	7	99P[a,b]
Fenoterol	8	6	159[b]
Trimetoquinol	9	9	17
Salbutamol	10	9	74P[b]
AH 12561	10	11	243P[b]
Terbutaline	29	34	257P[b]
Salmefamol	31	29	100P[b]
Orciprenaline	102	107	304[b]

All drugs administered intravenously. With the exception of (−)-isoprenaline the racemic form of each agonist was used.

[a] P, partial agonist compared to (−)-isoprenaline.

[b] Equipotent dose significantly higher than on the other responses ($P < 0.05$.)

resting blood pressure of the anesthetized guinea-pig is low, usually about 50 mmHg diastolic pressure. Blood pressure data, therefore, have not been reported. Nine β-adrenoceptor agonists with widely differing chemical structures were used (Apperley et al., 1976). Cumulative dose-response curves were determined for the agonists, isoprenaline being used as the reference drug in each experiment. Isoprenaline had an identical potency on tracheal segment and soleus muscle and a slightly lower potency on the heart. Two agonists, trimetoquinol and orciprenaline, were slightly less active on heart rate than on the other two responses. The other agonists were all markedly less active on heart rate than on the other two responses; and most, including salbutamol, were partial agonists compared to isoprenaline on heart rate. The potency of each of the nine agonists was virtually identical on tracheal segment and soleus muscle.

The potencies of propranolol; practolol; and H35/25, a β-adrenoceptor antagonist with apparently the opposite profile of selectivity to practolol (Levy, 1967), were determined against isoprenaline in the same experimental model (Table 3) (Apperley and Levy, 1975). Propranolol was virtually equipotent in blocking the three isoprenaline-induced responses. Practolol was clearly more potent in blocking heart rate responses than tracheal segment or soleus muscle responses to isoprenaline; H35/25 possessed exactly the opposite profile of blocking activity. There was no significant difference in the potency of practolol or H35/25 on tracheal segment and soleus muscle.

2. Cat   The effects of β-adrenoceptor agonists were determined on the lung, measured as an inhibition of 5-hydroxytryptamine–induced bron-

Table 3. Activities of β-adrenoceptor antagonists in the anesthetized guinea pig

	$ID_{50}{}^{a}$ (mg/kg i.v.) Against $(-)$-Isoprenaline		
Antagonist	Decrease in Tracheal Pressure	Decrease in Soleus Muscle Tension	Increase in Heart Rate
Propranolol	0.05	0.04	0.06
	(0.02–0.14)	(0.01–0.09)	(0.04–0.09)
Practolol	8	13	0.9
	(3–24)	(4–34)	(0.5–2)
H35/25	0.2	0.3	>10
	(0.1–0.4)	(0.2–0.4)	

The values quoted are means with 95% confidence limits in brackets.
[a] ID_{50}—dose of antagonist required to inhibit the response to $(-)$-isoprenaline by 50%.

chospasm, soleus muscle, blood pressure, and heart rate (Apperley et al., 1976) (Table 4). Once again, isoprenaline was used as the reference agonist in each experiment. The experimental design precluded estimation of EC_{50} values and of the maximum attainable responses. Nevertheless, isoprenaline was clearly unselective in its ability to inhibit 5-hydroxytryptamine–induced bronchospasm, decrease soleus muscle tension, decrease diastolic blood pressure, and increase heart rate. The slopes of the dose-response curves for the eight test agonists were parallel to those for isoprenaline on all four parameters. Trimetoquinol, like isoprenaline, was unselective in its action; but the other seven agonists each exhibited a significantly lower potency on heart rate than on the lung, soleus muscle, and blood pressure relative to

Table 4. Activities of β-adrenoceptor agonists in the anesthetized cat

	Equipotent Dose for			
Agonist	Inhibition of 5-Hydroxytryptamine-induced Bronchospasm	Decrease in Soleus Muscle Tension	Decrease in Diastolic Blood Pressure	Increase in Heart Rate
$(-)$Isoprenaline	1	1	1	1
Fenoterol	3	3	2	6^{a}
AH 4553	3	5	5	11^{a}
Trimetoquinol	3	3	4	4
AH 12561	4	4	5	18^{a}
Salmefamol	5	10	8	26^{a}
Salbutamol	9	9	9	27^{a}
Terbutaline	14	23	20	113^{a}
Orciprenaline	30	36	45	73^{a}

All drugs administered intravenously. With the exception of $(-)$-isoprenaline, the racemic form of each agonist was used.
[a] Equipotent dose significantly higher than on the other responses ($P < 0.05$).

isoprenaline. There was no significant difference in potency on the lung, soleus muscle, and blood pressure for any of the agonists.

In this respect our findings differ from those reported in the literature for several β-adrenoceptor agonists. Orciprenaline (Engelhardt, Hoefke, and Wick, 1961), fenoterol (O'Donnell, 1970), salbutamol, terbutaline (Wasserman and Levy, 1974), carbuterol (Wardell et al., 1974; Colella et al., 1977), and procaterol (OPC-2009) (Himori and Taira, 1977; Yabuuchi, Yamashita, and Tei, 1977; Yamashita, Takai, and Yabuuchi, 1978) have all been reported to be relatively less potent in lowering blood pressure than in preventing bronchospasm and/or in reducing soleus muscle tension in anesthetized cats or dogs; and these findings have led to the suggestion that the vascular β-adrenoceptor differs from the lung and soleus muscle β-adrenoceptors. We think that the difference between our results and the others arises because of methodological differences. In preliminary experiments in the anesthetized cat we noted that the longer-acting β-adrenoceptor agonists such as salbutamol caused desensitization of β-adrenoceptors in the vasculature but not elsewhere. To overcome this, isoprenaline and the test β-adrenoceptor agonist were administered alternately, beginning with doses selected for each drug to produce near-threshold responses and using threefold increases in dose in each case; not more than four dose levels of each drug were administered in any one experiment; and the interval between doses was at least 30 minutes and was sometimes as long as 1½ hours. If this procedure was not followed, the potency of the test agonist was always relatively lower on blood pressure than on the lung and soleus muscle. The fact that similar precautions were not taken in the other studies has resulted, in our opinion, in an underestimate of the relative potency of the previously mentioned agonists at the vascular β-adrenoceptor.

One observation that remains to be explained is the lower lung:heart selectivity of salbutamol and the other β-adrenoceptor agonists in cat than in guinea pig. A possible reason for this difference is discussed in Section IV A.

The potencies of propranolol, practolol, and H35/25 were also determined in the anesthetized cat (Table 5). Dose-response curves to isoprenaline were obtained for the lung, the soleus muscle, blood pressure, and heart rate before and after the intravenous administration of antagonist. Three or four dose levels of antagonist were tested in each cat. The results were analyzed by the method of Arunlakshana and Schild (1959) (Fig. 3). The antagonists all caused parallel displacements to the right of the isoprenaline dose-response curves on all four responses. The antagonist potency of propranolol was almost identical on the lung, the soleus muscle, and blood pressure and was only very slightly lower on the heart. In contrast, practolol was 10–12 times more potent on the heart than on the lung, the soleus muscle, and blood pressure; H35/25 possessed

Table 5. Activities of β-adrenoceptor antagonists in the anesthetized cat

Antagonist	Inhibition of 5-Hydroxytryptamine-Induced Bronchospasm		Decrease in Soleus Muscle Tension		Decrease in Diastolic Blood Pressure		Increase in Heart Rate	
	DR_{10}	Slope	DR_{10}	Slope	DR_{10}	Slope	DR_{10}	Slope
Propranolol	0.1 (0.08–0.2)[a]	1.1 (0.9–1.3)	0.1 (0.07–0.3)	1.0 (0.9–1.1)	0.1 (0.07–0.2)	1.0 (0.9–1.1)	0.2 (0.18–1.3)	1.1 (0.8–1.3)
Practolol	25 (11–59)	1.0 (0.7–1.2)	22 (14–35)	1.1 (0.9–1.4)	28 (24–33)	1.0 (0.9–1.1)	2 (1.6–3.2)	0.9 (0.8–1.0)
H35/25	4 (2–9)	1.1 (0.8–1.5)	5 (3–8)	1.2 (0.9–1.4)	5 (3–8)	1.4 (1.1–1.6)	>10	—

DR_{10}—dose of antagonist (mg/kg i.v.) to produce an isoprenaline dose ratio of 10.
Slope of regression obtained from plot of log (isoprenaline dose ratio—1) on log antagonist dose, (mg/kg i.v.).
[a] Figures in parentheses are 95% confidence limits.

ANAESTHETIZED CAT. PROPRANOLOL v ISOPRENALINE ON HEART RATE

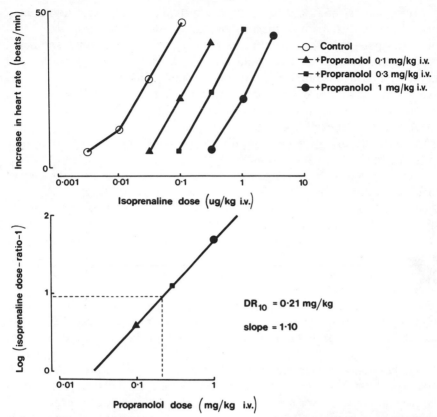

Figure 3. Interaction between propranolol and isoprenaline on the heart rate of the chlora-lose-anesthetized cat. DR_{10}—dose of antagonist (mg/kg i.v.) to produce an isoprenaline dose ratio of 10.

exactly the opposite profile of blocking activity. There was no significant difference in the antagonist potency of practolol or of H35/25 on the latter three responses.

The questions posed earlier in this section can now be reconsidered. Our results show that potency on the lung and the soleus muscle is the same for each of the nine β-adrenoceptor agonists tested. Corresponding studies with well over 100 β-adrenoceptor agonists synthesized in this laboratory (unpublished results) and with other β-adrenoceptor agonists reported in the literature (Bowman and Rodger, 1972; Gwee et al., 1972; Rodger, 1973) produced essentially the same finding. To date, there is only one β-adrenoceptor agonist, sulfonterol, for which a difference in potency on lung and soleus muscle has been claimed. Kaiser et al. (1975) reported that in the anesthetized cat, sulfonterol was 5 times less potent than isoprenaline on the lung, 30 times less potent on soleus muscle, 2,300 times less potent on blood pressure, and 34 times less potent on the heart. However, we could not confirm these results; in our anesthetized cat model, sulfonterol was 20–40 times less potent than isoprenaline on the lung, the soleus muscle, and blood pressure and several hundred times less potent on the heart (Apperley and Levy, unpublished results). Once again, we think it likely that differences in experimental procedure account at least in part for the different results. Empirically, then, it appears unlikely that the bronchodilating and tremor-enhancing properties of β-adrenoceptor agonists can be dissociated, at least when the drugs are given systemically. At present the problem is overcome by giving the drugs by inhalation.

Our results with both agonists and antagonists also strongly suggest that the β-adrenoceptors in the lung and the soleus muscle are of the same type. This conclusion is in agreement with that of a previous, more limited study (Bowman and Nott, 1970).

On the more general question to which this chapter is addressed, the pronounced differences in potency shown by both agonists and antagonists on the β-adrenoceptors in the heart, on the one hand; and in the lung, the soleus muscle, and the vasculature, on the other, provide further striking support for the dual β-adrenoceptor hypothesis. The results suggest that β-1 adrenoceptors mediate positive chronotropic responses and that β-2 adrenoceptors mediate bronchodilator, tremor-enhancing, and vasodepressor responses.

It has to be recognized, however, that the force of this conclusion is tempered by the fact that there are limitations to the interpretation of experiments *in vivo* over and above those already described for experiments *in vitro* (Furchgott, 1972). For example, the assumption that the increase in heart rate in our experiments is a direct measure of the positive chronotropic potency of β-adrenoceptor agonists would not be justified if there was a significant reflex component in response to the accompanying vasodepressor response. The reflex component is large in conscious animals (Dunlop and Shanks, 1968; Daly, Farmer, and Levy, 1971); but in the anesthetized cat and guinea pig, positive chronotropic responses to β-adrenoceptor agonists appear to be entirely direct in origin (Bowman and Rodger, 1972; Apperley and Levy, unpublished observations). The assumption that the fall in blood pressure caused by β-adrenoceptor agonists in the anesthetized cat is a direct measure of their potency at vascular β-adrenoceptors would also not be justified if the vasodepressor response was attenuated to a significant degree by an increase in cardiac output. We have no direct evidence on this point, but the finding that the vasodepressor responses to isoprenaline were unaltered after cardiac responses had been abolished by practolol (Table 5) suggests that there is no significant attenuation. In this context it is important to note that in our experiments vasodepressor responses were measured as changes in diastolic, rather than mean or systolic, blood pressure because diastolic blood pressure changes are less influenced by changes in cardiac output. Even assuming that the response measured does reflect accurately the degree of β-adrenoceptor activation in the particular organ or system, there are further problems with *in vivo* experiments. In the intact animal, it is not possible to control the distribution and disposition patterns of the administered drugs and it is often not possible to measure responses to agonists or antagonists under steady-state conditions. It is easy to see, given all these limitations, how differences in agonist or antagonist potency might arise *in vivo* even though the receptors mediating the observed responses were the same. Nevertheless, we believe that the striking and complementary patterns of selectivity obtained with the agonists and antagonists in our experiments are most unlikely to have arisen merely because of limitations in the experimental conditions and that they can be explained satisfactorily only by postulating two subtypes of β-adrenoceptor. This point is perhaps best illustrated with an example. Let us therefore attempt to explain our results in terms of differences in the distribution of the drugs examined. One would have to postulate that isoprenaline and propranolol were each distributed more or less uniformly; that salbutamol and the other selective β-adrenoceptor agonists were each distributed to the same extent in bronchial, soleus, and vascular muscle, but to a lesser extent in cardiac muscle; that the same happened to be true for practolol; but that the opposite happened to be true for H35/25. Now it cannot be stated for certain that this series of coincidences did not occur, but it seems to us that the idea of two subtypes of β-adrenoceptor is far more probable. Turning the proposition upside down, it can be argued with some justification that the fact that such clear patterns of selectivity were obtained *despite* the limitations of *in vivo* experiments actually strengthens the conclusion that the responses are mediated by two subtypes of β-adrenoceptor. Furthermore, the striking correlation between the selectivity profiles of practolol and salbutamol *in vivo* and *in vitro* makes it highly unlikely that the *in vivo* selectivities are merely artifacts that arise because of limitations in the experimental conditions.

In summary, then, it is our contention that the *in vitro* and *in vivo* results, when considered together, represent an impressive body of evidence in support of the dual β-adrenoceptor hypothesis.

C. Experiments on β-Adrenoceptor—Coupled Adenylate Cyclase

The enzyme adenylate cyclase is stimulated by β-adrenoceptor agonists in virtually all tissues in which β-adrenoceptors can be demonstrated pharmacologically. The consequent generation of cyclic AMP appears to mediate many, if not all, of the effects of β-adrenoceptor agonists (Lefkowitz et al., 1976). If there are in fact two subtypes of β-adrenoceptor, the ability of selective β-adrenoceptor agonists and antagonists to respectively stimulate and block the generation of cyclic AMP should parallel the selectivity observed in pharmacological experiments on intact preparations. Two studies reported in the literature suggest that this may be the case.

Burges and Blackburn (1972) examined the effects of some β-adrenoceptor agonists and antagonists on adenylate cyclase activity in homogenates of rat heart and lung. The order of potency of catecholamines for stimulation of adenylate cyclase in rat heart homogenates was isoprenaline > noradrenaline > adrenaline; salbutamol was inactive. In rat lung homogenates the catecholamine order of potency was isoprenaline > adrenaline > noradrenaline; salbutamol was an effective stimulator of adenylate cyclase, about 8 times less potent than isoprenaline. The ability of propranolol, practolol, and butoxamine (a β-2 selective antagonist) to antagonize isoprenaline-induced stimulation of heart and lung adenylate cyclase was also investigated. Propranolol was virtually unselective, practolol was about 15 times more potent on heart than on lung adenylate cyclase, and butoxamine was about 4 times more active on lung than on heart adenylate cyclase.

Lefkowitz (1975) determined the potencies of a range of β-adrenoceptor agonists and antagonists on adenylate cyclase activity in membranes from dog myocardium, skeletal muscle, liver, lung, and paraovarian fat and from frog erythrocytes. The order of potency of catecholamines for stimulation of adenylate cyclase in cardiac and adipose membranes was isoprenaline > noradrenaline > adrenaline; in the other tissues the order was isoprenaline > adrenaline > noradrenaline. Propranolol was the most potent antagonist of isoprenaline-induced stimulation of adenylate cyclase in all tissues. Practolol was a more potent antagonist than butoxamine in heart and adipose membranes, but the reverse was true in other tissues. Soterenol did not fit into the pattern established with the other drugs. However, although soterenol has been characterized as a selective β-2 adrenoceptor agonist (Apperley et al., 1976), we have also found in unpublished experiments that it possesses additional actions—for example, a depressant or desensitizing action on cardiac muscle—and as shown by Lefkowitz (1975), it has a lower efficacy than isoprenaline at β-adrenoceptors. It is not therefore a very suitable agent to use for the investigation of β-adrenoceptor subtypes.

The conclusion drawn from both of these investigations was that the results are in reasonable agreement with the dual β-adrenoceptor hypothesis. A criticism of both studies is that the antagonistic potencies were determined against a single dose of isoprenaline rather than against isoprenaline dose-response curves. It should also be noted that some of the limitations that apply to pharmacological experiments in isolated tissues (outlined in Section III A) also apply to the adenylate cyclase experiments.

IV. EVIDENCE THAT β-1 AND β-2 ADRENOCEPTORS CAN OCCUR TOGETHER IN A SINGLE ORGAN OR TISSUE

A. Evidence from Pharmacological Experiments

Although the results of our experiments provide a large body of evidence in support of the dual β-adrenoceptor hypothesis, there is still a considerable body of evidence that at first sight appears to be inconsistent with the hypothesis and that therefore requires explanation. We think, with the benefit of hindsight, that much of this evidence is invalid, either because it was obtained from inadequately designed experiments or because the results were inadequately analyzed. Nevertheless, even when evidence of this type is discounted, there remains a small but significant body of evidence that cannot easily be reconciled with the dual β-adrenoceptor hypothesis.

One example comes from a study in cat isolated atria by Cornish and Miller (1975). They showed that the order of potency of the catecholamines in causing increases in cardiac rate and force of contraction was isoprenaline > noradrenaline $\geq$ adrenaline and that practolol was a relatively potent antagonist of isoprenaline (pA_2 = 6.54). These results would appear to indicate that the responses are mediated by β-1 adrenoceptors. On the other hand, salbutamol was a full agonist, 20–40 times less potent than isoprenaline; this fact would appear to indicate that the responses are mediated by β-2 adrenoceptors. Another example concerns results obtained with a potent β-2 selective agonist, MJ 9184-1, on airway smooth muscle, which supposedly contains β-2 adrenoceptors. MJ 9184-1 was equipotent with isoprenaline in relaxing guinea pig isolated trachea and half as potent as isoprenaline as a bronchodilator in the anesthetized cat; yet it was 158 times less potent than isoprenaline in relaxing cat isolated trachea (Davey, Malta, and Raper, 1974).

We think that these and many other inconsistencies can be explained by the idea that β-1 and β-2 adrenoceptors can occur together in the same organ or tissue and can mediate the same response. This was first suggested in 1972 by Carlsson and coworkers (Carlsson et al., 1972). They showed that equal submaximal chronotropic responses of cat heart to β-adrenoceptor agonists were blocked to different extents by different β-adrenoceptor blocking drugs (Fig. 4). Propranolol produced a pronounced block of all responses. The β-1 selective practolol reduced the responses to different degrees, the order being noradrenaline > isoprenaline > adrenaline > salbutamol. The β-2 selective H35/25 also produced a differential blockade but in the reverse order: salbutamol > adrenaline >

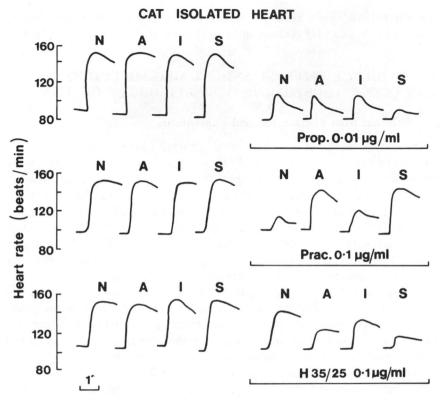

Figure 4. Cat isolated heart. Chronotropic responses to injected noradrenaline (N, 0.1–0.2 μg), adrenaline (A, 0.2–0.3 μg), isoprenaline (I, 0.01 μg) and salbutamol (S, 0.7–1 μg) before and during perfusion with propranolol (Prop.), practolol (Prac.), and H35/25. (Reproduced with permission from Carlsson et al., 1972.)

isoprenaline > noradrenaline. If it is assumed that isoprenaline is essentially nonselective, then, from the results presented in Section III A, it is clear that noradrenaline shows selectivity for β-1 adrenoceptors and adrenaline and salbutamol show selectivity for β-2 adrenoceptors. Carlsson and coworkers suggested, therefore, that the results could best be explained by assuming that *both* β1 and β-2 adrenoceptors mediate positive chronotropic responses in cat heart, the β-1 type constituting the major proportion and the β-2 type the minor proportion of the total population. In this situation the proportion of each type of receptor stimulated will depend both on the relative sensitivity of the agonist for β-1 and β-2 adrenoceptors and on the relative proportions of the two types of receptor. The chronotropic response to noradrenaline, for instance, seems to result mainly from β-1 adrenoceptor stimulation, as a consequence of the selectivity of noradrenaline for β-1 adrenoceptors and of the higher proportion of β-1 than β-2 adrenoceptors in the S-A node. On the other hand, despite the predominance of β-1 adrenoceptors, salbutamol appears to act mainly on β-2 adrenoceptors because of its very high degree of β-2 selectivity. Carlsson and coworkers have recently shown that the same pattern is obtained when dose-response curves to noradrenaline and adrenaline, instead of single doses, are examined in cat isolated heart. They showed that propranolol blocked noradrenaline and adrenaline positive chronotropic dose-response curves to about the same extent, that metoprolol (a β-1 selective antagonist) blocked noradrenaline dose-response curves to a greater extent than adrenaline dose-response curves, whereas butoxamine blocked adrenaline dose-response curves to a greater extent than noradrenaline dose-response curves (E. Carlsson, personal communication). Preliminary studies indicate that positive chronotropic responses of dog and human heart are also mediated by both β-1 and β-2 adrenoceptors, with β-1 adrenoceptors once again predominating (Ablad et al., 1975a).

Further support for this general idea has come from some elegant experiments carried out under carefully controlled conditions in guinea pig tracheal smooth muscle (Furchgott, 1976). Inhibitory concentration-response curves were obtained with both isoprenaline and noradrenaline in individual tracheal strips brought to a steady tone level with carbachol. In strips from 33 animals the molar potency ratio of isoprenaline: noradrenaline averaged 55, but it ranged from a low of 10 to a high of 300 in strips from different animals. It was postulated that variation of the isoprenaline: noradrenaline molar potency ratio resulted from variation of the β-1:β-2 adrenoceptor ratio, the molar potency ratio decreasing as the proportion of β-1 adrenoceptors increased. Support for this postulation was obtained by using practolol and isopropylmethoxamine (a β-2 selective antagonist). In strips with isoprenaline: noradrenaline molar potency ratios ranging from 10 to 45, the pA$_2$ for practolol was 6.06 against noradrenaline, 5.07 against isoprenaline, and 4.73 against salbutamol; whereas the pA$_2$ for isopropylmethoxamine was 5.04 against noradrenaline, 6.3 against isoprenaline, and 6.8 against salbutamol. On strips from one animal with an isoprenaline: noradrenaline molar potency ratio of 296 (practically all β-2 adrenoceptors) the pA$_2$ for practolol was 4.75 against both noradrenaline and isoprenaline. All these results are consistent with the hypothesis that tracheal smooth muscle of guinea pig has both β-1 and β-2 adrenoceptors, with predominance of the β-2 type but with ratios that vary from animal to animal.

Evidence reported mainly within the last three years indicates that the β-1:β-2 ratio can vary even between different regions of the same organ or tissue. For example, there appear to be differences in the proportions of β-1 and β-2 adrenoceptors in the sinus node and the myocardium of cat heart (Carlsson et al., 1977). Although the β-1 type is predominant in both regions, the proportion of β-2 adrenoceptors is higher in the sinus node than in the myocardium. The proportions of β-1:β-2 adrenoceptors also appear to vary in different regions of airways smooth muscle. For example, in cat lung strip the order of potency of the catecholamines in causing relaxation was isoprenaline > adrenaline > noradrenaline; salbutamol and terbutaline were potent agonists; and practolol was a relatively weak antagonist (pA$_2$ = 5.4). In contrast, in cat trachea the order of potency of the catecholamines was isoprenaline > noradrenaline > adrenaline, salbutamol and terbutaline were weaker agonists, and practolol was a more potent antagonist (pA$_2$ = 6.4) (Lulich, Mitchell, and Sparrow, 1976). Lulich et al. concluded that cat tracheal smooth muscle contains a predominance of β-1 adrenoceptors and cat lung smooth muscle a predominance of β-2 adrenoceptors. In a corresponding study in guinea pig airways, Zaagsma, Oudhof, and Van der Heijden (1978) showed that lung smooth muscle contains only β-2 adrenoceptors, whereas tracheal smooth muscle contains both β-1 and β-2 adrenoceptors, as was first demonstrated by Furchgott (see above). The vascular β-adrenoceptor was originally classified as β-2 (Lands et al., 1967a), and our results in the anesthetized cat (see Section III B) and dog (Daly, Flook, and Levy, 1975) show clearly that intravenously administered isoprenaline produces its vasodepressor response predominantly through β-2 adrenoceptors. Nevertheless, evidence is now available to suggest that β-1 adrenoceptors are present in certain vascular beds and that they can mediate vasodilatation. A clear example is shown in the investigation by Taira, Yabuuchi, and Yamashita (1977) of β-adrenoceptors mediating vasodilatation in femoral, superior mesenteric, and renal vascular beds of dogs pretreated with phenoxybenzamine. In the femoral and superior mesenteric beds salbutamol was about 15 times less potent than isoprenaline, whereas in the renal vascular bed it was about 240 times less potent. Vasodilator responses to isoprenaline in the femoral and superior mesenteric beds were unaffected by practolol, but those in the renal vascular bed were blocked by the same doses of practolol. In contrast, vasodilator responses to salbutamol in the renal vascular bed were unaffected by practolol. The authors concluded that the renal vascular bed contains both β-1 and β-2 adrenoceptors, whereas the femoral and superior mesenteric beds contain only β-2 adrenoceptors. Belfrage (1978b) obtained evidence to suggest that β-adrenoceptors mediating vasodilatation are mainly of the β-2 type in dog skeletal muscle but mainly of the β-1 type in dog subcutaneous adipose tissue. Edvinsson and Owman (1974), working with the middle cerebral artery isolated from the cat, and in which α-adrenoceptors, uptake$_1$, and uptake$_2$ were blocked, showed that the rank order of β-adrenoceptor agonist potency for causing vasodilatation was isoprenaline > noradrenaline = adrenaline > terbutaline. They concluded therefore that the receptors were of the β-1 subtype. There is a considerable amount of evidence that the β-adrenoceptor mediating vasodilatation in the coronary vascular bed is of the β-1 subtype; there is also a considerable amount of evidence to the contrary. We shall return to this problem shortly.

Last, we have obtained evidence of heterogeneity in the β-adrenoceptors that mediate inhibition of gastric acid secretion in the dog (Daly, Long, and Stables, 1978). Salbutamol was about 30 times less potent than isoprenaline in inhibiting pentagastrin-stimulated acid secretion. The antisecretory effect of isoprenaline was blocked by propranolol and practolol but not by H35/25, whereas the effect of salbutamol was blocked by propranolol and H35/25 but not by practolol. It was concluded that both β-1 and β-2 adrenoceptors can mediate inhibition of acid secretion in the dog, the β-1 adrenoceptors composing the major proportion and the β-2 adrenoceptors the minor proportion of the total population.

To summarize, it is now apparent that the β-1:β-2 ratio can vary (a) for the same organ between species (e.g., in cat trachea β-1 predominates, but in guinea-pig trachea β-2 predominates), (b) for different organs in the same species (e.g., in cat lung β-2 predominates, but in cat heart β-1 predominates), (c) for the same organ between individual animals of the same species (e.g., guinea-pig trachea), and (d) for different regions of the same organ (e.g., in cat airways, in the trachea β-1 predominates, but in the lung β-2 predominates).

The two examples outlined previously can now be reconsidered in the light of these new concepts. In cat isolated atria the order of potency of the catecholamines and the high blocking potency of practolol against isoprenaline are consistent with the presence of a major proportion of β-1 adrenoceptors; the relatively high potency of salbutamol is consistent with the presence of a minor, although significant, proportion of β-2 adrenoceptors. MJ 9184-1 has a relatively low potency in cat tracheal smooth muscle because of a predominance of β-1 adrenoceptors in this region of the airways; it has a relatively high potency in cat lung smooth muscle because of a predominance of β-2 adrenoceptors in this region of the airways.

Explanations for several other inconsistencies are now also forthcoming. First, the unusually high potency of noradrenaline relative to isoprenaline in guinea pig tracheal strip (Table 1) is very probably due to the presence of a minor although significant proportion of β-1 adrenoceptors. We predict that in the presence of an adequate β-1 adrenoceptor blocking concentration of practolol the isoprenaline:noradrenaline activity ratio would increase from the observed value of 24 to a value nearer to the 100–400 range obtained on preparations that contain an almost uniform population of β-2 adrenoceptors (see Table 1). Second, the lower lung:heart selectivity of the β-2 selective agonists in the anesthetized cat than in the anesthetized guinea pig could be due to differences in the proportions of β-1 and β-2 adrenoceptors in the S-A nodes of the two species. From data discussed above it is clear that the cat S-A node contains a minor although significant proportion of β-2 adrenoceptors and that the tachycardia produced by salbutamol (and presumably by the other β-2 selective agonists tested) in the cat is mediated almost entirely through these β-2 adrenoceptors. The interspecies difference in selectivity would be readily explained if the guinea pig S-A node were found to be devoid of β-2 adrenoceptors, or even if it were found to contain a significantly smaller proportion of β-2 adrenoceptors than the cat S-A node. Since Kaumann et al. (1978) have obtained evidence of two types of β-adrenoceptor in guinea pig isolated right atrium—a practolol-sensitive and practolol-insensitive receptor—the latter explanation seems more likely. Third, we will now return to the question of the subtype of β-adrenoceptor mediating coronary vasodilatation. The conclusion from three of the four published studies on isolated coronary arteries was that the β-1 adrenoceptor is involved (Drew and Levy, 1972; Baron, Speden, and Bohr, 1972; Johansson, 1973). In contrast, the conclusion from most of the studies *in vivo* was that that the β-2 adrenoceptor is involved (see Drew and Levy, 1972, for references). Analysis of direct responses to adrenoceptor agonists and antagonists in the coronary vascular bed *in vivo* is especially complicated because of the pronounced influence of accompanying changes in the mechanical and metabolic activity of the myocardium (Parratt, 1969). For this reason we were inclined to discount the *in vivo* evidence available up to 1972, but we were unable to discount the results of a later elegant *in vivo* study by Gross and Feigl (1975). These workers determined the direct effects of β-adrenoceptor agonists and antagonists on coronary vascular β-adrenoceptors in the potassium-arrested dog heart *in situ*. Salbutamol was 8 times less potent than isoprenaline in producing coronary vasodilatation and was clearly a full agonist. Propranolol was a potent antagonist of isoprenaline-induced coronary vasodilatation, whereas practolol was virtually inactive. It was concluded that the coronary vascular β-adrenoceptors are of the β-2 subtype. In the light of the evidence discussed in this section that suggests that variations can occur in the β-1 : β-2 ratio between different regions of the same organ or tissue, we think that the most likely explanation of the contradictory findings is that β-1 adrenoceptors predominate in the larger coronary arteries used for the *in vitro* experiments, whereas β-2 adrenoceptors predominate in the coronary arterioles that are the main site of the resistance changes measured *in vivo*. An almost exact analogy is provided by cat airways; as described above, the smooth muscle of the large airways contains predominantly β-1 adrenoceptors, whereas the smooth muscle of the fine airways contains predominantly β-2 adrenoceptors.

The presence of presynaptic β-adrenoceptors in noradrenergic nerve endings has recently been demonstrated. Activation of these receptors triggers a positive feedback mechanism leading to an increase in transmitter release (see Celuch, Dubocovich, and Langer, 1978, for references). The β-1 or β-2 nature of the presynaptic β-adrenoceptor is still uncertain. According to Dahlof et al. (1975), the presynaptic receptors in the noradrenergic nerves of the hind limb vasculature of the cat are of the β-1 subtype because they are blocked by metoprolol, a selective β-1 adrenoceptor antagonist. Yet the same group have proposed that the presynaptic β-adrenoceptors in the rat portal vein are mainly of the β-2 subtype because adrenaline is much more potent than noradrenaline in facilitating transmitter release (Dahlof, Ljung, and Ablad, 1978). Stjarne and Brundin (1976) suggest that the presynaptic β-adrenoceptors in human omental arteries and veins are of the β-2 subtype for two reasons: (a) because salbutamol and terbutaline enhanced transmitter release, whereas a β-1 adrenoceptor agonist, tazolol (H110/38), was without effect; and (b) because the enhancement of transmitter release caused by isoprenaline was blocked by H35/25 but not by practolol. Further studies like those of Stjarne and Brundin, using selective β-adrenoceptor agonists and antagonists, are required; but in the light of the new concepts discussed above, it would not be surprising if the presynaptic β-adrenoceptor were of the β-1 subtype in some regions and of the β-2 subtype in other regions, or if the two subtypes occurred together with the proportions varying from region to region.

B. Evidence from Receptor Binding Studies

The use of radiolabelled β-adrenoceptor antagonists to identify and characterize the β-adrenoceptor is now a well-established technique (Maguire, Ross, and Gilman, 1977). One of the commonly used radiolabelled ligands is ^{3}H-dihydroalprenolol (^{3}H-DHA). The specific binding of ^{3}H-DHA is of high affinity, reversible, and stereospecific and has pharmacological characteristics that indicate that the binding is to the β-adrenoceptor (Barnett, Rugg, and Nahorski, 1978). Nahorski and coworkers have determined the ability of selective and nonselective β-adrenoceptor agonists and antagonists to displace ^{3}H-DHA specific binding in membranes from a variety of tissues. The results provide evidence in support of the dual β-adrenoceptor hypothesis and for the presence of both β-1 and β-2 adrenoceptor subtypes in the same tissue.

In the rat lung, for example, the nonselective β-adrenoceptor antagonists, timolol, propranolol, and oxprenolol, all inhibited ^{3}H-DHA binding, producing smooth displacement curves that on Scatchard analysis were best described by single straight lines. In contrast, in a similar analysis for practolol the displacement curve clearly showed an inflection at lower concentrations of the antagonist. The Scatchard plot was best satisfied by two lines, suggesting the presence of two binding sites for practolol, one with a low affinity and the other with a high affinity. Similar results were obtained with two other β-1 selective antagonists, atenolol and paraoxprenolol. It was concluded that the lung membranes contained both β-1 and β-2 adrenoceptors. Further analysis of the Scatchard plots indicated that the β-1 and β-2 subtypes were present in a ratio of approximately 1:3 (Barnett et al., 1978). These conclusions were greatly strengthened by results obtained in rat lung membranes with the β-2 selective agonist, procaterol (Rugg, Barnett, and Nahorski, 1978). Scatchard analysis of displacement curves using this drug produced a mirror image of the picture obtained with practolol and the other β-1 selective antagonists. Procaterol appears to have a 20-fold greater affinity for β-2 than for β-1 adrenoceptors. Curiously, the β-2 selective agonists, salbutamol and terbutaline, each appear to have almost the same affinity for β-1 and β-2 adrenoceptors; the selectivity of these drugs must therefore be due to their higher efficacies at β-2 than at β-1 adrenoceptors.

The results of similar experiments on membranes from other tissues are summarized in Table 6. It is noteworthy that although the proportions of β-1 to β-2 sites are very different in different tissues, the inhibition constants for practolol for the two sites were remarkably similar throughout (Ki for the high affinity site $1.5 - 8 \times 10^{-7}$ M; Ki for the low affinity site $1.5 - 8 \times 10^{-5}$ M). Nahorski and coworkers concluded that their data provided strong evidence that only two β-adrenoceptor binding sites exist and that these two sites frequently coexist in the same tissue but that they vary in proportion between different tissues.

The use of the direct receptor binding technique in purified membrane fragments for receptor characterization is free from some of the potential

Table 6. Summary of results obtained from direct binding studies on the distribution of β-1 and β-2 adrenoceptors in various tissues

Tissue	Proportion of Adrenoceptors			Reference
Rat Lung	β-1 (25%)	:	β-2 (75%)	Barnett, Rugg, and Nahorski, 1978
Rat Heart	β-1 (>80%)			Barnett, Rugg, and Nahorski, 1978
Rabbit Lung	β-1 (60%)	:	β-2 (40%)	Rugg, Barnett, and Nahorski, 1978
Rat, Mouse, Rabbit, and Human Cerebral Cortex	β-1 (60%–70%)	:	β-2 (30%–40%)	Nahorski, 1978
Chick and Frog Cerebral Hemispheres	—		β-2 (100%)	Nahorski, 1978
Rat Parietal Cortex	β-1 (70%)	:	β-2 (30%)	Nahorski and Willcocks, 1978
Rat Striatum	β-1 (70%)	:	β-2 (30%)	Nahorski and Willcocks, 1978
Rat Hypothalamus	β-1 (30%)	:	β-2 (70%)	Nahorski and Willcocks, 1978
Rat Cerebellum and Medulla-Pons	—		β-2 (100%)	Nahorski and Willcocks, 1978

limitations of pharmacological experiments in intact tissues. For example, differences in tissue distribution of drugs possessing different physico-chemical properties and differing rates of equilibrium of drugs between bulk and receptor phases should not be a problem in receptor binding studies. There are certain disadvantages, however. In the final analysis it cannot be guaranteed that all of the "specific binding" is in fact binding specifically to the β-adrenoceptor. Uptake processes and enzymes often show as much hormone specificity as do the receptor sites, so it would not be surprising if a specific receptor antagonist also showed higher affinity for related removal processes. As noted in Section III, practolol inhibits catechol O-methyltransferase at slightly lower concentrations than are required to block the β-adrenoceptors in rat heart (Kenakin and Black, 1978). There have also been problems in determining the precise extent of the "specific binding," and these have led to some difficulties in the interpretation of results (Nahorski, personal communication). Last, without the use of cell separation techniques it is not possible to determine from receptor binding studies whether the β-1 and β-2 subtypes occur together on the same cell type and, therefore, whether they mediate the same response. This should not be a problem in pharmacological experiments.

Nevertheless, we are in little doubt that the evidence for the coexistence of β-1 and β-2 adrenoceptors in the same tissue is good when the data from the pharmacological studies or from the receptor binding studies are considered separately. When the evidence from these two independent sources is considered together, we believe that it is overwhelming.

V. FURTHER COMMENTS ON THE DUAL β-ADRENOCEPTOR HYPOTHESIS

A. Use of Noncatecholamine β-Adrenoceptor Agonists and β-Adrenoceptor Antagonists in Defining β-Adrenoceptor Subtypes

The dual β-adrenoceptor hypothesis was derived from data obtained with a series of catecholamines (Lands et al., 1967a). Because criticism of the hypothesis arose from results obtained with noncatecholamine β-adrenoceptor agonists or with β-adrenoceptor antagonists, it has been suggested that adrenoceptor classification be undertaken primarily with catecholamines and that noncatecholamine agonists or antagonists are useful only in a corroborative role (Arnold and McAuliff, 1971; Arnold, 1972; Grana, Lucchelli, and Zonta, 1974). We do not think that this argument is logical; if discrepancies exist, either the experimental evidence or the receptor classification is invalid. In any case, we believe that the evidence drawn together in this article shows that events have passed the argument by. The dual β-adrenoceptor hypothesis is in fact supported by data obtained with the catecholamines, with noncatecholamine β-adrenoceptor agonists, and with β-adrenoceptor antagonists.

B. Alternatives to the β-1 : β-2 Adrenoceptor Terminology

Ariens and Simonis (1976) suggested that since there are two adrenergic hormones—adrenaline released from the adrenal medulla and noradrenaline released from the noradrenergic nerves—the existence of two types of β-adrenoceptor (and two types of α-adrenoceptor as well) with differing sensitivities might have been predicted. According to Ariens and Simonis, organs with a noradrenergic innervation—for example, heart and gastrointestinal tract—contain β-adrenoceptors that are "primarily responsive" to noradrenaline (transmitter), whereas organs without a noradrenergic innervation—for example, uterus and striated muscle—contain β-adrenoceptors that are "primarily responsive" to adrenaline (hormone). Therefore, Ariens and Simonis proposed that the β-adrenoceptors in the innervated and noninnervated organs be termed β_T and β_H respectively—in effect, replacing the β-1 and β-2 terminology. We can envisage a number of problems with this proposal. Although β_H adrenoceptors do indeed respond primarily to adrenaline, it would be more accurate to describe β_T adrenoceptors as responding well to both noradrenaline and adrenaline (Table 1 of this article; Arnold, 1972; Grana et al., 1974), in which case, much of the justification for the β_T and β_H terminology disappears. The $\beta_T : \beta_H$ terminology also raises severe semantic problems. As has been described at length in section IV, many organs appear to contain both β-adrenoceptor subtypes. For example, both β-1 (β_T) and β-2 (β_H) adrenoceptors are found in the cat S-A node, a region with a dense noradrenergic innervation. The intriguing possibility exists that the β-1 (β_T) adrenoceptors are located in the immediate vicinity of the noradrenergic nerve endings and that the β-2 (β_H) adrenoceptors are located away from the nerve endings, although still within the S-A node region; but as yet there is no evidence for this. Also, as noted by Ariens and Simonis themselves, adrenaline is the neurotransmitter in frog heart (Burnstock, 1969); and the receptor that responds to the neurotransmitter is (not surprisingly) the β-2 (β_H) adrenoceptor. In this instance the definition of the innervated receptor as β_T breaks down completely. We consider, therefore, that there is no advantage to be gained by replacing the neutral β-1 and β-2 terminology with β_T and β_H and that there are good reasons for not doing so.

Grana et al. (1974) noted that noradrenaline and adrenaline were similar in potency on one set of β-adrenoceptors, whereas noradrenaline was considerably less potent than adrenaline on a second set of β-adrenoceptors. Because the relative potency on the first set was "closer to that on α-receptors," whereas the relative potency on the second set "approached that postulated by Ahlquist as characteristic of β-receptors," Grana et al. proposed the terms βα and ββ respectively. Inspection of the results of Grana et al. shows that βα and ββ adrenoceptors correspond to β-1 and β-2 adrenoceptors respectively. We prefer the β-1 : β-2 terminology.

C. Selectivity of β-Adrenoceptor Agonists and Antagonists in Man

Ablad et al. (1976) pointed out that the idea that β-1 and β-2 adrenoceptors can coexist in the same organ might explain the limited selectivity of β-adrenoceptor agonists and antagonists in man. For example, the bronchospasm caused by β-1 adrenoceptor antagonists in certain asthmatic patients could be due to the fact that β-1 adrenoceptors are important for bronchial smooth muscle relaxation in these patients. Bronchial smooth muscle relaxation in human beings is indeed mediated by both β-1 and β-2 adrenoceptors (Ablad et al., 1976). A consequence of the coexistence concept is that it will not be possible to develop β-adrenoceptor agonists and antagonists with absolute organ selectivity; indeed, it may not be possible even to improve on the clinical selectivity of presently available agents, because the limiting factor for selectivity is the proportion of the subordinate receptor in the organ in which the unwanted effect is produced rather than the difference in potency at β-1 and β-2 adrenoceptors.

Another consequence is that for prediction of selectivity in human beings it is necessary to select an animal species in which, ideally, the proportions of the two β-adrenoceptor subtypes in each organ correspond to those found in human beings. We agree with the conclusion of Bowman and Raper (1976) that the cat provides a more accurate prediction of the bronchodilator: positive chronotropic selectivity of β-adrenoceptor agonists in human beings than does the guinea pig.

VI. NATURE OF THE DIFFERENCE BETWEEN β-1 AND β-2 ADRENOCEPTORS

If it is accepted that there are only two subtypes of β-adrenoceptor and that they can occur together in the same organ or tissue and mediate the same response, certain deductions can be made about the nature of the difference between the two subtypes. In the discussion that follows, we have assumed for the sake of simplicity that α- and β-adrenoceptors are distinct entities (for discussion of this question see Benfey, this volume).

The β-adrenoceptor is a discrete binding site on a regulatory subunit, probably lipoprotein in character, that is located in the cell membrane in close proximity to the catalytic subunit of adenylate cyclase. There is now little doubt that the regulatory subunit is distinct from the catalytic subunit (Lefkowitz et al., 1976). The mechanism by which binding of agonist to the

β-adrenoceptor results in activation of adenylate cyclase—the "coupling" mechanism—is currently the subject of intense investigation (reviews by Levitzki, 1978, and Maguire et al., 1977).

The question under consideration can thus be formulated precisely as follows: What is the nature of the difference in the lipoprotein regulatory subunit that gives rise to β-1 and β-2 adrenoceptors?

Some of the authors who postulated that the β-adrenoceptor exists as a multiplicity of subtypes went on, quite reasonably, to suggest that the multiplicity might be due to the different "environments" in which the regulatory subunit finds itself in different tissues. If the different environments imposed slightly different conformations on the regulatory subunit, a spectrum of β-adrenoceptor binding sites with slightly different sensitivities to agonists and antagonists would be expected. However, this idea breaks down if there are only two subtypes of β-adrenoceptor and, in particular, if they can coexist in the same cell membrane.

We think that by far the most likely explanation of the difference between β-1 and β-2 adrenoceptors is the one put forward by Robison, Butcher, and Sutherland (1970). They suggested that the regulatory lipoprotein exists in two distinct forms that differ from one another in much the same way as one isoenzyme differs from another. The term *isoenzyme* is used to describe enzymes that exist in more than one structural form and that possess similar but not identical catalytic powers. Robison et al. (1970) coined the term *isoreceptor* for receptors with similar functional properties but different sensitivities to agonists and antagonists. The isoenzymic character of lactate dehydrogenase, one of the best understood examples of its kind, has its basis in the existence of two distinct polypeptide regulatory subunits differing slightly in their amino acid composition (Wilkinson, 1965). By analogy, the regulatory subunit containing the β-adrenoceptor could exist in two forms that differ only slightly in their amino acid composition.

Brittain, Jack, and Ritchie (1970) and Brittain, Dean, and Jack (1976) argued that the natural catecholamines, adrenaline and noradrenaline, differ only to a small extent in their sensitivity at β-1 and β-2 adrenoceptors and that selective stimulation or blockade of β-adrenoceptors is an unnatural phenomenon brought about by unnatural interactions with unnatural agonists or antagonists. In our view there is good evidence that one of the natural catecholamines, noradrenaline, *does* possess a significantly different sensitivity at β-1 and β-2 adrenoceptors. This difference was one of the main reasons why the dual β-adrenoceptor hypothesis was formulated in the first place (Arnold, 1972). Our results in Table 1 confirm that, relative to isoprenaline, noradrenaline is about 30 times more potent on β-1 than on β-2 adrenoceptors. Furchgott's (1976) analysis of data obtained on guinea pig trachea showed that noradrenaline has a 30-fold greater affinity for β-1 than for β-2 adrenoceptors. Since the efficacy of noradrenaline appears to be the same for activating either type of receptor (Furchgott, 1975, 1976), this difference in affinity represents a true difference in the sensitivity of noradrenaline for the two receptor subtypes. There is also clear evidence from direct ligand binding studies to suggest that noradrenaline has a higher affinity for β-1 than β-2 adrenoceptors (Rugg et al., 1978; Nahorski, 1978). Brittain et al. (1970) proposed that the physiological β-adrenoceptor—that is, the discrete site on the regulatory subunit with which noradrenaline and adrenaline combine—is the same from one tissue to another and that unnatural agonists or antagonists combine with the pharmacological receptor, an area encompassing the physiological receptor and exosites located in the surrounding membrane. The pharmacological receptor can differ from one tissue to another because the nature of the membrane exosites can differ chemically from one tissue to another, the difference being a reasonable consequence of tissue differentiation. In our opinion, however, the evidence with noradrenaline demonstrates unequivocally that there *is* a difference in the physiological β-adrenoceptor. The origin of the selectivity of unnatural agonists or antagonists then becomes an open question. It could still be due to differences in exosites. However, if both β-adrenoceptor subtypes do occur in the same cell membrane, it is difficult to see how a membrane difference could give rise to different exosites; the difference would be more likely to have its basis in a difference in the regulatory subunit outside the physiological receptor. Alternatively, it could be that the molecular modifications that confer selectivity in unnatural agonists or antagonists enable these drugs to recognize the same difference in the physiological receptor that is recognized by noradrenaline. We prefer this explanation because of its simplicity. Only one difference between β-1 and β-2 adrenoceptors need be invoked, and the requirement for physiological and pharmacological receptors disappears—at least as far as the explanation of selectivity is concerned. However, at present there seems to be no way of deciding which of the two alternatives is the correct one.

The regulatory subunit containing the β-adrenoceptor and the adenylate cyclase catalytic subunit are known to be products of separate genes (Insel et al., 1976). If the regulatory subunits containing β-1 and β-2 adrenoceptors do differ chemically from one another, they must also be the products of separate genes. There is some evidence in the literature that is consistent with this idea, although it is by no means conclusive. First, Lacombe et al. (1976) showed that the β-adrenoceptors in normal rat liver cells differed from those in tumor cells derived from rat liver cells (Zajdela hepatoma cells). In normal liver the order of potency for stimulating adenylate cyclase was protokylol (a selective β-2 adrenoceptor agonist) > isoprenaline > adrenaline > noradrenaline. In Zajdela hepatoma cells the order of potency was isoprenaline > protokylol > noradrenaline >

adrenaline. In normal liver the isoprenaline-stimulated cyclase was blocked by butoxamine but not by practolol; the opposite was true in the Zajdela hepatoma cells. It was concluded that the malignant transformation was accompanied by a switch of the adrenoceptor from the normal β-2 type to the β-1 type. Second, Richardson and Nahorski (1978) obtained evidence to suggest that both β-adrenoceptor subtypes are present in the estrogen-treated rat myometrium but that only the β-2 subtype is present in the progesterone-treated myometrium. This finding is of great interest in the present context because steroids are known to exert many of their actions by influencing gene expression (Thompson and Lippman, 1974).

VII. SUMMARY AND CONCLUSIONS

We believe that our wide-ranging experiments with β-adrenoceptor agonists and antagonists in isolated organs and in anesthetized guinea pigs and cats, together with the results of the ligand binding studies, constitute a consistent and compelling trend of evidence in support of the dual β-adrenoceptor hypothesis. The refinement of the hypothesis proposing that β-1 and β-2 adrenoceptors can coexist in a single tissue or organ and can mediate the same response resolves many of the inconsistencies in the literature. Evidence for the coexistence was obtained from pharmacological and ligand binding studies; there are also a few indications from experiments on β-adrenoceptor–coupled adenylate cyclase (Mayer, 1972; Coleman and Somerville, 1977). We believe that the case for coexistence of β-1 and β-2 adrenoceptors in the same cell type is strong; but it could be made even stronger if pharmacological, ligand binding, and adenylate cyclase studies could be carried out on the same tissue and also if the ligand binding and adenylate cyclase studies could be carried out in a homogeneous cell culture.

At the molecular level it seems to us that the simplest explanation of the difference between β-1 and β-2 adrenoceptors is that there is a minor chemical difference in the lipoprotein regulatory subunit and that this is manifested as a slight difference in the β-adrenoceptor binding site. This difference can be recognized by noradrenaline and by selective β-adrenoceptor agonists and antagonists. If this explanation is correct, β-1 and β-2 adrenoceptors must be the products of separate genes.

It is important to recognize that the only really direct way of answering the questions to which we have addressed ourselves—are there subtypes of β-adrenoceptor; if so, how many; and what is the nature of the difference between them?—is to isolate the macromolecule containing the β-adrenoceptor and to determine its chemical structure and conformation. Until this is achieved, we have no choice but to continue to rely on indirect methods of analysis, both pharmacological and biochemical. It is because of the indirect nature of the available methods that we have emphasized the need to establish *patterns* of activity when characterizing receptors, preferably using both agonists and antagonists with complementary profiles of selectivity. It is obvious in retrospect that both Ahlquist's and Lands' classifications depended upon the establishment of broad patterns of activity with the range of adrenoceptor agonists available at the time their studies were carried out. Now that a wider range of adrenoceptor agonists and antagonists is available and there is a better understanding of the potential variables and a greater ability to control them, we should expect the patterns to become more clearly defined. The search for such patterns must still continue, however. Since the introduction of the concept of β-adrenoceptor subtypes just over a decade ago, there seems to have been an almost compulsive desire on the part of many researchers in this field to attribute any variation in the relative potency of β-adrenoceptor agonists or in the potency of β-adrenoceptor antagonists to a receptor difference (and to be frank, we in this laboratory have not been blameless in this respect in the past). We hope that we have been able to convince people at least to hesitate before proposing additional β-adrenoceptor subtypes; if so, this chapter will have been worth the writing.

The conclusions in this chapter relate mainly to the β-adrenoceptors mediating "pharmacological" responses, but they may well have wider implications. There is evidence that β-1 and β-2 adrenoceptors can mediate metabolic responses (Lands et al., 1967a; Arnold, 1972; Loakpradit and Lockwood, 1977). These responses should now be reinvestigated in the expectation that in some cases both β-1 and β-2 subtypes will be found to mediate the same response. There is already evidence that the fat cells in dog adipose tissue contain both β-1 and β-2 adrenoceptors (Ablad et al., 1975b; Belfrage, 1978a). The conclusions are also likely to have relevance to other receptor systems. For example, there is now a considerable amount of evidence for more than one type of α-adrenoceptor. Bearing in mind the lessons to be learned from the β-adrenoceptor system, we suggest the following: that the best possible conditions for receptor classification studies be employed; that efforts be made to establish patterns of activity; that a neutral terminology be used—for example, α_1 and α_2—rather than one that seeks to indicate the site or function of the subtypes; and that the likelihood be considered that the subtypes coexist in the same tissue or organ and mediate the same response.

The questions posed in this chapter may be resolved in the not-too-distant future if progress toward the isolation of the β-adrenoceptor continues at its present rate. We look forward to this event; but, bearing in mind the associated threat of redundancy, we hope we will be understood if we end by echoing the plea of St. Augustine—"Lord . . . not just yet!"

VIII. REFERENCES

Åblad, B.; Borg, K.O.; Carlsson, E.; Ek. L.; Johnsson, G.; Malmfors, T.; Regardh, L.G.: A Survey of the Pharmacological Properties of Metoprolol in Animals and Man. Acta Pharmacol Toxicol [Suppl V] 36(1975a)7–23

Åblad, B.; Borjesson, I.; Carlsson, E., Johnsson, G.: Effects of Metoprolol and Propranolol on Some Metabolic Responses to Catecholamines in the Anaesthetized Dog. Acta Pharmacol Toxicol [Suppl V] 36(1975b)85–95

Åblad, B.; Carlsson, E.; Dahlof, C.; Ek, L.: Some Aspects of the Pharmacology of β-Adrenoceptor Blockers. Drugs 11 suppl 1(1976)100–111

Ahlquist, R.P.: A Study of the Adrenotropic Receptors. Am J Physiol 153(1948)586–600

Apperley, G.H.; Brittain, R.T.; Coleman, R.A.; Kennedy, I.; Levy, G.P.: Characterization of the β-Adrenoceptors in the Mesovarium of the Rat. Br J Pharmacol 63(1978)345P–346P

Apperley, G.H.; Daly, M.J.; Levy, G.P.: Selectivity of β-Adrenoceptor Agonists and Antagonists on Bronchial, Skeletal, Vascular and Cardiac Muscle in the Anaesthetized Cat. Br J Pharmacol 57(1976)235–246

Apperley, G.H.; Levy, G.P.: Characterisation of the β-Adrenoceptors of the Guinea-Pig Tracheobronchial, Skeletal and Cardiac Muscle. Br J Pharmacol 54(1975)260–261P

Ariens, E.J.; Simonis, A.M.: Receptors and Receptor Mechanisms. In: Beta-adrenoceptor Blocking Agents, pp. 3–27, ed. by P.R. Saxena, R.P. Forsyth. North Holland Publishing Company, Amsterdam, 1976

Arnold, A.: Differentiation of Receptors Activated by Catecholamines—III. Il Farmaco Ed Sci 27(1972)79–100

Arnold, A.; McAuliff, J.P.: Differentiation of Receptors Activated by Catecholamines. 2. Arch Int Pharmacodyn Ther 193(1971)287–293

Arunlakshana, O.; Schild, H.O.: Some Quantitative Uses of Drug Antagonists. Br J Pharmacol Chemother 14(1959)48–58

Barnett, D.B.; Rugg, E.L.; Nahorski, S.R.; Direct Evidence of Two Types of β-Adrenoceptor Binding Site in Lung Tissue. Nature 273(1978)166–168

Baron, G.D.; Speden, R.N.; Bohr, D.F.: Beta-adrenergic receptors in coronary and skeletal muscle arteries. Am J Physiol 223(1972)878–881

Barrett, A.M.; Carter, J.: Comparative Chronotropic Activity of β-Adrenoceptive Antagonists. Br J Pharmacol 40(1970)373–381

Belfrage, E.: Vasodilatation and Modulation of Vasoconstriction in Canine Subcutaneous Adipose Tissue Caused by Activation of β-Adrenoceptors. Acta Physiol Scand 102 (1978a)459–468

Belfrage, E.: Comparison of β-Adrenoceptors Mediating Vasodilatation in Canine Subcutaneous Adipose Tissue and Skeletal Muscle. Acta Physiol Scand 102(1978b)469–476

Bowman, W.C.; Nott, M.W.: Actions of Some Sympathomimetic Bronchodilator and Beta-Adrenoceptor Blocking Drugs on Contractions of the Cat Soleus Muscle. Br J Pharmacol 38(1970)37–49

Bowman, W.C.; Raper, C.: Sympathomimetic Bronchodilators and Animal Models for Assessing Their Potential Value in Asthma. J Pharm Pharmacol 28(1976)369–374

Bowman, W.C.; Rodger, I.W.: Actions of the Sympathomimetic Bronchodilator Rimiterol (R 798), on the Cardiovascular, Respiratory and Skeletal Muscle Systems of the Anaesthetized Cat. Br J Pharmacol 45(1972)574–583

Bowman, W.C.; Zaimis, E.: The Effects of Adrenaline, Noradrenaline and Isoprenaline on Skeletal Muscle Contractions in the Cat. J Physiol (Lond) 144(1958)92–107

Bristow, M.; Sherrod, T.R.; Green, R.D.: Analysis of β-Receptor Drug Interactions in Isolated Rabbit Atrium, Aorta, Stomach and Trachea. J Pharmacol Exp Ther 171(1970)52–61

Brittain, R.T.; Dean, C.M.; Jack, D.: Sympathomimetic Bronchodilator Drugs. Pharmacol Ther [B] 2(1976)423–462

Brittain, R.T.; Farmer, J.B.; Jack, D.; Martin, L.E.; Simpson, W.T.: Alpha—[(t-Butylamino)Methyl]-4-Hydroxy-m-Xylene-$\alpha^1\alpha^3$-Diol (AH 3365); a Selective β-Adrenergic Stimulant. Nature 219(1968)862–863

Brittain, R.T.; Farmer, J.B.; Marshall, R.J.: Some Observations on the β-Adrenoceptor Agonist Properties of the Isomers of Salbutamol. Br J Pharmacol 48(1973)144–147

Brittain, R.T.; Jack, D.; Ritchie, A.C.: Recent β-Adrenoceptor Stimulants. In: Advances in Drug Research, Vol. V, pp. 197-253, ed by N.J. Harper, A.B. Simmonds. Academic, London-New York, 1970

Burges, R.A.; Blackburn, K.J.: Adenyl Cyclase and the Differentiation of β-Adrenoceptors. Nature [New Biol] 235(1972)249-250

Burnstock, G.: Evaluation of the Autonomic Innervation of Visceral and Cardiovascular Systems in Vertebrates. Pharmacol Rev 21(1969)247-324

Carlsson, E.; Åblad, B.; Brandstrom, A.; Carlsson, B.: Differentiated Blockade of the Chronotropic Effects of Various Adrenergic Stimuli in the Cat Heart. Life Sci 11(1972)953-958

Carlsson, E.; Dahlof, C.G.; Hedberg, A.; Persson, H.; Tangstrand, B.: Differentiation of Cardiac Chronotropic and Inotropic Effects of β-Adrenoceptor Agonists. Naunyn-Schmiedebergs Arch Pharmacol 300(1977)101-105

Celuch, S.M.; Dubocovich, M.L.; Langer, S.Z.: Stimulation of Presynaptic β-Adrenoceptors Enhances [³H]-Noradrenaline Release during Nerve Stimulation in the Perfused Cat Spleen. Br J Pharmacol 63(1978)97-109

Colella, D.F; Chakrin, L.W.; Shetzline, A.; Wardell, J.R.: Characterization of the Adrenergic Activity of Carbuterol (SK&F 40 383-A). Eur J Pharmacol 46(1977)229-241

Coleman, A.J.; Somerville, A.R.: The Selective Action of β-Adrenoceptor Blocking Drugs and the Nature of β_1 and β_2-Adrenoceptors. Br J Pharmacol 59(1977)83-93

Cornish, E.J.; Miller, R.C.: Comparison of the β-Adrenoceptors in the Myocardium and Coronary Vasculature of the Kitten Heart. J Pharm Pharmacol 27(1975)23-30

Cullum, V.A.; Farmer, J. B.; Jack, D.; Levy, G.P.: Salbutamol: a New, Selective β-Adrenoceptive Receptor Stimulant. Br J Pharmacol 35(1969)141-151

Dahlof, C.; Åblad, B.; Borg, K.O., Ek. L.; Waldeck, B.: Prejunctional Inhibition of Adrenergic Nervous Vasomotor Control Due to β-Receptor Blockade. In: Chemical Tools in Catecholamine Research, Vol. II, pp. 201-210, ed. by O. Almgren, A. Carlsson, J. Engel. North Holland Publishing Company, Amsterdam, 1975

Dahlof, C.; Ljung, B.; Åblad, B.: Relative Potency of β-Adrenoceptor Agonists on Neuronal Transmitter Release in Isolated Rat Portal Vein. In: Recent Advances in the Pharmacology of Adrenoceptors, pp. 355-356, ed. by E. Szabadi, C.M. Bradshaw, P. Bevan. Elsevier/North Holland, Amsterdam, 1978

Daly, M.J.; Farmer, J.B.; Levy, G.P.: Comparison of the Bronchodilator and Cardiovascular Actions of Salbutamol, Isoprenaline and Orciprenaline in Guinea-Pigs and Dogs. Br J Pharmacol 43(1971)624-638

Daly, M.J.; Flook, J.J.; Levy, G.P.: The Selectivity of β-Adrenoceptor Antagonists on Cardiovascular and Bronchodilator Responses to Isoprenaline in the Anaesthetized Dog. Br J Pharmacol 53(1975)173-181

Daly, M.J.; Long, J.M.; Stables, R.: The Role of β_1- and β_2-Adrenoceptors in the Inhibition of Gastric Acid Secretion in the Dog. Br J Pharmacol 64(1978)153-157

Davey, T.; Malta, E.; Raper, C.: A Comparison of the Activities of the β-Adrenoceptor Agonists MJ 9184-1 and (−)-Isoprenaline in Guinea-Pig and Cat Preparations. Clin Exp Pharmacol Physiol 1(1974)43-52

Drew, G.M.; Levy, G.P.: Characterization of the Coronary Vascular β-Adrenoceptor in the Pig. Br J Pharmacol 46(1972)348-350

Dunlop, D.; Shanks, R.G.: Selective Blockade of Adrenoceptive Beta Receptors in the Heart. Br J Pharmacol Chemother 32(1968)201-218

Edvinsson, L.; Owman, C.: Pharmacological Characterization of Adrenergic Alpha and Beta Receptors Mediating the Vasomotor Responses of Cerebral Arteries in Vitro. Circ Res 35(1974)835-849

Engelhardt, A.; Hoefke, W.; Wick, H.: Zur pharmakologie des sympathomimeticums 1-(3,5-dihydroxy-phenyl)-1-hydroxy-2-isopropylamino-athane. Arztneim Forsch 11(1961)521-525

Furchgott, R.F.: The Pharmacological Differentiation of Adrenergic Receptors. Ann NY Acad Sci 139(1967)553-570

Furchgott, R.F.: The Classification of Adrenoceptors (Adrenergic Receptors). An Evaluation from the Standpoint of Receptor Theory. In: Handbook of Experimental Pharmacology, pp. 283-335, ed. by H. Blaschko, E. Muscholl. Springer, New York, 1972

Furchgott, R.F.: Postsynaptic Receptor Mechanisms. Blood Vessels 12(1975)337-338

384 / Michael J. Daly and Geoffrey P. Levy

Furchgott, R.F.: Postsynaptic Adrenergic Receptor Mechanisms in Vascular Smooth Muscle. In: Vascular Neuroeffector Mechanisms, pp. 131–142. Karger, Basel, 1976

Grana, E.; Lucchelli, A.; Zonta, F.: Selectivity of β-Adrenergic Compounds III—Classification of β-Receptors. Il Farmaco Ed Sci 29(1974)786–792

Gross, G.J.; Feigl, E.O.: Analysis of Coronary Vascular Beta Receptors in Situ. Am J Physiol 228(1975)1909–1913

Gwee, M.C.E.; Nott, M.W.; Raper, C.; Rodger, I.W.: Pharmacological Actions of a new β-Adrenoceptor Agonist, MJ-9184-1, in Anaesthetized Cats. Br J Pharmacol 46(1972)375–385

Himori, N.; Taira, N.: Assessment of the Selectivity of OPC-2009, a new β₂-Adrenoceptor Stimulant, by the Use of the Blood-Perfused Trachea in Situ and of the Isolated Blood-Perfused Papillary Muscle of the Dog. Br J Pharmacol 61(1977)9–17

Insel, P.A.; Maguire, M.E.; Gilman, A.G.; Bourne, H.R.; Coffino, P.; Melmon, K.L.: Beta Adrenergic Receptors and Adenylate Cyclase: Products of Separate Genes? Mol Pharmacol 12(1976)1062–1069

Jenkinson, D.H.: Classification and Properties of Peripheral Adrenergic Receptors. Br Med Bull 29(1973)142–147

Johansson, B.: The β-Adrenoceptors in the Smooth Muscle of Pig Coronary Arteries. Eur J Pharmacol 24(1973)218–224

Kaiser, C., Schwartz, M.S., Colella, D.F.; Wardell, J.R.: Adrenergic Agents 3. Synthesis and Adrenergic Activity of some Catecholamine Analogs Bearing a Substituted Sulfonyl or Sulfonylalkyl Group in the Meta Position. J Med Chem 18(1975)674–683

Kaumann, A.J.; Birnbaumer, L.; Wittmann, R.: Heart β-Adrenoceptors. In: Receptors and Hormone Action, Vol. III, pp 133–177, ed by O'Malley. Academic, New York, 1978.

Kenakin, T.P.; Black, J.W.: The Pharmacological Classification of Practolol and Chloropractolol. Mol Pharmacol 14(1978)607–623

Lacombe, M.L.; Rene, E.; Guellan, G.; Hanoune, J.: Transformation of the β₂-Adrenoceptor in Normal Rat Liver into a β₁ Type in Zajdela Hepatoma. Nature 262(1976)70–72

Lands, A.M.; Arnold, A., McAuliff, J.P.; Luduena, F.P.; Brown, T.G.: Differentiation of Receptor Systems Activated by Sympathomimetic Amines. Nature 214(1967a)597–598

Lands, A.M.; Luduena, F.P.; Buzzo, H.J.: Differentiation of Receptors Responsive to Isoproterenol. Life Sci 6(1967b)2241–2249

Lefkowitz, R.J.: Heterogeneity of Adenylate Cyclase-Coupled β-Adrenergic Receptors. Biochem Pharmacol 24(1975)583–590

Lefkowitz, R.J.; Limbird, L.E.; Mukherjee, C.; Caron, M.C.: The β-Adrenergic Receptor and Adenylate Cyclase. Biochim Biophys Acta 457(1976)1–39

Levitzki, A.: The Mode of Coupling of Adenylate Cyclase to Hormone Receptors and Its Modulation by GTP. Biochem Pharmacol 27(1978)2083–2088

Levy, B.: A Comparison of the Adrenergic Receptor Blocking Properties of 1-(4'-Methylphenyl)-2-Isopropylamino-Propanol-HCl and Propranolol. J Pharmacol Exp Ther 156 (1967)452–462

Loakpradit, T.; Lockwood, R.: Differentiation of Metabolic Adrenoceptors. Br J Pharmacol 59(1977)135–140

Lulich, K.M.; Mitchell, H.W.; Sparrow, M.P.: The Cat Lung Strip As an in Vitro Preparation of Peripheral Airways: A Comparison of β-Adrenoceptor Agonists, Autacoids and Anaphylactic Challenge on the Lung Strip and Trachea. Br J Pharmacol 58(1976)71–79

Maguire, M.E.; Ross, E.M.; Gilman, A.G.: β-Adrenergic Receptor: Ligand Binding Properties and the Interaction with Adenyl Cyclase. In: Advances in Cyclic Nucleotide Research, Vol. VIII, pp. 1–83, ed. by P. Greengard, G.A. Robison. Raven, New York, 1977

Marsden, C.D.; Meadows, J.C.: The Effect of Adrenaline on the Contraction of Human Muscle—One Mechanism Whereby Adrenaline Increases the Amplitude of Physiological Tremor. J Physiol (Lond) 194(1968)70P–71P

Marsden, C.D.; Meadows, J.C.: The Effect of Adrenaline on the Contraction of Human Muscle. J Physiol (Lond) 207(1970)429–448

Mayer, S.E.: Effects of Adrenergic Agonists and Antagonists on Adenylate Cyclase Activity of Dog Heart and Liver. J Pharmacol Exp Ther 181(1972)116–125

Moran, N.C.: Pharmacological Characterization of Adrenergic Receptors. Pharmacol Rev 18(1966)503–512

Nahorski, S.R.: Heterogeneity of Cerebral β-Adrenoceptor Binding Sites in Various Vertebrate Species. Eur J Pharmacol 51(1978)199–209

Nahorski, S.R.; Willcocks, A.L.: Identification of β-Adrenoceptor Subtypes in Various Regions of the Rat Brain. In: Recent Advances in the Pharmacology of Adrenoceptors, pp. 347–348, ed. by E. Szabadi, C.M. Bradshaw, P. Bevan. Elsevier/North Holland, Amsterdam, 1978

O'Donnell, S.R.: A Selective β-Adrenoceptor Stimulant (Th 1165a) Related to Orciprenaline. Eur J Pharmacol 12(1970)35–43

O'Donnell, S.R.; Wanstall, J.C.: Evidence That the Efficacy (Intrinsic Activity) of Fenoterol is Higher Than That of Salbutamol on β-Adrenoceptors in Guinea-Pig Trachea. Eur J Pharmacol 47(1978)333–340

Parratt, J.R.: Pharmacological Aspects of the Coronary Circulation. Prog Med Chem 6(1969)11–66

Patil, P.N.; Lapidus, J.B.; Tye, A.: Steric Aspects of Adrenergic Drugs. J Pharm Sci 59(1970)1205–1234

Richardson, A.; Nahorski, S.R.: Direct Identification of the β-Adrenoceptor in Rat Uterus. In: Recent Advances in the Pharmacology of Adrenoceptors, pp. 335–336, ed. by E. Szabadi, C.M. Bradshaw, P. Bevan. Elsevier/North Holland, Amsterdam, 1978

Robison, G.A.; Butcher, R.W.; Sutherland, E.W.: On the Relation of Hormone Receptors to Adenyl Cyclase. In: Fundamental Concepts in Drug-Receptor Interactions, pp. 59–91, ed. by J. F. Danielli, D.J. Triggle. Academic, London, 1970

Rodger, I.W.: Effects of Isoetharine on Airways Resistance, Heart Rate and Contractions of the Soleus Muscle of the Anaesthetized Cat. Eur J Pharmacol 24(1973)211–217

Rugg, E.L.; Barnett, D.B.; Nahorski, S.R.: Coexistence of Beta-1 and Beta-2 Adrenoceptors in Mammalian Lung: Evidence from Direct Binding Studies. Mol Pharmacol 14 (1978)996–1005

Schild, H.O.: Receptor Classification with Special Reference to β-Adrenergic Receptors. In: Drug Receptors, pp. 29–36, ed. by H.P. Rang. Macmillan, London, 1973

Stephenson, R.P.: A Modification of Receptor Theory. Br J Pharmacol Chemother 11(1956)379–393

Stjarne, L.; Brundin, J.: β_2-Adrenoceptors Facilitating Noradrenaline Secretion from Human Vasoconstrictor Nerves. Acta Physiol Scand 97(1976)88–93

Taira, N.; Yabuuchi, Y.; Yamashita, S.: Profile of β-Adrenoceptors in Femoral, Superior Mesenteric and Renal Vascular Beds of Dogs. Br J Pharmacol 59(1977)577–583

Thompson, E.B.; Lippman, M.E.: Mechanism of Action of Glucocorticoids. Metabolism 23(1974)159–202

Wardell, J.R.; Colella, D.F.; Shetzline, A.; Fowler, P.J.: Studies on Carbuterol (SK&F 40383-A), a New Selective Bronchodilator Agent. J Pharmacol Exp Ther 189(1974)167–184

Wasserman, M.A.; Levy, B.: Cardiovascular and Bronchomotor Responses to Selective Beta Adrenergic Receptor Agonists in the Anaesthetized Dog. J Pharmacol Exp Ther 189(1974)445–455

Wilkinson, J.H.: Isoenzymes, 1st ed. E. and F.N. Spon, London, 1965

Yabuuchi, Y.; Yamashita, S.; Tei, S.: Pharmacological Studies of OPC-2009, a Newly Synthetized Selective Beta Adrenoceptor Stimulant, in the Bronchomotor and Cardiovascular System of the Anaesthetized Dog. J Pharmacol Exp Ther 202(1977)326–336

Yamashita, S.; Takai, M.; Yabuuchi, Y.: Actions of Procaterol (OPC-2009), a New β_2-Adrenoceptor Stimulant, on Pulmonary Resistance, Contractions of the Soleus Muscle, and Cardiovascular System of the Anaesthetized Cat. J Pharm Pharmacol 30(1978)273–279

Zaagsma, J.; Oudhof, R.; Van der Heijden, P.J.C.M.: On the heterogeneity of β-Adrenoceptors in the Respiratory Tract. In: Proceedings of the Seventh International Congress of Pharmacology, ed. by J. R. Boissier, P. Lechat, p. 425. Pergamon, Oxford, 1978

The Identification and
Isolation of Adrenergic Receptors

David J. Triggle and John F. Moran

I. INTRODUCTION

The concept of the pharmacological receptor dates to the last century; and Langley's (1906) statement in reference to skeletal muscle, "It is convenient to have a term for the specially excitable constituent, and I have called it the receptive substance. It receives the stimulus, and by transmitting it, causes contraction" (p. 182), drew early attention to two major components of the drug-receptor interaction: recognition and initiation of biological response.

Until recently knowledge of receptors and drug-receptor interactions was derived almost entirely from analyses of dose-response curves. However, the dose-response curve is—even under the most favorable circumstances, where distribution, metabolism, and other modulating factors have been controlled or eliminated—a composite of two fundamental quantities: the affinity of the drug for the receptor and the ability of the drug-receptor complex to initiate response. Thus, the dose-response curve cannot be considered a priori a saturation curve. In the absence of direct evidence

This work was supported in part by a grant from the National Institutes of Health (HL 16003).

of the relationship between receptor occupancy (ligand binding) and biological response, interpretation of the dose-response curve is at best ambiguous. Such evidence is vital not only to the development of a basic understanding of drug-receptor interactions but also to the resolution of questions concerning the organization of recognition and amplification sites within the receptor, the presence or absence of receptors in tissues, the similarity or dissimilarity of receptors, changes in receptors in desensitized or supersensitized states, receptor development in cellular maturation, and changes in receptors in pathologic states. The direct measurement of ligand binding to receptors can, in principle, provide answers to the above general questions and serve as the vital first component of receptor isolation. Subsequent components can serve to isolate and characterize the macromolecules subserving the binding and amplification functions and ultimately to reconstitute receptor function.

The greatest success in isolation of a receptor has been with the nicotinic receptor from the electric organ of the electric eel, and this has depended to a great extent on the high receptor concentration in this tissue (picomoles per milligram of protein [Cohen and Changeux, 1975]), which is 10^2–10^3 times the concentration found in the adrenergic systems thus far investigated.

In this chapter we attempt to evaluate studies on ligand binding to adrenergic α and β receptors as they apply to eventual receptor isolation and to review reports dealing with the general questions referred to above. Several reviews dealing with catecholamine receptors are available (Haber and Wrenn, 1976; Kunos, 1978; Lefkowitz, 1974, 1976; Lefkowitz et al., 1976; Levitski, 1976; Maguire, Ross, and Gilman, 1977; Wolfe, Harden, and Molinoff, 1977). Studies on the β receptor are far more numerous than those on α receptors, doubtless because a biochemical response induced upon agonist binding to β receptors has been identified. This response of adenylate cyclase can be readily monitored and provides an assay *in vitro* that is not dependent upon cellular integrity. Yet in the strictest sense of the word there have been few attempts to isolate adrenergic receptors. However, there have been a large number of studies dealing with the quantitative characterization of ligand binding to both α and β receptors; and such studies are, of course, a prerequisite for actual isolation. In any event, the characterization of ligand binding has been more useful than strict isolation in answering fundamental questions concerning drug-receptor interactions and the nature of the receptor.

II. CRITERIA AND CONDITIONS FOR LIGAND BINDING STUDIES

The number of adrenergic agonists and antagonists that might be used in ligand binding studies to α and β receptors is enormous. However, a suitable ligand must fulfill certain criteria; and, as will be seen in the following discussion, many pitfalls exist if the criteria are not met. Further, it will become apparent that many unforeseen difficulties exist in attempting to choose an appropriate ligand for binding studies, since nonspecific interactions cannot be predicted. For example, nonspecific or nonreceptor binding accounts for 60%–80% of total binding of [^{3}H] propranolol, whereas with [^{3}H] dihydroalprenolol and [^{125}I] hydroxybenzylpindolol nonspecific binding is only 5%–25% of the total (Lefkowitz, 1976). Thus, despite the apparent pharmacological specificity and high affinity of a ligand, it does not necessarily follow that the same degree of specificity will be shown when binding is studied.

A. Saturation

The binding of a radiolabeled ligand should show saturation, since only a finite number of receptors exist. In order to fulfill this criterion, the concentration range of ligand used should ideally be varied over at least a 100-fold range and bracket the K_B of the ligand. Experiments carried out over narrow concentration ranges, particularly when a significant range of concentrations above the K_B is not used, may fail to show other lower affinity binding sites and can be misleading. Dihydroergocryptine, a ligand used to study α receptors (Williams, Mullikin, and Lefkowitz, 1976b), also binds to dopamine and serotonin receptors (Tittler, Weinreich, and Seeman, 1977). Although it is possible to analyze α receptors with this ligand at low concentrations, a complete saturation curve is required so that the sites can be characterized with respect to affinities and numbers. In this way, despite the lack of absolute specificity, one can determine the suitability of using a ligand concentration that will bind predominantly at the receptor under study; and by using appropriate antagonists, the specificity of the various binding sites may be determined.

As pointed out by Birnbaumer, Pohl, and Kaumann (1974), however, a linear Scatchard plot and Hill coefficient of 1.0 may be deceiving and do not necessarily rule out a heterogeneous receptor population, since two types of receptor could be present, one of high affinity and high capacity and the other of low affinity for the ligand and low capacity.

Early attempts at α receptor isolation using the irreversible α receptor antagonists Dibenamine (Yong et al., 1966), phenoxybenzamine (Lewis and Miller, 1966), and related 2-halogenoethylamines (May et al., 1967; Moran et al., 1967; Moran and Triggle, 1970; Yong and Nickerson, 1973) encountered major obstacles, because no evidence was found for saturability of binding in the concentration range in which these ligands produced their pharmacological effect. Further, although pharmacologic protection could be demonstrated with reversible agonists and antagonists, this protection was accompanied by small or insignificant protection against radioligand binding, and there was no correlation between the extent of protection and the activity of the protecting ligands at the α receptor. A survey of the several attempts to label α-adrenoceptors using agents of the Dibenamine type led to the conclusion that "while it is possible to obtain receptor protection and specificity of action with irreversible antagonists at the pharmacological level, it is not possible to obtain specificity of action at the chemical level with agents currently available" (Moran et al., 1967, p. 26).

B. Reversibility

When a reversible radiolabeled ligand is used, the bound compound should be completely dissociable when the ligand-hormone complex is diluted or upon the addition of excess unlabeled ligand. Further, the dissociated ligand should be chemically unchanged and bind to a receptor preparation with the same properties as the fresh ligand. In some cases, as with dihydro-ergocryptine binding to liver plasma membranes (Guellaen et al., 1978), the ligand is metabolized very rapidly, and the binding data thus obtained become suspect unless appropriate controls and corrections are applied. In the case of the early studies with [^{3}H] catecholamines (Aprille, Lefkowitz, and Warshaw, 1974; Bilezikian and Aurbach, 1973; Dunnick and Marinetti, 1971; Lefkowitz, Sharp, and Haber, 1973), it has been demonstrated that the catecholamine binding actually involved oxidative coupling of catecholamines to membrane nucleophiles (Cuatrecasas et al., 1974), thus accounting for the irreversible binding observed.

The ratio of the experimentally determined rate constants of association (k_1) and dissociation (k_{-1}) should be comparable to the dissociation constant (K_B) determined at equilibrium. With very high affinity ligands, which are usually antagonists, the rate of dissociation (k_{-1}) is slow, since k_1 generally approaches diffusion-controlled limits. A correlation between the kinetics of binding and the onset of effect should be obtained if the ligand is bound to functional receptor sites. Thus the rate of dissociation of bound antagonist should correlate with the appearance of responsiveness to an agonist. This need not be linear, if, for example, there exists a large receptor reserve; but the correlation should, on the other hand, give a good estimate of the receptor reserve.

In studies using [^{3}H] catecholamines, although saturable binding was demonstrable, binding was very slow and either irreversible or only slowly reversible. Thus, despite the fact that there was agreement between K_B (binding) and K_{AC} (adenylate cyclase) in several instances, the weight of other discrepancies demonstrates quite conclusively that receptor binding was at best a minor component of the total binding observed (for a review of these studies see Cuatrecasas et al., 1975; Levitzki, 1976).

C. Specificity

Specific binding of the radioligand should be inhibited by agents that activate or antagonize the receptor; and, conversely, compounds that are inactive at the receptor should not inhibit binding of the radioligand. The concentrations of an agonist that compete with the radioligand should be related to its potency as a stimulant. In the simplest case, the dissociation constant (K_B) determined by the inhibition of binding should be equal to the ED_{50} value determined by measuring a pharmacological effect or stimulation of adenylate cyclase if there is no receptor reserve. If spare receptors exist, the K_B should be greater than the ED_{50}. However, the K_B determined for antagonists is independent of the presence or absence of a receptor reserve, and agreement between these values should be found (Wolfe et al., 1977; Maguire et al., 1977).

The binding of ligands should be stereoselective, and preferential inhibition by catecholamines having the R configuration in the side chain should be observed. The order of potency should be the same as is found for pharmacologic activity. The stereoselectivity of agonist action that characterizes the pharmacological event was absent in the early binding studies on [^{3}H] catecholamines, and the concentrations of β-antagonist required to inhibit binding were substantially higher than those required for β-receptor blockade (Dunnick and Marinetti, 1971; Lefkowitz et al., 1973).

D. Methodology

1. Ligands Ligands used in adrenergic receptor studies are labeled with tritium, incorporated by catalytic reduction (Lefkowitz et al., 1974; Williams et al., 1976b) or catalytic exchange (Levitzki, Atlas, and Steer, 1974; Lefkowitz and Williams, 1977); or with iodine, using the Hunter and Greenwood (1962) procedure (Aurbach et al., 1976) or synthesis (Bobik et al., 1977). To date, the ligands shown in figure 1 have been successfully used. Iodination with ^{125}I provides ligands of high specific activity as compared to ^{3}H, as the theoretical specific activities when substituting 1 atom in a ligand are 2,200 C/mmole and 29 C/mmole respectively (Bayly and Evans, 1974). ^{125}I-labeled ligands permit the use both of less biological material and of low concentrations of ligand where nonspecific binding is minimized and rates of association can be more accurately measured. This advantage is not without risk, as the high specific activity can result in severe radiolysis. Degradation of purified [^{125}I] HYP can occur in minutes unless stored at $-20°C$ in the presence of phenol (Brown et al., 1976a). Further, the relatively rapid radioactive decay to products of unknown biological potency requires frequent synthesis of fresh ligand (Maguire et al., 1977).

2. Separation The choice of method to separate free and bound ligand must depend on a consideration of the kinetics of dissociation of the bound ligand. Filtration on glass fiber filters is generally preferred to microcentrifugation techniques (Rodbell et al., 1971) because of its rapidity ($\simeq$ 20 s), which is essential if the dissociation (k_{-1}) is relatively fast

α AGONIST

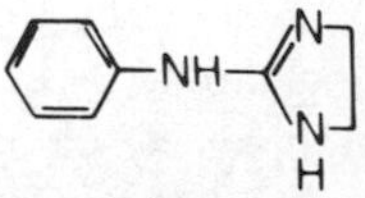

[³H]Clonidine
Greenberg et al., 1976

β AGONIST

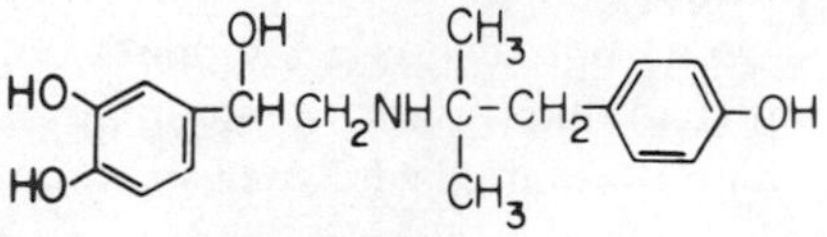

[³H]Hydroxybenzylisoproterenol ([³H]HBI)
Lefkowitz and Williams, 1977

α ANTAGONISTS

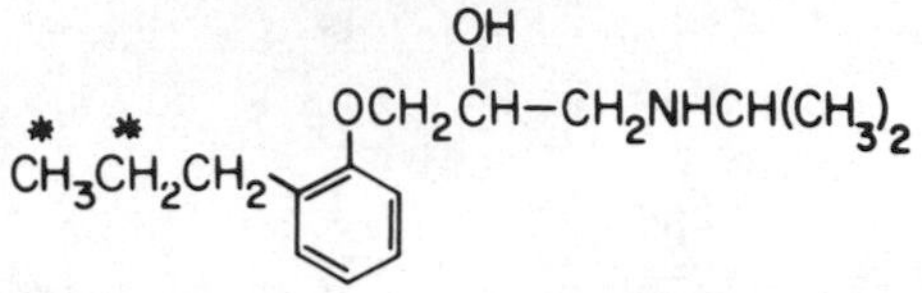

[³H]Dihydroergocryptine ([³H]DHE)
Williams et al., 1976

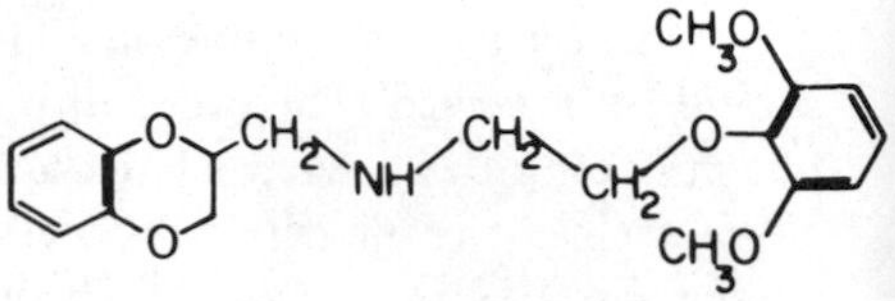

[³H]WB 4101
Greenberg et al., 1976

β ANTAGONISTS

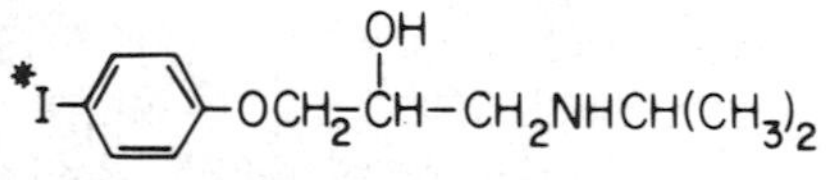

[¹²⁵I]3-(4-Iodophenoxy)-1-Isopropylaminopropan-2-ol ([¹²⁵I]IP)
Bobik et al., 1977

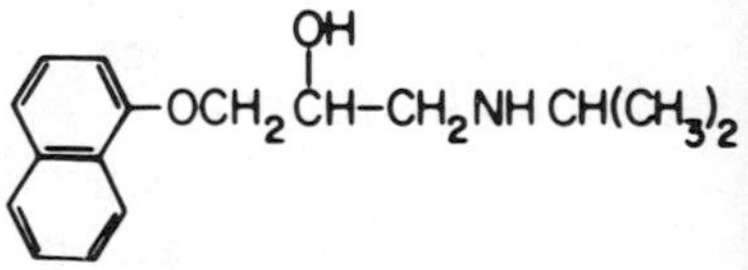

[³H]Propranolol
Levitzki et al., 1974

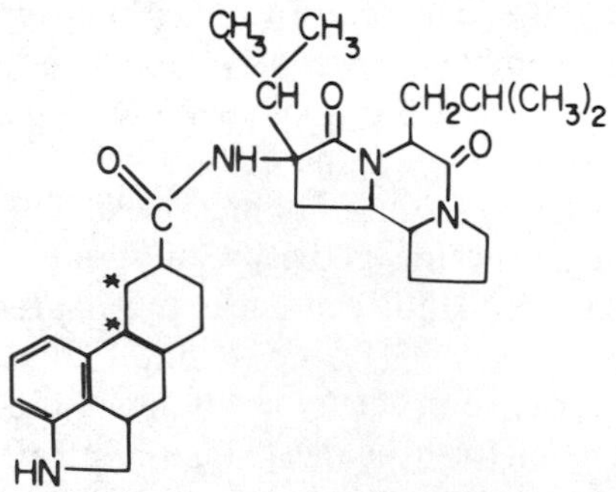

(−)-[³H]Dihydroalprenolol ([³H]DHA)
Lefkowitz et al., 1974

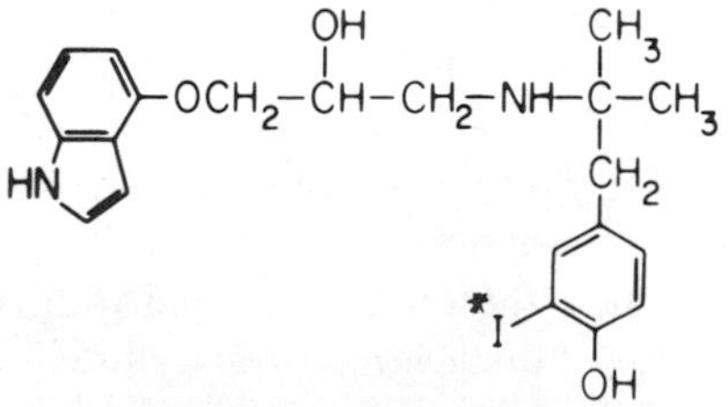

[¹²⁵I]Iodohydroxybenzylpindolol ([¹²⁵I]HYP)
Aurbach et al., 1976

Figure 1. Ligands used in studies on α and β receptors. Position of the radioisotope is indicated by an asterisk (*) unless the compound is generally labeled. The following have also been used as radioligands: [³H] epinephrine ([³H] E), [³H] norepinephrine ([³H] NE) and [³H] isoproterenol ([³H] ISO).

(Maguire et al., 1977). Nonspecific binding is lower by the filtration method than by centrifugation (Lefkowitz, 1976). Solubilization of the receptor requires different techniques and involves column chromatography (Caron and Lefkowitz, 1976a), equilibrium dialysis (Caron and Lefkowitz, 1976b), or precipitation techniques (Desbuquois and Aurbach, 1971; Haga, Haga, and Gilman, 1977a).

3. **Assay conditions** Binding has been assessed in a variety of media ranging from distilled water to physiological saline; Tris-HCl buffer is the most common medium. Variation in conditions can lead to significant artifacts. Thus, in one of the earliest reported receptor binding studies, Chagas (1959) claimed to have partially purified the cholinergic receptor. However, the equilibrium dialysis experiments were done in distilled water and the ligands bound to the protein simply as counterions (Ehrenpreis, Fleisch, and Mittag, 1969). It would appear that caution should be exercised concerning this point. Its potential importance in the study of α receptors can be assessed from the work of Ruffolo et al. (1976), who studied the binding of [^{3}H] dihydroazapetine to rat vas deferens in distilled water. Although many of the criteria of binding outlined previously could be demonstrated, inhibition of binding by catecholamines was not stereoselective.

Of more importance, however, is that the incubation conditions for determining binding and adenylate cyclase activity in β receptor systems are not in general identical, despite the importance of assessing the receptor-occupancy–adenylate-cyclase relationship. For example, inclusion of dithiothreitol in the cyclase reaction mixture, but not in the binding incubation, results in a 10-fold difference when comparing activation of adenylate cyclase to binding as the affinity is decreased in the presence of DTT (Lucas, Hanoune, and Bockaert, 1978).

Lefkowitz and Williams (1977) reported that the affinities for agonist are somewhat higher when determined with [^{3}H] HBI as compared to [^{3}H] DHA; but this difference was resolved when it was found that inclusion of pyrocatechol and ascorbate in the [^{3}H] HBI experiments was responsible: when included with agonist and [^{3}H] DHA, the values were comparable.

Maguire et al. (1977) have pointed out other difficulties, including the effects of purine nucleotides on binding and adenylate cyclase dose-response curves, refractoriness to adrenergic agonists, and the ability of ATP to mimic the effects of guanyl nucleotides in some cases. Lacking evidence to the contrary, it is therefore necessary to determine binding and response relationships under identical conditions; and it would be appropriate to do these studies under physiological conditions. This could also be of particular importance in relating the pharmacological potency of a series of compounds to their potency in competing with bound ligand, as the former activity is always assessed in physiological media. It is known, at least in some instances, that changes in ionic composition can affect the binding of α agonists (Tuttle and Moran, 1969) and high concentrations of Zn^{++}, Cu^{++} and Cd^{++} do inhibit binding of [^{3}H] DHE and [^{3}H] DHA to the adrenergic receptors of the hepatic plasma membrane (Guellaen et al., 1978), although Co^{++}, Mg^{++}, Ca^{++} and Mn^{++} had no effect at 10^{-3} M.

4. Nonspecific binding To determine nonspecific binding, assays are carried out in the presence of a competing agonist or antagonist at a concentration that will occupy essentially all the receptor sites. The assay should be carried out under conditions where the concentration of receptor in the assay is at least 10-fold lower than the K_B of the interaction under study or the classical reversible kinetics are not obtained (Cuatrecasas et al., 1975). Under these conditions the concentration of competing ligand can be readily calculated from the Michaelis-Menten equation. If the concentration of radioactive ligand is below the K_B value, displacement by a competing ligand employed at 100 times its respective K_B value should provide a good estimate of nonspecific binding. Higher concentrations of competing ligand can also compete at nonspecific sites (Molinoff, 1973), thus complicating the results. In some instances advantage is taken of the stereoselectivity of competing ligands where the difference in binding observed in the presence of competing "wrong" and "right" isomers is taken as the "specific binding." It is assumed in the case of the least potent isomer that only nonspecific competition occurs and that this will be equal to the nonspecific competition of the more potent isomer (Harden, Wolfe, and Molinoff, 1976b).

Clearly it is of great advantage to minimize the nonspecific binding, as is best illustrated by the use of pyrocatechol in the case of catecholamines. In contrast to earlier studies with [^{3}H] catecholamines, recent studies have demonstrated that specific binding with [^{3}H] catecholamines can be achieved in the presence of pyrocatechol and ascorbic acid, which eliminate nonspecific binding—presumably by blocking sites having high affinity for the catechol moiety and by preventing oxidation and the subsequent irreversible binding (Lefkowitz and Williams, 1977; Lefkowitz and Hamp, 1977). Although less dramatic, gains toward this end can also be achieved by prewetting filters and washing filters at 37°C.

In some cases it appears that the nonspecific binding is so great that the specific binding remains undetected. Thus iodination of hydroxyphenyl-KL-255 (I)* and hydroxyphenylalprenolol (II)* resulted in β antagonists that were of appreciably identical potency to iodinated hydroxybenzylpindolol (III)* but that unlike [^{125}I] HYP, did not demonstrate specific binding (Harden et al., 1976b). Calculations using Hansch II parameters demonstrate that the two ligands showing no specific binding are 10–50 times more hydrophobic and presumably partition sufficiently into the lipid bilayer to prevent detection of the specific component of binding.

---

* Fig. 2. See structural formulas on page 408.

III. RECEPTOR ISOLATION

According to the previous criteria, there are now a considerable number of successful studies characterizing α and β receptors by direct quantitative radioligand binding methods. An immediate conclusion from these studies is that the receptor concentration is relatively constant despite a diverse collection of tissues and varying degrees of purification (Table 1).

In only a very few instances, however, has the ligand binding study been carried to the stage of actual isolation of the receptor, and then only for the β receptor. To our knowledge there is no report of any successful *in vitro* reconstitution of either the α or the β receptor.

Table 1. Binding of ligands to α- and β-adrenergic receptors

Source of Membrane Preparation	Ligand*	K_B nM	Capacity† fmoles/mg Protein	Reference
β-Receptor				
Dog heart	[³H] DHA	11	350	Alexander, Williams, and Lefkowitz, 1975b
Rat adipocyte	"	12	240	Williams et al., 1976a
Rat cerebral cortex	"	7	180	Alexander, Davis, and Lefkowitz, 1975a; Mukherjee et al., 1976b
Frog erythrocyte	"	7.5	300	Mukherjee et al., 1975a
Frog erythrocyte	"	2	185‡	Caron & Lefkowitz, 1976a,b
Human lymphocyte	"	10	75	Williams et al., 1976c
Rat cerebral cortex	"	1.1	300	Bylund and Snyder, 1976
Rat pineal	"	18	600	Zatz et al., 1976
Turkey erythrocyte	"	3	100	Pike & Lefkowitz, 1978
Rat parotid	"	8	450	Au, Malbon, and Butcher, 1977
Turkey erythrocyte	[¹²⁵I] HYP	0.025	250	Brown et al., 1976a,b
Rat glioma (C₆)	"	0.250	75	Maguire et al., 1976
Mouse lymphoma (S49)	"	0.033	26	Insel et al., 1976; Ross et al., 1977
Rat heart	"	1.4	200	Harden et al., 1976
Rat liver	"	2.4	39	Wolfe, Harden, and Molinoff, 1976
Rat cerebral cortex	"	1.3	300	Sporn and Molinoff, 1976
Human fibroblasts	"	0.015	100	McGuire et al., 1976
Calf cerebellum	[³H] E	31	225§	U'Pritchard & Snyder 1977a
Guinea pig heart	[¹²⁵I] IP	22	800	O'Donnell & Woodcock, 1978
Frog erythrocyte	[³H] HBI	10	190	Lefkowitz and Williams, 1977

continued

Table 1—*continued*

Source of Membrane Preparation	Ligand*	K_B nM	Capacity† fmoles/mg Protein	Reference
α-Receptor				
Rabbit uterus	[³H] DHE	10	150	Williams et al., 1976b
Rat parotid	[³H] DHE	10.5	30	Strittmatter, Davis, and Lefkowitz, 1977a, b
Rat liver	[³H] DHE	4.9	1400	Guellaen et al., 1978
Dog aorta	[³H] DHE	10	145	Tsai and Lefkowitz, 1978
Human platelets	[³H] DHE	35	830	Kafka, Tallman, and Smith, 1977
Rat cerebral cortex	[³H] DHE	1.6	525§	Greenberg and Snyder, 1978
Rat brain	[³H] WB-4101	0.6	250§	Greenberg et al., 1976
Rat brain	[³H] clonidine	5	300§	Greenberg et al., 1976
Rat cerebral cortex	[³H] WB-4101		80	Skolnick et al., 1978
Calf cerebral cortex	[³H] NE	26	275§	U'Pritchard and Snyder, 1977a
	[³H] E	18	183§	
Calf cerebellum	[³H] E	5	100§	U'Prichard and Snyder, 1977b

* For abbreviations of ligands see Figure 1.

† The capacities are dependent upon the purity of the membrane preparation as well as upon the tissue concentration.

‡ Purified membrane preparations contain 1,760 fmoles/mg protein and a solubilized preparation 2,470 fmoles/mg protein.

§ These firures are calculated from the original data given in pmoles/gm wet weight assuming 40mg protein/gm tissue (Bylund and Snyder, 1976).

Probably the most important conclusion thus far from the β receptor isolation studies is that the β receptor ligand binding site and the adenylate cyclase moiety are separate species. Limbird and Lefkowitz (1977) have completely resolved β receptor binding and adenylate cyclase activity in frog erythrocytes by gel exclusion chromatography, and a corresponding separation in turkey erythrocytes has been achieved by affinity chromatography with agarose-alprenolol (Vauquelin et al., 1977). The β receptor binding site and adenylate cyclase activity have been separated from S49 mouse lymphoma cells (Haga et al., 1977a) to yield Lubrol-PX-associated proteins with estimated molecular weights of the receptor protein and the adenylate cyclase of 220×10^3 and 75×10^3 respectively. Of interest is that both the receptor protein and the adenylate cyclase associate with approximately 100 molecules of detergent, indicating that the binding and the catalytic components of the β-receptor-linked adenylate cyclase have significant hydrophobic components.

An indication that the β receptor binding protein may be oligomeric is suggested by the fact that the irreversible β antagonist N-[2-hydroxy-3-(1-naphthyloxy)propyl]-N'-bromoacetylethylenediamine (Atlas and Levitzki,

1976) labels, in apparently specific fashion, two distinct proteins of the turkey erythrocyte membrane with molecular weight in the range 37,000–41,000 (Atlas and Levitzki, 1978).

It should be noted that these few isolation studies have not yielded information concerning the molecular basis of adrenoceptor function. They have, however, established the important conclusion that, for the adenylate-cyclase-linked β receptor, the binding site and the catalytic sites are completely separate. The majority of studies on adrenoceptors have been concerned with quantification of ligand binding and have been directed at determining the relationship between receptor occupancy and response in elucidating the factors serving to regulate receptor function and in providing further criteria for the subclassification of receptors. It is these studies that have thus far been the more productive and the remaining sections of this chapter will be concerned primarily with a discussion of them and of their significance.

IV. RECEPTOR ORGANIZATION

A question for all pharmacological receptors is that of the relationship between the agonist binding site and the receptor catalytic or amplification site. For the adenylate-cyclase-linked β receptor, it has been generally agreed that the receptor and the cyclase components reside in opposite halves of the cell membrane; and recent studies using specific β receptor radioligands have demonstrated very directly the independent regulation and physical separability of the binding and catalytic sites (Greaves, 1975; Haga et al., 1977b; Ross and Gilman, 1977b).

Assaying for adenylate cyclase activity and β receptors by [^{125}I]-HYP binding in cultured mammalian cell lines has revealed that wild type S49 mouse lymphoma cells contain functional β-receptor-linked adenylate cyclase but that a variant clone of these cells (obtained by culture in the presence of isoproterenol and a phosphodiesterase inhibitor [Bourne, Coffino, and Tomkins, 1975]) lacks basal, F$^-$, and isoproterenol-sensitive adenylate cyclase activity (Insel et al., 1976). Yet both cell lines possess [^{125}I] HYP binding sites with properties consistent with β receptors in the same concentration and with the same affinity. These findings are complemented by the HC-1 cell line (derived from the HTC rat hepatoma), which is phenotypically similar to the adenylate-cyclase-negative S49 cell and also possesses [^{125}I] HYP sites but lacks adenylate cyclase activity.

That these findings are most consistent with the thesis that receptor and enzyme are products of distinct genes is indicated by several sets of cell fusion experiments. Fusion of parental clones responsive to β agonists with unresponsive clones produced hybrids with a greatly diminished β response and reduction of β receptor density. Fusion of two β-responsive clones produces a β-sensitive hybrid with normal receptor density (Brunton et al., 1977). Similar conclusions may be drawn from work showing that fusion of

N-ethylmaleimide or heat-treated turkey erythrocytes (adenylate cyclase lost) with Friend erythroleukemia or mouse adrenal tumor cells (which lack hormone-sensitive adenylate cyclase and possess no measurable [^{125}I] HYP binding capacity) produce isoproterenol-sensitive hybrids (Orly and Schramm, 1976; Schramm et al., 1977).

These reconstitution experiments *in vivo* are matched by reconstitution *in vitro*. When adenylate cyclase solubilized from mouse L cell membranes (lacking β binding sites) is mixed with β-receptor-containing, adenylate-cyclase-deficient S49 cell membranes, a catecholamine-sensitive adenylate cyclase system is generated whose specificity with regard to agonists and antagonists meets the pharmacological criteria of the β receptor (Ross and Gilman, 1977a).

These studies indicating the separate regulation of enzyme and binding sites are confirmed by studies using radioligand binding to demonstrate the physical separability of the two species. Thus, following treatment of frog erythrocyte or S49 membranes with Gpp(NH)p (to stabilize and activate adenylate cyclase; see Section VA), detergent solubilization and gel filtration or density-gradient ultracentrifugation yield distinct components that have either adenylate cyclase or specific [^{3}H] DHA or [^{125}I]-HYP binding only (Limbird and Lefkowitz, 1977; Haga et al., 1977a).

At this time nothing can be said about the constitution of the α receptor, though it will not be suprising if it is found that the receptor contains at least two distinct components.

V. OCCUPANCY AND RESPONSE

Clark's classical treatment of drug receptor interactions assumed that response is proportional to receptor occupancy (Clark, 1937). This assumption has been challenged by others, who have postulated the existence of a receptor reserve or spare receptors whereby fractional occupancy of receptors can elicit full response (Furchgott, 1955; Stephenson, 1956; Nickerson, 1956).

Ligand binding studies can provide a direct quantitative comparison between receptor occupancy and dose- response curves. In the simplest case, the dissociation constant of an agonist determined by binding (K_B)* should

---

* Through out this chapter K_B designates the ligand dissociation constant determined from binding experiments. This may be determined from direct binding of a radioligand or from the competition of an unlabeled agonist or antagonist with binding of a labeled ligand. These values should, in the simplest situation of ligand binding to a set of equivalent noninteracting sites, be identical. However, significant discrepancies have been observed under certain conditions. Thus an agonist dissociation constant determined by direct binding and by competition with a labeled antagonist may not be identical. Such a finding, which has been noted for a number of receptor systems, may indicate the existence of agonist and antagonist states of a single receptor or the existence of distinct receptor populations (sect. VI).

be equal to the ED_{50} value determined from dose-response curves. If a receptor reserve or a nonlinear relationship between occupancy and response exists, the K_B value should be different from the ED_{50} value. Regardless of the nature of the relationship between occupancy and response, however, the values of antagonists should be equal to the K_D values determined from dose-response relationships.

A. β-Adrenergic Receptors

In an elegant treatment of the β receptor system, Gilman and his colleagues have pointed out that there is a wide variation in the ratio of the dissociation constants for binding (K_B) to the dissociation constants determined for the activation of adenylate cyclase (K_{AC}) as summarized in Table 2 (Maguire et al., 1977). They have suggested that the ratio K_B/K_{AC} defines the efficiency of coupling: high values indicate maximal enzyme activity with minimal occupancy of receptors, whereas low ratios imply poor coupling where receptor occupation must be complete before full effects are seen.

Nucleotides (GTP, ITP) and analogues (GppNHp) improve coupling in S49 cells. In fact, in the absence of GTP, although isoproterenol binds to these cells, it does not have any effect on adenylate cyclase activity. In systems in which nucleotides have an effect, they shift K_B values to higher values, whereas K_{AC} is lowered in the presence of the analogue GppNHp (Maguire et al., 1977), resulting in a net increase in the ratio K_B/K_{AC}.

As can be seen in Table 2, the ratio K_B/K_{AC} for rat heart is considerably less than 1, particularly with isoproterenol, which is indicative of poor coupling. However, if one compares K_B to the ED_{50} for inotropic or chronotropic effects, the ratios are much larger for agonists and appreciably the same for the antagonist. This can be interpreted in several ways: it could indicate that coupling is lost on homogenization of tissues in preparation for binding studies, as suggested by Maguire et al. (1977). Thus, in intact tissue the coupling, and therefore the relationship between occupancy and

Table 2. Comparison of K_B/K_{AC} ratios for β receptor systems (Maguire et al., 1977)

Tissue	Ratio K_B/K_{AC}*
Rat heart	0.03
Rat liver	0.03
Turkey erythrocyte	0.16
Rat pineal	1.3
Frog erythrocyte	1.0
Rat adipocyte	0.26
Rat glioma	1.0
Mouse lymphoma	4.5

* The values of K_{AC} are "averaged" values for NE, E, and ISO (see Maguire et al., 1977, for further details).

Table 3.   Comparison of K_B, K_{AC} and ED_{50} values for cardiac β receptors

Ligand	[^{125}I]-HYP K_B, M	K_{AC}, M	K_B/K_{AC}	ED_{50}, M‡	K_B/ED_{50}
(−)-Norepinephrine	2.5×10^{-6}	2.5×10^{-5}* 1.0×10^{-5}†	0.1	2.5×10^{-7}	40
(−)-Epinephrine	5.0×10^{-8}	1.3×10^{-5}* 1.0×10^{-5}†	0.0048	1.5×10^{-7}	38
(−)-Isoproterenol	2.5×10^{-9}	6.3×10^{-7}* 6.0×10^{-7}†	0.004	6.3×10^{-9}	0.4
(−)-Propranolol	7.6×10^{-10}	1.3×10^{-9}	0.58	3.0×10^{-9}	0.2

* From Harden et al. (1976a)—rat heart.

† From Kaumann, Birnbaumer, and Yang, (1974)—kitten atria.

‡ ED_{50} values are estimates of the dose required for half maximal inotropic and chronotropic effects, since it was noted that they were 2–3 orders of magnitude less active in increasing adenylate cyclase then in producing inotropic or chronotropic effects (Kaumann et al., 1974).

response, could be more directly proportional. In agreement with this is the observation of Harden et al. (1976a) that K_B and K_{AC} are identical in intact astrocytoma cells, but on homogenization K_B remained constant, whereas K_{AC} increased 10-fold. Alternatively, poor coupling between receptor and cyclase as reflected in the K_B/K_{AC} value could be compensated for by efficient coupling between cyclase and the final effect as measured by the ED_{50} and reflected in the K_{AC}/EC_{50} ratios in Table 3. Thus, to gain further insight into the occupancy-response relationship, ligand binding studies must involve comparison of initial binding and both intermediate and final events in the sequence of biologic response.

B. α Receptors

Studies on binding in α receptor systems are limited; the data are summarized in Table 4. Values for K_B/EC_{50} are relatively constant, and it appears that there is not a significant receptor reserve and that coupling between receptor occupancy and response is near unity. Whether or not intermediate events, when measured, will show compensating coupling must await further investigations. The absence of a reserve is, however, consistent with results obtained by independent methods (May et al., 1967; Moran and Triggle, 1970).

VI.   RECEPTOR DIFFERENTIATION

The long-standing and fundamental division of adrenoceptors, derived from pharmacologic observations, into the α and β types has been amply confirmed by many studies of the direct binding of radiolabeled agonists and antagonists.

For β-adrenergic ligands the close structural similarity and identical stereoselectivity of agonists and antagonists is consistent with the simplest interpretation of the mutual competitive relationship seen in both binding and dose-response curves, namely interaction at a common binding site (Triggle and Triggle, 1977a). A division of β receptors into two subclasses, β_1 and β_2, has been proposed from pharmacological data on agonist and antagonist selectivities (Lands et al., 1967; Triggle and Triggle, 1977a), β_1 receptors being associated with adipose and cardiac tissue and β_2 receptors with liver, trachea, uterus, and skeletal muscle. Some controversy exists about the overall validity of this classification, arising in part from the well-known difficulties of receptor quantification by essentially indirect means.

However, direct binding experiments have provided clear support for the β_1/β_2 subclassification. Thus, in a comparison of the abilities of selective and nonselective β antagonists to inhibit [³H] DHA binding in rat heart and lung membranes, identical K_B values were found for nonselective antagonists in both tissues (Table 5; Barnett, Rugg, and Nahorski, 1978), and the binding curves were consistent with a single set of noninteracting sites. However, whereas β_1 selective antagonists showed only one set of sites in cardiac membranes, both low- and high-affinity sites were found in lung membranes; this finding is consistent with the latter tissue's containing two

Table 4. Comparison of K_B and ED_{50} values for various α receptor systems

Tissue	Ligand	K_B, M	ED_{50}	K_B/ED_{50}
Rabbit	[³H] DHE			
uterus[a]	NE	6.5×10^{-7}	4×10^{-6}	0.16
	E	2.3×10^{-7}	8×10^{-7}	0.3
	Phentolamine	1.5×10^{-8}	8×10^{-9}	1.9
Dog aorta[b]	[³H] DHE			
	NE	2.6×10^{-6}	1×10^{-8}	2.6
	E	1.0×10^{-6}	1×10^{-6}	1.0
	Phentolamine	5.3×10^{-8}	$14–30 \times 10^{-9}$	~2
Rat parotid[c]	[³H] DHE			
	NE	1×10^{-5}	1×10^{-5}	1.0
	E	3×10^{-5}	3×10^{-5}	1.0
	Phentolamine	3×10^{-7}	1×10^{-8}	3.0
Human	[³H] DHE			
platelets[d]	NE	2.5×10^{-7}	6×10^{-7}	0.4
	E	1.3×10^{-7}	1.7×10^{-7}	0.76
	Phentolamine	4.5×10^{-8}	3.4×10^{-8}	1.3

[a] Data from Williams et al. (1976b).

[b] Data from Tsai and Lefkowitz (1978).

[c] Data from Strittmatter et al. (1977a). Values represent concentration required to stimulate half maximal K^+ release from parotid cells.

[d] Data from Kafka et al. (1977). ED_{50} values represent the concentration of ligand required to cause 50% inhibition of PGE_1-stimulated cyclic AMP production or concentration of antagonist required to cause 50% reversal of l-norepinephrine stimulation.

Table 5. K_B values for adrenergic β-antagonist binding in rat lung, heart, and cerebral cortex (Barnett et al., 1978)

Antagonist	Lung	Heart K_B, M	Cerebral Cortex
A. Nonselective			
(−)-Propranolol	5×10^{-10}	3×10^{-10}	—
(+)-Propranolol	3×10^{-8}	4×10^{-8}	—
(−)-Timolol	1.5×10^{-9}	1.5×10^{-9}	—
B. Selective (β_1)			
Practolol	6×10^{-5}, 6.5×10^{-7}	8.6×10^{-7}	6.5×10^{-5}, 2.9×10^{-7}
Atenolol	2.9×10^{-5}, 5×10^{-7}	2.0×10^{-7}	—

distinct receptor populations, one of which is identical to that found in heart. Similar conclusions have been drawn for rat cerebral cortex, where β_1 antagonists show both high- and low-affinity binding.

The situation with respect to differentiation of α receptors is less clear. For α-adrenergic ligands the structural resemblance between agonists and antagonists is not striking, leading to suggestions that they may bind at distinct sites (Triggle and Triggle, 1977a). Furthermore, unlike the situation with peripheral β receptors, there is not clear-cut evidence for a subdivision of α receptors on postsynaptic membranes, although a difference between pre- and postsynaptic receptors does appear to exist on the basis of pharmacologic evidence (Starke, 1977; Wikberg, 1978).

However, several studies on CNS α receptors do suggest a heterogeneity of α receptor populations. Binding of labeled agonists ([^{3}H] NE, [^{3}H] E, and [^{3}H] clonidine) or antagonists ([^{3}H] WB 4101) reveals that both types of ligand show saturable specific binding with the ligand specificity characteristic of the α receptor (Greenberg, U'Prichard, and Snyder, 1976; U'Prichard and Snyder, 1977a, b, c; U'Prichard et al., 1977a, b; Greenberg and Snyder, 1978; Peroutka et al., 1978). It is found, however, that agonists are more potent in displacing bound agonist than bound antagonist, whereas the reverse holds true for antagonists. Furthermore, partial agonist ergot alkaloids display similar affinities for displacing either agonist or antagonist (Table 6).

Such data are consistent with a heterogeneity of receptors or with the postulate that receptors exist in agonist or antagonist states, the latter suggestion according with proposals made for other neurotransmitter systems and providing a basis for the differentiation of agonist and antagonist activity. However, several lines of evidence indicate that these populations of binding sites are not readily interconvertible. Hill plots for the displacement of [^{3}H] clonidine or [^{3}H] WB-4101 by agonists or antagonists have slopes of 1.0, as do the plots for mixed agonists-antagonists in competing

Table 6. Inhibition of clonidine and WB 4101 binding in rat
brain by α-adrenergic ligands (Greenberg and Snyder, 1978)

Ligand	[³H] Clonidine log K_B, nM	[³H] WB-4101 log K_B, nM
(−)-Epinephrine	0.77	2.77
(+)-Epinephrine	1.81	4.55
(−)-Norepinephrine	1.23	3.00
(+)-Norepinephrine	2.78	4.83
Clonidine	0.76	2.63
Phentolamine	1.34	0.56
WB 4101	2.30	−0.22
Indoramin	3.81	0.77
Ergotamine	1.08	1.08
Dihydroergotamine	0.38	0.54
Dihydroergocryptine	0.85	0.38

for [³H] DHE binding. However, slopes of plots for inhibition of [³H] DHE binding by pure agonists or antagonists have $n_h < 1.0$.

Further evidence for the discrete nature of these binding sites comes from studies of regional distribution in rat and calf brain (U'Prichard et al., 1977a, b). In cerebral cortex of both species [³H] DHE binding is equal to the sum of [³H] agonist and [³H] antagonist binding (Table 7A), suggesting that [³H] DHE can bind to sites preferentially labeled by either agonist or antagonist. In other brain regions, however, significant discrepancies occur in the regional distribution of [³H] ligand binding (Table 7B). Thus in cerebellar cortex there are very few antagonist-preferring sites, whereas in the pons there are few agonist-preferring sites.

The significance of these findings with respect to α receptor function or classification is not entirely clear. The apparent noninterconvertibility and discrepant regional distribution argue against a description in which the agonist and antagonist binding simply reflects alternate states of the same receptor. More plausible is the existence of distinct populations of α receptors, one having high and the other low affinity for α agonists. The possibility that these represent pre- and postsynaptic receptors seems unlikely, since binding of either [³H] clonidine or [³H] WB 4101 is not reduced by 6-

Table 7A. Ligand binding to rat and calf cerebral cortex (U'Prichard et al., 1977b)

	Ligand		
	[³H] Clonidine	[³H] WB 4101	[³H] DHE
Capacity,	14 ± 3	11 ± 1.0	21 ± 1.7 (Rat)
p mols/g tissue	8 − 9	8 − 9	15 − 17 (Calf)

Table 7B. Regional distribution of α-adrenergic ligand binding in calf brain (Peroutka et al., 1978)

Region	[³H] E pmols/g	%	[³H] NE pmols/g	%	[³H] WB 4101 pmols/g	%	[³H] DHE pmols/g	%
Frontal cortex	3.9	100	2.9	100	2.3	100	2.8	100
Cerebellar cortex	2.3	59	2.0	69	0	0	1.5	54
Pons	0.6	15	0.5	17	1.1	48	1.0	36

hydroxydopamine treatment (U'Prichard et al., 1977b). Although differences in ligand selectivity for peripheral pre- and postsynaptic receptors seem established (Starke, 1977), the possible subclassification of peripheral postsynaptic receptors is less well established (Triggle and Triggle, 1977a; Peroutka et al., 1978); and it is simply not possible now to conclude whether the apparent division of CNS α receptors corresponds to any peripheral division.

VII. RECEPTOR REGULATION

It has long been realized that tissue sensitivity to catecholamines can be modified by hormonal and neuronal influences. As early as 1906 Dale noted that the effect of epinephrine changed from inhibitory to excitatory according to whether the uterine tissue of the cat was in a virgin or a pregnant state. Similarly, it has been known for many years that an increase in chemosensitivity is a general consequence of denervation of an effector system (Cannon and Rosenblueth, 1949). Until recently, however, it has been possible to draw only indirect conclusions about any role of changes in adrenoceptor quantity and quality in such phenomena as desensitization, supersensitivity, neuronal maturation, or hormonal modulation of uterine and cardiovascular reactivity. Radioligand binding techniques have served to indicate that changes in adrenoceptors do play a role in the modulation of tissue sensitivity; moreover, similar work with other neurotransmitter and hormone and immune systems has served to illustrate the apparently general concept that modification of receptor concentration and/or binding properties is an important homeostatic regulatory mechanism in cell communication (Raff, 1976).

A. Desensitization

Exposure of an effector system to a stimulant frequently results in a reversible diminution of response to further stimulus. This process of desensitization may be classified, in pharmacological terms, as specific or nonspecific, according to the absence or presence respectively of desensitization to structurally dissimilar ligands (Barsoum and Gaddum, 1935; Triggle and Triggle, 1977b).

Desensitization to catecholamines in β receptor systems has been reported at tissue and cellular levels (Kebabian et al., 1975; Makman, 1971; Remold-O'Donnell, 1974; Mickey et al., 1976; Dismukes and Daly, 1976) and in clinical states such as the isoprenaline-refractory asthmatic (Greenacre, Schofield, and Conolly, 1978). In many instances the desensitization appears to be specific, as judged by lack of cross-desensitization; and such pharmacological studies suggest, but do not prove, that changes in adrenoceptors may be involved. However, since the process of specific β-adrenoceptor desensitization is mediated by agonists only, is directly proportional to the intrinsic activity of the agonists (Mukherjee and Lefkowitz, 1977), and does not occur in mutant cells containing β receptors but lacking adenylate cyclase (Shear et al., 1976) or in filipin-uncoupled systems (Mukherjee and Lefkowitz, 1977), it is also possible that it occurs as a result of the receptor activation process—possibly through changes in phosphodiesterase, protein kinase, or other activity dependent upon cAMP function (Johnson et al., 1978; Wolfe et al., 1977).

That specific desensitization includes a role for changes in the adrenoceptor itself is, however, indicated by a number of recent binding studies in β receptor systems (Table 8). A common finding is that receptor concentration, as measured by antagonist binding, is reduced by approximately 50% and that in the adenylate-cyclase-linked β receptor systems there is a generally good correlation between loss of cAMP formation and loss of receptor sites. The notable exception is for human astrocytoma cells, where a much larger reduction in adenylate cyclase V_{max} occurs relative to loss of binding sites. It should be noted, however, that in this instance isoproterenol produces cross-desensitization to PGE_1.

Although these studies provide valuable evidence that a reduction in receptor availability does occur in specific adrenoceptor desensitization, they nonetheless leave a number of very important questions unanswered. Thus, no more than a 50%–60% reduction in receptor availability is found; this must presumably represent a "masking" of receptors, since in general the process of desensitization is reversible and its recovery is facilitated by guanine nucleotides and is not prevented by inhibitors of protein synthesis. However, exceptions to these generalizations are known. Thus recovery from desensitization in human fibroblasts (Franklin, Morris, and Twose, 1975) and desensitization in RGC6 rat glioma cells are dependent upon protein synthesis (DeVellis and Brooker, 1974). How the receptors are masked to antagonist binding remains unclear. One possibility is that during desensitization conversion to a high-affinity agonist binding state occurs, as indicated by the binding of [³H] HBI and [³H] DHA to frog erythrocyte

Table 8. Desensitization of β-adrenoceptors

System	Ligand	Agonist	Receptor		Adenylate Cyclase		Reference
			Conc.	Affinity	V_{max}	Affinity	
Frog erythrocytes (in vivo)	[³H] DHA	(−)ISO 20 mg/kg 3x/24 h	50%↓	No change	77%↓	No change	Mukherjee et al., 1975b, 1976b
Frog erthrocytes (in vivo)	[³H] DHA	(−)ISO 10⁻⁴ M, > 5 h	50%↓	No change	70%↓	No change	Mickey, Tate, and Lefkowitz, 1975; Mickey et al., 1976
Frog erythrocytes membranes	[³H] DHA	(−)ISO 10⁻⁵ M, 1 h	60%↓	No change	60%↓	No change	Mukherjee and Lefkowitz 1976, 1977
Frog erythrocytes membranes	[³H] DHA	HBI 10⁻⁷ M, 15 m	60%↑	—			Williams and Lefkowitz, 1977
	[³H] HBI	HBI 10⁻⁷ M, 15 m	60%↑	—			
Rat pineal	[³H] DHA	Dark (12 h) inc. symp. act.	40%↓	No change	80%↓		Kebabian et al., 1975
	[³H] DHA	(−)ISO 5 mg/kg/2 h	45%↓	No change	80%↓		
Turkey erythrocyte reticulocytes	[¹²⁵I] HYP	(−)ISO 10⁻⁵ M, 5 h		No desensitization			Hanski and Levitski, 1978
Human astrocytoma cells	[¹²⁵I] HYP	(−)ISO 10⁻⁵ M, 2 h (nonspecific)	20%↓	—	80–90%↓ (whole cells) 35%–50%↓ (fragments)		Johnson et al., 1978
S49 mouse lymphoma cells	[¹²⁵I] HYP	(−)ISO 10⁻⁶ M, 2–5 h	25%–45%↓	No change	75%↓	No change	Shear et al., 1976

membranes, in which desensitization is accompanied by approximately equal and opposite changes in [³H] DHA and [³H] HBI binding (Williams and Lefkowitz, 1977). However, such a conversion does not appear to be involved with receptor desensitization produced in intact frog erythrocytes (Lefkowitz, Mullikin, and Williams, 1978)—a finding that serves to illustrate the differences in desensitization occurring in whole cells and membrane fragments. Desensitization in membrane fragments appears to be more rapid and more sensitive to reversal by guanine nucleotides, thus raising the possibility that the desensitization process seen in membrane fragments is unrelated to that seen in whole cells. Presumably the latter is more reflective of any physiological role for adrenoceptor desensitization. Nonetheless, a reduction in receptor availability for both agonist occupation and antagonist binding appears to be a common feature of the desensitization process.

B. Hormonal Regulation

Considerable similarity exists between the effects of excess sympathetic activity and the cardiovascular effects of hyperthyroidism (Spaulding and North, 1975). Despite early suggestions that specific sensitivity changes to catecholamines occur in the hyperthyroid state, the causal relationship between thyroid hormone and sympathetic function has remained obscure. Several recent studies have indicated, however, that one component of thyroid involvement is mediated through alterations in the adrenoceptor population (Table 9). T_4 or T_3 treatment produces a significant increase (approximately twofold) in β receptor concentration without change in ligand affinity, and thyroidectomy or propylthiouracil treatment produces a decrease in β receptor numbers. It is noteworthy that both T_4 *and* propylthiouracil produce decreases in the α receptor concentration, as is the fact that the α receptor concentration is some threefold higher than the β receptor concentration. In light of the known effects of thyroid hormone on DNA regulation and protein synthesis (Tata, 1968), it might be anticipated that the increase in β receptors represents newly synthesized material; and accordingly, T_4 did not affect β receptor binding when studied in myocardial membranes *in vitro* (Williams et al., 1977). However, a cycloheximide-insensitive increase in receptor number has been shown in ventricle slices supplemented with amino acids (Kempson, Marinetti, and Shaw, 1978), which finding may represent membranal incorporation of an internal pool of presynthesized receptors.

Thyroid hormone is known also to be involved in the control of lipolysis in adipose tissue, and fat cells from hypothyroid rats show reduced free fatty acid and cAMP responses to epinephrine (Debons and Schwartz, 1961; Correze et al., 1974). However, this impairment is not accompanied by significant changes in $(-)$-[³-H] DHA binding (Malbon et al., 1978),

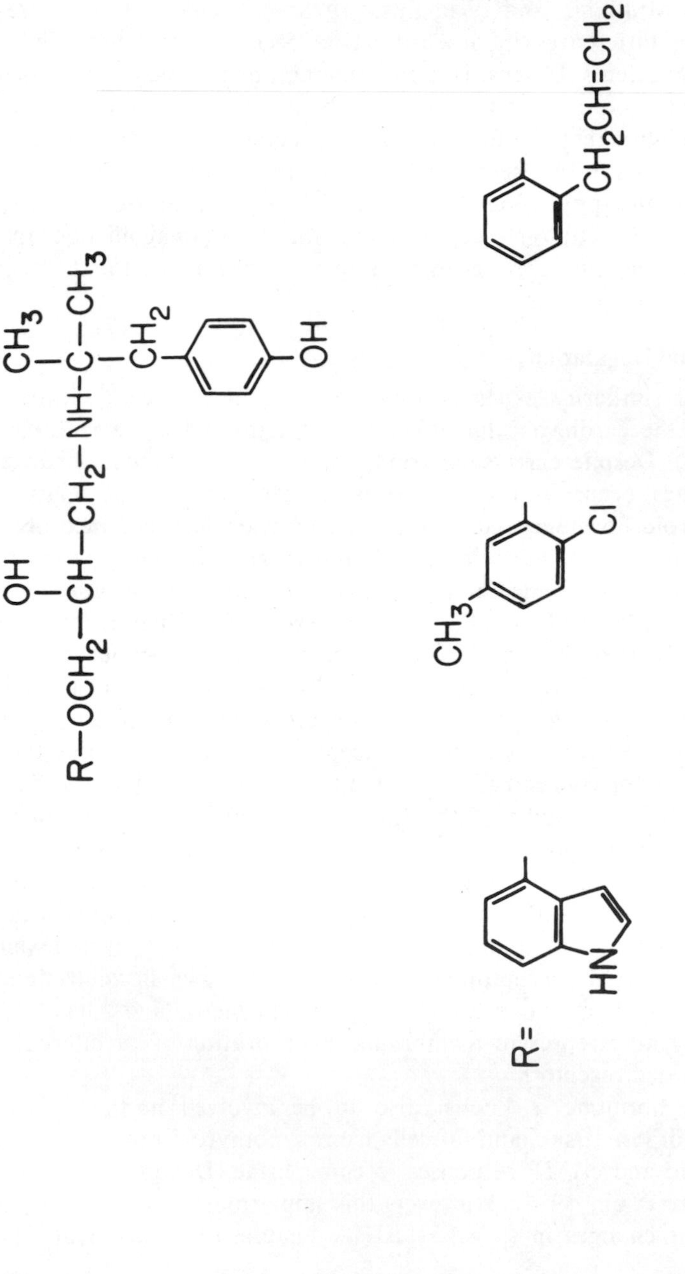
R—OCH₂—CH—CH₂—NH—C—CH₃
OH
CH₃
CH₂
OH
R=
HN
CH₃
Cl
CH₂CH=CH₂

I Hydroxybenzylpindolol

II Hydroxyphenyl KL-255

III Hydroxyphenylalprenolol

Figure 2.

indicating that the impairment occurs at a level other than the β-adrenergic recognition site itself. This would appear consistent with the finding that the lipolytic response to ACTH and glucagon is also impaired (Correze et al., 1974).

The glycogenolytic response of the liver appears to be under control of α or β receptors according to species and hormonal status (Exton and Harper, 1975; Exton et al., 1972). Chan and Exton (1977) have reported that the response of the rat liver to epinephrine changes, in terms of glucose production, from pure α to mixed α/β following adrenalectomy. Ligand binding studies have shown that this change in pharmacological response is accompanied by an increase in β receptors with no change in α receptor concentration (Table 10). Whether the relatively small change in the α/β ratio observed by Guellaen et al. (1978) is sufficient to account for the conversion of pharmacological response is unclear.

A most dramatic and long-recognized effect of hormones concerns gonadal hormone modulation of uterine sensitivity to catecholamines (Dale, 1906). Thus in estrogen-dominated human or rabbit uterus the α-adrenergic response dominates, whereas in pregnant or progesterone-dominated uterus the β response dominates (Miller, 1967). A change in the receptor population is an obviously attractive hypothesis to explain such findings; but in the absence of direct evidence, alternative explanations are equally possible, in view of the many effects of estrogen and progesterone on uterine tissue (Triggle and Triggle, 1977c). However, measurements by Roberts et al. (1977) have shown (Table 11) that the concentration of α receptors in rabbit uterus increases and decreases with estrogen and progesterone treatment respectively, but that no change in β receptors occurs. Whether this change in $\alpha:\beta$ ratio is sufficient to explain the reversal of response is not clear, but the data do serve to indicate that interconversion of α and β receptors is not the basis of the gonadal hormone effect and render less plausible the postulate that the α and β receptors are simply alternate configurations of the same structure interconvertible by temperature, hormones, and other modulating influences (Kunos, 1978).

C. Receptor Development

A central problem in neurobiology concerns the role of the neurotransmitter receptor in the control of the development, pattern, and maintenance of the neuron–effector-cell interaction. It is of importance to determine the relative roles of the neuron and of the effector cell in determining neuronal and receptor maturation.

Comparatively little is known concerning the development of the adrenoceptor and its role in the development and maintenance of the neuronal network. However, radioligand binding studies should provide answers to such questions as these: Does receptor development involve

Table 9. Thyroid modification of adrenoceptors

Tissue	Treatment	[³H] DHE K_B, M	Cap., pmol/mg-Prot	[³H] DHA K_B, M	Cap., pmol/mg/Prot	Reference
Rat heart	Control	—		1.5×10^{-9}	38	Banerjee and Kung, 1977
(Sprague-Dawley)	Thyroidectomized	—		1.2×10^{-9}	26	
Rat heart	Control	4.5×10^{-9}	307	6.2×10^{-9}	92	Ciaraldi and Marinetti, 1977
(Sprague-Dawley)	T4*	18.5×10^{-9}†	165	0.7×10^{-9}	302	
	Propylthiouracil‡	2.5×10^{-9}	52	4.3×10^{-9}	66	
Rat heart	Control			$12 \pm 5 \times 10^{-9}$	89 ± 5	Williams et al., 1977
(Cox-Wistar)	T4			$15 \pm 8 \times 10^{-9}$	196 ± 7	
	T3			$19 \pm 6 \times 10^{-9}$	180 ± 20	

* T4, 75 µg/100g b·w/sc, 17 days.
† Saturation of [³H] DHE binding not observed.
‡ 0.1% propylthiouracil in drinking water for 10 days.

Table 10. Corticosteroid modification of adrenoceptors

Tissue	Condition	[³H] DHE K_B	Cap., fmol/mg/p	[³H] DHA K_B	Cap., fmol/mg/p	[¹²⁵I] HYB K_B	Cap., fmol/mg/p	Ref.
Rat liver (Female, Wistar)	Control	2.7×10^{-9}	103.0 ± 60	4.4×10^{-9}	55	—		Guellaen et al., 1978
	Adrenalectomized	2.0×10^{-9}	105.0 ± 45*	2.2×10^{-9}	107†	—		
Rat liver (Male, Sprague-Dawley)	Control	—	—			$2.6 \pm 1.5 \times 10^{-9}$	188 ± 27	Wolfe et al., 1976
	Adrenalectomized	—	—			$5.4 \pm 3.3 \times 10^{-9}$	972 ± 158†	

* Not significantly different from control.
† Significantly different from control.

Table 11. Estrogen and progesterone modification of adrenoceptors in rabbit uterus (Roberts et al., 1977)

Animal status	[³H] DHE Binding		[¹²⁵I] HYP Binding	
	K_B	No. of Sites fmol mg DNA	K_B	Cap. fmol mg DNA
Estrogen	$5.1 \pm 1.1 \times 10^{-9}$	3400 ± 400	$2.1 \pm 0.3 \times 10^{-10}$	86 ± 11
Progesterone	$8.0 \pm 2.8 \times 10^{-9}$*	1000 ± 200†	$2.2 \pm 2 \times 10^{-10}$*	56 ± 9*

* Not significantly different.
† Significantly different (p < 0.001).

separate assembly of binding and catalytic sites? Do receptors control development of innervation, or does innervation control receptor development? What is the relationship between receptor development and maturation of the neuronal neurotransmitter machinery? What are the changes in receptors occurring in the absence of neuronal influences?

Harden et al. (1977a) have studied the development of β-adrenoceptors in the rat cerebral cortex. The very low density of [¹²⁵I] HYP binding sites present at days 1–7 after birth increases rapidly, reaching adult levels by day 14. This development parallels the development of β-responsive adenylate cyclase, although F⁻-sensitive activity is present at birth and has developed to 60% of maximum by day 6. These data suggest that it is the appearance of β-adrenergic recognition sites that initiates formation of the functional β receptor unit. This time course does not correspond with the time course of the development of presynaptic development, which is a much slower process. Thus for the rat cerebral cortex, receptor development appears as independent from neuronal activity. This is confirmed by studies in rats treated with 6-hydroxydopamine immediately after birth (Harden et al., 1977b), which chemical sympathectomy affects the time course of neither β receptor nor AC development, despite the virtually complete destruction of noradrenergic terminals.

A nonneuronal example of adrenoceptor changes during cell maturation is provided by the rat reticulocyte-erythrocyte transformation (Bilezikian et al., 1977a, b). Reticulocytes contain functionally coupled adenylate cyclase and β receptor binding sites. With maturation there is a progressive loss of both adenylate cyclase (isoproterenol and F⁻-sensitive) and β binding sites. However, the time course of loss of these properties is very different, indicating both the discrete character and the separate regulation of these two functions.

D. Supersensitivity

The increase in effector organ sensitivity following interruption of innervation has long been known (Cannon and Rosenblueth, 1949). In the case of the sympathetic nervous system, the supersensitive response has both pre- and postsynaptic components (Trendelenberg, 1972; Fleming, McPhillips, and Westfall, 1973). It appears probable that changes in the concentration of adrenoceptors is a contributing postsynaptic factor. This has already been noted for the pineal gland, which shows a diurnal rhythm in both sensitivity and β receptor concentration (Sect. VII). Similar conclusions have been drawn for other systems. Thus, 6-hydroxydopamine treatment augments the β-adrenoceptor sensitivity in rat cerebral cortex by $\sim$ 80%, and this is accompanied by a lesser but significant increase in β receptor number without change in affinity (Table 12; Sporn et al., 1976). A larger increase in β receptor density has been shown following 6-hydroxydopamine treatment of rats from day 1–4 after birth (Table 12; Harden et al., 1977b), perhaps reflecting the greater plasticity of the developing nervous system. A small increase ($\sim$ 20%) has been reported for β receptor density in rabbit iris rendered supersensitive by removal of the superior cervical ganglion. No change in α receptor density was found (Page and Neufeld, 1978). These latter findings are consistent with the thesis that denervation supersensitivity in smooth muscle is largely due to nonreceptor influences.

Increases in [³H] DHA binding of some 25% in rat cerebral cortex following 6-hydroxydopamine treatment have also been reported by Skolnick et al. (1978). This work also illustrates the independence of the β-receptor binding and catalytic sites, since, depending upon the strain, the increase in binding is (Sprague-Dawley) or is not (F 344) accompanied by hyperresponsiveness of the adenylate cyclase system.

Limited and conflicting data are available for α-adrenoceptor systems. In rat cerebral cortex Skolnick et al. (1978) found no change in [³H] WB 4101 binding following 6-hydroxydopamine, whereas small but significant increases of [³H] clonidine (23%) and [³H] WB 4101 (8%) binding were found when whole brain preparations were used (U'Prichard et al., 1977b).

Table 12. Effect of chemical denervation on β-receptors in rat cerebral cortex

Preparation	Age	K_B, M	Capacity fmol mg protein	% Increase in AC activity above control	Ref.
Control*		$1.1 \pm 0.1 \times 10^{-9}$†	290 ± 1	80%	Sporn et al., 1976
6-HOdopamine		$1.2 \pm 0.2 \times 10^{-9}$	380 ± 1		
Control‡	100 days	$9.3 \pm 0.5 \times 10^{-11}$§	56 ± 6.0	71%	Harden et al., 1977b
6-HOdopamine	100 days	$9.5 \pm 0.5 \times 10^{-11}$	95 ± 8.0		

* Sprague-Dawley rats injected on two successive days intraventricularly with 200 µg 6HODA and sacrificed 7–9 days later.

† Measured with a low specific activity preparation of [¹²⁵I] HYP (partially inactivated?)

‡ Sprague-Dawley rats (new born) injected with 100 µg/g.b.w. SC of 6-HODA and repeated on three successive days.

§ Measured with high specific activity [¹²⁵I] HYP.

VIII. CONCLUSIONS

In the strictest sense, there have been few attempts to purify, isolate, and characterize adrenergic receptors, although this area will no doubt receive much attention in the next several years. The great majority of current studies dealing with ligand binding have demonstrated the validity of using these compounds in receptor assays, and there is little doubt that binding is concerned with processes that satisfy the pharmacological definition of α or β receptors. The success of these studies has depended, as have similar studies on other receptor systems, upon the availability of suitable radioligands. The importance of binding studies carried out to date, although not directed specifically toward isolation, should not be underestimated, for they have permitted determination of receptor concentrations and ligand affinities. This has provided a more rational basis for structure-activity analyses and has permitted definitive answers to questions concerning receptor changes in a variety of physiologic and pharmacologic processes. Furthermore, these studies are facilitating approaches to the understanding of the most important question concerning receptor function, the linkage between receptor occupancy and biologic response.

It is clear, however, that our knowledge of adrenoceptor function is still seriously lacking, and further studies focusing directly on the isolation and purification of adrenergic receptors hold much promise. Isolation of the agonist binding component, together with identification and isolation of associated macromolecules necessary to generate the intracellular signal leading to response, will provide insight into the mechanisms involved in coupling and the opportunity to reconstitute the system.

IX. REFERENCES

Alexander, R.W.; Davis, J.N.; Lefkowitz, R.J.: Direct Identification and Characterization of β-Adrenergic Receptors in Rat Brain. Nature 258(1975a)437–439

Alexander, R.W.; Williams, L.T.; Lefkowitz, R.J.: Identification of Cardiac β-Adrenergic Receptors by (−) [³H] Alprenolol Binding. Proc Natl Acad Sci USA 72(1975b)1564–1568.

Aprille, J.R.; Lefkowitz, R.J.; Warshaw, J.B.: [³H] Norepinephrine Binding and Lipolysis by Isolated Fat Cells. Biochim Biophys Acta 373(1974)502–513

Atlas, D.; Levitzki, A.: An Irreversible Blocker for the β-Adrenergic Receptor. Biochem Biophys Res Comm 69(1976)397–403

Atlas, D; Levitzki, A.: Tentative Identification of β-Adrenoreceptor Subunits. Nature 272(1978)370–371

Au, D.K.; Malbon, C.C.; Butcher, F.R.: Identification and Characterization of Beta-Adrenergic Receptors in Rat Parotid Membranes. Biochim Biophys Acta 500(1977)361–371

Aurbach, G.D.; Brown, E.M.; Hauser, D.; Troxler, F.: β-Adrenergic Receptor Interactions. Characterization of Iodohydroxybenzopindolol As a Specific Ligand. J Biol Chem 251(1976)1232–1238

Aurbach, G.D.; Fedak, S.A.; Woodard, C.J.; Palmer, J.S.; Hauser, D.; Troxler, F.: β-Adrenergic Receptor: Stereospecific Interaction of Iodinated Blocking Agent with a High Affinity Site. Science 186(1974)1223–1224

Banerjee, S.P.; Kung, L.S.: β-Adrenergic Receptors in Rat Heart: Effects of Thyroidectomy. Eur J Pharmacol 43(1977)207–308

Barnett, D.B.; Rugg, E.L.; Nahorski, S.R.: Direct Evidence of Two Types of β-Adrenoceptor Binding Site in Lung Tissue. Nature 273(1978)166–168

Barsoum, G.S.; Gaddum, J.H.: Pharmacological Estimation of Adenosine and Histamine in Blood. J Physiol 85(1935)1–14

Bayly, R.J.; Evans, E.A.: Storage and Stability of Compounds Labeled with Radioisotopes, Review. Amersham/Searle Corporation, Arlington Heights, Ill., 1974

Bilezikian, J.P.; Aurbach, G.D.: A β-Adrenergic Receptor of the Turkey Erythrocyte. I. Binding of Catecholamine and Relationship to Adenylate Cyclase Activity. J Biol Chem 248(1973)5575–5583

Bilezikian, J.P.; Spiegel, A.M.; Brown, E.M.; Aurbach, G.D.: Identification and Persistence of Beta Adrenergic Receptors during Maturation of the Rat Reticulocyte. Mol Pharmacol 13(1977a)775–785

Bilezikian, J.P.; Spiegel, A.M.: Gammon, D.E.; Aurbach, G.D.: The Role of Guanyl Nucleotides in the Expression of Catecholamine-Responsive Adenylate Cyclase during Maturation of the Rat Reticulocyte. Mol Pharmacol 13(1977b)786–795

Birnbaumer L.; Pohl, S.L.; Kaumann, A.J.: Receptors and Acceptors: A Necessary Distinction in Hormone Binding Studies. Adv Cyclic Nucleotide Res 4(1974)239–281

Bobik, J.R.; Woodcock, E.A.; Johnson, C.I.; Funder, J.W.: The Preparation of 3-(4-Iodophenoxy)-1-Isopropylamino-2-Propanol-^{125}I, a β-Adrenergic Antagonist. J Labelled Comp 13(1977)605–610

Bourne, H.R.; Coffino, P.; Tomkins, G.M.: Selection of a Variant Lymphoma Cell Deficient in Adenylate Cyclase. Science 187(1975)750–752

Brown, E.M.; Aurbach, G.D.; Hauser, D.; Troxler, F.: β-Adrenergic Receptor Interactions. Characterization of Iosohydroxybenzylpindolol as a Specific Ligand. J Biol Chem 251(1976a)1232–1238

Brown, E.M.; Fedak, S.A.; Woodard, C.J.; Aurbach, G.D.; Rodbard, D.: β-Adrenergic Receptor Interactions, Direct Comparison of Receptor Interaction and Biological Activity. J Biol Chem 251(1976b)1239–1246

Brunton, L.L.; Maguire, M.E.: Anderson, H.J.; Gilman, A.G.: Expression of Genes for Metabolism of Cyclic Adenosine 3′:5′-monophosphate in Somatic Cells. β-Adrenergic and PGE$_1$ Receptors in Parental and Hybrid Cells. J Biol Chem 252(1977)1293–1302

Bylund, D.B.; Snyder, S.H.: Beta Adrenergic Receptor Binding in Membrane Preparations from Mammalian Brain. Mol Pharmacol 12(1976)568–580

Cannon, W.B.; Rosenblueth, A.: The Supersensitivity of Denervated Structures. MacMillan, New York, 1949

Caron, M.G.; Lefkowitz, R.J.: β-Adrenergic Receptors: Solubilization of (−) [^{3}H] Alprenolol Binding Sites from Frog Erythrocyte Membranes. Biochem Biophys Res Comm 68(1976a)315–322

Caron, M.G.; Lefkowitz, R.J.: Solubilization and Characterization of the β-Adrenergic Receptor Binding Sites of Frog Erythrocytes. J Biol Chem 251(1976b)2374–2384

Chagas, C.: Studies on the Mechanisms of Curarization. Ann NY Acad Sci 81(1959)345–357

Chan, T.M.; Exton, J.H.: Enhanced β-Adrenergic Activation of Glycogen Phosphorylase in Hepatocytes from Adrenalectomized Rats. Fed Proc 36(1977)384(Abs. 608)

Ciaraldi, T.; Marinetti, G.V.: Thyroxine and Propylthiouracil Effects In Vivo on Alpha and Beta Adrenergic Receptors in Rat Heart. Biochem Biophys Res Comm 74(1977)984–991

Clark, A.J.: General Pharmacology. In: Handbuch der Experimentellen Pharmakologie, pp. 1–222, ed. by A. Heffter, N. Heubner. Vol. IV. Springer, Berlin, 1937

Cohen, J.B.; Changeux, J.P.: The Cholinergic Receptor Protein in its Membrane Environment. Ann Rev Pharmacol 15(1975)83–103

Correze, C.; Laudat, M.H.; Laudat, P.; Nunez, J.: Hormone-dependent Lipolysis in Fat-cells from Thyroidectomized Rats. Mol Cell Endocrinol 1(1974)309–327

Cuatrecasas, P.; Hollenberg, M.D.; Chang, K.J.; Bennett, V.: Hormone Receptor Complexes and their Modulation of Membrane Function. Rec Prog Hormone Res 31(1975)37–84

Cuatrecasas, P.; Tell, G.P.E.; Sica, V.; Parikh, I.; Chang, K.J.: Noradrenaline Binding and the Search for Catecholamine Receptors. Nature 247(1974)92–97

Dale, H.H.: On Some Physiological Actions of Ergot. J Physiol 34(1906)163–206

DeVellis, J.; Brooker, G.: Reversal of Catecholamine Refractoriness by Inhibitors of RNA and Protein Synthesis. Science 186(1974)1221-1223

Debons, A.F.; Schwartz, I.L.: Dependence of the Lipolytic Action of Epinephrine *In Vitro* Upon Thyroid Hormone. J Lip Res 2(1961)86-91

Desbuquois, B.; Aurbach, G.D.: Use of Polyethylene Glycol to Separate Free and Antibody-bound Peptide Hormones in Radioimmunoassays. J Clin Endocrin Metab 33(1971)732-738

Dismukes, R.K.; Daly, J.W.: Adaptive Responses of Brain Cyclic AMP-generating Systems to Alterations in Synaptic Input. J Cyc Nuc Res 2(1976)321-336

Dunnick, J.K.; Marinetti, G.V.: Hormone Action at the Membrane Level. III. Epinephrine Interaction with the Rat Liver Plasma Membrane. Biochim Biophys Acta 249(1971)122-134

Ehrenpreis, S.; Fleisch, J.H.; Mittag, T.W.: Approaches to the Molecular Nature of Pharmacological Receptors. Pharmacol Rev 21 (1969)131-181

Exton, J.H.; Friedman, N.; Wong, E.; Brineaux, J. P.; Corbin, J.D.; Park, C.R.: Interaction of Glucocorticoids with Glucagon and Epinephrine in the Control of Gluconeogenesis and Glycogenolysis in Liver and of Lipolysis in Adipose Tissue. J Biol Chem 247(1972) 3579-3588

Exton, J.H.; Harper, S.C.: Role of Cyclic AMP in the Actions of Catecholamines on Hepatic Carbohydrate Metabolism. Adv Cyc Nucl Res 5(1975)519-532

Fleming, W.W.; McPhillips, J.J.; Westfall, D.P.: Postjunctional Supersensitivity and Subsensitivity of Excitable Tissues to Drugs. Ergeb Physiol 68(1973)55-119

Franklin, T.J.; Morris, W.P.; Twose, P.A.: Desensitization of *Beta*-adrenergic Receptors in Human Fibroblasts in Tissue Culture. Mol Pharmacol 11(1975)485-491

Furchgott, R.F.: Pharmacology of Vascular Smooth Muscle. Pharmacol Rev., 7(1955) 183-265.

Greaves, M.F.: Membrane Receptor-adenylate Cyclase Relationships. Nature 265(1975) 681-683

Greenacre, J.K.; Schofield, P.; Conolly, M.E.: Desensitization of the β-Adrenoceptor of Lymphocytes from Normal Subjects and Asthmatic Patients *In Vitro*. Br J Clin Pharmacol 5(1978)199-206

Greenberg, D.A.; Snyder, S.H.: Pharmacological Properties of [3H] Dihydroergocryptine Binding Sites Associated with *Alpha* Noradrenergic Receptors in Rat Brain Membranes. Mol Pharmacol 14(1978)38-49

Greenberg, D.A.; U'Prichard, D.C.; Snyder, S.H.: *Alpha*-Noradrenergic Receptor Binding in Mammalian Brain: Differential Labeling of Agonist and Antagonist States. Life Sci 19(1976)69-76

Guellaen, G.; Yates-Aggerbeck, M.; Vauquelin, G.; Strosberg, D.; Hanoune, J.: Characterization with [3H] Dihydroergocryptine of the α-Adrenergic Receptor of the Hepatic Plasma Membrane. Comparison with the β-Adrenergic Receptor in Normal and Adrenalectomized Rats. J Biol Chem 253(1978)1114-1120

Haber, E.; Wrenn, S.: Problems in Identification of the *Beta*-Adrenergic Receptor. Physiol Rev 56(1976)317-338

Haga, T.; Haga, K.; Gilman, A.G.: Hydrodynamic Properties of the β-Adrenergic Receptor and Adenylate Cyclase from Wild Type and Variant S49 Lymphoma Cells. J Biol Chem 252(1977a)5776-5782

Haga, T.; Ross, E.M.; Anderson, H.J.; Gilman, A.G.: Adenylate Cyclase Permanently Uncoupled from Hormone Receptors in a Novel Variant of S49 Mouse Lymphoma Cells. Proc Natl Acad Sci USA 74(1977b)2016-2020

Hanski, E.; Levitzki, A.: The Absence of Desensitization in the *Beta* Adrenergic Receptors of Turkey Reticulocytes and Erythrocytes and Its Possible Origin. Life Sci 22(1978)53-60

Harden, T.K.; Wolfe, B.B.; Johnson, G.L.; Perkins, J.P.; Molinoff, P.B.: β-Adrenergic Receptors of Intact and Broken Human Astrocytoma Cells. Trans Am Soc Neurochem 7(1976a)231

Harden, T.K.; Wolfe, B.B.; Molinoff, P.B.: Binding of Iodinated *Beta* Adrenergic Antagonists to Proteins Derived from Rat Heart. Mol Pharmacol 12(1976b)1-15

Harden, T.K.; Wolfe, B.B.; Sporn, J.R.; Perkins, J.P.; Molinoff, P.B.: Ontogeny of β-Adrenergic Receptors in Rat Cerebral Cortex. Brain Res 125(1977a)99-108

Harden, T.K.; Wolfe, B.B.; Sporn, J.R.; Poulos, B.K.; Molinoff, P.B.: Effects of 6-

Hydroxydopamine on the Development of the *Beta* Adrenergic Receptor/Adenylate Cyclase System in Rat Cerebral Cortex. J Pharmacol Exp Ther 203(1977b)132–143.

Hunter, W. M.; Greenwood, F.C.: Preparation of Iodine-131 Labelled Human Growth Hormone of High Specific Activity. Nature 194(1962)495–496

Insel, P.A.; Maguire, M.E.; Gilman, A.G.; Bourne, H.R.; Coffino, P.; Melmon, K.L.: *Beta* Adrenergic Receptors and Adenylate Cyclase: Products of Separate Genes? Mol Pharmacol 12(1976)1062–1069

Johnson, G.L.; Wolfe, B.B.; Harden, T.K.; Molinoff, P.B.; Perkins, J.P.: Role of β-Adrenergic Receptors in Catecholamine-induced Desensitization of Adenylate Cyclase in Human Astrocytoma Cells. J Biol Chem 253(1978)1472–1480

Kafka, M.S.; Tallman, J.F.; Smith, C.C.: *Alpha*-adrenergic Receptors on Human Platelets. Life Sci 21(1977)1429–1438

Kauman, A.J.; Brinbaumer, L.; Yang, P.C.: Studies on Receptor-mediated Activation of Adenylyl Cyclases. IV. Characteristics of the Adrenergic Receptor Coupled to Myocardial Adenylyl Cyclase. J Biol Chem 249(1974)7874–7885

Kebabian, J.W.; Zatz, M.; Romero, J.A.; Axelrod, J.: Rapid Changes in Rat Pineal β-Adrenergic Receptor: Alterations in *l* ³H Alprenolol Binding and Adenylate Cyclase. Proc Natl Acad Sci USA 72(1975)3735–3739

Kempson, S.; Marinetti, G.V.; Shaw, A.: Hormone Action at the Membrane Level. VII. Stimulation of Dihydroalprenolol Binding to *Beta*-Adrenergic Receptors in Isolated Rat Heart Ventricle Slices by Triiodothyronine and Thyroxine. Biochim Biophys Acta 540(1978)320–329

Kunos, G.: Adrenoceptors. Ann Rev Pharmacol Toxicol 18(1978)291–311

Lands, A.M.; Arnold, A.; McAuliff, J.P.; Luduena, F.P.; Brown, T.G.: Differentiation of Receptor Systems Activated by Sympathomimetic Amines. Nature 214(1967)597–598

Langley, J.N.: On Nerve Endings and on Special Excitable Substances in Cells. Proc R Soc LXXVII B (1906)170–194

Lefkowitz, R.J.: Molecular Pharmacology of *Beta*-Adrenergic Receptors—A Status Report. Biochem Pharmacol 23(1974)2069–2076

Lefkowitz, R.J.: The β-Adrenergic Receptor. Life Sci 18(1976)461–472

Lefkowitz, R.J.; Hamp, M.: Comparison of Specificity of Agonist and Antagonist Radioligand Binding to β-Adrenergic Receptors. Nature 268(1977)453–454

Lefkowitz, R.J.; Limbird, L.E.; Mukherjee, C.; Caron, M.G.: The β-Adrenergic Receptor and Adenylate Cyclase. Biochim Biophys Acta 457(1976)1–39

Lefkowitz, R.J.; Mukherjee, C.; Coverstone, M.; Caron, M.G.: Stereospecific (³H) (−)-Alprenolol Binding Sites, β-Adrenergic Receptors and Adenylate Cyclase. Biochem Biophys Res Comm 60(1974)703–709

Lefkowitz, R.J.; Mullikin, D.; Williams, L.T.: A Desensitized State of the *Beta* Adrenergic Receptor not Associated with High-Affinity Agonist Occupancy. Mol Pharmacol 14(1978)376–380

Lefkowitz, R.J.; Sharp, G.W.G.; Haber, E.: Specific Binding of β-Adrenergic Catecholamines to a Subcellular Fraction from Cardiac Muscle. J Biol Chem 248(1973)342–349

Lefkowitz, R.J.; Williams, L.T.: Catecholamine Binding to the β-Adrenergic Receptor. Proc Natl Acad Sci USA 74(1977)515–519

Levitzki, A.: Catecholamine Receptors. In: Receptors and Recognition, Series A, Vol. II, pp. 200–229, ed. by P. Cuatrecasas, M.F. Greaves. Wiley, New York, 1976

Levitzki, A.; Atlas, D.; Steer, M.L.: The Binding Characteristics and Number of β-Adrenergic Receptors in the Turkey Erythrocyte. Proc Natl Acad Sci USA 71(1974)2773–2776

Lewis, J.E.; Miller, J.W.: The Use of Tritiated Phenoxybenzamine for Investigating Receptors. J Pharmacol Exp Ther 154(1966)46–55

Limbird, L. E.; Lefkowitz, R.J.: Resolution of β-Adrenergic Receptor Binding and Adenylate Cyclase Activity by Gel Exclusion Chromatography. J Biol Chem 252(1977)799–802

Lucas, M.; Hanoune, J.; Bockaert, J.: Chemical Modification of the Beta Adrenergic Receptors Coupled with Adenylate Cyclase by Disulfide Bridge-Reducing Agents. Mol Pharmacol 14(1978)227–236

Maguire, M.E.; Ross, E.M.; Gilman, A.G.: β-Adrenergic Receptor: Ligand Binding Properties and the Interaction with Adenyl Cyclase. In: Advances in Cyclic Nucleotide Research, pp. 1-83, ed. by P. Greengard, G.A. Robison. Raven, NY, 1977

Maguire, M.E.; Wiklund, R.A.; Anderson, H.J.; Gilman, A.G.: Binding of ^{125}I Iodohydroxybenzylpindolol to Putative β-Adrenergic Receptors of Rat Glioma Cells and Other Cell Clones. J Biol Chem 251(1976)1221-1231

Makman, M.H.: Conditions Leading to Enhanced Response to Glucagon, Epinephrine, or Prostaglandins by Adenylate Cyclase of Normal and Malignant Cultured Cells. Proc Natl Acad Sci USA 68(1971)2127-2130

Malbon, C.C.; Moreno, F.J.; Cabelli, R.J.; Fain, J.N.: Fat Cell Adenylate Cyclase and β-Adrenergic Receptors in Altered Thyroid States. J Biol Chem 253(1978)671-677

May, M.; Moran, J.F.; Kimelberg, H.; Triggle, D.J.: Studies on the Noradrenaline α-Receptor. II. Analysis of the "Spare-Receptor" Hypothesis and Estimation of the Concentration of α-Receptor in Rabbit Aorta. Mol Pharmacol 3(1967)28-36

Mickey, J.; Tate, R.; Lefkowitz, R.J.: Subsensitivity of Adenylate Cyclase and Decreased β-Adrenergic Receptor Binding After Chronic Exposure to (-)-Isoproterenol In Vitro. J Biol Chem 250(1975)5727-5729

Mickey, J.V.; Tate, R.; Mullikin, D.; Lefkowitz, R.J.: Regulation of Adenylate-Cyclase-Coupled Beta Adrenergic Receptor Binding Sites by Beta Adrenergic Catecholamines In Vitro. Mol Pharmacol 12(1976)409-419

Miller, J.W.: Adrenergic Receptors in the Myometrium. Ann NY Acad Sci 139(1967)788-798

Molinoff, P.B.: Methods of Approach for the Isolation of β-Adrenergic Receptors. In: Frontiers in Catecholamine Research, pp. 357-360, ed. by E. Usdin, S.H. Snyder. Pergamon, New York, 1973

Moran, J.F.; May, M.; Kimelberg, H.; Triggle, D.J.: Studies on the Noradrenaline α-Receptor. I. Techniques of Receptor Isolation. The Distribution and Specificity of Action of N-(2-Bromoethyl)-N-ethyl-l-napthylmethylamine, a Competitive Antagonist of Noradrenaline. Mol Pharmacol 3(1967)15-27

Moran, J.F.; Triggle, D.J.: Approaches to the Quantitation and Isolation of Pharmacological Receptors. In: Fundamental Concepts in Drug Receptor Interactions, pp. 133-176, ed. by J.F. Danielli, J.F. Moran, D.J. Triggle. Academic, New York, 1970

Mukherjee, C.; Caron, M.G.; Coverstone, M; Lefkowitz, R.J.: Identification of Adenylate Cyclase-coupled β-Adrenergic Receptor in Frog Erythrocytes with (-) [^{3}H] alprenolol. J Biol Chem 250(1975a)4869-4876

Mukherjee, C.; Caron, M.G.; Lefkowitz, R.J.: Catecholamine-Induced Subsensitivity of Adenylate Cyclase Associated with Loss of β-Adrenergic Receptor Binding Sites. Proc Natl Acad Sci USA 72(1975b)1945-1949

Mukherjee, C.; Caron, M.G.; Lefkowitz, R.J.: Regulation of Adenylate Cyclase Coupled β-Adrenergic Receptors by β-Adrenergic Catecholamines. Endocrinol 99(1976a)347-357

Mukherjee, C.; Caron, M.; Mulliken, D.; Lefkowitz, R.J.: Structure-Activity Relationships of Adenylate Cyclase-Coupled Beta Adrenergic Receptors: Determination by Direct Binding Studies. Mol Pharmacol 12(1976b)16-31

Mukherjee, C.; Lefkowitz, R.J.: Desensitization of β-Adrenergic Receptors by Beta-Adrenergic Agonists in a Cell-free System: Resensitization by Guanosine 5'-(β,γ-imino)triphosphate and other Purine Nucleotides. Proc Natl Acad Sci USA 73(1976)1494-1498

Mukherjee, C.; Lefkowitz, R.J.: Regulation of Beta Adrenergic Receptors in Isolated Frog Erythrocyte Plasma Membranes. Mol Pharmacol 13(1977)291-303

Nickerson, M.; Receptor Occupancy and Tissue Response. Nature 178(1956)697-698

O'Donnell, S.R.; Woodcock, E.A.: A Comparison of the Binding Constant (K_D) of ^{125}I-labeled 3-(4-Iodophenoxy)-1-Isopropylamino-Propan-2-ol Obtained on β-Adrenoceptors in Guinea Pig Myocardial Membranes, with its Dissociation Constants (K_B) Obtained on Guinea-Pig Isolated Atria and Trachea. J Pharm Pharmacol 30(1978)96-100

Orly, J.; Schramm, M.: Coupling of Catecholamine Receptor from One Cell with Adenylate Cyclase from Another Cell by Cell Fusion. Proc Natl Acad Sci USA 73(1976)4410-4414

Page, E.D.; Neufeld, A.H.: Characterization of α- and β-Adrenergic Receptors in Membranes Prepared from the Rabbit Iris Before and After Development of Supersensitivity. Biochem Pharmacol 27(1978)953-958

Peroutka, S.J.; Greenberg, D.A.; U'Prichard, D.C.; Snyder, S.H.: Regional Variations in Alpha Adrenergic Receptor Interactions of [³H] Dihydroergocryptine in Calf Brain: Implications for a Two-site Model of Alpha Receptor Function. Mol Pharmacol 14(1978)403–412

Pike, L.J.; Lefkowitz, R.J.: Agonist-specific Alterations in Receptor Binding Affinity Associated with Solubilization of Turkey Erythrocyte Membrane *Beta* Adrenergic Receptors. Mol Pharmacol 14(1978)370–375

Raff, M.: Self Regulation of Membrane Receptors. Nature 259(1976)265–266

Remold-O'Donnell, E.: Stimulation and Desensitization of Macrophage Adenylate Cyclase by Prostaglandins and Catecholamines. J Biol Chem 249(1974)3615–3621

Roberts, J.M.; Insel, P.A.; Goldfien, R.D.; Goldfien, A.: α-Adrenoceptors but not β-Adrenoceptors Increase in Rabbit Uterus with Oestrogen. Nature 270(1977)624–625

Rodbell, M.; Krans, H.M.J.; Pohl, S.L.; Birnbaumer, L.: The Glucagon-sensitive Adenyl Cyclase System in Plasma Membranes. III. Binding of Glucagon: Method of Assay and Specificity. J Biol Chem 246(1971)1861–1871

Ross, E.M.; Gilman, A.G.: Reconstitution of Catecholamine-sensitive Adenylate Cyclase Activity. Interaction of Solubilized Components with Receptor-replete Membrane. Proc Natl Acad Sci USA 74(1977a)3715–3719

Ross, E.M.; Gilman, A.G.: Resolution of Some Components of Adenylate Cyclase Necessary for Catalytic Activity. J Biol Chem 252(1977b)6966–6969

Ross, E.M.; Maguire, M.E.; Sturgill, T.W.; Biltonen, R.L.; Gilman, A.G.: Relationship Between the β-Adrenergic Receptor and Adenylate Cyclase. J Biol Chem 252(1977) 5761–5775

Ruffolo, R.R.; Fowble, J.W.; Miller, D.D.; Patil, P.N.: Binding of [³H] Dihydroazapetine to *Alpha*-Adrenoreceptor-Related Proteins from Rat Vas Deferens. Proc Natl Acad Sci USA 73(1976)2730–2734

Schramm, M.; Orly, J.; Eimerl, S; Korner, M.: Coupling of Hormone Receptors to Adenylate Cyclase of Different Cells by Cell Fusion. Nature 268(1977)310–313

Shear, M.; Insel, P.A.; Melmon, K.L.; Coffino, P.: Agonist-specific Refractoriness Induced by Isoproterenol. Studies with Mutant Cells. J Biol Chem 251(1976)7572–7576

Sholnick, P.; Stalvey, L.P.; Daly, J.W.; Hoyler, E.; Davis, J.N.: Binding of α- and β-Adrenergic Ligands to Cerebral Cortical Membranes: Effect of 6-Hydroxydopamine Treatment and Relationship to the Responsiveness of Cyclic AMP-Generating Systems in Two Rat Strains. Eur J Pharmacol 47(1978)201–210

Spaulding, S.W.; North, R.H.: Thyroid-catecholamine Interactions. Med Clin N Amer 59(1975)1123–1131

Sporn, J.R.; Harden, T.K.; Wolfe, B.B.; Molinoff, P.B.: β-Adrenergic Receptor Involvement in 6-Hydroxydopamine-induced Supersensitivity in Rat Cerebral Cortex. Science 194(1976)624–626

Sporn, J.R.; Molinoff, P.B.: β-Adrenergic Receptors in Rat Brain. J Cyc Nuc Res 2(1976)149–161

Starke, K.: Regulation of Noradrenaline Release by Presynaptic Receptor Systems. Rev Physiol Biochem Pharmacol 77(1977)1–124

Stephenson, R.P.: A Modification of Receptor Theory. Br J Pharmacol 11(1956)379–393

Strittmatter, W.J.; Davis, J.N.; Lefkowitz, R.J.: α-Adrenergic Receptors in the Rat Parotid Gland. I. Correlation of [³H] Dihydroergocryptine Binding and Catecholamine-stimulated Potassium Efflux. J Biol Chem 252(1977a)5472–5477

Strittmatter, W.J.; Davis, J.N.; Lefkowitz, R.J.: α-Adrenergic Receptors in Rat Parotid Cells. II. Desensitization of Receptor Binding Sites and Potassium Release. J Biol Chem 252(1977b)5478–5482

Tata, J.R.: Coordinated Formation of Membranes and Biosynthetic Activity during Growth and Development. In: Regulatory Functions of Biological Membranes, pp. 222–235, ed. by J. Järnefelt. American Elsevier, New York, 1968

Tittler, M.; Weinreich, P.; Seeman, P.: New Detection of Brain Dopamine Receptors with [³H]-Dihydroergocryptine. Proc Natl Acad Sci USA 74(1977)3750–3753

Trendelenburg, U.: Factors Influencing the Concentration of Catecholamines at the Receptors. In: Handbook of Experimental Pharmacology, Vol. XXXIII, pp. 726–761, ed. by H. Blashko and E. Muscholl. Springer, Berlin, 1972

Triggle, D.J.; Triggle, C.R.: Chemical Pharmacology of the Synapse. Chapter 2. Academic, London and New York, 1977a

Triggle, D.J.; Triggle, C.R.: Chemical Pharmacology of the Synapse. Chapter 3. Academic, London and New York, 1977b

Triggle, D.J.; Triggle, C.R.: Chemical Pharmacology of the Synapse. Chapter 4. Academic, London and New York, 1977c

Tsai, B.S.; Lefkowitz, R.J.: [^{3}H] Dihydroergocryptine Binding to Alpha Adrenergic Receptors in Canine Aortic Membranes. J Pharmacol Exp Ther 204(1978)606–614

Tuttle, R.R.; Moran, N.C.: The Effect of Calcium Depletion on the Combination of Agonists and Competitive Antagonists with Alpha Adrenergic and Histaminergic Receptors of Rabbit Aorta. J Pharmacol Exp Ther 169(1969)255–263

U'Prichard, D.C.; Greenberg, D.A.; Sheehan, P.; Snyder, S.H.: Regional Distribution of α-Noradrenergic Receptor Binding in Calf Brain. Brain Res 138(1977a)151–158

U'Prichard. D.C.; Greenberg, D.A.; Snyder, S.H.: Binding Characteristics of a Radiolabeled Agonist and Antagonist at Central Nervous System Alpha Noradrenergic Receptors. Mol Pharmacol 13(1977b)454–473

U'Prichard, D.C.; Snyder, S.H.: Binding of [^{3}H] Catecholamines to α-Noradrenergic Receptor Sites in Calf Brain. J Biol Chem 252(1977a)6450–6463

U'Prichard, D.C.; Snyder, S.H.: Differential Labelling of α and β-Noradrenergic Receptors in Calf Cerebellum Membranes with [^{3}H] Adrenaline. Nature 270(1977b)261–263

U'Prichard, D.C.; Snyder, S.H.: [^{3}H] Epinephrine and [^{3}H] Norepinephrine Binding to α-Noradrenergic Receptors in Calf Brain Membranes. Life Sci 20(1977c)527–534

Vauquelin, G.; Geynet, P.; Hanoune, J.; Strosberg, A.D.: Isolation of Adenylate Cyclase-free β-Adrenergic Receptor from Turkey Erythrocyte Membranes by Affinity Chromatography. Proc Natl Acad Sci USA 74(1977)3710–3714

Wikberg, J.E.S.: Pharmacological Desensitization of Adrenergic α-Receptors in the Guinea-pig. Nature 273(1978)164–166

Williams, L.T.; Jarett, L.; Lefkowitz, R.J.: Adipocyte β-Adrenergic Receptors. Identification and Subcellular Localization by (−)-[^{3}H] Dihydroalprenolol Binding. J Biol Chem 251(1976a)3096–3104

Williams, L.T.; Lefkowitz, R.J.: Slowly Reversible Binding of Catecholamine to a Nucleotide-Sensitive State of the β-Adrenergic Receptor. J Biol Chem 252(1977)7207–7213

Williams, L.T.; Lefkowitz, R.J.; Watanabe, A.M.; Hathaway, D.R.; Besch, H.R.: Thyroid Hormone Regulation of β-Adrenergic Receptor Number. J Biol Chem 252(1977)2787–2789

Williams, L.T.; Mullikin, D.; Lefkowitz, R.J.: Identification of α-Adrenergic Receptors in Uterine Smooth Muscle Membranes by [^{3}H] Dihydroergocryptine Binding. J Biol Chem 251(1976b)6915–6923

Williams, L.T.; Snyderman, R.; Lefkowitz, R.J.: Identification of β-Adrenergic Receptors in Human Lymphocytes by (−)-[^{3}H]-Alprenolol Binding. J Clin Inves 57(1976c)149–155

Wolfe, B.B.; Harden, T.K.; Molinoff, P.B.: β-Adrenergic Receptors in Rat Liver: Effects of Adrenalectomy. Proc Natl Acad Sci USA 73(1976)1343–1347

Wolfe, B.B.; Harden, T.K.; Molinoff, P.B.: In Vitro Study of β-Adrenergic Receptors. Ann Rev Pharmacol Toxicol 17(1977)575–604

Yong, M.S.; Nickerson, M.: Dissociation of Alpha Adrenergic Receptor Protection from Inhibition of [^{3}H] phenoxybenzamine Binding in Vascular Tissue. J Pharmacol Exp Ther 186(1973)100–108

Yong, M.S.; Parulekar, M.R.; Wright, J.; Marks, G.S.: Studies of the Chemical Nature of the α-Adrenergic Receptor. Biochem Pharmacol 15(1966)1185–1195

Zatz, M.; Kebabian, J.W.; Romero, J.A.; Lefkowitz, R.J.; Axelrod, J.: Pineal Beta Adrenergic Receptor: Correlation of Binding of [^{3}H]-l-alprenolol with Stimulation of Adenylate Cyclase. J Pharmacol Exp Ther 196(1976)714–722

Cyclic AMP and Myocardial Contraction

John H. McNeill

I. INTRODUCTION

The concept of cyclic AMP as a "second messenger" mediating the effects of many drugs and hormones is now familiar to anyone who has taken a course in biology. The subject has been reviewed many times, and the interested reader is referred to the most recent reviews (e.g., Greengard and Robison, 1977). The history of cyclic AMP and cardiac function goes back only to 1965, when it was first measured by two groups of workers independently (Robison et al., 1965; Cheung and Williamson, 1965) following injection of epinephrine into rat heart. Before 1965, however, lines of investigation had been moving toward the involvement of cyclic AMP, even though it was not recognized at the time.

In 1959 Ellis, in a review, implicated glycogenolysis in the inotropic effect of drugs such as epinephrine. This was followed by an intensive investigation, beginning with Hess and Haugaard (1958), of the effects of drugs on the enzyme glycogen phosphorylase. Phosphorylase exists in two interconvertible forms in the heart, phosphorylase *a* and phosphorylase *b*. Phosphorylase *a*, an active form of the enzyme, is involved in the breakdown of glycogen. Phosphorylase *b*, an inactive form, and will catalyze the breakdown of glycogen only when the intracellular level of 5'-AMP is elevated to a high level. Hess and Haugaard (1958) and Kukovetz et al. (1959) reported that adrenergic amines that increased contractile force also increased phosphorylase activity; α-adrenergic amines that did not increase force also did not increase the activity of the enzyme. The relative order of potency of the catecholamines was the same whether contractile force or

Original work of the author was supported by grants from the Medical Research Council (Canada) and the Canadian Heart Foundation.

phosphorylase activity was measured. Isoproterenol, for example, was the most potent agent on either parameter.

Further evidence showing a correlation between phosphorylase activity and cardiac function was provided by Mayer and Moran (1960). These workers showed an increase in cardiac phosphorylase activity resulting from both epinephrine and electrical stimulation of the cardioaccelerator nerves in the open-chest dog. The increase was blocked by dichloroisoproterenol, the only β-adrenergic blocker available at the time.

Beginning with the report of Mayer, Cotton, and Moran (1963), doubts began to be cast on the involvement of phosphorylase in the inotropic response. In that report it was noted that small doses of epinephrine could produce increases in force but did not increase phosphorylase a activity. The end of the phosphorylase theory came in 1965 when Robison et al. (1965) and Cheung and Williamson (1965) both reported that phosphorylase activation in epinephrine-injected rat hearts did not increase until after the inotropic response had begun. Thus, activation of the enzyme and the subsequent breakdown of glycogen could not be responsible for the initiation of the inotropic response. The debate, however, persisted for some years following the above two reports and an earlier one by Øye et al. (1964).

Concomitant with the studies just mentioned, Sutherland and Rall had made their Nobel-Prize-winning discovery of a heat-stable factor in liver that increased following the use of epinephrine and was involved in glycogenolysis (Rall, Sutherland, and Berthet, 1957; Rall and Sutherland, 1958; Sutherland and Rall, 1958). From this beginning the now famous second messenger hypothesis was formulated, and the actions of a wide variety of drugs and hormones (the "first messengers") are now attributed to their ability to elevate tissue cyclic AMP levels (Robison, Butcher, and Sutherland, 1971).

Enzymes for the synthesis of cyclic AMP (adenylate cyclase) and for the breakdown of the nucleotide (phosphodiesterases) were soon discovered and characterized (Murad et al., 1962; Butcher and Sutherland, 1962; Sutherland, Rall, and Menon, 1962). It was at this time that Sutherland drafted his now famous four criteria that must be met in order to implicate cyclic AMP in the action of a drug or hormone. They are as follows:

1. Demonstration of a response to the hormone (drug) in a washed broken-cell preparation. That is, the drug or hormone must be capable of stimulating adenylate cyclase from the tissue or organ involved.
2. The agent must be able to increase cyclic AMP in intact cells. This criterion should be further clarified by stating that the increase in cyclic AMP should occur before any other response and in a dose-dependent manner. It should not be possible to produce the desired response in the tissue or organ with doses of the hormone that do not increase cyclic AMP.

3. Drugs affecting phosphodiesterase should potentiate or inhibit the hormone action.

4. Exogenous cyclic AMP or its derivatives should mimic the effect of the hormone.

Many, if not all, of the criteria have been met for several drugs that affect the heart; the evidence is reviewed in the following sections. Recent experiments have indicated that the criteria, now more than fifteen years old, may no longer be adequate in order to state with certainty that the actions of a drug are definitely mediated through cyclic AMP. The evidence will be considered for each drug category separately.

II. ADRENERGIC AMINES

In 1962 Murad et al. provided the first evidence that cyclic AMP might be involved in the cardiac actions of drugs. These workers, working with dog heart adenylate cyclase, found that the order of potency of the catecholamines for stimulating the enzyme was the same as that noted in the inotropic effect. In 1965 Robison et al. and Cheung and Williamson reported on their experiments, in which epinephrine was injected into perfused rat hearts. It was found that cyclic AMP increased prior to the increase in force and that phosphorylase activation lagged behind the other two events. These results have been confirmed many times with many β-adrenergic drugs in a variety of cardiac preparations and in a number of species; they, at least, are not in dispute (Drummond, Duncan, and Hertzman, 1966; Namm and Mayer, 1968; Namm, Mayer, and Maltbie, 1968; Kukovetz, Pöch, and Wurm, 1973; Drummond and Hemmings, 1973b; Schümann, Endoh, and Brodde, 1975; Dobson, Ross, and Mayer, 1976; Polson, Goldberg, and Shideman, 1977; McNeill and Verma, 1973; Martinez and McNeill, 1977a; McNeill, 1978). It has also been reported (Rall and West, 1963) that the methylxanthines, agents known to inhibit phosphodiesterase, will enhance the cardiac actions of the catecholamines. Whether this action of theophylline and like drugs can be wholly ascribed to the affects of the drugs on phosphodiesterase is a subject of some debate; it is dealt with more fully under part VI of this chapter. The effect of cyclic AMP or its dibutyryl derivative on the heart can mimic the actions of the catecholamines (part III; also see Tsien, 1977). Thus all Sutherland's criteria for the involvement of cyclic AMP in the inotropic responses to the catecholamines have been met. The evidence, interpreted in another way, would also indicate that cyclic AMP is involved in controlling or modulating force changes in the heart. How the nucleotide might do this is beyond the scope of this review. The general view now held is that cyclic AMP, by activating a protein kinase enzyme which in turn can phosphorylate other proteins, can perhaps alter the permeability of membranes to calcium.

Other possibilities involve the phosphorylation of sarcoplasmic reticulum, troponin, and a number of other intracellular structures that would alter either the binding or the response of the structures to calcium. The net effect would initially be an increase in the free intracellular level of calcium, leading to a positive inotropic response and an increased rate of calcium binding, which would lead in turn to an increased rate of relaxation (Tsien, 1977). Catecholamines are known to affect calcium influx and binding, to produce a positive inotropic response, and to increase the rate of relaxation of cardiac muscle. The evidence at present favors a role for cyclic AMP in these responses, but definitive proof is lacking at this point.

There are several reports in the literature that claim to have dissociated the effect of adrenergic amines on cyclic AMP from the effect on force. Early reports (Benfey, 1971) that claimed a dissociation based on the effects of phenylephrine can now be discounted on the base of the fact that phenylephrine produces much of its inotropic response through the stimulation of α-adrenergic receptors (Osnes and Øye, 1975; Verma and McNeill, 1976a; Starke, 1972; Schümann, Endoh, and Wagner, 1974; Endoh, Brodde, and Schümann, 1976; Martinez and McNeill, 1977a). Cyclic AMP increases do not occur following α-receptor stimulation, and some other mechanism is certainly involved (Endoh et al., 1976; Martinez and McNeill, 1977a).

It has also been suggested that α and β receptors are, in fact, one receptor that can modify into one form or another, depending on certain conditions such as temperature (Benfey, Kunos, and Nickerson, 1974; Kunos and Nickerson, 1976, 1977). Since α receptor stimulation does not result in an increase in cyclic AMP, and since the α receptor, according to this theory, is a form of the β receptor, then cyclic AMP cannot be involved. A recent review by Benfey (1977) has concluded that the evidence for receptor interconversion is not strong. Recent reports (Martinez and McNeill, 1977b) tend to support the latter argument. (See also Benfey in this volume.)

Older work questioning the involvement of cyclic AMP in the inotropic action of adrenergic amines has been reviewed (Sobel and Mayer, 1973). The evidence presented claiming a dissociation is not strong. A further review of such data is provided by Tsien (1977) and will not be commented on further.

Very recent work has seriously questioned the cyclic AMP theory of drug action in the heart. In fact, the data, which will now be discussed, make completely untenable the original hypothesis that cyclic AMP must increase in all or most of the cells of the heart in order to produce a response. Venter and coworkers at the University of California (San Diego) began in 1972 to study the effect of isoproterenol covalently bound to glass beads (Venter et al., 1972). The beads, which are really glass chips rather than beads, vary in size (20–300 μm diameter) and are associated with 1–10 picomoles of isoproterenol/bead. The drug is linked to the glass by means of a silicon-propylamido-phenyldiazo side chain attached to the catechol ring on the 6 position. When the beads are placed directly on the cardiac preparation (papillary muscle), a dose-dependent (number of beads vs. response) increase in contractile force occurs without an increase in cyclic AMP. The increase in force noted is similar to that obtained when isoproterenol was placed in the bath. In the latter case, of course, cyclic AMP levels rose markedly (Venter, Arnold, and Kaplan, 1975). Similarly, Ingebretsen et al. (1977) observed that both isoproterenol and isoproterenol bound to glass beads produced an inotropic effect on guinea pig heart partially depolarized with 22 mM K$^+$. No increase in cyclic AMP was noted with the bound isoproterenol, although phosphorylase activity did increase. It appears that the initiation of the response comes from the point of contact of the bead with the muscle and is propagated from there (Venter et al., 1972, 1973; Ingebretsen et al., 1977; Venter et al., 1975; Verlander et al., 1976).

The possibility that the drug is not bound to the glass in toto and that the response is due to a leakage of isoproterenol has been raised (Yong, 1973; Yong and Richardson, 1974, 1975) and denied (Venter and Kaplan, 1974). If the beads did leak, a relatively high concentration of isoproterenol could occur in the area of the receptor when the bead was placed on the muscle. For the purposes of the involvement of cyclic AMP in the response, however, whether or not the beads leak makes very little difference. The point is that an inotropic response results when the beads are placed in contact with the muscle and that whole tissue cyclic AMP levels do not increase. It is possible, of course, that cyclic AMP increases only in the cells that are in contact with the bead. In that case, when cyclic AMP was measured in the entire muscle, it would be difficult to detect the small change in nucleotide levels. If this did occur, the cyclic AMP theory would have to be reformulated to state that a change in cyclic AMP in one or a few cells would result in the propagation of the response throughout the entire muscle. Such an interpretation is quite feasible; but, if true, it would require that most proposals involving the action of cyclic AMP on sarcolemma, sarcoplasmic reticulum, and troponin be altered considerably. If cyclic AMP is causing a propagated response in cardiac muscle, it is not readily apparent, given the present state of knowledge, how the response occurs. In his most recent paper (Hu and Venter, 1978) Venter used isoproterenol diazotized to a 12,800 mol wt random copolymer of hydroxypropylglutamine with p-aminophenylalanine. Referred to as copoly-Iso, the compound is soluble in physiological solutions but diffuses less rapidly than does isoproterenol because of its size. With this compound the whole muscle is exposed to the drug, and thus the contact at one point that is found in the glass bead experiments does not occur. Copoly-Iso produced an inotropic response in cat papillary muscle without an increase in cyclic AMP. Isoproterenol alone increased both force and cyclic AMP in the study. The authors conclude that the copoly-Iso response, and probably the isoproterenol response itself, results from an interaction of the drugs at β-adrenergic receptors on the surface of the muscle. Following receptor activation at the cell surface, the response is propagated throughout the muscle.

Studies using bound isoproterenol clearly demonstrate that mechanical changes can occur in the heart without detectable changes in cyclic AMP. The data can be interpreted in a number of ways. The most simple explanation is that cyclic AMP is not involved in the inotropic response but is involved in metabolic effects of the catecholamines, such as glycogenolysis. A second interpretation is that cyclic AMP changes in only a few cells but is still responsible for the propagation of the response. This interpretation, as stated previously, would require a total overhaul of the proposed effects of cyclic AMP on calcium metabolism, since such theories require that cyclic AMP increase in each cell. Such a possibility could be represented as follows:

$$\text{Drug} \rightarrow \underset{\text{Activation}}{\beta \text{ receptor}} \rightarrow \uparrow\text{cAMP (some cells)} \rightarrow \underset{\text{Response}}{\text{Inotropic}}$$

A third possibility is that cyclic AMP is normally involved in the inotropic response. Under certain conditions the cell is capable of responding to the drug and the final effect is the same; however, a different pathway could be used to arrive from point A (receptor stimulation) to point B (final response). This possibility is represented in the following scheme:

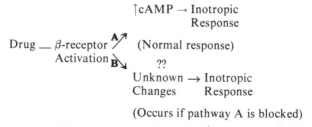

Redundancy is not unknown in nature, and the latter interpretation remains a possibility. Experimental data are needed, however, before the latter two interpretations can be classed at a higher level than speculation.

The remaining drugs to be discussed are histamine, glucagon, the phosphodiesterase inhibitors, and derivatives of cyclic AMP. It should be kept in mind that experiments such as those carried out by Venter and his colleagues have not been carried out with these drugs. Indeed, in the case of the last two groups of compounds such experiments would be impossible, since such drugs must penetrate the cell in order to be effective. It must be remembered that the data cited, when positive, merely associate cyclic AMP with the inotropic effect of the drugs. In no case has a cause-and-effect relationship been determined.

III. CYCLIC AMP AND ITS ANALOGUES

Cyclic AMP itself normally does not penetrate into the heart; therefore a positive inotropic effect is not usually noted. In sarcolemma-free ("skinned") cardiac muscle fibers cyclic AMP can produce a relaxation (Fabiato and Fabiato, 1975). Dibutyryl cyclic AMP, a more lipid-soluble cyclic AMP analogue, has been shown to produce a positive inotropic effect in perfused hearts (Kukovetz and Pöch, 1970; Ahren, Hjalmarson, and Isaksson, 1971; Drummond and Hemmings, 1973a; McNeill, 1977), papillary muscles (Skelton, Levey, and Epstein, 1970; Wilkerson, Paddock, and George, 1976), electrically driven atria (Meinertz, Nawrath, and Scholz, 1972; 1973a, b; Meinertz et al., 1974), spontaneously beating atria (Drummond and Hemmings, 1973a), and cultured heart cells (Krause et al., 1970). Like the catecholamines, dibutyryl cyclic AMP decreases the time to peak tension and accelerates the rate of relaxation in papillary muscles of the cat (Meinertz, Nawrath, and Scholz, 1975, 1976; Kaumann, 1977). The onset of the drug is slow and doses required are high, but these facts may be explained on the basis that the compound penetrates cells slowly and that most of the drug does not get to its site of action. Data obtained with cyclic AMP and its derivatives tend to support the theory involving the nucleotide in inotropic responses.

IV. HISTAMINE

The positive inotropic effect of histamine in the heart was reported in 1910 (Dale and Laidlaw, 1910). Trendelenburg (1960) showed that histamine had inotropic and chronotropic effects on cat, guinea pig, and rabbit atria. Pöch and Kukovetz (1967) and Dean (1968) both noted the similarities between histamine and epinephrine on guinea pig heart and suggested that cyclic AMP might be involved in the actions of the drug. Klein and Levey (1971) and McNeill and Muschek (1972) demonstrated that histamine could stimulate cardiac adenylate cyclase at a site different from that used by catecholamines. Later work from McNeill's laboratory (McNeill and Verma 1974a, b) showed that histamine and two histamine analogues could stimulate adenylate cyclase and increase force of contraction, phosphorylase, and cyclic AMP in the guinea pig heart. The order of potency was the same for all events, and all actions could be blocked by the newly discovered H_2 receptor blocking agent burimamide. Thus an H_2 receptor appeared to be involved. It was also noted that the increase in cyclic AMP preceded the onset of the inotropic response.

Several workers later reported that the guinea pig left atrium contained only H_1 receptors (Reinhardt, Wagner, and Schümann, 1974; Steinberg and Holland, 1975). Verma and McNeill (1977) confirmed these results but were also able to show that stimulation of H_1 receptors did not result in an increase of cyclic AMP, whereas stimulation of H_2 receptors always did. There is considerable variability between species. The rabbit heart, in contrast to the guinea pig heart, contains predominantly H_1 receptors; H_2 receptors occur only in the right atrium of that species. Again cyclic AMP changes occurred only in response to H_2 receptor stimulation. Cyclic GMP did not change under any circumstances (McNeill and Verma, 1979). Verma and McNeill (1976b) pointed out that β and H_2 agonists produced similar effects both on force and on cyclic AMP and that α and H_1 agonists were like each other as well. This similarity has recently been examined on the electrophysiological effects of the agents. Both β and H_2 agonists increase the slow inward current in guinea pig ventricle, but α and H_1 agonists do not (Tenner et al., 1978; Inoue, McNeill, and Puil, 1978).

The H_1 cardiac actions of histamine are not associated with cyclic AMP. Recently Tenner and McNeill (1978) examined the effects of H_1 receptor stimulation in guinea pig left atria. The experimental conditions were modified in order to increase the basal developed force of the atria. Conditions such as lowering the temperature, increasing the external calcium concentration, and increasing the frequency of stimulation to an optimal level were found to increase basal developed force. Under such conditions the H_1 inotropic effect of histamine was markedly decreased or abolished. Responses to isoproterenol, on the other hand, were generally enhanced by these procedures. A similar finding had previously been reported by Endoh et al. (1975) when the inotropic effect of phenylephrine was studied under conditions of reduced temperature. Again the similarity between α and H_1 effect is apparent. Endoh et al. (1975) reported that α agents appeared to depend more on the external Ca^{++} concentration for their inotropic effects relative to the β-adrenergic agents. A similar finding may occur when H_1 agonists are compared with H_2 agents in this regard. Tenner and McNeill (1978) did point out that the agent that increased cyclic AMP (in this case isoproterenol) had its actions enhanced by conditions that increased basal developed force. They speculated that cyclic AMP might provide some added factor in the response to such agents.

The actions of histamine are enhanced by theophylline (McNeill, Coutinho, and Verma, 1974). Further comments on this interaction are to be found in part VI.

The H_2 actions of histamine on cyclic AMP have not been dissociated from the inotropic effect of the drug. As stated previously, a cause-and-effect relationship has not been established at this time.

V. GLUCAGON

It was demonstrated in 1960 by Farah and Tuttle that glucagon can produce an inotropic response. The increase in force produced by glucagon is a direct effect and is not due to the release of endogenous catecholamines, since it is not decreased by β-adrenergic blocking agents (Glick et al., 1968; LaRaia, Craig, and Reddy, 1968; Lucchesi, 1968; Spieka, 1970; Hammer, Sriussadaporn, and Freis, 1973; Brunt and McNeill, 1978). Glucagon will also increase the activity of cardiac glycogen phosphorylase and stimulate glycogenolysis in the heart (Cornblath et al., 1963; Williams and Mayer, 1966; Mayer, Namm, and Rice, 1970). The effects noted are much like those of epinephrine; and Mayer et al. (1970) have demonstrated that the epinephrine; and Mayer et al. (1970) have demonstrated that the glucagon response, like that of epinephrine, is dependent on calcium availability. It has also been demonstrated that glucagon can increase the activity of adenylate cyclase prepared from the hearts of rats (Murad and Vaughan, 1969), cats and humans (Levey and Epstein, 1969), and dogs (Entman, Levey, and Epstein, 1969).

These findings are, of course, similar to those previously reported for agonists such as the catecholamines; and many of the authors cited speculated that glucagon produced its cardiac effects by increasing tissue levels of cyclic AMP. Early attempts to demonstrate such a relationship were unsuccessful. In both beating hearts (LaRaia et al., 1968) and heart slices (LaRaia and Reddy, 1969) it was reported that glucagon did not increase cyclic AMP. A later study by Mayer et al. (1970) using perfused rat heart did demonstrate a glucagon-induced increase in cyclic AMP. It was not demonstrated that cyclic AMP increased before the inotropic event. In 1975 Henry, Dobson, and Sobel were able to increase cyclic AMP in the perfused rat heart in a dose-dependent manner, using the same doses of glucagon that produced an inotropic effect. Brunt and McNeill (1978) reported that injection of glucagon into perfused rat hearts produced dose-dependent increases in force and cyclic AMP. Time reponse studies indicated that cyclic AMP increased prior to the inotropic event. When hearts were perfused with theophylline at a concentration that inhibited phosphodiesterase, the actions of glucagon on cyclic AMP, force of contraction, and phosphorylase activity were all enhanced. In the rat heart, then, glucagon meets the criteria of Sutherland as being a drug that produces its effects through cyclic AMP.

There are data, however, that do not support the involvement of cyclic AMP in the cardiac actions of glucagon. Sobel and Mayer (1973), in a literature review, point out that glucagon, unlike the catecholamines, does not decrease the time to reach peak tension and, in fact, actually increases it. Thus, although the biochemical and force changes may be similar, the two drugs appear to differ when more subtle parameters are measured.

There are other reports that indicate that glucagon can decrease time to peak tension. Kobayashi, Nakayama, and Kimura (1971) and Greef (1976) have found a decrease in guinea pig heart, and Epstein, Levey, and Skelton et al. (1971) and Prasad (1975) in cat and dog heart, respectively.

Henry et al. (1975) have published strong evidence against the involvement of cyclic AMP in the cardiac glucagon response. Using the guinea pig isovolumic left heart preparation, these workers have clearly demonstrated an inotropic effect of glucagon that is not accompanied by a change in cyclic AMP. Rat hearts, prepared in the same manner as was used for guinea pig hearts, did show an increase in force and cyclic AMP. Tsien (1977), in reviewing the data, felt that perhaps other effects of glucagon, such as the inhibition of Na^+, K^+ ATP-ase, as reported by Prasad (1975), might play a role in the actions of the drug in some species but that the action on cyclic AMP might still be involved in other species. The suggestion may be plausible in that other cardiac stimulant drugs—for example, histamine—can produce inotropic effects in different species through entirely different mechanisms. Of interest here as well is the finding that in Langendorff-perfused guinea pig hearts, glucagon does not appear to produce an inotropic effect, (McNeill, unpublished observations, 1969; H.R. Besch, personal communication, 1971). Unless, however, the data of Henry et al. (1975) can be explained more adequately, the causal involvement of cyclic AMP in the cardiac actions of glucagon is questionable.

VI. PHOSPHODIESTERASE INHIBITORS

The use of drugs that inhibit phosphodiesterase *in vitro* in experiments designed to demonstrate that cyclic AMP is involved in a particular response is widespread. It is not unusual to see drugs such as the methylxanthines or papaverine used in an attempt to enhance the action of a second agonist. A positive interaction between the two drugs is usually interpreted as meaning that both drugs act through cyclic AMP, one by inhibiting the breakdown of cyclic AMP and one by increasing the formation of the nucleotide by stimulating adenylate cyclase. Very often the effect of the drugs on cyclic AMP or adenylate cyclase is not measured; the changes are simply assumed to occur. Forgotten also in such experiments are known facts concerning other effects of the drugs that could also explain the responses obtained.

The methylxanthines, particularly theophylline, have been the most widely studied phosphodiesterase inhibitors as far as investigations in the heart are concerned. These drugs are known to inhibit phosphodiesterase (Butcher and Sutherland, 1962). In addition, the order of potency of four methylxanthines (theophylline, caffeine, theobromine, and isobutylmethylxanthine) in inhibiting cardiac phosphodiesterase and enhancing the inotropic and phosphorylase-activating effects of norepinephrine in perfused guinea pig hearts was found to be the same (McNeill, Brenner, and Muschek, 1973). There are numerous reports in the literature pointing out that theophylline can enhance the cardiac actions of drugs known to stimulate adenylate cyclase and in addition possesses certain apparent β-adrenergic-like properties such as positive inotropic and smooth muscle relaxing effects (cf. Sutherland and Robison, 1966; Kukovetz et al., 1973; McNeill et al., 1974; Dönges Heitmann, and Jungbluth, 1977). It is clear that the methylxanthines can enhance the inotropic and phosphorylase-activating effects of norepinephrine, histamine, and glucagon (McNeill et al., 1974; Brunt and McNeill, 1978). It is also clear that the various methylxanthines can produce a positive inotropic effect in various cardiac preparations (Rall and West, 1963; McNeill et al., 1974; Dönges et al., 1977; Martinez and McNeill, 1977c). When cyclic AMP levels have been measured, however, it has also been clear that the methylxanthines can produce these effects without increasing cyclic AMP. In perfused rat or guinea pig hearts injections of theophylline increased the force of contraction approximately 25% without increasing cyclic AMP. Injections of other agonists known to stimulate adenylate cyclase, when given in doses that produced similar changes in force did produce measurable increases in nucleotide levels (McNeill et al., 1974). Similarly, perfusion of hearts with theophylline for brief periods (8 m) followed by the injection of either histamine or norepinephrine resulted in an enhancement of the inotropic and phosphorylase-activating effect without an enhancement of the effect on cyclic AMP. In rat atria theophylline produced an inotropic response and a modest increase in cyclic AMP. When the animals were pretreated with reserpine, the inotropic response was not significantly affected, but the cyclic AMP increase was abolished. In non-reserpine-treated atria both norepinephrine and theophylline increased cyclic AMP. When both drugs were combined, however, the effects were merely additive; no potentitation was noted (Martinez and McNeill, 1977c). The conclusion from these studies was that theophylline produced its inotropic effect and enhanced the actions of histamine and norepinephrine by means of a mechanism that did not involve cyclic AMP. The cyclic AMP increases that were noted with theophylline were apparently due to the release of endogenous norepinephrine. It is apparent that exposure of cardiac preparations to theophylline in sufficient concentrations for a sufficient period of time will result in an increase in cyclic AMP (Dönges et al., 1977; Brunt and McNeill, 1978). In the experiments of Dönges et al. (1977) the effect of theophylline on isolated guinea pig auricles was tested. Theophylline produced dose-dependent increases in both cyclic AMP and force of contraction, and the effects were not blocked by propranolol. The authors reported that they could not dissociate the increase in cyclic AMP from the increase in force. Contrary data were obtained by Martinez and McNeill (1977c) in rat atria. Differences in species may account for the apparent discrepancy in results. It appears, however, that the cardiac actions and interactions of theophylline can occur without detectable changes in whole tissue levels of cyclic AMP.

The similarities between the effects of the methylxanthines and the β-adrenergic effects of the catecholamines may be more apparent than real. The inotropic effect produced by the two groups of drugs differs considerably, for example. Caffeine prolongs the active state of cardiac muscle (de Gubareff and Sleator, 1965; Gibbs, 1967) and increases the duration of the action potential duration (de Gubareff and Sleator, 1965). Catecholamines decrease the time to peak tension and increase the rate of relaxation; methylxanthines have the opposite effect (Blinks et al., 1972).

Blinks et al. (1972) have reviewed the actions of the xanthines on calcium metabolism. Xanthines increase the influx of calcium and decrease the rate of calcium sequestration (Scholz, 1971a, b; Shine and Langer, 1971). Efflux of calcium is reduced by caffeine (Shine and Langer, 1971). More calcium is thus available for excitation contraction coupling, and a positive inotropic effect results. More calcium would also be available to interact with drugs that stimulate adenylate cyclase, thus enhancing their effect on both contractile force and phosphorylase activation (McNeill et al., 1974). Other effects of the xanthines that differ from the catecholamines include cardiac contracture at high doses (Fabiato and Fabiato, 1975). Cyclic AMP and adrenergic amines do not produce this response. Xanthines enhance and catecholamines reduce potassium-induced contractures (Meinertz et al., 1976).

Dönges et al. (1977) feel that the above discrepancies can be resolved if it is considered that the xanthines produce two effects. One effect would occur through the inhibition of phosphodiesterase and the subsequent increase in cyclic AMP, resulting in a cyclic-AMP-induced increase in intracellular calcium, which would then result in the inotropic response. The differences between xanthine and catecholamine responses, according to Dönges et al. (1977), can be explained by a second direct effect of the xanthines on calcium metabolism.

The data for these drugs are controversial and do not resolve the discrepancies at present. Some laboratories report xanthine effects without nucleotide changes; others do not. The only point upon which everyone does agree is that the effects of the xanthines on the heart are not entirely due to the inhibition of phosphodiesterase.

Reports on the cardiac actions of other phosphodiesterase inhibitors are equally controversial. Papaverine is probably the most widely used nonxanthine phosphodiesterase inhibitor. A positive inotropic effect has been reported for papaverine by some workers (Klaus, Krebs, and Seitz,

1970; Endoh and Schümann, 1975) but not by others (McNeill et al., 1973; Henry et al., 1975). Both McNeill and coworkers and Henry and coworkers reported that the drug increased cyclic AMP but that force did not increase. Although these results could be interpreted as dissociating cyclic AMP from the inotropic response, it must be remembered, as Tsien (1977) has pointed out, that papaverine has effects in addition to blocking phosphodiesterase. The drug can produce negative inotropic effects and appears to block the slow calcium current (Tsien, 1977). This view has been reinforced by a recent very thorough study of the cardiac effects of papaverine on guinea pig atria (Reinhardt et al., 1977). The controversy regarding phosphodiesterase inhibition and inotropy will probably not be resolved until relatively specific phosphodiesterase inhibitors possessing relatively minimal complicating additional effects are developed. Korth (1978) has recently reported that isobutylmethylxanthine fits this criterion, because he could mimic the action of isoproterenol on guinea pig papillary muscle with regard to relaxation time, total contraction time, and time to peak tension. Theophylline and papaverine, on the other hand, had the opposite effect on these parameters; and all three drugs enhanced the inotropic action of isoproterenol.

VII. ROLE OF CYCLIC GMP IN CARDIAC FUNCTION

Cyclic GMP has received much less attention than cyclic AMP in most tissues, and the heart is no exception. It was suggested by Goldberg and his colleagues (1975) that cyclic GMP may have a function in the cell that is opposite to that of cyclic AMP: decreases or increases in the levels of one nucleotide would be accompanied by the opposite change in the other, and an increase in cyclic GMP would produce an effect opposite to that noted when cyclic AMP was increased. This was referred to as the yin-yang hypothesis. In a series of paper beginning in 1970 George and his colleagues (George et al., 1970; George, Wilkerson, and Kadowitz, 1973; George et al., 1975; Fink et al., 1976) were able to demonstrate that exposure of heart to acetylcholine or vagal stimulation resulted in a marked negative inotropic effect. The mechanical response was accompanied by increases in cyclic GMP, and a correlation between the two events was noted. Cyclic AMP decreased as well, but there was a stronger relationship between the levels of cyclic GMP and the force response than was noted with cyclic AMP. Watanabe and Besch (1975) reported that dibutyryl cyclic GMP antagonized the inotropic effect of isoproterenol in guinea pig heart. A negative inotropic effect of 8-bromo cyclic GMP on both left and right isolated atria has also been reported (Nawrath, 1976).

All the above data supported the hypothesis that cyclic GMP is a mediator of the negative inotropic effect of cholinergic drugs. Because of technical difficulties in measuring changes in cyclic GMP, the early studies cited above used large doses of drug. Such doses produced marked negative inotropic responses. More recent assay methods (Harper and Brooker, 1975) have made the measurement of previously undetectable levels of cyclic GMP routine. Recent studies have completely dissociated cyclic GMP levels from the inotropic state of the heart.

Diamond, Ten Eick, and Trapani (1977) reasoned that if cyclic GMP levels controlled or affected cardiac force, any agent that increased cardiac cyclic GMP level should produce a negative inotropic effect. Cut atrial strips were exposed to either sodium nitroprusside or various doses of acetylcholine. Sodium nitroprusside produced a remarkable 1700% increase in the levels of cyclic GMP but also produced an 11% *increase* in force of contraction. With acetylcholine the maximum increase in cyclic GMP observed was only 350% and was accompanied by a 63% decrease in force. Two low doses of acetylcholine, which decreased force by 14.9% and 19.5%, had no effect on cardiac cyclic GMP. There thus did not appear to be any relationship between cyclic GMP levels and force in cat atria. Cyclic AMP levels were also monitored and did not change with either drug.

In another recent study, Brooker (1977) demonstrated that carbachol could increase cyclic GMP in guinea pig left atria, but only at a dose that decreased force of contraction by nearly 100%. The data from the laboratories of Diamond et al. and Brooker are quite clear, and it can be stated that at the present time no known relationship exists between cardiac cyclic GMP levels and force of contraction. As Brooker (1977) has stated, "cyclic GMP has been a cyclic nucleotide in search of a function."

VIII. CYCLIC AMP DURING NORMAL CONTRACTION

Changes in cyclic AMP levels during the contraction cycle have been recorded and have been cited as evidence supporting the role of this cyclic nucleotide in modulating contractile force. Brooker (1973) reported that cyclic AMP increased in electrically stimulated frog ventricle strips, with occurrence of the peak early in systole. An independent study by Wollenberger et al. (1973) confirmed these results and also demonstrated a decrease in cyclic GMP concomitant with the increased cyclic AMP level. The significance of these findings is made doubtful, however, by the more recent report of Krause and Wollenberger (1976), who demonstrated that depletion of catecholamines by 6-hydroxydopamine or the presence of a β-adrenergic blocking agent prevented the oscillations in cyclic nucleotides from occurring. The effect noted previously, then, was probably due to release of endogenous catecholamines. The oscillations have been noted only in amphibian myocardium. Dobson and his colleagues (1976) were unable to find cyclic AMP change throughout the contractile cycle in guinea pig papillary muscle. Using the spontaneously contracting uterus, where it may be easier to detect changes because of the length of the contraction cycle, Johansson and Andersson (1975) have reported that cyclic AMP and cyclic GMP levels oscillate. However, two other laboratories, using a paired experimental design rather than comparing nucleotide values from different experiments, have failed to confirm this observation (Diamond and Hartle, 1974; Meisheri and McNeill, 1977). Present evidence, then, does not lend support to the proposed role of cyclic nucleotides in spontaneously contracting muscle.

IX. SUMMARY AND CONCLUSIONS

In summary, an attempt has been made to review critically the evidence that has led to the hypothesis that cyclic AMP and cyclic GMP are involved in the inotropic effect of drugs. The conclusions reached in this review are that although a great deal of evidence suggests that cyclic AMP is involved in the inotropic effect of several drugs, no causal relationship between cyclic AMP and inotropy has been established. More recent studies indicate that inotropic effect can be produced by drugs such as the catecholamines without increases in whole tissue cyclic AMP levels. These data may indicate that cyclic AMP is not involved in the inotropic effect or that cyclic AMP changes occur only in certain cellular compartments in concentrations too small to be detected. It may also mean that under appropriate conditions pathways other than those involving cyclic AMP may be stimulated by drugs, thus leading to the positive inotropic event.

The initial data involving cyclic GMP in the negative inotropic effect of cholinergic drugs now seem to have been contradicted by more sophisticated studies that have dissociated the mechanical from the biochemical actions of such compounds. The function of cyclic GMP in the heart must be stated to be unknown at this point.

The concept that cyclic nucleotides are involved in the effects of cardiac drugs may or may not stand the tests of time and rigorous scientific investigation. However, the concept will have served its purpose, whether correct or not, in stimulating a tremendous number of studies that have revealed a great deal about the physiology and biochemistry of cardiac tissue.

X. REFERENCES

Ahren, K.; Hjalmarson, A.; Isaksson, O.: Inotropic and Metabolic Effects of Dibutyryl Cyclic Adenosine 3′,5′-monophosphate in the Perfused Rat Heart. Acta Physiol Scand 82(1971)79–90
Benfey, B.G.: Lack of Relationship between Myocardial Cyclic AMP Concentrations and Inotropic Effects of Sympathomimetic Amines. Br J Pharmacol 43(1971)757–763

Benfey, B.G.: Cardiac Adrenoceptors at Low Temperature: What is the Experimental Evidence for the Adrenoceptor Interconversion Hypothesis. Fed Proc 36(1977)2575–2579

Benfey, B.G.; Kunos, G.; Nickerson, M.: Dissociation of Cardiac Inotropic and Adenlyate Cyclase Activating Receptors. Br J Pharmacol 51(1974)253–257

Blinks, J.R.; Olson, C.B.; Jewell, B.R.; Bravený, P.: Influence of Caffeine and Other Methylxanthines on Mechanical Properties of Isolated Mammalian Heart Muscle. Evidence for a Dual Mechanism of Action. Circ Res 30(1972)367–392

Brooker, G.: Oscillation of Cyclic Adenosine Monophosphate Concentration during the Myocardial Contraction Cycle. Science 182(1973)933–934

Brooker, G.: Dissociation of Cyclic GMP from the Negative Inotropic Action of Carbachol in Guinea Pig Atria. J Cyclic Nuc Res 3(1977)407–413

Brunt, M.E.; McNeill, J.H.: The Effect of Glucagon on Rat Cardiac Cyclic AMP, Phosphorylase a and Force of Contraction. Arch Int Pharmacodyn 233(1978)42–52

Butcher, R.W.; Sutherland, E.W.: Adenosine 3',5'-phosphate in Biological Materials. I. Purification and Properties of Cyclic 3',5'-nucleotide Phosphodiesterase and Use of this Enzyme to Characterize Adenosine 3',5'-phosphate in Human Urine. J Biol Chem 237(1962)1244–1250

Cheung, W.Y.; Williamson, J.R.: Kinetics of Cyclic Adenosine Monophosphate Changes in Rat Heart Following Epinephrine Administration. Nature 207(1965)979–981

Cornblath, M.; Randle, P.J.; Parmeggiani, A.; Morgan, H.E.: Regulation of Glycogenolysis in Muscle. Effects of Glucagon and Anoxia on Lactate Production, Glycogen Content, and Phosphorylase Activity in the Perfused Isolated Rat Heart. J Biol Chem 238(1963)1592–1597

Dale, H.H.; Laidlaw, P.P.: The Physiological Action of β-Iminazolethylamine. J Physiol (Lond) 41(1910)318–344

Dean, P.M.: Investigation into the Mode of Action of Histamine on the Isolated Rabbit Heart. Br J Pharmac Chem 32(1968)65–77

de Gubareff, T.; Sleator, W. Jr.: Effects of Caffeine on Mammalian Atrial Muscle and its Interaction with Adenosine and Calcium. J Pharmacol Exp Ther 148(1965)202–214

Diamond, J.; Ten Eick, R.E.; Trapani, A.J.: Are Increases in Cyclic GMP Levels Responsible for the Negative Inotropic Effects of Acetylcholine in the Heart? Biochem Biophys Res Comm 79(1977)912–918

Diamond, J.; Hartle, D.K.: Cyclic Nucleotide Levels during Spontaneous Uterine Contractions. Can J Physiol Pharmacol 52(1974)763–767

Dobson, J.G. Jr.; Ross, J. Jr.; Mayer, S.E.: The Role of Cyclic Adenosine 3',5'-monophosphate and Calcium in the Regulation of Contractility and Glycogen Phosphorylase Activity in Guinea Pig Papillary Muscle. Circ Res 39(1976)388–395

Dönges, C.; Heitmann, M.; Jungbluth, H.; Meinertz, T.; Schmelzle, B.; Scholz, H.: Effectiveness of Theophylline to Increase Cyclic AMP Levels and Force of Contraction in Electrically Paced Guinea Pig Auricles: Comparison with Isoprenaline, Calcium and Ouabain. Naunyn Schmiedebergs Arch Pharmacol 301(1977)87–97

Drummond, G.I.; Duncan, L.; Hertzman, E.: Effect of Epinephrine on Phosphorylase b Kinase in Perfused Rat Hearts. J Biol Chem 241(1966)5899–5903

Drummond, G.I.; Hemmings, S.J.: Inotropic and Chronotropic Effects of Dibutyryl Cyclic AMP. Advan Cyclic Nuc Res 1(1973a)307–316

Drummond, G.I.; Hemmings, S.J.: Role of Adenylate Cyclase-Cyclic AMP in Cardiac Actions of Adrenergic Amines. In: Recent Advances in Studies on Cardiac Structure and Metabolism, vol. III, pp. 213–222, ed. by N.S. Dhalla. University Park Press, Baltimore, 1973(b)

Ellis, S.: Relation of Biochemical Effects of Epinephrine to Its Muscular Effects. Pharmacol Rev 11(1959)469–479

Endoh, M.; Brodde, O.E.; Schümann, H.J.: Relationship between the Level of cAMP and the Contractile Force under Stimulation of α and β-Adrenoceptors by Phenylephrine in the Isolated Rabbit Papillary Muscle. Naunyn Schmiedebergs Arch Pharmac 295(1976)109–115

Endoh, M.; Schümann, H.J.: Effects of Papaverine on Isolated Rabbit Papillary Muscle. Eur J Pharmacol 30(1975)213–220

Endoh, M.; Wagner, J.; Schümann, H.J.: Influence of Temperature on the Positive Inotropic

Effects Mediated by α and β-Adrenoceptors in the Isolated Rabbit Papillary Muscle. Naunyn Schmiedebergs Arch Pharmacol 287(1975)61–72

Entman, M.L.; Levey, G.S.; Epstein, S.E.: Mechanism of Action of Epinephrine and Glucagon on the Canine Heart: Evidence for Increase in Sarcotubular Calcium Stores Mediated by Cyclic 3',5'-AMP. Circ Res 25(1969)429–438

Epstein, S.E.; Levey, G.S.; Skelton, C.L.: Adenyl Cyclase and Cyclic AMP. Circulation 43(1971)437–450

Fabiato, A.; Fabiato, F.: Relaxing and Inotropic Effects of Cyclic AMP on Skinned Cardiac Cells. Nature 253(1975)556–558

Farah, S.; Tuttle, R.: Studies on the Pharmacology of Glucagon. J Pharmacol Exp Ther 129(1960)49–55

Fink, G.D.; Paddock, R.J.; Rodgers, G.M.; Busuttil, R.W.; George, W.J.: Elevated Cyclic GMP Levels in Rabbit Atria Following Vagal Stimulation and Acetylcholine Treatment. Proc Soc Exp Biol Med 153(1976)78–82

George, W.J.; Ignarro, L.J.; Paddock, R.J.; White, L.; Kadowitz, P.J.: Oppositional Effects of Acetylcholine and Isoproterenol on Isometric Tension and Cyclic Nucleotide Concentrations in Rabbit Atria. J Cyclic Nuc Res 1(1975)339–347

George, W.J.; Polson, J.B.; O'Toole, A.g.; Goldberg, N.D.: Elevation of Guanosine 3',5'-Cyclic Phosphate in Rat Heart after Perfusion with Acetylcholine. Proc Natl Acad Sci USA 66(1970)398–403

George, W.J.; Wilkerson, R.D.; Kadowitz, P.J.: Influence of Acetylcholine on Contractile Force and Cyclic Nucleotide Levels in the Isolated Perfused Rat Heart. J Pharmacol Exp Ther 184(1973)228–235

Gibbs, C.L.: Role of Catecholamines in Heat Production in the Myocardium. Circ Res Suppl III 3(1967)223–230

Glick, G.; Parmley, W.; Wechsler, A.; Sonnenblick E.: Glucagon. Its Enhancement of Cardiac Performance in the Cat and Dog and Persistence of its Inotropic Action Despite Beta-Receptor Blockade with Propranolol. Circ Res 22(1968)789–799

Goldberg, N.D.; Haddox, M.K.; Nicol, S.E.; Glass, D.B.; Sanford, C.H.; Kuehl, F.A.; Estensen, R.: Biological Regulation through Opposing Influences of Cyclic GMP and Cyclic AMP: The Yin Yang Hypothesis. Advan Cyclic Nuc Res 5(1975)307–330

Greeff, K.: Einfluss von Pharmaka auf die Kontraktilität des Herzens. Verh Dtsch Ges Kreislaufforsch 42(1976)80–92

Greengard, P.; Robison, G.A. (eds.): Advances in Cyclic Nucleotide Research, Vol. VIII. Raven, New York, 1977

Hammer, J.; Sriussadaporn, S.; Freis, E.D.: Effect of Glucagon on Heart Muscle Contractility. Clin Pharmacol Ther 14(1973)51–61

Harper, J.F.; Brooker, G.: Femtomole Sensitive Radioimmunoassay for Cyclic AMP and Cyclic GMP after 2'0 Acetylation by Acetic Anhydride in Aqueous Solution. J Cyclic Nucleotide Res 1(1975)207–218

Henry, P.D.; Dobson, J.G.; Sobel, B.E.: Dissociations between Changes in Myocardial Cyclic Adenosine Monophosphate and Contractility. Circ Res 36(1975)392–400

Hess, M.; Haugaard, N.: The Effect of Epinephrine and Aminophylline on the Phosphorylase Activity of Perfused Contracting Heart Muscle. J Pharmacol Exp Ther 122(1958)169–175

Hu, E.H.; Venter, J.C.: Adenosine Cyclic 3',5'-monophosphate Concentrations during the Positive Inotropic Response of Cat Cardiac Muscle to Polymeric Immobilized Isoproterenol. Mol Pharmacol 14(1978)237–245

Ingebretsen, W.R.; Becker, E.; Friedman, W.F.; Mayer, S.E.: Contractile and Biochemical Responses of Cardiac and Skeletal Muscle to Isoproterenol Covalently-Linked to Glass Beads. Circ Res 40(1977)474–484

Inoue, F.; McNeill, J.H.; Puil, E.: Cardiac Histamine Receptors: Electrical Responses in Partially Depolarized Guinea Pig Heart Muscle. Proc Can Fedn Biol Soc 21(1978)559

Johansson, S.; Andersson, R.G.G.: Variations of Cyclic Nucleotide Monophosphate Levels during Spontaneous Uterine Contractions. Experientia 31(1975)1314–1315

Kaumann, A.J.: Relaxation of Heart Muscle by Catecholamines and by Dibutyryl Cyclic Adenosine 3',5'-Monophosphate. Naunyn Schmiedebergs Arch Pharmacol 296(1977)205–215

Klaus, W.; Krebs, R.; Seitz, N.: Über die Dissoziation von Funktion und Stoffwechsel des

Isolierten Meerschweinchenherzens unter der Einfluss von Phosphiodiesterase Hemmstoffen. Naunyn Schmiedebergs Arch Pharmacol 267(1970)99–113

Klein, I; Levey, G.S.: Activation of Myocardial Adenyl Cyclase by Histamine in Guinea Pig, Cat and Human Heart. J Clin Invest 50(1971)1012–1015

Kobayashi, T.; Nakayama, R.; Kimura, K.: Effects of Glucagon, Prostaglandin E_1 and Dibutyryl Cyclic 3′,5′-AMP upon the Transmembrane Action Potential of Guinea Pig Ventricular Fiber and Myocardial Contractile Force. Jpn Circ J 35(1971)807–819

Korth, M.: Effects of Several Phosphodiesterase Inhibitors on Guinea Pig Myocardium. Naunyn Schmiedebergs Arch Pharmacol 302(1978)77–86

Krause, E-G.; Halle, W.; Kallabis, E.; Wollenberger, A.: Positive Chronotropic Response of Cultured Isolated Rat Heart Cells to $N^6,2′$-0-Dibutyryl-3′,5′-Adenosine Monophosphate. J Mol Cell Cardiol 1(1970)1–10

Krause, E-G.; Wollenberger, A.: Cyclic Nucleotides and Heart. In: Cyclic Nucleotides: Mechanisms of Action, pp. 229–250, ed. by H. Cramer, J. Schultz. Wiley, New York, 1976

Kukovetz, W.R.; Hess, M.E.; Shenfeld, J.; Haugaard, N.: The Action of Sympathomimetic Amines on the Isometric Contraction and Phosphorylase Activity of the Isolated Rat Heart. J Pharmacol Exp Ther 127(1959)122–127

Kukovetz, W.R.; Pöch, G.: Cardiostimulatory Effects of Cyclic 3′,5′-Adenosine Monophosphate and its Acylated Derivatives. Naunyn Schmiedebergs Arch Pharmacol 266 (1970)236–254

Kukovetz, W.R.; Pöch, G.; Wurm, A.: Effect of Catecholamines, Histamine and Oxyfedrine on Isotonic Contraction and Cyclic AMP in the Guinea Pig Heart. Naunyn Schmiedebergs Arch Pharmacol 278(1973)403–424

Kunos, G.; Nickerson, M.: Temperature Induced Interconversion of α- and β-Adrenoceptors in the Frog Heart. J Physiol (Lond) 256(1976)23–40

Kunos, G.; Nickerson, M.: Effects of Sympathetic Innervation and Temperature on the Properties of Rat Heart Adrenoceptors. Br J Pharmacol 59(1977)603–614

LaRaia, P.; Craig, R.; Reddy, W.J.: Glucagon: Effect on Adenosine 3′,5′-Monophosphate in the Rat Heart. Amer J Physiol 215(1968)968–970

LaRaia, P.; Reddy, W.J.: Hormonal Regulation of Myocardial Adenosine 3′,5′-Monophosphate. Biochem Biophys Acta 177(1969)189–195

Levey, G.S.; Epstein, S.E.: Activation of Adenyl Cyclase by Glucagon in Cat and Human Heart. Circ Res 24(1969)151–156

Lucchesi, B.R.: Cardiac Actions of Glucagon. Circ Res 22(1968)777–787

McNeill, J.H.: The Effect of Dibutyryl Cyclic AMP on Cardiac Phosphorylase a Activity in Euthyroid and Hyperthyroid Hearts. Proc West Pharmacol Soc 20(1977)405–408

McNeill, J.H.: The Effect of Dobutamine on Rat Cardiac Cyclic AMP, Phosphorylase a and Force of Contraction. Res Comm Chem Path Pharmacol 20(1978)597–600

McNeill, J.H.; Brenner, M.J.; Muschek, L.D.: Interaction of Four Methylxanthine Compounds and Norepinephrine on Cardiac Phosphorylase Activation and Cardiac Contractility. Recent Adv Stud Card Struct Metab 3(1973)261–274

McNeill, J.H.; Coutinho, F.E.; Verma, S.C.: Lack of Interaction between Norepinephrine or Histamine and Theophylline on Cardiac Cyclic AMP. Can J Physiol Pharmacol 52(1974)1095–1101

McNeill, J.H.; Muschek, L.D.: Histamine Effects on Cardiac Contractility, Phosphorylase and Adenyl Cyclase. J Mol Cell Cardiol 4(1972)611–624

McNeill, J.H.; Verma, S.C.: Phenylephrine Induced Increases in Cardiac Contractility, Cyclic AMP and Phosphorylase a. J Pharmacol Exp Ther 187(1973)296–299

McNeill, J.H.; Verma, S.C.: Blockade by Burimamide of the Effects of Histamine and Histamine Analogs on Cardiac Contractility, Phosphorylase Activation and Cyclic Adenosine Monophosphate. J Pharmacol Exp Ther 188(1974a)180–188

McNeill, J.H.; Verma, S.C.: Blockade of Cardiac Histamine Receptors by Promethazine. Can J Physiol Pharmacol 52(1974b) 23–27

McNeill, J.H.; Verma, S.C.: Cardiac Histamine Receptors and Cyclic AMP: Differences between Guinea Pig and Rabbit Heart, In: "Histamine Receptors," Yellin, T.O. (Ed), Spectrum, New York, 1979

Martinez, T.T.; McNeill, J.H.: Cyclic AMP and the Positive Inotropic Effect of Norepinephrine and Phenylephrine. Can J Physiol Pharmacol 55(1977a)279–287

Martinez, T.T.; McNeill, J.H.: The Effect of Temperature on Cardiac Adrenoceptors. J Pharmacol Exp Ther 203(1977b)457–466

Martinez, T.T.; McNeill, J.H.: The Effect of Theophylline on Amine-Induced Cardiac Cyclic AMP and Cardiac Contractile Force. Can J Physiol Pharmacol 55(1977c)98–104

Mayer, S.E.; Cotton, M. deV.; Moran, N.C.: Dissociation of the Augmentation of Cardiac Contractile Force from the Activation of Myocardial Phosphorylase by Catecholamines. J Pharmacol Exp Ther 139(1963)275–282

Mayer, S.E.; Moran, N.C.: Relation between Pharmacologic Augmentation and Cardiac Contractile Force and the Activation of Myocardial Glycogen Phosphorylase. J Pharmacol Exp Ther 129(1960)271–281

Mayer, S.E.; Namm, D.; Rice, L.: Effects of Glucagon on Cyclic 3',5'-AMP, Phosphorylase Activity and Contractility of Heart Muscle of the Rat. Circ Res 26(1970)225–233

Meinertz, T.; Nawrath, H.; Scholz, H.: Über die Positiv Inotrope Wirkung von Dibutyryl-3',5'-AMP an Isolierten Rattenvorhöfen. Pflügers Arch 333(1972)197–212

Meinertz, T.; Nawrath, H.; Scholz, H.: Dibutyryl Cyclic AMP and Adrenaline Increase Contractile Force and ^{45}Ca Uptake in Mammalian Cardiac Muscle. Naunyn Schmiedebergs Arch Pharmacol 277(1973a)107–112

Meinertz, T.; Nawrath, H.; Scholz, H.: Stimulatory Effects of DBcAMP and Adrenaline on Myocardial Contraction and ^{45}Ca Exchange. Naunyn Schmiedebergs Arch Pharmacol 279(1973b)327–338

Meinertz, T.; Nawrath, H.; Scholz, H.: Relaxant Effects of Dibutyryl Cyclic AMP on Mammalian Cardiac Muscle. J Cyclic Nuc Res 1(1975)31–36

Meinertz, T.; Nawrath, H.; Scholz, H.: Possible Role of Cyclic AMP in the Relaxation Process of Mammalian Heart: Effects of Dibutyryl Cyclic AMP Theophylline on Potassium Contractures in Cat Papillary Muscle. Naunyn Schmiedebergs Arch Pharmacol 293 (1976)129–137

Meinertz, T.; Nawrath, H.; Scholz, H.; Winter, K.: Effect of DBcAMP on Mechanical Characteristics of Ventricular and Atrial Preparations of Several Mammalian Species. Naunyn Schmiedebergs Arch Pharmacol 282(1974)143–153

Meisheri, K.D.; McNeill, J.H.: Cyclic Nucleotide Levels in Spontaneously Contracting Rat Uterine Strips. Proc West Pharmacol Soc 20(1977)139–142

Murad, F.; Chi, Y.M.; Rall, T.W.; Sutherland, E.W.: Adenyl Cyclase: III. The Effect of Catecholamines and Choline Esters on the Formation of Adenosine 3',5'-Phosphate by Preparations from Cardiac Muscle and Liver. J Biol Chem 237(1962)1233–1238

Murad, F.; Vaughan, M.: Effect of Glucagon on Rat Heart Adenyl Cyclase. Biochem Pharmacol 18(1969)1053–1059

Namm, D.H.; Mayer, S.E.: Effects of Epinephrine on Cardiac 3',5'-AMP, Phosphorylase Kinase, and Phosphorylase. Mol Pharmacol 4(1968)61–69

Namm, D.H.; Mayer, S.E.; Maltbie, M.: The Role of Potassium and Calcium Ions in the Effect of Epinephrine on Cardiac Cyclic Adenosine 3',5'-Monophosphate, Phosphorylase Kinase and Phosphorylase. Mol Pharmacol 4(1968)522–530

Nawrath, H.: Cyclic AMP and Cyclic GMP May Play Opposing Roles in Influencing Force of Contraction in Mammalian Myocardium. Nature 262(1976)509–511

Osnes, J.B.; Øye, I.: Relationship between Cyclic AMP Metabolism and Inotropic Response of Perfused Rat Hearts to Phenylephrine and Other Adrenergic Amines. Advan Cyclic Nuc Res 5(1975)415–433

Øye, I.; Butcher, R.W.; Morgan, M.E.; Sutherland, E.W.: Epinephrine and Cyclic 3',5'-AMP Levels in Working Rat Heart. Fed Proc 23(1964)262

Pöch, G.; Kukovetz, W.R.: Drug-Induced Release and Pharmacodynamic Effects of Histamine in the Guinea Pig heart. J Pharmacol Exp Ther 156(1967)522–527

Polson, J.B.; Goldberg, N.D.; Shideman, F.E.: Norepinephrine- and Isoproterenol-Induced Changes in Cardiac Contractility and Cyclic Adenosine 3',5'-Monophosphate Levels during Early Development of the Embryonic Chick. J Pharmacol Exp Ther 200(1977)630–637

Prasad, K.: Glucagon Induced Changes in the Action Potential, Contraction and Na$^+$, K$^+$-ATPase of Cardiac Muscle. Cardiovasc Res 9(1975)355–365

Rall, T.W.; Sutherland, E.W.: Formation of a Cyclic Adenine Ribonucleotide by Tissue Particles. J Biol Chem 232(1958)1065–1076

Rall, T.W.; Sutherland, E.W.; Berthet, J.: The Relationship of Epinephrine and Glucagon on the Reactivation of Phosphorylase in Liver Homogenates. J Biol Chem 224(1957)463–475

Rall, T.W.; West, R.C.: The Potentiation of Cardiac Inotropic Responses to Norepinephrine by Theophylline. J Pharmacol Exp Ther 139(1963)269–274

Reinhardt, D.; Roggenbach, W.; Brodde, O-E.; Schümann, H.J.: Influence of Papaverine and Isoproterenol on Contractility and Cyclic AMP Level of Left Guinea Pig Atria at Different Rates of Beat. Naunyn Schmiedebergs Arch Pharmacol 299(1977)9–15

Reinhardt, D.; Wagner, J.; Schümann, H.J.: Differentiation of H_1 and H_2-Receptors Mediating Positive Chrono- and Inotropic Responses to Histamine on Atrial Preparations of the Guinea Pig. Agents and Actions 4(1974)217–221

Robison, G.A.; Butcher, R.W.; Øye, I.; Morgan, H.E.; Sutherland, E.W.: The Effect of Epinephrine on Adenosine 3',5'-Phosphate Levels in the Isolated Perfused Rat Heart. Mol Pharmacol 1(1965)168–177

Robison, G.A.; Butcher, R.W.; Sutherland, E.W.: Cyclic AMP. Academic, New York, 1971

Scholz, H.: Über den Mechanismus der Positiv Inotropen Wirkung von Theophyllin am Warmblüterherzen. II. Wirkung von Theophyllin auf Aufnahme und Abgabe von ^{45}Ca. Naunyn Schmiedebergs Arch Pharmacol 271(1971a)396–409

Scholz, H.: Über den Mechanismus der Positiv Inotropen Wirkung von Theophyllin am Warmblüterherzen. III. Wirkung von Theophyllin auf Kontraktion und Ca-abhängige Membranpotentialänderungen. Naunyn Schmiedebergs Arch Pharmacol 271(1971b)410–429

Schümann, H.J.; Endoh, M.; Brodde, O-E.: The Time Course of the Effects of α- and β-Adrenoceptor Stimulation by Isoprenaline and Methoxamine on the Contractile Force and cAMP Level of the Isolated Rabbit Papillary Muscle. Naunyn Schmiedebergs Arch Pharmacol 289(1975)291–302

Schümann, H.F.; Endoh, M.; Wagner, J.: Positive Inotropic Effects of Phenylephrine in the Isolated Rabbit Papillary Muscle Mediated by α- and β-Adrenoceptors. Naunyn Schmiedebergs Arch Pharmacol 284(1974)133–148

Shine, K.I.; Langer, G.A.: Caffeine Effects upon Contraction and Calcium Exchange in Rabbit Myocardium. J Mol Cell Cardiol 3(1971)255–270

Skelton, C.L.; Levey, G.S.; Epstein, S.E.: Positive Inotropic Effects of Dibutyryl Cyclic Adenosine 3',5'-monophosphate. Circ Res(1970)35–43

Sobel, B.E.; Mayer, S.E.: Cyclic Adenosine Monophosphate and Cardiac Contractility. Circ Res 32(1973)407–414

Spilker, B.: Comparison of the Inotropic Response to Glucagon, Ouabain and Noradrenaline. Br J Pharmacol 40(1970)382–395

Starke, K: Alpha Sympathomimetic Inhibition of Adrenergic and Cholinergic Transmission in the Rabbit heart. Naunyn Schmiedebergs Arch Pharmacol 274(1972)18–45

Steinberg, M.I.; Holland, D.R.: Separate Receptors Mediating the Positive Inotropic and Chronotropic Effect of Histamine in Guinea Pig Atria. Eur J Pharmacol 34(1975)95–104

Sutherland, E.W.; Rall, T.W.: Fractionation and Characterization of a Cyclic Adenine Ribonucleotide Formed by Tissue particles. J Biol Chem 232(1958)1077–1091

Sutherland, E.W.; Rall, T.W.; Menon, T.: Adenylate Cyclase I. Distribution, Preparation and Properties. J Biol Chem 237(1962)1220–1227

Sutherland, E.W.; Robison, G.A.: The Role of Cyclic 3',5'-AMP in Responses to Catecholamines and Other Hormones. Pharmacol Rev 18(1966)145–161

Tenner, T.E. Jr.; Inoue, F.; Puil, E.; McNeill, J.H.: Inotropic and Electrophysiological Responses to Adrenergic and Histaminergic Receptor Stimulation in the Heart. Pharmacologist 20(1978)459

Tenner, T.E. Jr.; McNeill, J.H.: Characterization of the Inotropic Response Induced by Stimulation of β-Adrenergic and H_1 Histaminergic Receptors in Guinea Pig Left Atria. Can J Physiol Pharmacol 56(1978)926–933

Trendelenburg, U.: The Action of Histamine and 5-Hydroxytryptamine on Isolated Mammalian Atria. J Pharmacol Exp Ther 130(1960)450–460

Tsien, R.W.: Cyclic AMP and Contractile Activity in Heart. In: Advances in Cyclic

Nucleotide Research, Vol. VIII, pp. 363–420, ed. by P. Greengard, G.A. Robison. Raven, New York, 1977

Venter, J.C.; Arnold, L.J.; Kaplan, N.O.: The Structure and Quantitation of Catecholamines Covalently Bound to Glass Beads. Mol Pharmacol 11(1975)1–9

Venter, J.C.; Dixon, J.E.; Maroko, P.R.; Kaplan, N.O.: Biologically Active Catecholamines Covalently Bound to Glass Beads. Proc Natl Acad Sci USA 69(1972)1141–1145

Venter, J.C.; Kaplan, N.O.: Stability of Catecholamines Immobilized on Glass Beads. Science 185(1974)459–460

Venter, J.C.; Ross, J.; Dixon, J.E.; Mayer, S.E.; Kaplan, N.O.: Immobilized Catecholamine and Cocaine Effects on Contractility of Heart Muscle. Proc Natl Acad Sci USA 70(1973)1214–1217

Verlander, M.S.; Venter, J.C.; Goodman, M.; Kaplan, N.O.; Saks, B.: Biological Activity of Catecholamines Covalently Linked to Synthetic Polymers: Proof of Immobilized Drug Theory. Proc Natl Acad Sci USA 73(1976)1009–1013

Verma, S.C.; McNeill, J.H.: Biochemical and Mechanical Effects of Phenylephrine on the Heart. Eur J Pharmacol 36(1976a)447–450

Verma, S.C.; McNeill, J.H.: Cardiac Histamine Receptors and Cyclic AMP. Life Sci 19(1976b)1797–1801

Verma, S.C.; McNeill, J.H.: Cardiac Histamine Receptors: Differences between Left and Right Atria and Right Ventricle. J Pharmacol Exp Ther 200(1977)352–362

Watanabe, A.M.; Besch, H.R.: Interaction between Cyclic Adenosine Monophosphate and Cyclic Guanosine Monophosphate in Guinea Pig Ventricular Myocardium. Circ Res 37(1975)309–317

Wilkerson, R.D.; Paddock, R.J.; George, W.: Effects of Derivatives of Cyclic AMP and Cyclic GMP on Contraction Force of Cat Papillary Muscles. Eur J Pharmacol 36(1976)247–251

Williams, J.B.; Mayer, S.E.: Hormonal Effects on Glycogen Metabolism in the Rat Heart in Situ. Molec Pharmacol 2(1966)454–464

Wollenberger, A.; Babskii, E.B.; Krause, E-G.; Genz, S.; Blohm, D.; Bogdanova, E.V.: Cyclic Changes in Levels of Cyclic AMP and Cyclic GMP in Frog Myocardium during the Cardiac Cycle. Biochem Biophys Res Commun 55(1973)446–452

Yong, M.S.: Stability of Catecholamines and Propranolol Covalently Bound to Sepharose and Glass Beads. Science 182(1973)157–158

Yong, M.S.; Richardson, J.B.: Stability of Catecholamines Immobilized on Glass Beads. Science 185(1974)460–461

Yong, M.S.; Richardson, J.B.: Stability and Biological Activity of Catecholamines and 5-Hydroxytryptamine Immobilized to Sepharose and Glass Beads. Can J Physiol Pharmacol 53(1975)616–628

Intracellular Sources of Calcium for Activation of Smooth Muscle

Edwin E. Daniel, Denis J. Crankshaw, and Chiu-Yin Kwan

I. EVALUATION OF METHODS FOR ESTABLISHING A ROLE FOR SEQUESTERED CALCIUM

Is Ca^{2+} sequestered inside smooth muscle cells ever released to initiate contraction? This is the primary question we will address. A secondary, related question is: Does Ca^{2+} sequestered inside smooth cells contribute

Research dealt with in the review from this laboratory was supported by the Medical Research Council and by the Ontario Heart Foundation.

normally to the coupling between excitation and contraction? If the answer to the first two questions is yes, what is the site of sequestration?

But first, how can unequivocal answers to these questions be obtained? Definition of terms is essential in dealing with these questions. First, what is meant by "sequestered inside smooth muscle cells"?

A. Criteria for Participation of Sequestered Calcium

Operationally, we will define intracellular sequestered Ca^{2+} as that unavailable to Ca^{2+} complexing agents which are themselves confined to the extracellular space. Any contractile response to excitation that is not rapidly blocked by a complexing agent like EGTA at pH 7 may use intracellular sequestered Ca^{2+}. Since diffusion of Ca^{2+} and EGTA in interstitial spaces may be delayed by geometric and electrostatic constraints, it is difficult to predict how rapidly extracellular Ca^{2+} should be removed by EGTA. A response believed to depend on extracellular Ca^{2+} is often used as a standard of comparison—e.g., K^+-induced tonic contraction in vascular smooth muscle. However, it is conceivable that the Ca^{2+} may be bound to extracellular sites associated with basement membrane glycoprotein or sialic acid residues associated with the external face of the plasmalemma and not removed by EGTA. If this Ca^{2+} is somehow released on excitation by an agonist and becomes preferentially available to the cell membrane rather than to the interstitial spaces, it might allow an EGTA-resistant contraction. How excitation could release this Ca^{2+} is unclear. We are ignorant of the relations between basement membrane and plasmalemma, but excitation might release it near or into the membrane channels or ionophores for Ca^{2+}. If there are barriers to free diffusion between membrane caveolae and interstitial spaces, or if the caveolae space is an unstirred compartment, Ca^{2+} bound within caveolae might in a similar fashion become available for excitation-contraction coupling. Relations between solvent and solute in the caveolae compartment and those constituents of interstitial fluid are unknown; studies of uptake of ferritin into caveolae have usually been made in fixed dead cells.

Operationally, by our definition, such Ca^{2+} would be included with intracellular Ca^{2+}. So far there is little direct evidence about the extent to which Ca^{2+} is bound to the external plasma membrane surface or about the release of such Ca^{2+} on excitation. However, the preceding discussion shows that our operational definition of intracellular sequestered Ca^{2+} does not necessarily imply localization only to intracellular organelles, such as endoplasmic reticulum, mitochondria, nucleus, or Golgi apparatus.

We can further restrict our operational definition of intracellular sequestered Ca^{2+} by adding the criterion that it is the Ca^{2+} which permits excitation-contraction coupling after selective inhibition of calcium influx via membrane channels or ionophores by Ca^{2+} channel blocking agents, e.g., Mn^{2+}, Co^{2+}, lanthanide ions, verapamil, or its methoxy derivative (D600), nefidipine, possibly SKF 525A, etc.[1] As with utilization of Ca^{2+} complexation above, response to one mode of excitation (e.g., K^+-induced depolarization) is shown to be inhibited by Ca^{2+} channel blocker, whereas response to another (e.g., catecholamine-induced) depolarization and contraction remains intact or partially so. The locus of Ca^{2+} channels and hence of the site of action of selective Ca^{2+} channel blocking agents has been shown to be the plasma membrane of cardiac muscle and Aplysia neurons (Bassingthwaighte and Reuter, 1972; Reuter, 1973; Fleckenstein, 1977; Kohlhardt et al., 1975; Goldman, 1976; Reuter and Scholz, 1977) and appears to be the same in the membrane in smooth muscles (Haeusler, 1971; Lammel and Golenhofen, 1971; Golenhofen & Lammel, 1972; Mayer, Van Breemen, and Casteels, 1972; Godfraind, Kaba, and Van Dorsser, 1972; Godfraind, Kaba, and Rojas, 1973; Van Breemen et al., 1973; Van Breemen, Hwang, and Siegel, 1977; Kroeger and Marshall, 1974; Riemer et al., 1974; Casteels and Van Breemen, 1975; Blowers, Ticku, and Triggle, in press; Deth, 1978; Fox and Daniel, accepted 1979; Crankshaw et al., in press; Golenhofen & Hermstein, 1975; Rosenberger and Triffle, 1978, but other sites of action are not yet excluded (Haeusler, 1971; Fleckenstein, 1977; Lammel, 1977). The classification of Ca^{2+} sources resulting from use of an operational definition of resistance to blockade by selective Ca^{2+} channel blockers ought to correspond to that using resistance to an extracellular calcium complexing agent.

One possible reason why this correspondence may be imperfect is that extracellular or superficial Ca^{2+} (removed by EGTA) may be necessary for some event in the sequence prior to release of sequestered Ca^{2+}. For example, superficial Ca^{2+} may be necessary to maintain a conformation of membrane receptor appropriate for combination with mediator, hormone, or other agonist; or it may be necessary for coupling of receptor occupation to initiation of response. Thus failure of a response to be resistant to deple-

---

[1] Ca channels with properties expected in a Hodgkin-Huxley system of permeability (voltage- and time-dependent activation and inactivation) have been demonstrated in heart muscle. The evidence for their existence in other excitable tissues has been summarized by Rosenberger and Triggle (1978) as follows:

(a) Ca-dependent membrane currents and potential changes can be seen in Na-free solutions, in TTX-containing solutions, or in preparations where Na channels have been inactivated preferentially by partial depolarization.
(b) The Ca currents are selectively inhibited by Mg^{2+}, Mn^{2+}, Ca^{2+}, La^{3+}, verapamil, D600, or nefidipine, but not by TTX or TEA (which inactivate Na or K channels respectively).
(c) In some systems Sr^{2+} or Ba^{2+} can substitute for Ca^{2+} in carrying currents.
(d) The threshold voltage- or time-dependent parameters for opening and closing of these channels differ from the parameters that apply to the Na channel.

In smooth muscle, the evidence for currents borne by Ca^{2+} is limited insofar as it depends on voltage-clamp data, which are somewhat controversial. Therefore, most of the evidence such as that in (b) is based on mechanisms of action established in other tissues.

tion of extracellular and superficial Ca^{2+} does not eliminate the possibility that it uses sequestered Ca^{2+}. Furthermore, there may be more than one membrane channel available for Ca^{2+} entry into cells. Thus failure of a given response to be inhibited by a Ca^{2+} channel blocking agent does not prove that it depends on sequestered Ca^{2+}. Positive evidence that a response is selectively resistant to Ca^{2+} depletion or to a variety of Ca^{2+}-channel blocking agents provides stronger support for the hypothesis of use of sequestered Ca^{2+} than negative evidence provides for that of dependence on extracellular Ca^{2+}. Furthermore, the finding that a given response is resistant to both procedures strengthens this positive evidence considerably, since Ca^{2+} depletion will probably affect its entrance by any type of Ca^{2+} channel, whereas Ca^{2+} channel blocking agents ought to spare the responses leading up to release of sequestered Ca^{2+}.

B. Exchange between Sequestered and Free Calcium

In most cases, contractile responses resistant to extracellular Ca^{2+} complexing agents or to Ca^{2+} channel blockers are only relatively resistant; i.e., with continued exposure to complexers or with a higher dose of channel blockers, the response is lost. Apparently, this occurrence is due to the fact that the sequestered Ca^{2+} must normally be resupplied from the extracellular pool. There is no evidence that Ca^{2+} channel blocking agents inhibit sequestration of Ca^{2+} at concentrations that block contractions attributed to release of sequestered Ca^{2+} (Rosenberger and Triggle, 1978; Crankshaw et al., 1978).

This raises two questions. To what degree is the internal sequestered calcium that is released on excitation recycled on relaxation directly to its binding site, and to what degree does it mix with the free intracellular Ca^{2+}? If it mixes freely with the intracellular free Ca^{2+}, application of a stimulus for release from sequestration during Ca^{2+} depletion should accelerate loss of the associated contractile response. At the other extreme, if Ca^{2+} that has been sequestered is totally recaptured by the same binding site after its release, there should never be any loss of contractile response to releasing agents despite the absence of external calcium. Such a case has not been reported, and the physical arrangement of compartments necessary for full recycling is hard to imagine. The experimental results to date suggest that the real situation approximates fairly extensive mixing of released sequestered Ca^{2+} with free intracellular Ca^{2+}.

In many cases, only one or two responses are obtained before sequestered Ca^{2+} is depleted (Van Breemen, 1969; Van Breemen and McNaughton, 1970; Van Breemen et al., 1972, 1973, 1977; Mayer et al., 1972; Goodman and Weiss, 1971a, b; Freeman and Daniel, 1973) though it persists for long periods in the absence of stimulation. There may be a dynamic equilibrium between intracellular free Ca^{2+} and sequestered Ca^{2+} or between sequestered Ca^{2+} and extracellular Ca^{2+}. Uptake of Ca^{2+} into sequestered intracellular Ca^{2+} probably depends on active, energy-requiring processes and requires adequate Ca^{2+} concentrations in some compartment that is depleted along with extracellular Ca^{2+}. Since intracellular Ca^{2+} levels during relaxation of smooth muscle are probably no more than 10^{-7} M, entrance of extracellular Ca^{2+} from a concentration of 10^{-3} M would not require any energy supply. On the other hand, to keep Ca^{2+} sequestered within the cell might require a continuous input of energy, especially since there must be a means of release and recapture of Ca^{2+}; so irreversible binding to a site of constant chemical structure would be inappropriate. So far we are aware of no studies that have given clear insight into the energy dependence of sequestration of calcium released for excitation-contraction coupling or the pathways involved in its restoration after release.

C. Other Approaches to Establishing Support of Contraction by Sequestered Ca^{2+}

Voltage-clamping techniques might provide evidence that release of sequestered Ca^{2+} is involved in a given response. For example, a given contracting agent might be demonstrated to cause no Ca^{2+} inward current or to cause a smaller increase in influx of Ca^{2+} than would be required to activate the contractile mechanism appropriately. Then it could be argued that all or part of the Ca^{2+} that actually evoked contraction was derived from internal stores. This would be a valid conclusion if Ca^{2+} currents could be identified and measured quantitatively by voltage-clamp techniques in smooth muscle.

Voltage-clamp techniques lead to valid conclusions insofar as it can be demonstrated that they provide for uniform voltage control (a constant membrane current density) across all the membranes in the clamped node. In most multicellular preparations a major problem seems to be a resistance in series with the clamp current which is not across the membrane itself. Control of membrane voltage may be difficult or impossible, because this series resistance is not distributed so that it contributes equally to the total resistance across all membranes at all points. A further problem is the reduction in space constants that accompany any permeability increase on activation of smooth muscle. This will increase the difficulty of maintaining constant current density across cells within the clamped region. For these reasons voltage clamping has not led to straightforward evidence for release of sequestered Ca^{2+} on excitation-contraction coupling.

Compartmental analysis of Ca^{2+} influx and/or efflux, on first consideration, seems an attractive way to obtain evidence that at least Ca^{2+} is sequestered in different intracellular compartments. Theoretically, at least, this approach could be used to show that uptake into or release from a particular sequestered (i.e., slowly exchanging) compartment was selectively affected by a given stimulant. This series of findings would provide strong circumstantial support for the hypothesis that the stimulant in question used sequestered Ca^{2+}. It would have the advantage that no nonphysiological interventions are required (e.g., Ca^{2+} depletion or Ca-channel blocking agents), and it could not be criticized on the grounds that the procedure interfered in some nonspecific way with excitation-contraction coupling.

An interpretation of compartments in real physical terms (Daniel and Robinson, 1970; Daniel, 1975) requires that evidence be available to show the following:

1. That the analysis itself (usually curve fitting of flux data to a sum of exponential) leads to fitting of each exponential term to a single homogenous compartment rather than to an approximation of two or more compartments by a single exponential. There are no unique solutions to curve fitting of sums of exponentials to empirical data.

2. That the use of a single lumped parameter (one exponential rate constant) can appropriately describe fluxes into and out of a single class of compartments obtained in millions of varying smooth muscle cells.

3. That the exchange between the various cellular compartments is markedly slower than exchange between the bath and extracellular binding sites and so can be appropriately represented by models of compartments in series or parallel without unresolvable interactions between Ca^{2+} emerging from cells and from noncellular sites.

In the opinion of these reviewers, the above criteria have never been fulfilled in studies of Ca^{2+} compartments asserted to be intracellular and related to excitation-contraction coupling. Late in its efflux from a variety of smooth muscles, Ca^{2+} is not emerging from a single compartment, since the rate constant for the decrease in total radioactive Ca^{2+} is always less than the rate constant for decrease in the rate of efflux. If efflux from only one compartment is occurring, these two rate constants are the same (Daniel, 1975). Instead, there are additional very slow or tightly bound compartments of Ca^{2+} (Van Breemen and Daniel, 1966; Van Breemen, Daniel, and Van Breemen, 1966). Efflux from Ca^{2+} bound to these can be estimated (Daniel and Robinson, 1970), but the errors involved in this and the subsequent compartmental analysis are large. If the last (slowest) component of efflux or influx is simply fitted empirically to the best straight line as is often done, the subsequent curve peeling procedures, whether graphic or by computer, must provide compartments that are empirically useful but unrelated to any physical compartments.

Another major difficulty relates to number 3 above. This is the case for a variety of reasons, including the following: (a) the intracellular calcium content is only about 1/10 to 1/50 of the total tissue Ca^{2+} and tends to become lost in the variation associated with other Ca^{2+} fluxes; (b) intracellular calcium may not be the slowest exchanging fraction. Extracellular bound Ca^{2+} may exchange very slowly. In addition, emerging cellular calcium probably interacts with sites in the external matrix and basement membrane and thereby acquires the same exchange kinetics as Ca^{2+} at these sites, if this process is slow relative to exchanges between cellular compartments.

The existence of $^{45}Ca^{2+}$ at external sites late in efflux is established by the fact that EGTA or La^{3+} increase the rate of late $^{45}Ca^{2+}$ efflux (Krejci and Daniel, 1970a, b; Weiss, 1972; Freeman and Daniel, 1973; Van Breemen and Casteels, 1974; Weiss and Goodman, 1975). When this increase is transient, it may reflect only removal of Ca^{2+} still bound at superficial sites. Often the increase is prolonged (Krejci and Daniel, 1970a, b; Freeman and Daniel, 1973). This prolonged increase could be a result of prevention of reuptake of emerging $^{45}Ca^{2+}$ by superficial sites or from increased rates of exchange at superficial sites. In either case, some $^{45}Ca^{2+}$ emerging at the time was associated with those sites and was being resupplied from another compartment directly or via an unstirred layer at this cell surface. The prolonged increase could also be a result of increased membrane permeability or membrane pumping of Ca^{2+}, but these latter explanations are unlikely; La^{3+} (see the section following concerning lanthanum method), which is believed to "seal in" intracellular Ca^{2+}, does not increase membrane leakiness or enhance membrane pumping on initial application.

Smooth muscles may lose weight when they contract (Potter and Sparrow, 1968; Krejci and Daniel, 1970a, b); and their surface membranes become contorted, because the actin filaments that carry the strain are attached only at certain points to the plasmalemma (Gabella, 1976, 1977). The origin of this lost water is probably less cellular and more extracellular, but this origin has not been fully analyzed. Contraction thus may result in the following: (a) an altered diffusion path for extracellular Ca^{2+} during contraction, with slowing of efflux (see Krejci and Daniel, 1970a, b); (b) uncertainty regarding what reference value (wet weight, dry weight, volume of cellular water, etc), should be used to normalize $^{45}Ca^{2+}$ contents at various times; (c) alteration in the surface-area-to-volume ratio of cells, causing difficulty in assigning a value to transmembrane flux per unit surface membrane. The net result is introduction of a number of artifactual changes in rate constants and compartmental sizes. All in all, Ca^{2+} flux studies have provided little valid and reliable information about internal sites of Ca^{2+} sequestration.

The lanthanum method has been advocated to overcome the problems associated with compartmental analysis. Van Breemen and his colleagues (Van Breemen and De Wier, 1971; Van Breemen and McNaughton, 1970; Van Breemen and Lesser, 1971; Van Breemen et al., 1972, 1977) suggested that ions of the lanthanide series had properties that would avoid these difficulties, i.e., by occupying the same membrane ion exchange sites as Ca^{2+} as a consequence of possessing similar ionic radii, and doing so with a higher affinity than Ca^{2+} as a consequence of their greater charge, lanthanide ions would prevent transmembrane exchange of Ca^{2+} and would also displace Ca^{2+} from the extracellular matrix. Furthermore, the La^{3+} ion, it was hoped, would have such a high affinity for exchange sites as to be unable itself to pass through the membrane by exchange diffusion. If these expectations were borne out, lanthanides would seal in intracellular Ca^{2+} and displace extracellular Ca^{2+} without entering cells or altering intracellular Ca^{2+} distribution. Then intracellular Ca^{2+} or $^{45}Ca^{2+}$ could be measured easily.

Unfortunately, Ca^{2+} does not pass the membrane exclusively by exchange diffusion. In some and perhaps most cells, it carries a current across the membrane (e.g., heart, neurons, smooth muscle [Baker et al., 1969; Baker, 1972; Bassingthwaighte and Reuter, 1972; Reuter, 1973; Inomata and Kao, 1976; Kohlhardt et al., 1975]); in others it leaves by a Na-Ca exchange system that may be electrogenic and ATP dependent (Baker, 1972); and in still others it is pumped by a Ca^{2+} pump, usually involving a Ca^{2+}-ATPase (Schatzmann, 1966, 1978; Raemaekers et al, 1974; Wei et al., 1976 a, b; Janis, Crankshaw, and Daniel, 1977; Daniel et al., 1977; Matlib et al., 1978; Kwan et al., 1979). Lanthanides appear to block the Ca^{2+} current-carrying channels as well as channels formed by ionophores and Na-Ca exchange (Van Breemen et al., 1973, 1977; Rosenberger et al., 1978), at least in some cases. There is little convincing evidence consistent with the existence of a major Na-Ca exchange component to transmembrane flux in smooth muscle (Raeymaekers et al., 1974; Daniel and Janis, 1975; Van Breeman et al., 1977; Brading, 1978), and the plasma membranes of smooth muscles possess ATP-dependent, Na^+-independent Ca^{2+} transport ability (Wei et al., 1976; Janis et al., 1977; Kwan et al., 1979; Matlib et al., 1979). This transport function is not prevented by La^{3+} (Crankshaw et al., 1978).

In rabbit aorta, Deth (1978) has reported that 10 mM La^{3+} failed to block extra $^{45}Ca^{2+}$ efflux induced by dinitrophenol or caffeine and that exposure to 10 mM La^{3+} at 4°C left a La^{3+}-resistant fraction 2 times larger than after exposure at 37°C. He concluded that there was cellular Ca^{2+} loss (presumably active transport) that was not blocked by La^{3+} at 37°C. Palaty (1977) has found similar results in rat tail arteries; see also Godfraind (1977).

Ca^{2+} efflux via the pump explains why in some smooth muscles (Freeman and Daniel, 1973; Hodgson and Daniel, 1973; Godfraind, 1976; Deth, 1978) even 10^{-2} M La^{3+} does not complete block $^{45}Ca^{2+}$ efflux. Over time, the La^{3+} concentration used to block loss of cellular Ca^{2+} has increased from 0.5 mM (Van Breemen, 1969) to 50 mM (Van Breemen et al., 1977), but the "lanthanum-resistant" fraction of Ca^{2+} has always been found to decrease with increasing exposure time (Palaty, 1977; Deth, 1978).

Van Breemen et al., (1977) have argued that 10 mM La^{3+} does block active efflux of Ca^{2+}; they base their argument on the finding that in rabbit aorta it inhibited the extra late $^{45}Ca^{2+}$ efflux produced by CN- or rotenone-induced inhibition of mitochondrial function. Since these cells retained some ATP and remained relaxed, but capable of contraction in response to high K^+ or norepinephrine, Van Breemen suggested that the extra intracellular Ca^{2+} released by mitochondrial inhibitors was being actively extruded. Therefore, La^{3+} inhibition of this extra efflux would amount to inhibition of active Ca^{2+} transport. However, both in guinea pig tenia coli and in rabbit aorta Van Breemen and colleagues (1977) have demonstrated an extra calcium efflux produced by iodoacetate plus dinitrophenol or iodoacetate plus cyanide, which is also partially blocked by 10 mM La^{3+}. In these cases no ATP remains; therefore active transport of Ca^{2+} is impossible. Whatever its mechanism, the increased Ca^{2+} efflux produced by CN or rotenone is unlikely to be by active transport, since similar increases are produced by IAA, DNP, CN, and combinations thereof that eliminate ATP.

The mechanism of increased $^{45}Ca^{2+}$ efflux after metabolic inhibition is puzzling. Van Breemen et al. (1977) report that the extra $^{45}Ca^{2+}$ efflux is partially independent, in both tenia coli and aorta, of influx of extracellular Ca^{2+}; and it may not depend on Na^+ and Ca^{2+} exchange. If $^{45}Ca^{2+}$ were released intracellularly by metabolic inhibition, the increased efflux could not represent increased efflux down an electrochemical gradient, but would have to result from continued or increased exchange of some external cation for internal Ca^{2+} of increased specific activity. If exchange for external Ca^{2+} or Na^+ is not necessary, then decreased specificity of the exchange system may be involved. Alternately, if ATP-dependent sites of Ca^{2+} binding or accumulation in the plasma membrane were altered by metabolic inhibitors, this Ca^{2+} might be released preferentially to the outside of the cell. Garfield and Daniel (1977a, b) have shown that rapid ATP depletion leads to swelling and eventual disappearance of membrane caveolae in smooth muscle; loss from such a depot would not depend on external Na^+ or Ca^{2+}.

In some smooth muscles La^{3+} does enter cells (Hodgson, Kidwai, and Daniel, 1972); and in others it may do so under some conditions, such as prolonged exposure or metabolic inhibition (Van Breemen et al., 1973; 1977; Brading, 1978; Triggle and Triggle, 1976). Inside cells, it may displace Ca^{2+} (Van Breemen et al., 1973; 1978).

If lanthanides behaved as claimed, they should, on application during contraction by an agent that increases Ca^{2+} entry, "freeze" the cell in the state of contracture. Any subsequent change (e.g., relaxation) would have to be attributed either to Ca^{2+} extrusion; to translocations within the cell (despite La^{3+}); or to secondary events such as depletion of ATP, ionic shifts, or interference by lanthanides with intracellular Ca^{2+} function. In many cases, addition of lanthanides during contraction does not prevent subsequent relaxation.

Despite the strong evidence that La^{3+} does not completely inhibit Ca efflux and may enter cells, the method has been extensively used to estimate intracellular Ca^{2+}. In our opinion, such values are serious underestimates. The lanthanum method has recently been improved (Palaty, 1977; Deth, 1978) by cooling to 4°C during the La^{3+} rinse so as to inhibit the Ca^{2+} pump. Thus, in the more recent version, it involves exposure of the tissue to 10 to 50 mM of lanthanide ion in a Ca-free Ringer solution at 4°C for 30 to 60 m. Use of the modified La^{3+} method (at 4°C) may aid in distinguishing intracellular Ca^{2+} from other sources, provided that (a) its ability to completely inhibit Ca^{2+} uptake and efflux has been demonstrated or any failures of inhibition taken into account; (b) its ability to displace all extracellular Ca^{2+} has been established; (c) its failure to enter cells and to alter intracellular sequestration or transport of Ca^{2+} has been demonstrated; and (d) its selectivity in affecting Ca^{2+} binding and transport through the membrane has been established. So far only a portion of these requirements have been met—most fully by Van Breemen, Deth, and colleagues (see above).

Dyes and electron opaque markers for Ca^{2+} have also been tried for the purpose of localizing Ca^{2+} and its intracellular sites of sequestration. If valid, such localization would resolve questions about the existence and function of such sites. A number of dyes have been used with the light microscope to this end, but light microscopy cannot resolve details of location in relation to organelles. With the electron microscope a number of agents have been used (e.g., pyroantimonate) that supposedly complex with Ca^{2+} and provide electron-opaque deposits at its binding sites (but see Garfield et al., 1972). In addition, since precipitates of Ca^{2+} may themselves be electron opaque, substances like oxalate that complex Ca have been used (Popescu et al., 1974; Popescu, 1974). Sometimes electron microprobe X-ray analysis has been used to confirm the presence of Ca^{2+}; e.g., Somlyo et al. (1978); Gupta and Hall (1978). The rationale for use of oxalate is unclear. The Ca^{2+} oxalate complex involves coordination of Ca^{2+} with oxalate. This would seem to be impossible if the Ca^{2+} is bound. Furthermore, if the total Ca^{2+} concentration is unchanged locally by oxalate, why is the presence of oxalate necessary to make it electron opaque? If the oxalate is intended to complex free Ca^{2+} contained inside an intracellular compartment, what is the reason to expect oxalate to leave the total Ca^{2+} concentration inside the compartment unchanged while lowering the activity of that Ca^{2+} to that consistent with the Ca^{2+} oxalate solubility product? In addition, what is the evidence that oxalate penetrates into all compartments in smooth muscle? In general, it seems unlikely that oxalate will demonstrate any bound Ca^{2+}, uncertain that it will reach all Ca^{2+} in internal compartments, and improbable that it will leave unaffected the Ca^{2+} concentration inside compartments. Moreover, it is probable that in cases where OsO_4 staining was used after oxalate, the OsO_4 was taken up at the sites in question and contributed to electron opacity. Clearly, to substantiate these methods, a number of criteria must be met.

First, the agents in question must be specific or highly selective for interaction with Ca^{2+}, and the degree of selectivity must be such that under the experimental conditions used other interfering substances can be ruled out as contributing to the color of electron opacity. Direct evidence of the Ca^{2+} content of the dye or opacity (e.g., with an electron probe) is desirable.

Second, it must be shown that both during exposure to the complexing agent and subsequently, cell Ca^{2+} is neither gained, lost, nor translocated between sites. Since fulfillment of the demand for proof that translocation has not occurred is equivalent to having prior knowledge of the location and concentrations of Ca^{2+} at intracellular sites (i.e., the same information that is being sought by staining intracellular substances), this criterion has never been met. Surprisingly, there have been few attempts to show even that total cellular Ca^{2+} is neither gained nor lost (Garfield et al., 1972).

Third, since sequestered Ca^{2+} may be bound by electrostatic or coordinate bonds to intracellular sites, it is essential that it be demonstrated that any proposed dye or complexing agent be able to compete effectively for Ca^{2+} with intracellular sites without leading to translocation or release of Ca^{2+} from these sites. Further, any such agent must be able to penetrate to all intracellular compartments. Few attempts have been made to fulfill this requirement.

Fourth, the detection limits of the dye-Ca^{2+} complex or electron-opaque Ca^{2+} deposit must be known so that false negative results can be eliminated. These detection limits may depend upon Ca^{2+} concentration, availability of Ca^{2+} coordination bonds, or other matters. Little attention has been paid to this requirement.[2]

D. Direct Study of Cell Organelles

Release of intracellular calcium from binding, based on demonstration of an increase in efflux associated with a contractile response to a given agonist, could provide a reasonable argument for dependence of that agonist on the released Ca^{2+} for excitation-contraction coupling. However, difficulties in

---

[2] Rose and Lowenstein (1975) showed that when aequorin and then Ca^{2+} were injected into large cells, the diffusion of Ca^{2+} through the cytoplasm (assessed by induction of aequorin luminescence) was severely restricted until metabolic inhibition prevented Ca uptake into sinks. Application of this technique has not been reported in smooth muscle. It could indicate potential Ca^{2+} sinks; and if luminescence could be followed during contraction, it could indicate intracellular Ca^{2+} sources.

interpreting Ca^{2+} efflux from smooth muscle cells have been mentioned. An alternative approach is to isolate putative sequestration sites as organelles and study Ca^{2+} binding and transport by them.

Isolation of membrane organelles (vesicles of plasma membrane, or endoplasmic reticulum, mitochondria, nuclei, etc.) provides an opportunity to obtain direct evidence of a capacity for sequestration of Ca^{2+}. Combined with evidence for release of Ca^{2+} from such sites of sequestration by appropriate stimuli, this could provide cogent necessary evidence for a role for sequestered Ca^{2+} in excitation-contraction coupling. Additional evidence would be required to establish that similar mechanisms operate in intact cells.

This approach is only now being tried because there are difficulties in obtaining and demonstrating the existence of relatively pure membrane fractions. Demonstration of purity requires use of valid markers for each membrane. Fractions containing 75% to 90% plasma membranes are now available (Janis et al., 1977; Matlib et al., 1979; Kwan et al., 1979), and these have been shown to accumulate Ca^{2+} in the presence of ATP (Matlib et al., 1979) and independent of Na^+ (Kwan et al. 1979; Janis et al., 1977). So far, release or alteration of transport of Ca^{2+} from plasma membrane by various agents supposed to release intracellular Ca^{2+} has not been demonstrated.

Mitochondria have also been isolated and seem by electron microscopic examination to be relatively pure (Vallieres et al., 1975). Isolated mitochondria accumulate Ca^{2+}, though not very effectively from concentrations less than or equal to 10^{-7} M (Vallieres et al., 1975; Janis et al., 1977). However, mitochondria *in situ* do not accumulate Ca^{2+} (Somlyo et al., 1978) except when cells are damaged. In addition, release of Ca^{2+} from smooth muscle mitochondria by excitants of smooth muscle or by the intracellular messengers they release has not been demonstrated.

Other cell organelles of smooth muscle (endoplasmic reticulum, Golgi membranes, or nuclear membranes) have never been isolated in sufficient purity for any conclusions to be drawn about their ability to accumulate or release Ca^{2+}. Microsomal fractions isolated from smooth muscle by ultracentrifugation—unlike those from liver, skeletal muscle, or cardiac muscle—do not contain a majority of membranes from endoplasmic reticulum (ER). Plasma membrane invariably makes a major contribution to the total membrane (Matlib et al., 1979; Kwan et al., 1979). Even denser fractions isolated from sucrose gradients are heavily contaminated with plasma membrane. Furthermore, no membrane marker for smooth muscle endoplasmic reticulum has been established, and markers from liver endoplasma reticulum (e.g., glucose-6-phosphatase) may have very low activities or may not be confined to ER (e.g., NADH oxidase). Recently, NADPH cytochrome-c reductase has been proposed as a marker (Daniel *et al.*, 1977;

Matlib *et al.*, 1979; Kwan *et al.*, 1979). Its distribution is consistent with its occurrence mainly in endoplasmic reticulum and possibly in outer mitochondrial membrane but with lesser activity.

Isolation of ER membrane with improved purity and with positive markers for membrane components will be necessary before this technique can support a role for these membranes. Even if substantial improvement in purity is not obtained, correlation between Ca^{2+} uptake or release and activity of an established marker for endoplasmic reticulum would provide some evidence supporting a possible role for this organelle in Ca^{2+} sequestration.

E. Release of Sequestered Calcium

Additional support for the existence of sequestered Ca^{2+} in smooth muscle cells could derive from experiments in which all contractile responses were eliminated by depleting calcium or blocking its entry. If another divalent cation, itself incapable of directly activating smooth muscle actomyosin, restored responses to some agonist, the simplest explanation would be that sequestered Ca^{2+} was released by the stimulant and that the divalent ion restored the mechanism for release. This approach has proved very fruitful in striated muscle (Frank, 1962). A similar interpretation applies in striated muscle to agents, like caffeine, that can induce contracture after Ca^{2+} depletion. Caffeine is believed to enter cells and release Ca^{2+} from sarcoplasmic reticulum (Frank, 1962; Endo, 1975). In most smooth muscles the actions of methylxanthines are primarily to inhibit contractile activity, but whether by phosphodiesterase inhibition and an increase in cAMP leading to an effect on Ca^{2+} sequestration, or by some other means such as depolarization block, is obscure (Ito and Kuriyama, 1971). In a few instances, contractions have been elicited by caffeine (Ito and Kuriyama, 1971) and interpreted as in skeletal muscle.

F. Localization of Sequestered Calcium

The demonstration that a particular stimulant, which fulfilled other criteria for dependence on internal sequestered Ca^{2+}, depleted Ca^{2+} from a particular intracellular site following application of that stimulant in the absence of external Ca^{2+} would constitute very strong evidence for excitation-contraction coupling dependent upon sequestered Ca^{2+}. The problem would be how to localize the Ca^{2+} released to a particular internal site (see below).

One way would be to isolate various cell organelles, study their ability to sequester Ca^{2+}, and then show that a particular stimulant under appropriate circumstances released that Ca^{2+}.

To sum up, the following evidence would provide strong support for a role of sequestered Ca^{2+} in excitation-contraction coupling: relative independence of an agonist-induced contraction from extracellular calcium removable by a complexing agent like EGTA, and resistance to blockade by selective Ca^{2+}-channel blocking agents, along with evidence that Ca^{2+} sequestered in internal organelles is released by that particular agonist. Other approaches are possible, but then limitations must be carefully considered in interpreting the results.

We have applied thse considerations to an analysis of the role of sequestered Ca^{2+} in three types of smooth muscle.

II. VASCULAR SMOOTH MUSCLE (VSM)

A. Classification of Excitation-Contraction Coupling Mechanisms

Vascular smooth muscle has been generally classified into two types on the basis of its electrical properties. One type generates action potentials upon excitation and the other responds to an excitatory agent by gradual depolarization and contraction and can contract without depolarization. The excitation-contraction coupling in these types of vascular smooth muscle has been termed electromechanical and pharmacomechanical coupling, respectively (Somlyo and Somlyo, 1968). The characteristics of each are shown in Table 1.

Identity of the ions involved in charge carrying during electromechanical coupling has not been established conclusively in vascular smooth muscle; but Ca and/or Na ions are usually assumed to be carriers of the inward current during the action potential, as in other smooth muscles (see section I-C). Channels selectively mediating calcium transloca-

Table 1. Excitation-contraction coupling

Property of Vessel	Electromechanical	Pharmacomechanical
Electrical property	Respond to excitation by generating spike response with changes in membrane potential	Respond to excitation by generating graded response without a necessary change in membrane potential
Mechanical property	Display only phasic K^+ contraction	Display more tonic K^+ contraction (some phasic contraction may occur first)
Morphological property	Small volume of endoplasmic reticulum; may have gap junctions and "single unit" behavior	Large volume of endoplasmic reticulum; may have few or no gap junctions, but show "multiunit" behavior despite good electrical coupling
Vessel type	Small arteries and veins	Large elastic arteries

tion have been observed in a variety of vascular smooth muscle systems (e.g., see Golenhofen and Hermstein, 1975; Bilek *et al.*, 1974; Schumann *et al.*, 1975) when Ca^{2+} antagonists have been used as experimental tools.

B. E-C Coupling in Arteries

Hinke et al. (1964, 1965) demonstrated that the noradrenaline-induced contraction of rat tail artery was less dependent on extracellular Ca^{2+} than was the K^+-induced contraction during Ca^{2+} withdrawal and required lower concentrations of Ca^{2+} for full restoration of contraction. He postulated that noradrenaline contraction used calcium released from intracellular sequestered stores, whereas potassium contraction required influx of extracellular calcium. In some cases (e.g., rabbit aorta or pulmonary artery) noradrenaline seems to be able to release intracellular Ca^{2+} without causing depolarization (Somlyo and Somlyo, 1968; Hinke, 1965; also see below) and perhaps does not require entrance of activator Ca^{2+}, in contrast to K^+-induced contractions (Shibata, 1969). Conclusions similar to Hinke's were drawn by Van Breemen and McNaughton (1970), Van Breemen *et al.*, (1972, 1973), and Freeman and Daniel (1973) for the phasic contraction to noradrenaline in rabbit aorta; by Haeusler (1972) for noradrenaline contraction of rabbit main pulmonary artery; by Peiper *et al.* (1971) and Bilek *et al.*, (1974) for noradrenaline contraction of rat aorta; and by Golenhofen and Hermstein (1973) for noradrenaline contraction of guinea pig aorta. These studies used Ca^{2+}-free solutions or Ca^{2+} antagonists such as La^{3+} or verapamil and compared noradrenaline to K^+-induced contraction.

Godfraind and Kaba (1969, 1972) and Massingham (1973) showed that the phasic component of the response of rat aorta and rabbit mesenteric artery to noradrenaline was resistant to Ca^{2+}-free solution and to Ca^{2+} antagonists, in contrast to K^+ contractions. However, the tonic contractions were abolished in Ca^{2+}-free solutions and by Ca^{2+} antagonists such as cinnarizine, which also blocked contractions from addition of Ca^{2+} to a depolarized Ca^{2+}-free preparations. Schumann et al. (1975) obtained similar results in rabbit aorta and mesenteric artery using verapamil.

Kalsner et al. (1970) showed that SKF 525A selectively blocked K^+-induced contractions of rabbit aorta—both those induced by K^+ in the presence of Ca^{2+} and those induced by Ca^{2+} in the presence of K^+—leaving noradrenaline-induced contractions more or less intact. SKF 525A also partially spared contractions to 5-HT, histamine, and angiotensin, in agreement with Van Breemen's findings. Neomycin (Goodman et al., 1974), like SKF 525A, selectively inhibited high K^+-induced contractions compared to contractions induced by noradrenaline, histamine, angiotensin, and 5-HT. However, it was more effective in relaxing a maintained contraction previously induced by these agents than it was in relaxing a K^+-induced contraction. Since it inhibited $^{45}Ca^{2+}$ uptake and increased its efflux, except when superficial Ca^{2+} had been removed by EDTA, these authors suggested that it prevented binding of Ca^{2+} at superficial sites. This superficial Ca^{2+} was considered to supply Ca^{2+} for coupling of the initial phasic contraction to high K^+ and the tonic phase of contraction to other agonists. Goodman and Weiss (1971a, b) had found similar results with La^{3+}. In most cases there was competition between Ca^{2+} antagonists and Ca^{2+} when it was used to initiate contraction in the presence of high K^+, but the antagonism of Ca^{2+} antagonists to noradrenaline and related agonists was noncompetitive. Thus the rat, rabbit, and guinea pig aortas and mesenteric arteries are similar in having an initial phasic contraction to noradrenaline and to agonists other than high K^+, which appears to use intracellular Ca^{2+}.

Van Breemen and his colleagues introduced the lanthanum method to measure intracellular Ca^{2+} in VSM (usually rabbit aorta). That method and its limitations have been discussed above (Sect. I-C; see also Weiss and Goodman, 1976). Using the La^{3+} method, they have found that angiotensin and histamine contract vascular smooth muscle in a way similar to that of noradrenaline (Devine et al., 1972; Deth and Van Breemen, 1977) and probably use the same intracellular Ca^{2+} source.

C. E-C Coupling in Veins

Excitation-contraction coupling in veins differs from that in large arteries. In portal vein of guinea pig, Golenhofen and Hermstein (1975) found that Ca^{2+}-free solutions inhibited noradrenaline-induced contractions similarly whether the drug initiated action potentials or was unable to do so after use of verapamil or D600. Both mechanisms were easily inhibited by and seemed equally sensitive to La^{3+}. This suggested that noradrenaline caused Ca^{2+} entry by two mechanisms or channels, one that involved action potentials and was susceptible to organic Ca^{2+} antagonists and one that did not involve spikes and was less suceptible to organic Ca^{2+} antagonists. In some veins, e.g., rat portal veins (Savino and Taquini, 1977), low concentrations of La^{3+} can inhibit spontaneous activity without abolishing contractile responses to various agonists and to high K^+. However, Bilek et al. (1974) found that contractions of rat portal vein in response to high K^+ or to noradrenaline were similarly inhibited by verapamil. Similar results were obtained by Mikkelsen et al. (1978) in studying effects of verapamil on human saphenous vein.

The anterior mesenteric portal vein of the rabbit similarly showed dependence on external Ca^{2+} for spontaneous electrical and mechanical activity and for contractions in response to a variety of agonists (Collins et al., 1972a). Further La^{3+} and Mn^{2+} similarly inhibited spontaneous activity and contractions in response to noradrenaline, histamine, 5-HT, procaine, and KCl; and there was little difference in susceptibility to inhibition between the phasic and tonic phases of contraction (Collins et al., 1972b).

Elevated Ca^{2+} concentrations were partially competitive against Mn^{2+} inhibition, but in high concentrations Ca^{2+} appeared to act as a membrane stabilizer. Thus, all who have studied them agree that large veins depend primarily upon entrance of extracellular Ca^{2+} for excitation-contraction coupling and have minimal intracellular Ca^{2+} stores. This raises the question, How is it that large arteries have stores of intracellular Ca^{2+} for excitation-contraction coupling but large veins do not?

D. Morphology and E-C Coupling

The volume content of endoplasmic reticulum varies in different types of smooth muscle, and there appears to be a positive correlation between the contractility of smooth muscles in the absence of extracellular calcium and their volume content of endoplasmic reticulum (Devine et al., 1972).

The rabbit main pulmonary artery, containing 7.5% by volume of ER, displays sizable contraction upon addition of acetylcholine and noradrenaline even in the absence of extracellular calcium (in 4 mM EGTA solution), whereas rabbit mesenteric vein, containing only 2% ER, contracts only minimally under the same condition.

However, the proportion of ER versus other potential stores for sequestered Ca^{2+} (plasmalemma) has not been studied in most blood vessels, and the determinants of Ca^{2+} sources for excitation-contraction coupling may be more subtle than the presence or absence of a certain quantity of endoplasmic reticulum.

E. E-C Coupling under Physiological Conditions

In rabbit main pulmonary artery (Su et al., 1964; Casteels et al., 1977) a mechanical response can be elicited without depolarization of the membrane, but this type of E-C coupling occurs only at low concentrations of noradrenaline. Casteels et al. (1977) found that these low noradrenaline concentrations (2×10^{-8} to 10^{-7} M) did not elicit a contraction in a Ca^{2+}-free medium and that the rising phase of the tension increase in a Ca^{2+}-containing solution was slow. There was increased $^{45}Ca^{2+}$ uptake into the La^{3+} resistant fraction but no increase in Ca^{2+} efflux. This phenomenon suggested that these low concentrations of noradrenaline acted by increasing the Ca^{2+} influx unaccompanied by depolarization. However, higher noradrenaline concentrations induced a contraction in Ca^{2+}-free medium. The tension developed faster than with lower noradrenaline concentrations, and increased $^{45}Ca^{2+}$ influx and efflux occurred. Casteels et al. attributed these results to the release of cellular Ca^{2+}, but how the release of intracellular Ca^{2+} is triggered at high concentrations of noradrenaline remains unclear. They concluded that the excitation-contraction coupling in the main pulmonary artery depends on the entry of external Ca^{2+} under physiological conditions, whereas the release of intracellular Ca^{2+} seems to be a phenomenon that occurs during exposure to pharmacological concentrations of noradrenaline.

F. Ca^{2+} Flux Studies

The possible existence of intracellularly bound Ca^{2+} and its participation in excitation-contraction coupling has also been investigated through $^{45}Ca^{2+}$ efflux studies. Conflicting results with regard to the effect of noradrenaline on $^{45}Ca^{2+}$ efflux (Hudgins and Weiss, 1968; Hudgins, 1969; Seidel and Bohr, 1971; Keatinge, 1972) were reported from several laboratories as a result of difficulties and problems involved in $^{45}Ca^{2+}$ efflux measurements, pointed out previously (sect. I-C). Van Breemen and his colleagues (1977) have studied the $^{45}Ca^{2+}$ efflux from rabbit aorta strips into a solution containing Ca-EGTA to circumvent the problem arising from the substantial amounts of $^{45}Ca^{2+}$ remaining bound in the extracellular space, as well as to avoid the possible deleterious effect on the permeability of cell membrane caused by using EGTA alone. They found that 10^{-5} M noradrenaline caused an increased rate of efflux, which is much more marked in Ca-EGTA medium than in Ca^{2+}-free medium. This was not due to increased Ca^{2+}-Ca^{2+} exchange, because a 15-fold difference in free extracellular Ca^{2+} concentration (0.1 to 1.5 mM) had no effect on the noradrenaline-enhanced efflux rate in the presence of EGTA. They concluded that noradrenaline released intracellular Ca^{2+} from a sequestered site.

They showed that noradrenaline-released intracellular Ca^{2+} is distinct from the intracellular Ca^{2+} removed during relaxation by showing that only the first of two contractions in response to noradrenaline during an efflux study released $^{45}Ca^{2+}$. Apparently, once released, Ca^{2+} does not recycle to the release site. One possible explanation is that Ca^{2+} released by noradrenaline is not located in the sites, which removes Ca^{2+} during relaxation. One source for the noradrenaline-releasable Ca^{2+} might be the cytoplasmic side of the plasma membrane. If $^{45}Ca^{2+}$ at this site were released by noradrenaline to initiate contraction and then either sequestered elsewhere or actively pumped from the cell, it would not be available for a second release. Furthermore, Ca^{2+} to be accumulated at this site could readily be resupplied by influx from the extracellular fluid—except when that influx is blocked by La^{3+} or other agents.

Caffeine depolarized the smooth muscle cells from rabbit main pulmonary artery and reduced its membrane resistance (Casteels et al., 1977). However, 10 mM caffeine does not induce a contraction of the pulmonary artery, even though it releases cellular Ca^{2+} (increased $^{45}Ca^{2+}$ efflux) in a way similar to that of noradrenaline at high concentrations (10^{-6} M). The mechanisms and site of Ca^{2+} release by caffeine are still obscure following this study.

G. Ca²⁺ Handling by
Isolated Subcellular Membranes of Vascular Smooth Muscle

Since the localization of an ATP-dependent Ca^{2+} accumulation system in the microsomal fraction of vascular smooth muscle was first reported by Hurwitz and his colleagues (1972, 1973), it was possible to obtain direct evidence of a Ca^{2+} accumulation capacity of intracellular organelles. Vascular subcellular membranes have been isolated from different vascular segments of various species, as shown in table 2. Most of these studies have isolated a microsomal fraction in the form of membrane vesicles and have shown that they accumulate Ca^{2+} via an ATP-dependent process. Since the microsomal fraction contains plasma membrane, endoplasmic reticulum and minor amounts of fragmented mitochondria in unknown proportions and since the yield of each organelle is unknown, the possible contribution to Ca^{2+} sequestration *in vivo* by a given organelle is difficult to assess. However, attempts have been made to correlate the distribution of Ca^{2+} uptake of microsomal fraction from rabbit and rat aorta on a continuous sucrose density gradient with the corresponding distribution of 5-nucleotidase activity and NADH oxidase activity (Hurwitz et al., 1973; Moore et al., 1975). It was concluded that both plasma membranes and endoplasmic reticulum vesicles can sequester Ca^{2+} in the presence of ATP. Ca^{2+} uptake activity appeared to be mainly associated with endoplasmic reticulum, assuming NADH oxidase is a marker for endoplasmic reticulum.

Although there is ample evidence that 5'-nucleotidase is a valid marker for smooth muscle plasma membrane, a valid marker for smooth muscle endoplasmic reticulum was not firmly established. (NADH oxidase, for example, is also present in mitochondrial membranes [Sottacassa, 1971]). It is unsafe to extrapolate the enzyme markers used for ER to striated muscle or other nonmuscle cells, such as liver, for example (see sect. II-G). Recently, NADPH cytochrome-c reductase distribution in subcellular membranes from rat myometrium has been found to be consistent with its occurrence primarily in endoplasmic reticulum and has been proposed as a valid marker in smooth muscle (Daniel *et al.*, 1977; Matlib et al., 1979). In vascular smooth muscle, NADPH cytochrome-c reductase activity is low and relatively unstable compared to that in myometrium smooth muscle. It was necessary to assay for this activity in freshly obtained membrane fractions and to increase assay temperature from 30°C to 37°C, using shorter preincubation times, to obtain relatively consistent and reproducible activities (Kwan et al., 1979).

It should be pointed out that a slight shift of the correlation between Ca^{2+} uptake activity and enzyme marker activity profiles does not necessarily indicate that the Ca^{2+} uptake capacity is not associated with the membranes defined by the enzyme marker used. It is possible that the Ca^{2+}

Table 2. Subcellular membrane preparation from vascular smooth muscle

Species	Vessels	Subcellular Membrane Studied	Homogenization Method	Fractionation Method	Enzyme Markers	References
Rabbit	Aorta	Mitochondria	Potter homogenizer	Differential centrifugation	5'-nucleotidase (PM)	Fitzpatrick et al., 1972
		Microsome			NADH oxidase (ER)	Hurwitz et al., 1973
Rabbit	Aorta	Microsome	Potter homogenizer	Differential centrifugation	Cytochrome c oxidase (MITO) No marker used for PM or ER	Baudouin and Meyer, 1972
Cattle	Aorta	Mitochondria	Potter homogenizer	Differential centrifugation	Cytochrome c oxidase (MITO)	Hess and Ford, 1974
		Microsome			5'-nucleotidase (PM) Na^+K^+-ATPase (PM) Ca^{++}/Mg^{++}/ATPase (ER)	
Pig	Coronary artery	Microsome	Potter homogenizer	Differential centrifugation	Na^+/K^+-ATPase (PM) Succinate dehydrogenase (MITO)	Zelck et al., 1974
Human	Umbilical artery	Mitochondria	Potter homogenizer	Differential centrifugation	Markers not reported	Clyman et al., 1976
Dog	Aorta	Microsome	Polytron homogenizer	Differential centrifugation	Markers not reported	Allen, 1977

Rat	Aorta	Microsome	Potter homogenizer	Differential centrifugation	5'-nucleotidase (PM) NADH oxidase (ER)	Moore et al., 1975
Rat	Aorta	Plasma membrane	Polytron homogenizer	Differential centrifugation and discontinuous sucrose density gradient centrifugation	5'-nucleotidase Phosphodiesterase I Ouabain-sensitive, K^+-stimulated phosphatase (PM) Cytochrome c oxidase (MITO)	Wei et al., 1976a
Rat	Mesenteric artery	Plasma membrane	Polytron homogenizer	Differential centrifugation and discontinuous sucrose density gradient centrifugation	5'-nucleotidase Phosphodiesterase I Ouabain-sensitive, K^+-sensitive, K^+-activated phosphatase Alkaline phosphatase (PM) Cytochrome c oxidase (MITO)	Wei et al., 1976b
Rat	Mesenteric artery	Plasma membrane	Polytron homogenizer	Differential centrifugation and discontinuous sucrose density gradient centrifugation	5'-nucleotidase Alkaline phosphatase (PM) NADPH cytochrome c reductase (ER) Cytochrome c oxidase (MITO) Rotenone-sensitive NADH cytochrome c reductase (outer MITO membrane)	Daniel et al., 1977 Kwan et al., 1978

uptake capacity associated with a given membrane could be underestimated because of the presence of membrane fractions that do not elicit Ca^{2+} uptake ability, such as mitochondrial outer membranes. Kwan et al. (1978) observed significant amounts of rotenone-insensitive NADH cytochrome-c reductase activity in the lightest membrane fraction of rat mesenteric artery on a discontinuous sucrose gradient, indicating some contamination of plasma membrane by mitochondrial outer membranes as well as by endoplasmic reticulum. This may explain why the Ca^{2+} uptake capacity is usually slightly less in this fraction, which has the highest 5'-nucleotidase activity, than in a slightly denser fraction (Daniel et al., 1977; Kwan et al., 1979). Unfortunately, detailed evaluation of the purity of isolated membrane fractions has not yet been carried out in other vascular smooth muscle systems.

A plasma-membrane-enriched fraction has been obtained from rat aorta and mesenteric artery by a series of differential centrifugations of the tissue homogenate followed by further membrane fractionation on a sucrose density gradient. The Ca^{2+} uptake by the plasma-membrane-enriched fraction is similar to (in aorta) or higher than (in mesenteric artery) the endoplasmic-reticulum-containing fractions and is well correlated with 5'-nucleotidase activity and other plasma membrane marker enzyme activities. Approximately 75%–90% pure plasma membrane fraction (see Matlib et al., 1979, for assumptions and calculations) has been obtained from vascular smooth muscle (Kwan et al., 1979), but the endoplasmic reticulum fractions isolated from rat aorta and mesenteric arteries were highly heterogeneous. In fact, most of the Ca^{2+} uptake activity can be accounted for by the contaminating plasma membranes.

The major difficulties in getting a pure endoplasmic reticulum in vascular smooth muscle may be as follows: 1) its limited content in vascular smooth muscle (Somlyo and Somlyo, 1968); 2) physical continuity between endoplasmic reticulum and fragments of plasma membrane (Devine et al., 1972), which might tend to alter the sedimentation pattern of endoplasmic reticulum (this may also explain the small contamination of plasma membrane by endoplasmic reticulum); 3) physical continuity between mitochondria and endoplasmic reticulum, since these two membrane systems are usually found close together near the nucleus; 4) rough-surfaced endoplasmic reticulum comigrates with mitochondria fragments.

There is no evidence that oxalate can enhance the Ca^{2+} uptake in the plasma-membrane-enriched fraction of vascular smooth muscle (Wei et al., 1976a; Kwan, 1979); however, the microsomal fractions from various vascular smooth muscles show oxalate-enhanced Ca^{2+} uptake activity. It is tempting to attribute the enhanced Ca^{2+} uptake to endoplasmic reticulum. However, lack of an oxalate effect has also been reported in some microsome preparations (Baudouin and Meyer, 1973; Allen, 1977) and in endoplasmic-reticulum-containing fractions of mesenteric artery (Kwan et al., 1978).

The Ca^{2+} sequestered by isolated aortic microsomal fractions can be significantly inhibited by 100 mM of K^+ and Na^+ (Baudouin and Meyer, 1972; Allen, 1977). Ca^{2+} sequestration by the plasma membrane fraction from rat mesenteric artery was not affected by 100 mM K^+ or 10 mM Na^+, but 100 mM Na^+ did cause 20%–30% inhibition. However, the uptake of Ca^{2+} in the presence of 10–100 mM Na^+ was not appreciably affected by the Na^+-specific ionophore monensin (10 μm); and Mg ATP produced as much Ca^{2+} accumulation as Na_2ATP, suggesting that the inhibition of Ca^{2+} sequestration by Na^+ is not mediated by Na^+-Ca^{2+}-coupled transport. Note that a Na^+-Ca^{2+} exchange mechanism has been proposed as an alternative route for the translocation of Ca^{2+} from cytosol or intracellular binding site to extracellular space (Sitrin and Bohr, 1971; Reuter et al., 1973).

A23187 and X537A, proposed Ca^{2+} ionophores, which induce contraction of aortic strips (Pressman, 1972, 1973) and release Ca^{2+} from loaded vesicles of sarcoplasmic reticulum (Scarpa et al., 1972), also inhibit Ca^{2+} sequestration by plasma membrane vesicles from rat aorta (Wei *et al.*, 1976) and mesenteric artery (Wei et al., 1976; Kwan et al., 1979) as well as releasing Ca^{2+} from preloaded plasma membrane vesicles of mesenteric arteries (Kwan, unpublished observation, 1978).

Baudouin and Meyer (1973) have reported that 10^{-7} M angiotensin and noradrenaline inhibit the Ca^{2+} accumulation by rabbit aortic microsomal fraction in the presence and in the absence of ATP. The inhibition by noradrenaline was antagonized by 10^{-4} M phenoxybenzamine. Adrenaline, on the other hand, increased Ca^{2+} accumulation in the presence and in the absence of ATP, and this enhancement of Ca^{2+} accumulation was suppressed by 10^{-4} M of the β-adrenoceptor blocking agent, LB-46. These results have not been confirmed.

Zelek et al. (1974) reported that 10^{-6} M bradykinin reduced the uptake of Ca^{2+} and increased the release of Ca^{2+} from the microsomal fraction of pig coronary artery preloaded with Ca^{2+} for 20 m. However, 10^{-6} M angiotensin had no effect on Ca^{2+} accumulation.

Allen (1977) has recently reported that La^{3+}, caffeine, isoproterenol, and adrenaline did not affect Ca^{2+} accumulation by canine aortic microsomes. It is difficult to draw a firm conclusion about the mechanism of action of these excitatory agents and Ca^{2+} antagonists on Ca^{2+} sequestration by vascular membranes from these studies using isolated subcellular membrane fractions, for the following reasons: (a) these studies were performed using microsomal fractions, so the site of release of Ca^{2+} by intracellular membranes could not be unequivocally determined; (b) different vascular segments from different species were used for membrane preparation; (c) different experimental conditions were set up.

The role of mitochondria in the regulation of cellular Ca^{2+} concentration during contraction-relaxation of vascular smooth muscle is rather obscure. Isolation of pure, functionally and structurally intact mitochondria from vascular smooth muscle is difficult. Most studies on Ca^{2+} sequestration by mitochondria from vascular smooth muscle cell were carried out with impure, fragmented mitochondria. The rate, capacity, and other properties of the Ca^{2+} sequestration by those mitochondrial fractions varies from one laboratory to another (Hurwitz et al., 1973; Hess and Ford, 1974; Clyman et al., 1976; Wei et al., 1976a, b). In their early studies of K^+ depolarized vascular smooth muscle using the electron probe, Somlyo and his colleagues observed substantial Ca^{2+}, Sr^{2+}, and Ba^{2+} accumulation in mitochondria (Somlyo et al., 1974; Somlyo, 1975; also see Somlyo and Somlyo, 1971). It was later realized that such massive uptake into mitochondria is a property of damaged cells. These workers failed to observe Ca^{2+} accumulation when they used electron probe analysis in mitochondria of undamaged vascular smooth muscle cells (Somlyo et al., 1978). Under normal physiological conditions mitochondria do not seem to be an essential sink or source of Ca^{2+} for excitation-contraction coupling.

Several other general problems are associated with studies of Ca^{2+} handling by isolated subcellular membrane from vascular and other smooth muscles; a summary of these problems follows.

1. The capacity for Ca^{2+} sequestration is dependent upon tissue handling, the composition of homogenization medium, the extent of tissue disruption, and the purity and stability of the isolated membrane fractions. For example, the adventitial layer of rabbit aorta, which contains mostly connective tissue and is mechanically separable from the medial smooth muscle layer, contributes almost one fifth of the total Ca^{2+} sequestration capacity of the aorta (Fitzpatrick, 1973). Rat mesenteric artery vascular tree contains large amounts of mesenteric connective tissues and fat cells, which also yield membrane vesicles capable of accumulating Ca^{2+} in the presence of ATP after tissue homogenization (Daniel et al., 1977; Kwan et al., 1979). EDTA has been widely used in subcellular membrane isolations, but it interferes with further fractionation of the microsomal fraction of mesenteric artery on a sucrose density gradient (Kwan et al., 1979).

2. The relative proportion of inside-out and right-side-out vesicles in the plasma membrane fraction has not been determined. The observed Ca^{2+} uptake therefore represents only a fraction of the full capacity.

3. No evidence is available to decide whether the spatial association between the cell membrane and the endoplasmic reticulum (Devine et al., 1972) is preserved or lost during isolation procedure. If membrane

permeability to or pumping of Ca^{2+} depend on this spatial association, differences in Ca^{2+} regulation in intact cells and in isolated membrane vesicles may occur.

4. To measure the concentration gradient for Ca^{2+} across the isolated plasma membrane, we need to know the content of Ca^{2+} and the size of vesicles. Since most isolated membrane fractions usually contain vesicles with heterogeneous size distributions and with various membrane orientations, extrapolation and comparison of the Ca^{2+} accumulation by isolated membrane vesicles to the fluxes of Ca^{2+} across the cell membrane require great caution.

It appears that both extracellular and intracellular Ca^{2+} may contribute to the excitation-contraction coupling in blood vessels. The importance of intracellular sequestered Ca^{2+} is minimal in veins and small arteries but may be greater in large arteries. A better understanding about the source of Ca^{2+} for excitation-contraction coupling in vascular smooth muscle clearly awaits further systematically pursued studies of various types of vascular smooth muscle.

III. INTESTINAL SMOOTH MUSCLE

A. E-C Coupling in Intestinal Muscle

Early work by Hurwitz and coworkers (1967, 1969) on guinea pig ileum (longitudinal muscle) suggested that sudden exposure of the tissue to Ca-free solution (with 5×10^{-6} M EGTA) caused a transient contraction similar to that earlier noted in the uterus and attributed (Daniel and Irwin, 1965b) to release of Ca^{2+} from a cellular source. After this contraction, contractility to a variety of agents gradually disappeared. The magnitude and duration of the contraction of ileum on Ca^{2+} withdrawal was increased by exposure to high Ca^{2+} solutions and by addition of acetylcholine (earlier shown to be relatively independent of extracellular Ca^{2+}). It was postulated that Ca^{2+} located at a superficial but intracellular depot might be involved. Entrance of Ca^{2+} into cell cytosol from this cellular depot was facilitated by removal of extracellular Ca.$^{2+}$ Evidence was presented that this site could supply calcium to maintain contractile tension, but that Ca^{2+} could also enter via another site, either down its electrochemical gradient or via superficial membrane sites. Subsequent studies (Hurwitz et al., 1969) were interpreted to indicate that the depot Ca^{2+} was in solution in a biophase, not bound to a saturable set of sites, and that some restraint other than a simple diffusion barrier limited the rate of Ca^{2+} movement from depot to cytoplasm. However, the locus of this depot has not subsequently been elucidated, and no data decisively exclude the possibilities that it is extracellular, associated with membrane caveolae, or basement membrane. Study of the sensitivity of this response to Ca^{2+}-channel blocking agents would clarify whether the depot Ca^{2+} must cross the cell membrane to initiate contractions.

B. Phasic and Tonic Contractions

Triggle and his coworkers (Triggle and Triggle, 1976; see also Swamy et al., 1976; Rosenberger et al., 1979; Blowers et al., 1979) have carefully studied Ca^{2+} sources in guinea pig ileum. They showed that contractions from both high K^+ and a potent, cholinesterase-stable, cholinergic agonist were markedly dependent on external Ca^{2+}. However, each agent caused an initial phasic contraction followed by partial relaxation and then by a slow tonic contraction that reached its maximum in 3 to 5 m after addition of the agonists. When duration of Ca^{2+} depletion was measured from the time of removal of Ca^{2+} to the time of addition of agonist, the tonic component seemed to be more sensitive to Ca^{2+} depletion: loss ($> 90\%$) of the phasic component required 3 to 10 m, compared to less than 1 m for the tonic component. However, when their data are used to make a measurement from the time of removal of Ca^{2+} to the time of maximum response in each phase, the distinction is less striking. After 10 m the phasic component was 5% or 16% of control (with high K^+ and cholinergic agonist respectively), whereas the tonic component after 6 to 8 m was 4% or 2% of control (Swamy et al., 1976). Insofar as the phasic component was more resistant to Ca^{2+} depletion than was the tonic component, these workers attributed it to dependence on Ca^{2+} bound at the external surface of the plasma membrane rather than on Ca^{2+} free in the interstitial space.

These conclusions are at variance with those reached by Imai and Takeda (1967), who studied potassium contractures of guinea pig tenia coli. Using Ca-EGTA buffers to fix external Ca^{2+} concentrations, they showed that phasic contractions were abolished by 10^{-7} M Ca^{2+}, whereas a reduced tonic contraction persisted even at 10^{-8} M Ca^{2+}. They also reported that the residual tonic contraction, after phasic contractions were abolished in a Ca^{2+}-free (no EGTA) medium, was augmented by $Cd^{2+} > Co^{2+} > Ni^{2+} > Mg^{2+}$. These ions (5 mM) also completely inhibited the phasic contractions obtained in normal Ca^{2+} media but only diminished the tonic contractions. Since phasic contractions were always associated with spikes, whereas tonic contractions were not, these authors concluded that phasic contractions were initiated by Ca^{2+} entrance during spikes, whereas tonic contractions depended in part on entrance of Ca^{2+} without spiking and partly on release of sequestered Ca^{2+}. The divalent ions were suggested to block Ca^{2+} influx but release sequestered Ca^{2+}. Whether these differing conclusions result from different Ca^{2+} mechanisms in different tissues is unclear. Recently, Magaribuchi et al. (1976) reported that La^{3+} suppressed tonic and phasic

K^+ contractions of tenia coli nearly equally, whereas an organic Ca^{2+} antagonist (diltrazem) suppressed tonic contractions selectively. They interpret the results in terms of equivalent effects of the two agents on Ca^{2+} influx and differential effects on release of Ca^{2+} from intracellular stores triggered by Ca^{2+} influx.

C. Cholinergic Agonists

Triggle and colleagues (Blowers et al., 1979) showed that both divalent (Mn^{2+}, Co^{2+}) and thulium (Tm^{3+}, a lanthanide ion) ions inhibited contractions of guinea pig ileum (longitudinal muscle) in response to a cholinergic muscarinic agonist and were slightly more potent against the tonic component of the contraction. In addition, organic Ca^{2+}-channel blocking agents such as D600 or nefedipine (Ba-1040) were effective antagonists and appeared to be competitive with external Ca^{2+}. Again, each was somewhat more potent against the tonic than against the phasic component of contraction. Studies of combined antagonism by D600, nefedipine, and Tm^{3+} revealed that the two organic Ca^{2+} channel blockers acted at the same site, but at a site different from Tm^{3+}. Associated with the phasic cholinergic contraction, there was no significant increase in $^{45}Ca^{2+}$ content, estimated either by total $^{45}Ca^{2+}$ uptake or by uptake into the Tm^{3+}-resistant fraction. By the first method, a decrease in $^{45}Ca^{2+}$ content occurred during partial relaxation following phasic contraction, and by both methods an increase occurred during the tonic contraction. Failure to see increased $^{45}Ca^{2+}$ uptake during the phasic contraction may have resulted from slow exchange between the $^{45}Ca^{2+}$ in the bath fluid and the interstitial and superficial Ca^{2+} that supplied this contraction. Contraction itself probably slowed this exchange by increasing the length or tortuosity of the diffusion path. This would explain why preequilibration with $^{45}Ca^{2+}$ for 60 m (shorter periods were not investigated) prior to exposure to the agonist revealed a significant increase (0.38 mmoles/kg wet weight) in Ca^{2+} content estimated by the Tm^{3+} method during phasic contraction. This increase was prevented by atropine, D600, and Tm^{3+} in concentrations that prevented the contraction.

A decrease in tissue weight associated with contraction could explain these results. However, we have calculated that a weight decrease of 30% during phasic contraction would be required to explain the observed gain; such a decrease seems very unlikely. Further, the increase in $^{45}Ca^{2+}$ was probably underestimated, since the Tm^{3+}-resistant fractions were estimated at 37°C rather than at 4°C (see above). The concentration of Tm^{3+} sufficient to block contraction (10^{-6} M), however, had no effect on Ca^{2+} uptake in the absence of the cholinergic agonist, even though 10^{-2} M Tm^{3+} appeared to completely exclude Ca^{2+} from cellular sites. This might imply that Ca^{2+} channels for entry associated with muscarinic stimulation have a higher affinity for Tm^{3+} than do other Ca^{2+} sites related to Ca^{2+} entry.

The diversity of Ca^{2+} sites in ileal muscle was further emphasized by studies (Swamy et al., 1976) with derivatives (e.g. 2-chloro) of SKF 525A and of parethoxycaine. Some of these selectively blocked phasic and tonic responses to the cholinergic agonist, leaving the responses to high potassium more or less intact. These findings were interpreted to mean that, even though Ca^{2+} channels could be opened either by depolarization or by occupation of cholinergic receptors and inhibited by displacement of membrane Ca^{2+} or inhibition of entry of Ca^{2+}, the process of Ca^{2+} channel opening by muscarinic agonists involves a specific Ca pool affected selectively by the above antagonists.

Whether these above results should be interpreted to mean that these are intracellular sites of Ca^{2+} associated with the phasic contractions of ileal longitudinal muscle and with responses to muscarinic agonists depends on the operational definition of *intracellular*. By the definition we have used (Sect. IA), these sites would be considered intracellular; and this is not inconsistent with the postulation by Triggle et al. (1976) that the sites are associated with the plasma membrane.

D. Other Approaches

Van Breemen and coworkers (1973, 1977) have attempted to delineate the intracellular Ca^{2+} content and its regulation by ATP-dependent Ca^{2+} extrusion in guinea pig tenia coli using the lanthanum method at 37°C (see above). They have shown (Raeymaekers et al., 1974) that when ATP is present the maintenance of the Ca^{2+} transmembrane gradient can be independent of the Na gradient (i.e., does not depend upon a simple Na-Ca exchange mechanism[3]). They also showed that high K increased the inward Ca^{2+} leak and that this was prevented by La^{3+} and D600. So far this group has not reported a classification of excitants based on their differing dependence on influx of extracellular Ca^{2+} or release of sequestered Ca^{2+}. Their work has been discussed above in relation to the lanthanum method.

Popescu et al. (1974) and Popescu (1974, 1977) have used Ca oxalate precipitation to localize Ca^{2+} within internal organelles of guinea pig tenia coli. They exposed guinea pig tenia to 140 mM KCl plus 40 mM potassium oxalate for 10 m at 22°C. Then tissues were fixed in 2.5% glutaraldehyde and postfixed as OsO_4 (2%). The potassium oxalate was present in all solu-

---

[3] Brading (1978) has presented evidence that there may also be a Na-Ca exchange system in tenia coli. This is based chiefly on the finding that reversal of the Na gradient causes a nonspecific increase in membrane permeability associated with entrance of Ca^{2+} into cells. There is also delayed increase in permeability associated with Ca^{2+} entrance following ATP depletion. Brading showed that this can be accelerated by reversing the Na gradient, and she interprets this as being due to a more rapid increase in intracellular Ca^{2+} in the absence of Na-Ca exchange. No measurements of Ca gain in ATP-depleted tissues with and without the Na gradient were reported.

tions until the dehydration steps. Opaque deposits were found in the endoplasmic reticulum, the mitochondria, the sarcolemma and associated cavaolae, and the nuclear mambrane. Identification of the electron-dense precipitates as calcium oxalate was based on previous studies of striated muscle rather than electron probe analysis of the smooth muscle itself. Osmium tetroxide clearly contributed to these deposits.

Proof of the validity of the method (see above) was not provided; e.g., no measurements were reported of total tissue Ca^{2+} with and without oxalate exposure and at various stages of fixation and dehydration. Cellular fractions (nuclear, mitochondrial, and microsomal) were isolated by centrifugation and their Ca^{2+} contents measured, but no attempt was made to determine the degree to which Ca^{2+} was gained or lost during isolation. The composition of the isolation medium was unclear, but it probably contained Ca^{2+} and no ATP. The effects of ATP on organelle Ca^{2+} content were not determined, even though ATP would be present in cells. Estimates by morphometry of volumes occupied by cellular organelles were obtained; but their Ca^{2+} contents were estimated by using the above data on Ca^{2+} content, which probably represent passive Ca^{2+} binding after exchange during isolation.

In evaluating these data on Ca^{2+} as estimated by Popescu et al. (1974), it should be noted that the total Ca^{2+} in these cellular sites was many times the amount of intracellular Ca^{2+} estimated as the La^{3+}-resistant fraction (Van Breemen et al., 1977). Most is probably bound rather than accumulated behind a barrier (since homogenization probably disrupts organelle integrity and no ATP was present). Thus it appears difficult to relate these data to physiological Ca^{2+} compartments. In contrast to these findings, Somlyo et al. (1978) find no evidence of Ca^{2+} accumulation by electron probe analyses in mitochondria of undamaged cells (high K^+, low Na^+) of vascular smooth muscle. In damaged cells (high Na^+, low K^+) massive uptake into mitochondria occurred. In muscles depolarized for 30 m by K^+ to increase Ca^{2+} influx, Ca^{2+} would be detected in the perinuclear membrane and associated endoplasmic reticulum. However, in polarized cells, Ca^{2+} could not be detected in these organelles with the sensitivity of detection currently available. These results imply that mitochondria and endoplasmic reticulum have the potential to be Ca^{2+} sequestering sites inside cells, but they do not provide any evidence that they function as such during normal excitation-contraction coupling. Furthermore, no evidence has been provided showing that release of Ca^{2+} from these sites occurs during excitation. Only increases in internal Na^+ or inorganic PO_4 have so far been demonstrated to be plausible physiological release mechanisms for mitochondrial Ca^{2+} (Carafoli and Crompton, 1978). Even uncouplers of phosphorylation, which should release any Ca^{2+} accumulated in mitochondria, do not usually cause contraction of intestinal or other muscle. Thus the

Ca^{2+} available from the mitochondria for excitation-contraction coupling is probably very small or rapidly removed on release.

E. Actions of
Different Mediators and Agonists on Excitation-Contraction Coupling

A few studies have shown that a variety of intestinal smooth muscles can still respond to muscarinic agonists in Ca^{2+}-free or Ca^{2+}-poor media, even after they have lost the ability to respond to elevation of K^+ (Ohashi et al., 1974) or electrical depolarization (toad stomach muscle: Sparrow and Simmonds, 1965). In the longitudinal muscle of guinea pig stomach, PGE_1-induced contractions were not inhibited by varapamil concentrations (10^{-5} M) that suppressed high K^+ contractions (Ishizawa and Miyazaki, 1977). Usually the resistance to depletion of the Ca^{2+} pools usable by these agonists for E-C coupling was only relative—i.e., they did become depleted in time, and depletion was accelerated by stimulation.

Ba^{2+}-induced contraction, on the other hand, seemed to depend on extracellular Ca^{2+} slightly less than did high K^+ contractions in some cases (Karaki et al., 1967), but in others it was resistant to Ca^{2+} depletion (Yukisada and Ebashi, 1961; Cheng, 1976). The ability of Ba^{2+} to release nerve mediators and the effects of Ca^{2+} on such release have not been fully explored.

Fox and Daniel (1979) have showed that the resting active tension of the lower esophageal sphincter of the opposum was somewhat more susceptible to Ca^{2+} depletion than "off" contractions of carbachol-induced contractions. In addition, this effect was more susceptible to inhibition by verapamil or nefedipine. On the other hand, nitroprusside was able to inhibit active tone nearly completely without markedly affecting off or carbachol-induced contractions. This was suggested to be a result of increased Ca^{2+} extrusion by nitroprusside. Active tension was attributed to an inward leak of extracellular Ca^{2+}; off contraction and carbachol-induced contractions were attributed to release of sequestered Ca^{2+} along with increased Ca^{2+} inward leak.

It is clear that generalizations about sources of Ca^{2+} for E-C coupling in intestinal muscle are impossible. The sources vary with the tissue, the species, the agonist, and even the phase of contraction. So far, there is no satisfying evidence that release of intracellular Ca^{2+} is involved in excitation-contraction coupling under physiological (in contrast to pharmacological) conditions.

IV. MYOMETRIUM

A. E-C Coupling in Myometrium

Isolated organ bath studies in which the extracellular Ca^{2+} concentration is manipulated, or in which various Ca^{2+} antagonists are applied, have failed to demonstrate unequivocally an intracellular source of Ca^{2+} for contraction. Evans et al. (1958) showed that rat uterus depolarized by immersion in a high K^+ solution at 20°C still contracted to addition of acetylcholine (Ach) or oxytocin (Ot). Edman and Schild (1962) showed that these responses of depolarized muscles were dependent upon the Ca^{2+} concentration in the medium. Furthermore, the isolated rat uterus contracted very briefly when transferred from normal Tyrode solution to Ca^{2+}-free K_2SO_4 Ringer at 20°C and then relaxed to baseline. The subsequent addition of Ca^{2+} to the medium caused a slow, sustained, and fully reversible contraction. When Ca^{2+} was absent from the medium, the response to ACh was slowly lost in both normal and depolarizing solutions. Frequent stimulation enhanced the rate of loss of response. ACh responses could still be elicited when responsiveness to K^+ was lost. Therefore, ACh was able to use a source of Ca^{2+} that was inaccessible to K^+ and was perhaps bound or slowly exchangeable at some undetermined site. Contractile responses to oxytocin (Marshall and Csapo, 1961), 5-HT, and noradrenaline (Paton, 1969) in the estrogenized rat uterus and to adrenaline in the rabbit uterus (Edman and Schild, 1963) were all shown to be dependent upon a fairly slowly exchanging Ca^{2+} pool that could be depleted more quickly in the presence of EDTA (Paton, 1969). A component of the response to ACh of the isolated uterus from estrogen-treated guinea pig was still present after 55 m immersion in a Ca^{2+}-free medium (Szurszewski and Bulbring, 1973), and this was claimed as evidence for the involvement of an intracellular store in this tissue in response to ACh; however, the effects of chelating agents on this residual response were not determined. It is possible that the Ca^{2+} was supplied from a slowly equilibrating extracellular pool.

The experiments of Daniel (1963), which studied the ability of Ba^{2+} and Sr^{3+} to replace Ca^{2+} in supporting contraction of the isolated rat uterus, further supported the involvement of a bound fraction of Ca^{2+} in producing contraction. After removal of extracellular Ca^{2+}, loss of contractile responses was slow but could be restored by Sr^{2+} (partially by Ba^{2+}). However, the loss of this response on removal of Sr^{2+} or Ba^{2+} was much more rapid, suggesting that Sr^{2+} was functioning only at an extracellular or superficial site, in contrast to Ca^{2+}, which also supported contraction by release from a sequestered site. The fairly long exposure to Ca^{2+}-free solution required to deplete the bound store of Ca^{2+} was attributed to binding of Ca^{2+} at the cell membrane (precise location not specified). Daniel and Irwin (1965a, b) showed that the rat uterus responded to the addition of EDTA in excess of all Ca^{2+} and Mg^{2+} present in the bath with a contraction that could be abolished by prior prolonged exposure to Ca^{2+}-free medium. It was concluded that EDTA acts by removing an inhibitory influence exerted by Mg^{2+} and by withdrawing Ca^{2+} from surface binding sites, at which it exerts a stabilizing influence. Since even very large excesses of EDTA provoked contraction before leading to inhibition of contraction, it has since been argued (Daniel, 1965) that a second binding site for Ca^{2+} is present in the uterus. Ca^{2+} bound at this second site is assumed to be initially unaffected by changes in external Ca^{2+} concentrations and is inaccessible to EDTA. When EDTA removes Ca^{2+} from the more superficially bound site, Ca^{2+} is mobilized from the second, or sequestered, site to promote a contraction. Whether this fraction is used by other stimulants is not known.

Several agents, which have been claimed to act by blocking Ca^{2+} influx, antagonize the contractile responses of the uterus—e.g., La^{3+} (Hodgson and Daniel, 1973; Szurszewski and Bulbring, 1973), SKF 525A, chlorpromazine (Hodgson and Daniel, 1973), and tetracaine (Feinstein, 1966). No convincing evidence has been presented that these agents act by a single mechanism, and the absence of a response in their presence does not prove that an intracellular Ca^{2+} store is not involved in the generation of a response (see Sect. IA).

The most universally accepted inhibitors of Ca^{2+} influx, D600 and verapamil, are both capable of inhibiting agonist-induced contractions of the isolated rat uterus (Fleckenstein et al., 1971). At a concentration of 5 × 10^{-6} M, both these agents inhibited the responses to KCl, ACh, carbachol, OT, and $BaCl_2$ "more or less completely." The effects of these agents were markedly reduced when the Ca^{2+} concentration of the medium was increased. The fact that responses were not completely abolished at the concentrations tested raises the question, Is there a part of the response to all these agents that is totally insensitive to the blockade of Ca^{2+} influx? However, it has never been established that these antagonists can block all Ca^{2+} influx into the myometrium; furthermore, the specificity of these agents against influx has not been shown to be absolute. In high concentrations, they inhibit ATP-dependent Ca^{2+} transport by plasma membrane vesicles (Crankshaw et al., 1977).

The evidence summarized above does not present a conclusive case for the participation of an intracellular Ca^{2+} store in the contractile response of the uterus. The strongest evidence, initiation of contraction on withdrawal of the divalent ion, could be explained in an alternate fashion.

B. Other Approaches

Most voltage-clamp studies on excitation of uterine smooth muscle that have been conducted with the use of the double sucrose gap technique have been interpreted to indicate that an inward current is, in part at least, carried by Ca^{2+} (Anderson et al., 1971; Mironneau and Lenfant, 1971; Vassort, 1975); but Kao (1975, 1977) has drawn contrary conclusions from his careful studies. If Ca^{2+} influx does occur, it is consistent with the role of Ca^{2+} influx from the extracellular space in activation of the muscle. Mironneau (1973), however, has obtained evidence that also supports a role for intracellular Ca^{2+} in excitation of the muscle. In the presence of Mn^{2+},

La^{3+}, or D600, contractile responses to brief depolarizations were abolished, and no slow inward current could be detected. Larger depolarizing steps (greater than $+40$ mV and duration longer than 200 ms), although producing no inward current (and hence no influx of Ca^{2+}), provoked a delayed contraction of the muscle. The source of Ca^{2+} for this delayed contraction would seem to be intracellular. Oxytocin increased the slow inward current but did not modify the second component of the response, believed to be due to intracellular Ca^{2+} release, and thus appeared to act solely by increasing Ca^{2+} influx (Mironneau, 1976). Prostaglandin E_1, however, at a low dose, had no effect upon the slow inward current. When the Ca^{2+} component of the current was blocked with D600, a tonic contraction was still produced. At the maximum effective dose, PGE_1 produced a large contracture that was unaffected by replacing the external medium with one containing no Ca^{2+} but 1 mM EGTA. The inward current at this high dose was reduced (Grosset and Mironneau, 1977). The results strongly suggest that PGE_1 releases Ca^{2+} from intracellular stores.

There is a wealth of evidence to show that isolated organelles from the myometrium are capable of sequestering Ca^{2+} under appropriate conditions. Organelles that can accumulate Ca^{2+} include the plasma membrane (Janis et al., 1975, 1976, 1977; Rangachari et al., 1976; Matlib et al., 1979), the endoplasmic reticulum (Janis et al., 1977; Matlib et al., 1979), and the mitochondria (Batra, 1973; Wikstrom et al., 1975; Janis et al., 1977; Malmstrom and Carafoli, 1977; Sakai et al., 1978), as well as microsomal fractions that are mixtures of several types of membrane, predominantly plasma membrane and endoplasmic reticulum (Carsten, 1969; Batra and Daniel, 1971). Most authors have concluded that the Ca^{2+}-accumulating properties observed in isolation represent Ca^{2+} sequestering capabilities in the viable muscle and that these various organelles can act to "take up" Ca^{2+} and promote relaxation of the muscle. What happens to the Ca^{2+} after it has been taken up by the various organelles is a moot point, which, important though it is, has received very little attention. The important question from our point of view is, Can any stimulus release Ca^{2+} from these supposed sequestering sites? To our knowledge the only stimulants that have been used to try to answer this question in the myometrium are oxytocin (OT) and prostaglandins.

Carsten has claimed that $PGF_{2\alpha}$, PGE_2, and OT can release large amounts of Ca^{2+} from microsomal fractions of uteri from different sources (Carsten 1973a, 1973b, 1974; Carsten and Miller, 1977); and the hypothesis would appear to be proved. However, studies with myometrial homogenates (Kimball et al., 1975; Crankshaw et al., submitted 1979) have shown that PGE_2 receptors present in this muscle are almost completely saturated at a concentration of less than 100 ng ml^{-1} and that $PGF_{2\alpha}$ has approximately 10 times lower affinity for the receptor than does PGE_2. The effects found by Carsten were still increasing at 100 μg ml^{-1} concentrations of either PG; and no great potency differences were noted, although such differences are seen *in vitro* and *in vivo* (Kimball et al., 1975). There is as yet no proof of the subcellular location of PG receptors in the myometrium, though the results of Grosset and Mironneau (1977) suggest that they are intracellular. Analogy with other systems, e.g., corpus luteum (Powell et al., 1976) and liver (Okamura and Terayama, 1977), suggests a site on the plasma membrane. If this were the case, a plasma-membrane-enriched preparation ought to show a clearer response to PGs than a microsomal fraction. Rangachari et al. (1976), however, were unable to demonstrate any effect of a high dose of PGF$_{2\alpha}$ (5 $\times$ 10^{-6} M) on Ca^{2+} uptake or release by such a preparation. The effects of PGs observed by Carsten seem to be nonspecific.

All evidence obtained about the mechanism of action of oxytocin (summarized above) suggests that it acts to increase the influx of extracellular Ca^{2+} to the cell; a majority (if not all) of the receptors for oxytocin are present in the plasma membrane (Crankshaw et al., 1978), there being no evidence for an intracellular site of action of the hormone. It is therefore difficult to relate the findings (Carsten, 1974; Carsten and Miller, 1977) that OT can release Ca^{2+} from microsomal fractions to the role of intracellularly bound Ca^{2+} in the normal response to this hormone. In summary, the release of Ca^{2+} from an intracellular binding site by a contractile agent under physiological conditions has not been demonstrated in myometrium. However, under pharmacological conditions, such release may occur.

V. CONCLUSIONS

1. The methods of studying the possible contribution of sequestered Ca^{2+} excitation-contraction coupling in smooth muscle are varied. The simplest involved use of Ca^{2+} sequestering agents and Ca^{2+}-channel blocking agents. Other methods are more sophisticated but must be applied with great care. None of these methods alone provides conclusive results.

2. There is clear evidence that some contractile responses of large arteries can use sequestered Ca^{2+}, but no evidence establishes such participation in contraction of veins or small arteries or establishes that excitants present in physiological amounts can use sequestered Ca^{2+} in any vascular smooth muscle.

3. There is substantial evidence that some intestinal muscle contractions depend upon a superficial but not free extracellular source of Ca^{2+}. However, Ca^{2+} from this source apparently must cross the cell membrane before initiating contraction. No major role of sequestered Ca^{2+} in excitation-contraction coupling was established.

4. There is evidence that sequestered Ca^{2+} may contribute to initiation of certain contractions of uterine muscle, but no physiological role for such Ca^{2+} has been established.

VI. REFERENCES

Adams, D.J.; Gage, P.W.: Gating Currents Associated with Sodium and Calcium Currents in an Aplysia Neuron. Science 192(1976)783–784

Allen, J.C.: Ca^{++}-Binding Properties of Canine Aortic Microsomes: Lack of Effect of c-AMP. Blood Vessels 14(1977)91–104

Anderson, N.C.; Ramon, F.; Snyder, A.: Studies on Calcium and Sodium in Uterine Smooth Muscle Excitation under Current-Clamp and Voltage-Clamp Conditions. J Gen Physiol 58(1971)322–339

Baker, P.F.: Transport and Metabolism of Calcium Ions in Nerve. Prog Biophys Mol Biol 24(1972)172–223

Baker, P.F.; Blaustein, M.P.; Hodgkin, A.L.; Steinhardt, R.O.: The Influence of Calcium on Sodium Efflux in Squid Axons. J Physiol (Lond) 200(1969)431–458

Bassingthwaighte, J.B.; Reuter, H.: Calcium Movements and Excitation-Contraction Coupling in Cardiac Cells. In: Electrical Phenomena in the Heart, pp. 354–395, ed. by W.C. DeMello. Academic, New York, 1972

Batra, S.: The Role of Mitochondrial Calcium Uptake in Contraction and Relaxation of the Human Myometrium. Biochim Biophys Acta 305(1973)428–432

Batra, S.C.; Daniel, E.E.: Dissociation of the Downhill Calcium Movements from Sodium and Potassium Movements in Rat Uterus. Can J Physiol Pharmacol 48(11)(1970)768–773

Batra, S.C.; Daniel, E.E.: ATP-Dependent Ca Uptake by Subcellular Fractions of Uterine Smooth Muscle. Comp Biochem Physiol 38A(1971)369–385

Baudouin, M.; Meyer, P.; Fermandjian, S.; Morgat, J.L.: Calcium Release Induced by Interaction of Angiotensin with Its Receptors in Smooth Muscle Cell Microsomes. Nature 235(1972)336–338

Baudouin-Legros, M.; Meyer, P.: Effects of Angiotensin Catecholamines and Cyclic AMP on Ca^{2+} Storage in Aortic Microsomes. Brit J Pharmacol 47(1973)377–385

Bilek, I.; Laven, R.; Peiper, U.; Regnat, K.: The Effect of Verapamil on the Response to Noradrenaline or to Potassium-Depolarization in Isolated Vascular Strips. Microvasc Res 7(1974)181–189

Blowers, L.; Ticku, M.K.; Triggle, D.J.: Calcium Movements in Antagonism in Guinea-Pig Intestinal Smooth Muscle Contraction. Can J Physiol Pharmacol (in press)

Brading, A.F.: Calcium-Induced Increase in Membrane Permeability in the Guinea-Pig Taenia Coli: Evidence for Involvement of a Sodium-Calcium Exchange System. J Physiol (Lond) 275(1978)65–84

Brading, A.F.; Widdicombe, J.N.: The Use of Lanthanum to Estimate the Numbers of Extracellular Cation-Exchanging Sites in the Guinea-Pig's Taenia Coli, and Its Effects on Transmembrane Monovalent Ion Movements. J Physiol (Lond) 266(1977)255–273

Burton, J.; Godfraind, T.: Sodium-Calcium Sites in Smooth Muscle and Their Accessibility to Lanthanum. J Physiol (Lond) 241(1974)287–298

Carafoli, E.; Crompton, M.: The Regulation of Intracellular Calcium by Mitochondria. Ann NY Acad Sci 307(1978)269–284

Carsten, M.E.: Role of Calcium Binding by Sarcoplasmic Reticulum in the Contraction and Relaxation of Uterine Smooth Muscle. J Gen Physiol 53(1969)414–426

Carsten, M.E.: Sarcoplasmic Reticulum from Pregnant Bovine Uterus. Prostaglandins and Calcium. Gynec Invest 4(1973a)95–105

Carsten, M.E.: Prostaglandins and Cellular Calcium Transport in the Pregnant Human Uterus. Am J Obstet Gynecol 117(1973b)824–832

Carsten, M.E.: Prostaglandins and Oxytocin: Their Effects on Uterine Smooth Muscle. Prostaglandins 5(1974)33–40

478 / Edwin E. Daniel, Denis J. Crankshaw, and Chiu-Yin Kwan

Carsten, M.E.; Miller, J.D.: Effects of Prostaglandin and Oxytocin on Calcium Release from Uterine Microsomal Fraction. J Biol Chem 252(1977)1576–1581

Casteels, R.; Kitamura, K.; Kuriyama, H.; Suzuki, H.: Excitation-Contraction Coupling in the Smooth Muscle Cells of the Rabbit Main Pulmonary Artery. J Physiol (Lond) 271(1977)63–79

Casteels, R.; Van Breemen, C.: Active and Passive Ca^{2+} Fluxes across Cell Membranes of the Guinea-Pig Taenia Coli. Pfluegers Arch 359(1975)197–207

Cheng, J.-T.: Calcium-Induced Release of Calcium in Rectal Smooth Muscle of Mice. Japan J Pharmacol 26(1976)73–78

Clyman, R.I.; Manganiello, V.C.; Lovell-Smith, C.J.; and Vaughan, M.: Ca^{2+} Uptake by Subcellular Fractions of Human Umbilical Artery. Am J Physiol 231(1976)1074–1081

Collins, G.A.; Sutter, M.C.; Teiser, J.C.: Calcium and Contraction of the Anterior Mesenteric-Portal Vein. Can J Physiol Pharmacol 50(1972a)289–299

Collins, G.A.; Sutter, M.C.; Teiser, J.C.: The Effect of Manganese on the Rabbit Anterior Mesenteric-Portal Vein. Can J Physiol Pharmacol 50(1972b)300–309

Crankshaw, D.J.; Branda, L.A.; Matlib, M.A.; Daniel, E.E.: Localization of the Oxytocin Receptor in the Plasma Membrane of Rat Myometrium. Eur J Biochem 86(1978)481–486

Crankshaw, D.J.; Janis, R.A.; Daniel, E.E.: The Effects of Ca^{2+} Antagonists on Ca^{2+} Accumulation by Subcellular Fractions of Rat Myometrium. Can J Physiol Pharmacol 55(1977)1028–1032

Daniel, E.E.: On Roles of Calcium, Strontium and Barium in Contraction and Excitability of Rat Uterine Muscle. Arch Int Pharmacodyn 146(1963)298–349

Daniel, E.E.: Attempted Synthesis of Data Regarding Divalent Ions in Muscle Function. In: Muscle, pp 295–313, ed. by W.M. Paul, E.E. Daniel, C.M. Kay, G. Marcklan, Pergamon Press, New York, 1965.

Daniel, E.E.: Influx and Efflux Measurements. In: Methods in Pharmacology, Vol. 3 Smooth Muscle, pp 699–721, ed. by E.E. Daniel; D.M. Paton. Plenum Press, New York, 1975

Daniel, E.E.; Irwin, J.: On the Mechanism whereby Certain Nucleotides Produce Contractions of Smooth Muscle. Can J Physiol Pharmacol 43(1965a)89–105

Daniel, E.E.; Irwin, J.: On the Mechanisms whereby EDTA, EGTA, DPTA, Oxalate, Desferrioxamine and 1,10,-Phenantholine Affect Contractility of Rat Uterus. Can J Physiol Pharmacol 43(1965b)111–136

Daniel, E.E.; Janis, R.: Calcium Regulation in the Uterus. Pharmac Therap 1(4)(1975)695–729

Daniel, E.E.; Kwan, C.Y.; Matlib, M.A.; Crankshaw, D.; Kidwai, A.: Characterization and Ca^{2+}-Accumulation by Membrane Fractions from Myometrium and Artery. In: Excitation-Contraction Coupling in Smooth Muscle, pp 181–188, ed by R. Casteels et al., Elsevier/North-Holland, Amsterdam, 1977

Daniel, E.E.; Robinson, K.: Sodium Exchange and Net Movement in Rat Uteri at 25°C. Can J Physiol Pharmacol 48(1970)598–624

Deth, R.; Van Breemen, C.: Agonist Induced Release of Intracellular Ca^{2+} in the Rabbit Aorta. J Membrane Biol 30(1977)363–380.

Deth, R.C.: Effect of Lanthanum and Reduced Temperature on ^{45}Ca Efflux from Rabbit Aorta. Am J Physiol 234(1978)C139–C145.

Devine, C.E.; Somlyo, A.V.; Somlyo, A.P.: Sarcoplasmic Reticulum and Excitation-Contraction Coupling in Mammalian Smooth Muscle. J Cell Biol 52(1972)690–718

Edman, K.A.P.; Schild, H.O.: The Need for Calcium in the Contractile Responses Induced by Acetylcholine and Potassium in the Rat Uterus. J Physiol (Lond) 161(1962)424–441

Edman, K.A.P.; Schild, H.O.: Calcium and the Stimulant and Inhibitory Effect of Adrenaline in Depolarized Smooth Muscle. J Physiol (Lond) 169(1963)404–411

Endo, M.: Mechanisms of Action of Caffeine on the Sarcoplasmic Reticulum of Skeletal Muscle. Proc Japan Acad 51(1975)479–484

Evans, D.H.L.; Schild, H.O.; Thesleff, S.: Effects of Drugs on Depolarized Plain Muscle. J Physiol (Lond) 143(1958)474–485

Feinstein, M.B.: Inhibition of Contraction and Calcium Exchangeability in Rat Uterus by Local Anesthetics. J Pharm Exp Ther 152(1966)516–524

Fitzpatrick, D.F.; Landon, E.J.; Debbas, G.; Hurwitz, L.: A Calcium Pump In Vascular Smooth Muscle. Science 176(1972)305–306

Fleckenstein, A.: Specific Pharmacology of Calcium in Myocardium, Cardiac Pacemakers, and Vascular Smooth Muscle. Ann Rev Pharmacol Toxicol 17(1977)149–166

Fleckenstein, A.; Grün, G.; Tritthart, H.; Byon, K.: Uterus-Relaxation durch Nochaktive Ca^{++}-antagonistische Hemmstoffe der elektro-mechanischen Koppelung wie Isoptin (Verpamil, Iproveratril) SubstanzD600 und Segontin (Prenylamin). Klin Wochenschr 49(1971)32–41

Fox, J.E.T.; Daniel, E.E.: The Role of Ca^{2+} in the Genesis of Lower Esophageal Sphincter Tone and Contraction. Amer J Physiol (accepted 1979)

Frank, G.B.: Utilization of Bound Calcium in the Action of Caffeine and Certain Multivalent Cations on Skeletal Muscle. J Physiol (Lond) 163(1962)254–268

Freeman, D.J.; Daniel, E.E.: Calcium Movements in Vascular Smooth Muscle and Its Detection Using Lanthanum as a Probe. Can J Physiol Pharmacol 51(1973)900–913

Gabella, G.: The Force Generated by a Visceral Smooth Muscle. J Physiol (Lond) 263(1976)199–213

Gabella, G.: Arrangement of Smooth Muscle Cells and Intramuscular Septa in the Taenia Coli. Cell Tiss Res 184(1977)195–212

Garfield, R.E.; and Daniel, E.E.: Relation of Membrane Vesicles to Volume Control and Na$^+$-Transport in Smooth Muscle: Effect of Metabolic and Transport Inhibition on Fresh Tissues. J Mechanochem Cell Motil 4(2)(1977a)113–155

Garfield, R.E.; Daniel, E.E.: Relation of Membrane Vesicles to Volume Control and Na$^+$-Transport in Smooth Muscle: Studies on Na$^+$-Rich Tissues. J Mechanochem Cell Motil 4(2)(1977b)157–176

Garfield, R.E.; Henderson, R.M.; Daniel, E.E.: Evaluation of the Pyroantimonate Technique for Localization of Tissue Sodium. Tissue and Cell 4(1972)575–589

Godfraind, T.: Calcium Exchange in Vascular Smooth Muscle, Action of Noradrenaline and Lanthanum. J Physiol (Lond) 260(1976)21–35

Godfraind, T.: The Lanthanum-Resistant Calcium Fraction. In: Excitation-Contraction Coupling in Smooth Muscle, pp 289–295, ed. by R. Casteels et al., Elsevier/North Holland Biomedical Press, Amsterdam, 1977

Godfraind, T.; Kaba, A.: Actions phasique et tonique de l'adrenaline sur un muscle lisse vasculaire et leur inhibition par des agents pharmacologiques. Arch Internat Pharmacol 178(1969)488–491

Godfraind, T.; Kaba, A.: The Role of Calcium in the Action of Drugs on Vascular Smooth Muscle. Arch Int Pharmacodyn Ther 196Suppl.(1972)35–49

Godfraind, T.; Kaba, A.; Rojas, R.: Inhibition by Cinnarazine of Calcium Channels Opening in Depolarized Smooth Muscle. Brit J Pharmacol 49(1973)164–165

Godfraind, T.; Kaba, A.; Van Dorsser, W.: The Action of Cinnarazine on the Contraction Induced by Calcium in Depolarized Arterial and Intestinal Smooth Muscle Preparations. Arch Int Pharmacodyn Ther 197(1972)399–400

Goldman, L.: Kinetics of Channel Gating in Excitable Membranes. Quart Rev Biophys 9(1976)491–526

Golenhofen, K.; Hermstein, N.: Spike-Free Activation Mechanism in Portal Vein and Aortic Smooth Muscle. Pfluegers Arch 339Suppl.(1973)R56

Golenhofen, K.; Hermstein, N.: Differentiation of Calcium Activation Mechanisms in Vascular Smooth Muscle by Selective Suppression with Verapamil and D600. Blood Vessels 12(1975)21–37

Golenhofen, K.; Lammel, E.: Selective Suppression of Some Components of Spontaneous Activity in Various Types of Smooth Muscle by Iproveratril (Verapamil). Pfluegers Arch 331(1972)233–243

Goodman, F.R.; Weiss, G.B.: Dissociation by Lanthanum of Smooth Muscle Responses to Potassium and Acetylcholine. Am J Physiol 220(1971a)759–766

Goodman, F.R.; Weiss, G.B.: Effects of Lanthanum on ^{45}Ca Movements and on Contractions Induced by Norepinephrine, Histamine and Potassium in Vascular Smooth Muscle. J Pharm Exp Ther 177(1971b)415–425

Goodman, F.R.; Weiss, G.B.; Adams, H.R.: Alterations by Neomycin of ^{45}Ca Movements and Contractile Responses in Vascular Smooth Muscle. J Pharmacol 188(1974)472–480

Grosset, A.; Mironneau, J.: An Analysis of the Actions of Prostaglandin E_1 on Membrane Currents and Contraction in Uterine Smooth Muscle. J Physiol (Lond) 270(1977)765–784

Gupta, B.L.; Hall, T.A.: Electron Microprobe X-Ray Analysis of Calcium. In: Calcium Transport and Cell Function, ed. by A. Scarpa and E. Carafoli. Ann N.Y. Acad Sci 301(1978)28–51

Haeusler, G.: The Effects of Verapamil on the Contractility of Smooth Muscle and on Excitation-Secretion Coupling in Adrenergic Nerve Terminals. Angiol 8(1971)156–160

Haeusler, G.: Differential Effect of Verapamil on Excitation-Contraction Coupling in Smooth Muscle and on Excitation-Secretion Coupling in Adrenergic Nerve Terminals. J Pharmacol 180(1972)672–682

Hess, M.L.; Ford, G.D.: Calcium Accumulation by Subcellular Fractions from Vascular Smooth Muscle. J Molec Cell Cardiol 6(1974)275–282

Hinke, J.A.M.: Calcium Requirements for Noradrenaline and High Potassium Ion Concentration in Arterial Smooth Muscle. In: "Muscle", ed. by W.M. Paul, E.E. Daniel, C.M. Kay, G. Monckton, 269–285, Pergamon Press, Oxford, 1965

Hinke, J.A.M.; Wilson, M.C.; Burnham, S.C.: Calcium and the Contractility of Arterial Smooth Muscle. Am J Physiol 206(1964)211–217

Hodgson, B.J.; Daniel, E.E.: Studies Concerning the Source of Calcium for Contraction of Rat Myometrium. Can J Physiol Pharmacol 51(1973)914–932

Hodgson, B.J.; Kidwai, A.M.; Daniel, E.E.: Uptake of Lanthanum by Smooth Muscle. Can J Physiol Pharmacol 50(1972)730–733

Hudgins, P.M.: Some Drug Effects on Calcium Movement in Aortic Strips. J Pharm Exp Ther 170(1969)303–310

Hudgins, P.M.; Weiss, G.B.: Differential Effects of Calcium Removal upon Vascular Smooth Muscle Contraction Induced by Norepinephrine, Histamine and Potassium. J Pharm Exp Ther 159(1968)91–97

Hudgins, P.M.; Weiss, G.: Characteristics of ^{45}Ca Binding in Vascular Smooth Muscle. Am J Physiol 217(1969)1310–1315

Hurwitz, L.; Fitzpatrick, D.F.; Debbas, G.; Landon, E.S.: Localizations of Calcium Pump Activity in Smooth Muscle. Science 179(1973)384–386

Hurwitz, L.; Joiner, P.D.: Excitation-Contraction Coupling in Smooth Muscle. Fed Proc 28(1969)1629–1633

Hurwitz, L.; Joiner, P.D.; Von Hagen, S.: Calcium Pools Utilized for Contraction in Smooth Muscle. Am J Physiol 213(1967)1299–1304

Imai, S.; Takeda, K.: Actions of Calcium and Certain Multivalent Cations on Potassium Contracture of Guinea-Pig Taenia Coli. J Physiol (Lond) 190(1967)155–169

Inomata, H.; Kao, C.Y.: Ionic Currents in the Guinea-Pig Taenia Coli. J Physiol (Lond) 255(1976)347–378

Ishizawa, M.; Miyazaki, E.: Calcium and the Contractile Response to Prostaglandin in the Smooth Muscle of Guinea-Pig Stomach. Experientia 33(1977)366–377

Ito, Y.; Kuriyama, H.: Caffeine and Excitation Contraction Coupling in the Guinea Pig Taenia Coli. J Gen Physiol 57(1971)448–463

Janis, R.A.; Crankshaw, D.J.; Daniel, E.E.: Control of Intracellular Ca^{2+} Activity in Rat Myometrium. Am J Physiol 232(1977)C50–C58

Janis, R.A.; Daniel, E.E.: Ca^{++} Transport by Subcellular Fractions from Smooth Muscle. Proc. Symp. Biochemistry of Smooth Muscle, Winnipeg, Canada; ed. by N.L. Stephens; pp. 653–674. University Park Press, Baltimore, 1975

Janis, R.A.; Lee, E.Y.; Allan, J.; Daniel, E.E.: The Role of Sarcolemma and Mitochondria in Regulating Ca^{2+} Movements in Human Myometrium. Pfluegers Arch 365(1976)171–176

Kalsner, S.; Nickerson, M.; Boyd, G.N.: Selective Blockade of Potassium Induced Contractions of Aortic Strips by β-Diethylamineoethyldiphenyl-propylacetate (SKF 525-A). J Pharm Exp Ther 174(1970)500–508

Kao, C.Y.: Recent Experiments in Voltage-Clamp Studies on Smooth Muscles. In Excitation Contraction Coupling in Smooth Muscle, pp. 91–96. ed. by R. Casteels et al., Elsevier/North Holland, Biomedical press, Amsterdam 1977

Kao, C.Y.; McCollough, J.R.: Ionic Currents in the Uterine Smooth Muscle. J Physiol (Lond) 246(1975)1–36

Karaki, H.; Ikeda, M.; Urakawa, N.: Effects of External Calcium and Metabolic Inhibitors on

Barium-Induced Tension Changes in Guinea Pig Taenia Coli. J Pharm Exp Ther 17(1967)603–612

Keatinge, W.R.: Mechanical Response with Reversed Electrical Response to Noradrenaline by Ca-Deprived Arterial Smooth Muscles. J Physiol (Lond) 224(1972)21–34

Kimball, F.E.; Kirton, K.T.; Spilman, C.H.; Wyngarden, L.J.: Prostaglandin E₁ Specific Binding in Human Myometrium. Biol Reprod 13(1975)482–489

Kohlhardt, M.; Krause, H.; Kübler, M.; Herdey, A.: Kinetics of Inactivation and Recovery of the Slow Inward Current in the Mammalian Ventricular Myocardium. Pfluegers Arch 355(1975)1–17

Krejci, I.; Daniel, E.E.: Effect of Contraction on Movements of Calcium 45 into and out of Rat Myometrium. Am J Physiol 219(1970a)256–262

Krejci, I.; Daniel, E.E.: Effects of Altered External Calcium Contractions on Fluxes of Calcium 45 in Rat Myometrium. Am J Physiol 219(1970b)263–269

Kroeger, E.A.; Marshall, J.M.: Beta Adrenergic-Effects on Myometrium. Role of Cyclic AMP. Am J Physiol 226(1974)1298–1303

Kwan, C.Y.: Garfield, R.; Daniel, E.E.: An Improved Procedure for the Isolation of Plasma Membranes from Rat Mesenteric Arteries. J Molec & Cell Cardiol 11(1979)639–660

Lammel, E.: ⁴⁵Ca Uptake of Stomach Smooth Muscle during Different Modes of Activation. In: Excitation Contraction Coupling in Smooth Muscle, pp. 273–277, ed. by R. Casteels et al., Elsevier/North Holland Biomedical Press, Amsterdam, 1977

Lammel, E.; Golenhofen, K.: Messungen der ⁴⁵Ca-Aufnahme an intestin aler glatter Muskulatur zur Hypothese eines von Ca-Ionen getragenesn Aktionsstromes. Pfluegers Arch 329(1971)269–282

Magaribuchie, T.; Nakajima, H.; Kryomoto, A.: Effects of Diltiazem and Lanthanum Ion on the Potassium Contraction of Isolated Guinea Pig Smooth Muscle. Japan J Pharmacol 27(1977)333–339.

Malmström, K.; and Carafoli, E.: The Interaction of Ca²⁺ with Mitochondria from Human Myometrium. Arch Biochem Biophys 182(1977)657–666

Marshall, J.M.; and Csapo, A.I.: Hormonal and Ionic Influences on the Membrane Activity of Uterine Smooth Muscle Cells. Endocrinol 68(1961)1026–1035

Massingham, R.: A Study of Compounds which Inhibit Vascular Smooth Muscle Contraction. Europ J Pharmacol 22(1973)75–82

Matlib, M.A.; Crankshaw, J.; Garfield, R.E.; Crankshaw, D.J.; Kwan, C.Y.; Branda, L.A.; Daniel, E.E.: Characterization of Membrane Fractions and Isolation of Purified Plasma Membrane from Rat Myometrium. J Biol Chem 254(1979)1834–1840

Mayer, C.J.; Van Breemen, C.; Casteels, R.: The Action of Lanthanum and D600 on the Calcium Exchange in the Smooth Muscle Cells of the Guinea-Pig Taenia Coli. Pfluegers Arch 337(1972)333–356

Mikkelsen, E.; Andersson, K.-E.; Bengtsson, B.: Effects of Verapamil and Nitroglycerin on Contractile Responses to Potassium and Noradrenaline in Isolated Human Peripheral Veins. Acta Pharmacol Toxicol 42(1978)14–22

Mironneau, J.: Excitation-Contraction Coupling in Voltage Clamped Uterine Smooth Muscle. J Physiol 233(1973)127–141

Mironneau, J.: Effects of Oxytocin on Ionic Currents Underlying Rhythmic Activity and Contraction in Uterine Smooth Muscle. Pflug Arch 363(1976)113–118

Mironneau, J.; Lenfant, J.: Analyse des réponses électriques de la fibre musculaire lisse d'uterus de ratte: Mise en évidence d'un courant lent calciosodique. CR Acad Sci Paris 272(1971)436–439

Moore, L.; Hurwitz, L.; Davenport, G.R.; Landon, E.J.: Energy-Dependent Calcium Uptake Activity of Microsomes from the Aorta of Normal and Hypertensive Rats. Biochim Biophys Acta 413(1975)432–443

Ohashi, H.; Takewaki, T.; Okada, T.: Calcium and the Contractile Effect of Carbachol in the Depolarized Guinea-Pig Taenia Caecum. Japan J Pharmacol 24(1974)601–611

Okamura, N.; Terayama, H.: Prostaglandin Receptor-Adenylate Cyclase System in Plasma Membranes of Rat Liver and Ascites Hepatomas, and the Effect of GTP upon It. Biochim Biophys Acta 465(1977)54–67

Palatý, V.: The Lanthanum-Resistant Fraction of Calcium in the Rat Tail Artery. In: Excitation-Contraction Coupling in Smooth Muscle, pp 297–302, ed. by R. Casteels *et al.*, Elsevier/North Holland Biomedical Press, Amsterdam, 1977

Paton, D.M.: The Contractile Response of the Isolated Rat Uterus to Noradrenaline and 5-Hydroxytryptamine. Eur J Pharmacol 3(1969)310–315

Peiper, U.; Griebel, L.; Wende, W.: Activation of Vascular Smooth Muscle of Rat Aorta by Noradrenaline and Depolarization—Two Different Mechanisms. Pfluegers Arch 330(1971)74–89

Popescu, L.M.: Conceptual Model of the Excitation-Contraction Coupling in Smooth Muscle: The Possible Role of the Surface Microvesicles. Studia Biophysica 44(1974)141–153

Popescu, L.M.: Cytochemical Study of the Intracellular Calcium Distribution in Smooth Muscle. In: Excitation-Contraction Coupling in Smooth Muscle, pp 13–23, ed. by R. Casteels *et al.*, Elsevier/North Holland Biomedical Press, Amsterdam, 1977

Popescu, L.M.; Diculescu, I.; Zelck, U.; Ionescu, N.: Ultrastructural Distribution of Calcium in Smooth Muscle Cells of Guinea-Pig Taenia Coli. Cell Tiss Res 154(1974)357–378

Potter, J.M.; Sparrow, M.P.: The Relationship between the Calcium Content of Depolarized Mammalian Smooth Muscle and Its Contractility in Response to Acetylcholine. Aust J Exp Biol Med Sci 46(1968)435–446

Powell, W.S.; Hammerström, S.; Samuelsson, B.: Localization of a Prostaglandin $F_{2\alpha}$ Receptor in Bovine *Corpus Luteum* Plasma Membranes. Eur J Biochem 61(1976)605–611

Pressman, B.C.: Carboxylic Ionophore as Mobile Carriers for Divalent Ions. In: The Role of Membranes in Metabolic Regulation, pp 149–164, ed. by M.A. Mehlman, R.W. Hanson, Academic Press, New York, 1972

Pressman, B.C.: Properties of Ionophores with Broad Range Cation Selectivity. Fed Proc 32(1973)1688–1703

Raeymaekers, L.; Wuytack, F.; Casteels, R.: Na-Ca Exchange in Taenia Coli of the Guinea Pig. Pfluegers Arch 347(1974)329–346

Rangachari, P.K.; Pernollet, M.G.; Worcel, M.: Calcium Uptake by Myometrial Membranes: Effect of A 23187, a Calcium Ionophore. Eur J Pharmacol 40(1976)291–294

Reuter, H.: Divalent Cations as Charge Carriers in Excitable Membranes. Prog Biophys Mol Biol 26(1973)1–43

Reuter, H.; Blaustein, M.P.; Haeusler, G.: Na-Ca Exchange and Tension Development in Arterial Smooth Muscle. Philos Trans R Soc Lond (Biol Sci) 265(1973)87–94

Reuter, H.; Scholz, H.: A Study of the Ion Selectivity and the Kinetic Properties of the Calcium Dependent Slow Inward Current in Mammalian Cardiac Muscle. J Physiol (Lond) 264(1977)17–43

Riemer, J.; Dörflu, F.; Mayer, C.-J.; Ulbrecht, G.: Calcium-Antagonistic Effects on the Spontaneous Activity of Guinea-Pig Taenie Coli. Pfluegers Arch 351(1974)241–258

Rose, B.; Lowenstein, W.R.: Calcium Ion Distribution in Cytoplasm Visualized by Aequorin: Diffusion in the Cytosol Is Restricted Due to Energized Sequestering. Science 190(1975)1204–1206

Rosenberger, L.B.; Ticku, M.K.; Triggle, D.J.: The Effects of Ca^{2+} Antagonists on Mechanical Responses and Ca^{2+} Movements in Guinea-Pig Ileal Longitudinal Smooth Muscle. Can J Physiol Pharmacol 57(1979)333–347

Rosenberger, L.; Triggle, D.J.: Calcium, Calcium Translocation and Specific Calcium Antagonists. In: Calcium in Drug Action, pp 3–31, ed. by G. Weiss, Plenum Press, New York, 1978

Sakai, K.; Takayanagi, I.; Uchida, K.; Takagi, K.: Effect of Papaverine on Ca^{2+} Uptake by a Mitochondrial Fraction Isolated from Rat Uterine Smooth Muscle. Eur J Pharmacol 50(1978)131–136

Savino, E.A.; Taquini, A.C.; Jr.: Effects of Adrenalin, Angiotensin, Potassium and Calcium on Lanthanum Treated Portal Veins. Arch Int. Pharmacodyn. 226(1977)100–108

Scarpa, T.; Bablassare, J.; Inesi, G.: The Effect of Calcium Ionophores on Fragmented Sarcoplasmic Reticulum. J Gen Physiol 60(1972)735–749

Schatzmann, H.J.: ATP-Dependent Ca^{++}-Extrusion from Human Red Cells. Experientia 22(1966)364–365

Schatzmann, H.J.; Bürgin, H.: Calcium in Human Red Blood Cells. Ann NY Acad Sci 307(1978)125–147

Schümann, H.J.; Görlitz, B.D.; Wagner, J.: Influence of Papaverine, D-600 and Nifedipine on the Effects of Noradrenaline and Calcium on the Isolated Aorta and Mesenteric Artery of the Rabbit. Naunym-Schmied Arch Pharmacol 289(1975)409–418

Seidel, C.L.; Bohr, D.F.: Calcium and Vascular Smooth Muscle Contraction. Circ Res 28–29Suppl. II(1971)88–95

Shibata, S.: Effect of Mn^{++} on ^{45}Ca Content and Potassium-Induced Contraction of the Aortic Strip. Can J Physiol Pharmacol 47(1969)827–829

Sitrin, M.D.; Bohr, D.F.: Ca and Na Interaction in Vascular Smooth Muscle Contraction. Am J Physiol 110(1971)1124–1128

Somlyo, A.V. and Somlyo, A.P.: Electromechanical and Pharmaco-Mechanical Coupling in Vascular Smooth Muscle. J Pharm Exp Ther 159(1968)129–145

Somlyo, A.V.; Somlyo, A.P.: Strontium Accumulation by Sarcoplasmic Reticulum and Mitochondria in Vascular Smooth Muscle. Science 174(1971)955–958

Somlyo, A.P.; Somlyo, A.V.; Devine, C.E.; Peters, P.D.; Hall, T.A.: Electron Microscopy and Electron Probe Analysis of Mitochondrial Cation Accumulation in Smooth Muscle. J Cell Biol 61(1974)723–742

Somlyo, A.P.; Somlyo, A.V.; Schuman, H.; Sloane, B.; Scarpa, A.: Electron Probe Analysis of Calcium Compartments in Cryo Sections of Smooth and Striated Muscles. In: Calcium Transport and Cell Fucntion, ed. by A. Scarpa, E. Carafoli, Ann NY Acad Sci 307(1978)523–544

Sottacassa, G.L.; Similarities and Dissimilarities between Outer Mitochondrial Membrane and Endoplasmic Reticulum. Adv Exp Med Biol 14(1971)229–244

Sparrow, M.P.; Simmonds, W.J.: The Relationship of the Calcium Content of Smooth Muscle to Its Contractility in Response to Different Modes of Stimulation. Biochim Biophys Acta 109(1965)503–511

Sperelakis, N.: Ca^{45} and Sr^{89} Movements with Contraction of Depolarized Smooth Muscle. Am J Physiol 203(1962)860–866

Su, C.; Bevan, J.A.; Ursillo, R.C.: Electrical Quiescence of Pulmonary Artery Smooth Muscle during Sympathomimetic Stimulation. Circ Res 15(1964)20–27

Swamy, V.C.; Triggle, C.R.; Triggle, D.J.: The Effects of Lanthanum and Thulium on the Mechanical Responses of the Rat Vas Deferens. J Physiol 254(1976)55–62

Szurszewski, J.H.; Bulbring, E.: The Stimulant Action of Acetylcholine and Catecholamines on the Uterus. Phil Trans R Soc Lond B 265(1973)149–156

Triggle, C.R.; Triggle, D.J.: An Analysis of the Action of Cations of the Lanthamide Series on the Mechanical Responses of Guinea-Pig Ileal Longitudinal Muscle. J Physiol (Lond) 254(1976)39–54

Vallieres, J.; Scarpa, A.; Somlyo, A.P.: Subcellular Fractions of Smooth Muscle. I. Isolation substrate utilization and Ca^{++} transport by main pulmonary artery and mesenteric vein mitochondria. Arch Biochem Biophys 170(1975) 659–669

Van Breemen, C.: Blockade of Membrane Calcium Fluxes by Lanthanum in Relation to Vascular Smooth Muscle Contractility. Arch Internat Physiol Biochem 77(1969)710–716

Van Breemen, C.; Casteels, R.: The Use of Ca-EGTA in Measurements of ^{45}Ca Efflux from Smooth Muscle. Pfluegers Arch 348(1974)239–245

Van Breemen, C.; Daniel, E.E.: The Influence of High Potassium Depolarization and Acetylcholine on Calcium Exchange in Rat Uterus. J Gen Physiol 49(1966)1299–1317

Van Breemen, C.; Daniel, E.E.; Van Breemen, D.: Calcium Distribution and Exchange in the Rat Uterus. J Gen Physiol 49(1966)1265–1297

Van Breemen, C.; De Wier, P.: Lanthanum Inhibition of ^{45}Ca Efflux from Squid Giant Axon. Nature (Lond) 226(1970)760–761

Van Breemen, C.; Farinas, B.R.; Casteels, R.; Gerba, P.; Wuytack, F.; Deth, R.: Factors Controlling Cytoplasmic Ca^{2+} Concentration. Philos Trans R Soc [Lond] Biol 265(1973)57–71

Van Breemen, C.; Farnias, B.R.; Gerba, P.; McNaughton, E.D.: Excitation-Contraction Coupling in Rabbit Aorta. Studied by the Lanthanum Method for Measuring Cellular Calcium Influx. Circ Res 30(1972)44–54

Van Breemen, C.; Hwang, O.; Siegel, B.: The Lanthanum Method. In: Excitation-Contraction Coupling in Smooth Muscle, pp. 243–252, ed. by R. Casteels et al., Elsevier/North Holland Biomedical Press, Amsterdam, 1977

Van Breemen, C.; Lesser, P.: The Absence of Increased Membrane Calcium Permeability during Norepinephrine Stimulation of Arterial Muscle. Microvasc Res 3(1971)113–114

Van Breemen, C.; McNaughton, E.: The Separation of Cell Membrane Calcium Transport from Extracellular Calcium Exchange in Vascular Smooth Muscle. Biochem Biophys Res Comm 39(1970)567–574

Vassort, G.: Voltage-Clamp Analysis of Transmembrane Ionic Currents in Guinea-Pig Myometrium: Evidence for an Initial Potassium Activation Triggered by Calcium Influx. J Physiol (Lond) 252(1975)713–734

Wei, J.W.; Janis, R.A.; Daniel, E.E.: Calcium Accumulation and Enzymatic Activities of Subcellular Fractions from Aortas and Ventricles of Genetically Hypertensive Rats. Circ Res 39(1976a)133–140

Wei, J.W.; Janis, R.A.; Daniel, E.E.: Isolation and Characterization of Plasma Membrane from Rat Mesenteric Arteries. Blood Vessels 13(1976b)279–292

Weiss, G.B.: Alterations in ^{45}Ca Distribution and Movements in Ileal Longitudinal Muscle. Agents and Actions 2(1972)246–256

Weiss, G.B.; Goodman, F.R.: Interactions between Several Rare Earth Ions and Calcium Ion in Vascular Smooth Muscle. J Pharmacol Exp Ther 195(1975)557–564

Weiss, G.B.; Goodman, F.R.: Distribution of a Lanthanide (^{147}Pm) in Vascular Smooth Muscle. J Pharmacol Exp Ther 198(1976)366–374

Wikström, M.; Ahonen, P.; Luukkainen, T.: The Role of Mitochondria in Uterine Contractions. FEBS letters 56(1975)120–123

Yaram, R.; Chandler, J.A.: Electron Probe Microanalyses of Skeletal Muscle. J Histochem Cytochem 22(1974)147–154

Yukisada, N.; Ebashi, F.: Role of Calcium in Drug Action on Smooth Muscle. Japan J Pharmacol 11(1961)46–53

Zelek, U.; Konya, L.; Albrecht, E.: ATP Dependent Calcium Uptake of $^{45}Ca^{2+}$ by Microsomal Fraction of Pig Coronary Artery and Its Dependence on Bradykinin and Angiotensin II. Acta Biol Med Ger 32(1974)K1–K5

Index

485